The Overactive Bladder

The Overactive Bladder

Evaluation and Management

Edited by

KARL KREDER MD
Professor
Department of Urology
University of Iowa Hospitals and Clinics
Iowa City, IA
USA

ROGER DMOCHOWSKI MD
Professor
Department of Urologic Surgery
Vanderbilt University Medical Center
Nashville, TN
USA

Foreword by

PAUL ABRAMS MD FRCS
Professor
Bristol Urological Institute
Southmead Hospital
Bristol
UK

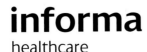

First published in the United Kingdom in 2007 by Informa Healthcare, Telephone House, 69-77 Paul Street, London ECZA 4LQ. Informa Healthcare is a trading division of Informa UK Ltd. Registered Office, 37/41 Mortimer Street, London W1T 3JH. Registered in England and Wales number 1072954.

Tel: +44 (0)20 7017 5000
Fax: +44 (0)20 7017 6336
Website: www.informahealthcare.com

A CIP record for this book is available from the British Library.
Library of Congress Cataloging-in-Publication Data

Data available on application

ISBN-10: 1 84184 630 9
ISBN-13: 978 1 84184 630 9

Distributed in North and South America by
Taylor & Francis
6000 Broken Sound Parkway, NW, (Suite 300)
Boca Raton, FL 33487, USA

Within Continental USA
Tel: 1 (800) 272 7737; Fax: 1 (800) 374 3401
Outside Continental USA
Tel: (561) 994 0555; Fax: (561) 361 6018
E-mail: orders@crcpress.com

Distributed in the rest of the world by
Thomson Publishing Services
Cheriton House
North Way
Andover, Hampshire SP10 5BE, UK
Tel: +44 (0)1264 332424
E-mail: tps.tandfsalesorder@thomson.com

Composition by Exeter Premedia Services Private Ltd., Chennai, India

Printed and bound in India by Replika Press Pvt Ltd.

Front cover image supplied by © 2007 A.D.A.M., Inc.

Contents

List of contributors   vii

Foreword   xi

Acknowledgments   xiii

Colour plates   xv

Introduction

1. Nomenclature   *Jerry G Blaivas*   3

2. The neurophysiology of lower urinary tract function   *William C de Groat*   11

3. Diagnosis of overactive bladder   *Eric S Rovner and Melissa Walls*   27

4. Measuring overactive bladder syndrome symptoms   *Rufus Cartwright and Linda Cardozo* . .   37

5. Nocturia   *Jeffrey P Weiss and Jerry G Blaivas*   51

6. Urodynamics   *Melissa C Fischer and Victor W Nitti*   63

7. Urgency–frequency syndrome and pelvic pain, and interstitial cystitis   *Harris E Foster Jr* . .   75

8. Pelvic floor muscle exercises and behavioral therapy   *Kathryn L Burgio and
    Diane F Borello-France*   87

Pharmacology

9. Overactive bladder: basic pharmacology   *Karl-Erik Andersson*   97

10. Drug delivery and intravesical instillation   *Pradeep Tyagi and Michael B Chancellor*   115

11. Pioneering agents: immediate release   *Philippe E Zimmern*   125

12. Tricyclic antidepressants   *Daniel Dugi and Gary E Lemack*   139

13. Propiverine hydrochloride in the treatment of idiopathic and neurogenic detrusor
    overactivity: efficacy, tolerability, and safety profile   *Manfred Stöhrer, Gerd Mürtz,
    Guus Kramer, and Herbert Rübben*   145

14. Extended release oral oxybutynin   *Rodney A Appell*   163

15. Tolterodine in the management of overactive bladder
    Jonathan S Starkman, Karl J Kreder, and Roger R Dmochowski   171

16. Trospium chloride   *David R Staskin*   189

17. Darifenacin   *Christopher R Chapple*   203

18. Solifenacin succinate   *Karl J Kreder and Roger R Dmochowski*   219

19. Transdermal oxybutynin (Oxytrol™)   *G Willy Davila*   229

20. Strategies for data comparison for drugs used in the treatment of overactive bladder
    Alan J Wein and Roger R Dmochowski 239

21. Pharmacotherapy of overactive bladder in bladder outlet obstruction
    Jonathan Sullivan and Paul Abrams 253

22. Botulinum toxin (Botox®)   *Christopher P Smith and George T Somogyi* 261

23. Acupuncture for treatment of overactive bladder   *Mary P FitzGerald* 277

24. Fesoterodine   *Roger R Dmochowski and Karl J Kreder* 283

Neuromodulation

25. Neuromodulation: mechanisms of action   *Tomas L Griebling* 293

26. Sacral nerve stimulation for overactive bladder symptoms
    Suzette E Sutherland and Steven W Siegel 303

27. The bion® microstimulator   *Jerome L Buller and Kenneth M Peters* 319

28. The Miniaturo™-I device: a new implantable electrostimulation system for the treatment of
    voiding dysfunction   *Ruud Bosch* 329

Surgical therapy

29. Transvaginal denervation   *Jorge Arzola and R Duane Cespedes* 339

30. Autoaugmentation   *Jerilyn M Latini* 345

31. Augmentation cystoplasty for overactive bladder   *Anthony R Stone and Dana K Nanigian* . 359

Special considerations

32. Overactive bladder in children   *Kenneth G Nepple and Christopher S Cooper* 373

33. Geriatric population   *Pat D O'Donnell* 385

34. Late breaking information   *Jean Jacques Wyndaele* 395

Index 409

Contributors

Paul Abrams MD FRCS
Professor
Bristol Urological Institute
Southmead Hospital
Bristol
UK

Karl-Erik Andersson MD PhD
Professor
Wake Forest Institute for Regenerative
  Medicine
Wake Forest University School of Medicine
Winston Salem, NC
USA

Rodney A Appell MD FACS
Professor
Division of Voiding Dysfunction
Scott Department of Urology
Baylor College of Medicine
Houston, TX
USA

Jorge Arzola MD
Resident
Department of Urology (MCSU)
Wilford Hall Medical Center
Lackland AFB, TX
USA

Jerry G Blaivas MD
Professor
Weill-Cornell College of Medicine
Urocenter of New York
New York, NY
USA

Diane F Borello-France PT PhD
Associate Professor
Department of Physical Therapy
Rangos School of Health Sciences
Duquesne University
Pittsburgh, PA
USA

Ruud Bosch MD PhD
Professor and Chairman
Department of Urology
University Medical Center Utrecht
Utrecht
The Netherlands

Jerome L Buller MD FACOG
Lieutenant Colonel, Medical Corp, US Army
Division Director and Associate Fellowship
Director, Female Pelvic Medicine and
Reconstructive Surgery
Department of Obstetrics and Gynecology
Walter Reed Army Medical Center
Washington, DC
USA

Kathryn L Burgio PhD
Professor of Medicine
University of Alabama at Birmingham
Department of Medicine
Geriatric Research, Education, and
Clinical Center
Birmingham VA Medical Center
Birmingham, AL
USA

Linda Cardozo MD FRCOG
Professor and Head
Department of Urogynaecology
King's College Hospital
London
UK

Rufus Cartwright MA MBBS
Senior Clinical Fellow
Department of Urogynaecology
King's College Hospital
London
UK

R Duane Cespedes MD
Associate Professor and Director
Female Urology and Urodynamics
Department of Urology (MCSU)
Wilford Hall Medical Center
Lackland AFB, TX
USA

Michael B Chancellor MD
Professor
Department of Urology
University of Pittsburgh
Pittsburgh, PA
USA

Christopher R Chapple MD FRCS (Urol)
Professor
Department of Urology
Royal Hallamshire Hospital
Sheffield
UK

Christopher S Cooper MD
Associate Professor
Department of Urology
Children's Hospital of Iowa
University of Iowa Hospitals and Clinics
Iowa City, IA
USA

G Willy Davila MD
Chairman
Department of Gynecology
Section of Urogynecology and Reconstructive
Pelvic Surgery
Cleveland Clinic
Weston, FL
USA

Roger R Dmochowski MD
Professor
Department of Urologic Surgery
Vanderbilt University Medical Center
Nashville, TN
USA

Daniel Dugi MD
Resident
Department of Urology
University of Texas
Southwestern Medical Center at Dallas
Dallas, TX
USA

Melissa C Fischer MD
Clinical Fellow
Department of Urology
New York University School of Medicine
New York, NY
USA

Mary P FitzGerald MD
Associate Professor
Division of Female Pelvic Medicine and
Reconstructive Surgery
Loyola University Medical Center
Maywood, IL
USA

Harris E Foster Jr MD
Professor
Section of Urology
Yale University School of Medicine
New Haven, CT
USA

Tomas L Griebling MD FACS FGSA
Associate Professor and Vice-Chair
Department of Urology
The University of Kansas
The Landon Center on Aging
Kansas City, KS
USA

William C de Groat PhD
Professor of Pharmacology
Department of Pharmacology
University of Pittsburgh School of Medicine
Pittsburgh, PA
USA

Guus Kramer
Biophysicist
Kennemerbeekweg
Bennebroek
Netherlands

Karl J Kreder MD
Professor
Department of Urology
University of Iowa Hospitals and Clinics
Iowa City, IA
USA

Jerilyn M Latini MD
Assistant Professor
Department of Urology
University of Michigan
Ann Arbor, MI
USA

Gary E Lemack MD
Associate Professor
Department of Urology
University of Texas Southwestern
    Medical Center at Dallas
Dallas, TX
USA

Gerd Mürtz MD
Medical Consultant of Apogepha
    Arzneimittel GmbH
Dresden
Germany

Dana K Narigian MD
Resident
University of California Davis Medical Center
Sacramento, CA
USA

Kenneth G Nepple MD
Resident
Department of Urology
Children's Hospital of Iowa
University of Iowa Hospitals and Clinics
Iowa City, IA
USA

Victor W Nitti MD FACS
Associate Professor and Vice Chairman
Department of Urology
New York University School of Medicine
New York, NY
USA

Pat D O'Donnell MD
Professor
Division of Urology
Southern Illinois University School of Medicine
Springfield, IL
USA

Kenneth M Peters MD
Director of Research
Ministrelli Program for Urologic Research and
    Education
Department of Urology
William Beaumont Hospital
Royal Oak, MI
USA

Eric S Rovner MD
Associate Professor
Department of Urology
Medical University of South Carolina
Charleston, SC
USA

Herbert Rübben MD PhD
Professor and Chairman
Department of Urology
University Hospital Essen
Essen
Germany

Steven W Siegel MD
Metro Urology
Centers for Continence Care and Female
Urology
St Paul, MN
USA

Christopher P Smith MD
Assistant Professor
Scott Department of Urology
Baylor College of Medicine
Houston, TX
USA

George T Somogyi MD PhD
Professor and Director
Neurourology Laboratory
Scott Department of Urology
Baylor College of Medicine
Houston, TX
USA

Jonathan S Starkman MD
Clinical Instructor
Department of Urologic Surgery
Vanderbilt University Medical Center
Nashville, TN
USA

David R Staskin MD
Associate Professor and Director
Female Urology and Urodynamics
Weill-Cornell Medical College
New York, NY
USA

Manfred Stöhrer MD PhD
Professor and Consultant
Department of Urology
University of Essen
Essen
Germany

Anthony R Stone MD
Professor
Department of Urology
University of California Davis Medical Center
Sacramento, CA
USA

Jonathan Sullivan
Consultant
Department of Urology
Worcestershire Acute Hospitals NHS Trust
Kidderminister
UK

Suzette E Sutherland MD
Metro Urology
Centers for Continence Care and Female
Urology
St Paul, MN
USA

Elizabeth B Takacs MD
Assistant Professor
Department of Urology
University of Iowa Hospitals and Clinics
Iowa City, IA
USA

Pradeep Tyagi MSc PhD
Postdoctoral Fellow
Department of Urology
University of Pittsburgh
Pittsburgh, PA
USA

Melissa Walls MD
Resident
Department of Urology
Medical University of South Carolina
Charleston, SC
USA

Alan J Wein MD PhD (HON)
Professor and Chief
Division of Urology
University of Pennsylvania
Philadelphia, PA
USA

Jeffrey P Weiss MD
Weill-Cornell College of Medicine
Urocenter of New York
New York, NY
USA

Jean Jacques Wyndaele MD DSci PhD FEBU
FISCOS
Professor and Chair
Department of Urology
University of Antwerp
Belgium

Philippe E Zimmern MD FACS
Professor
Department of Urology
University of Texas Southwestern
  Medical Center at Dallas
Dallas, TX
USA

Foreword

The overactive bladder is *not* a new disease or a term invented for those wishing to sell pills to patients. The term was coined by Alan Wein and myself when we were asked to organize a meeting on "The Unstable Bladder" on an unrestricted educational grant by Pharmacia in 1996.[1] We pointed out that unstable bladder was a urodynamic diagnosis and we usually treated patients with the symptoms of frequency, urgency, urgency incontinence and nocturia without a urodynamics diagnosis, in the first instance. We also pointed out that we wished to include discussion of patients with neurological disease, who would be excluded by the term "unstable bladder", as this only applied to those without an obvious cause for their detrusor overactivity. Pharmacia were most unhappy about our insistence on using the term "overactive bladder" as the title for the meeting. This was because Pharmacia only had "unstable bladder" as an indication for the use of their antimuscarinic drug. Nevertheless, Alan and I insisted and Pharmacia acquiesced. Subsequently, the term has become accepted worldwide and is, of course, used to market all products for the condition. The origin of the term overactive bladder is described in an article in Urology[2].

Once the term was coined it had to be defined, and after several iterations the ICS (2002) Standardisation Report defined the overactive bladder as urgency, with or without urgency incontinence, usually with frequency and nocturia.[3] It was also necessary to exclude other conditions such as urinary infection and inadequately controlled diabetes as causes of the same symptoms. However, despite these definitions which are essentially medical, there is still a need for clarity of thought when looking at these definitions in patient terms. It is confusing to patients to talk about urge and urgency and furthermore, it is unnecessary. The ICS (2002) suggested that urge means need and therefore is easily confused with urgency, and should not be used. There is very little point in asking patients whether they have urgency or urgency incontinence. Of much more use are questions such as "do you have to drop everything and rush to the toilet, otherwise you might leak urine?"

Karl Kreder and Roger Dmochowski are to be complimented on assembling this comprehensive book on Overactive Bladder (OAB) written by a distinguished group of clinicians and scientists. Unusually for a text book, it includes not only accepted treatments but also discusses new treatments, still in the development stage, such as implanted pudendal nerve stimulation and the new antimuscarinic fesoterodine. The inclusion of chapters on particularly problematic patient groups, such as children and the elderly, is most welcome, as the importance and implications of OAB in these two important sections of our society are greater than for independently living young to middle aged adults.

The book is an excellent update on Overactive Bladder, the theories behind its genesis, its assessment and its management from behavioural therapy to augmentation cystoplasty.

Paul Abrams MD FRCS
Professor of Urology
Bristol Urological Institute
Bristol
UK

REFERENCES

1. Abrams P, Wein AW. The overactive bladder. Urology 50, Suppl. 6A.
2. Abrams P. Describing bladder storage function: overactive bladder syndrome and detrusor overactivity. Urology 2003; 62 (Suppl. 5B): 28–37.
3. Abrams P, Cardozo L, Fall M et al. The standardisation of terminology of lower urinary tract function: report from the Standardisation Subcommittee of the International Continence Society. Neurourol Urodynam 2002; 21: 167–178.

Acknowledgments

The editors would like to thank Kristina K. Greiner for her editorial assitance.

Color Plates

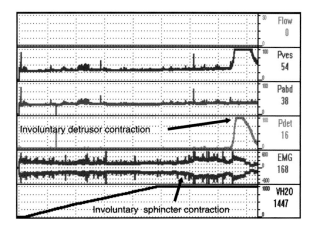

Figure 1.1 Terminal detrusor overactivity in a man with type 1 detrusor external sphincter dyssynergia (EMG relaxes after onset of detrusor contraction). During this examination he was incontinent and voided to completion, but the examination was performed in the supine position, so uroflow was not measured. Flow, uroflow; Pves, vesical pressure; Pabd, abdominal pressure; Pdet, detrusor pressure; EMG, sphincter electromyography; VH2O, infused bladder volume.

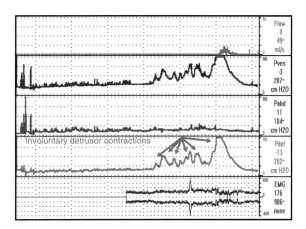

Figure 1.2 Phasic detrusor overactivity in a 53-year-old man with prostatic obstruction. Flow, uroflow; Pves, vesical pressure; Pabd, abdominal pressure; Pdet, detrusor pressure; EMG, sphincter electromyography.

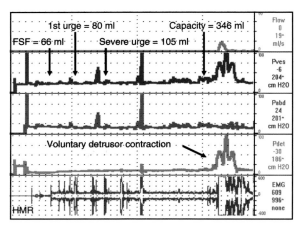

Figure 1.3 Type 1 overactive bladder (OAB). This is a 54-year-old woman with mild exacerbating–remitting multiple sclerosis who complains of urinary frequency, urgency, and urge incontinence. *Urodynamic tracing:* first sensation of bladder filling (FSF) = 66 ml, 1st urge = 80 ml; severe urge = 105 ml; bladder capacity = 346 ml. Although she complains of urge incontinence, there are no involuntary detrusor contractions and she has a voluntary detrusor contraction at 346 ml. The apparent increase in EMG activity during the detrusor contraction is artifact. Unintubated peak uroflow (Q_{max}) = 20 ml/s. Flow, uroflow; Pves, vesical pressure; Pabd, abdominal pressure; Pdet, detrusor pressure; EMG, sphincter electromyography.

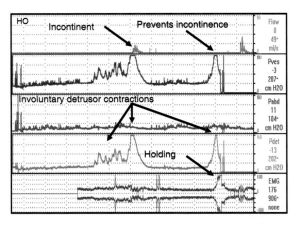

Figure 1.4 Type 2 overactive bladder (OAB) and prostatic obstruction in a 53-year-old man with a 20-year history of refractory urgency, urge incontinence, and enuresis. *Urodynamic tracing*. During bladder filling he is instructed to neither void nor prevent micturition and to report his sensations to the examiner. There are a series of poorly sustained involuntary detrusor contractions (arrows) that he perceives as a severe urge to void and then there is a sustained voiding contraction whence he relaxes his sphincter and is incontinent. The bladder is filled again and there is another involuntary detrusor contraction. This time he is instructed to try to hold. He contracts his sphincter, obstructing the urethra, the detrusor contraction subsides, and he is not incontinent. Flow, uroflow; Pves, vesical pressure; Pabd, abdominal pressure; Pdet, detrusor pressure; EMG, sphincter electromyography.

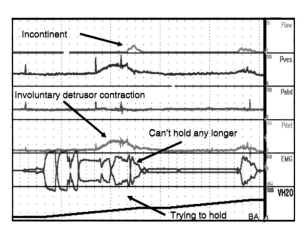

Figure 1.5 Type 3 overactive bladder (OAB) in a 42-year-old woman with refractory urge incontinence. *Urodynamic study*. A strong urge is felt at a bladder volume of 50 ml and she contracts her sphincter to prevent incontinence. At a volume of 275 ml, she develops an involuntary detrusor contraction and is able to continue contracting her sphincter, preventing incontinence. At 350 ml, she can no longer hold and she voids involuntarily. Flow, uroflow; Pves, vesical pressure; Pabd, abdominal pressure; Pdet, detrusor pressure; EMG, sphincter electromyography; VH2O, infused bladder volume.

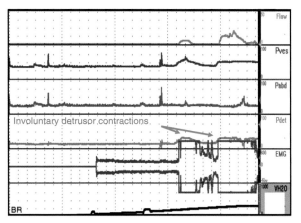

Figure 1.6 Type 4 overactive bladder (OAB) in an otherwise normal woman with refractory urge incontinence. *Urodynamic tracing*. There are two involuntary detrusor contractions; each time she voids involuntarily without control. The apparent increase in EMG activity is artifact, likely due to poor contact of the EMG electrodes, possibly due to urine leakage. Flow, uroflow; Pves, vesical pressure; Pabd, abdominal pressure; Pdet, detrusor pressure; EMG, sphincter electromyography; VH2O, infused bladder volume.

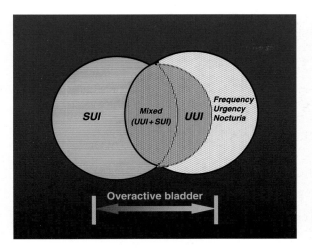

Figure 3.1 Spectrum of overactive bladder (OAB). OAB and stress incontinence may coexist. In addition, the OAB symptom complex includes those patients with irritative voiding symptoms such as urinary frequency, urgency, and nocturia, as well those with urgency incontinence and mixed (stress and urgency) incontinence. UUI, urgency incontinence; SUI, stress incontinence.

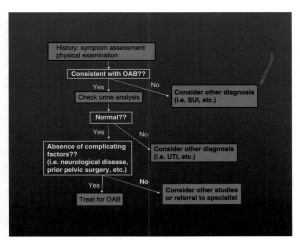

Figure 3.2 Algorithm for evaluation of overactive bladder (OAB). SUI, stress incontinence; UTI, urinary tract infection.

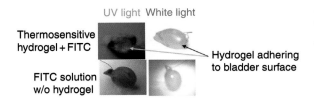

Figure 10.4 Photographs of a rat bladder instilled with thermosensitive hydrogel. Thermosensitive hydrogel was localized in the rat bladder by loading the hydrogel with a fluorescent probe that appears green in ultraviolet (UV) light 48 hours after instillation. Rat bladder instilled with a fluorescent probe without any hydrogel did not show any green color of the probe under UV light. FITC, fluorescein isothiocyanate.

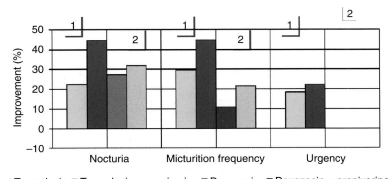

Figure 13.4 Improvement (%) of clinical symptoms following treatment with 0.2 mg/day tamsulosin monotherapy and in combination with 20 mg/day propiverine (1, from reference 29, with permission) and treatment with 4 mg/day doxazosin monotherapy and in combination with 20 mg/day propiverine (2, from reference 30).

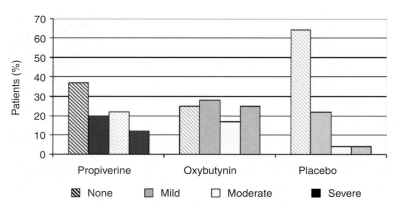

Figure 13.5 Severity of dryness of the mouth in 366 patients with urgency/urge incontinence following a 4-week treatment with propiverine 15 mg three times daily (tid), oxybutynin 5 mg twice daily (bid), or placebo. (From reference 14, with permission)

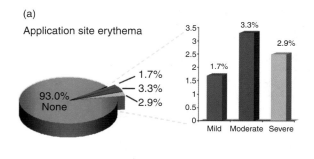

Figure 15.3 Tolterodine ER release as a function of pH.

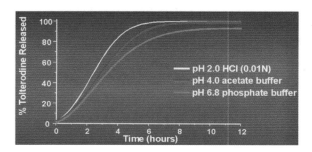

Figure 19.8 Skin erythema (a) and pruritis (b) occur in a small percentage of patients.

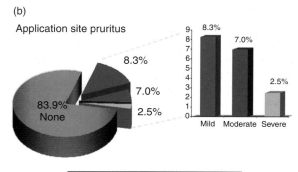

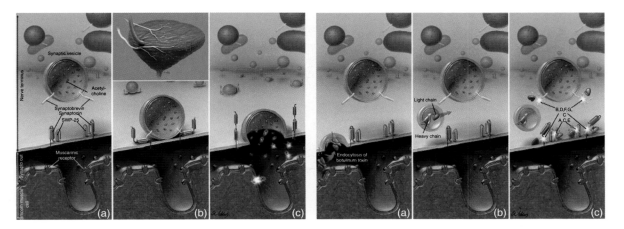

Figure 22.3 Schematic diagram demonstrating: (1) normal fusion and release of acetylcholine from nerve terminals via interaction of SNARE (soluble *N*-ethylmaleimide-sensitive fusion attachment receptor) proteins (left panel, a–c) and (2) binding, internalization, and cleavage of specific SNARE proteins by botulinum neurotoxins A–G (right panel, a–c).

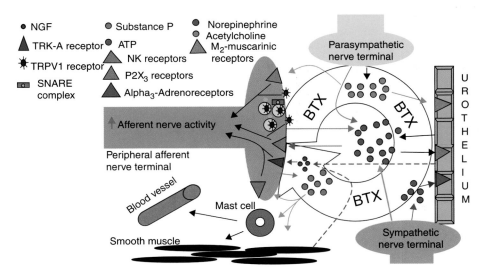

Figure 22.4 Illustration mechanisms of action of botulinum toxin (BTX) in suppressing detrusor overactivity that include: (1) inhibiting acetylcholine or adenosine triphosphate (ATP) or norepinephrine release from parasympathetic nerves, sympathetic nerves, afferent nerves, or bladder urothelium; (2) blocking neuropeptide release such as calcitonin gene related peptide (CGRP) or substance P from afferent nerves; (3) diminishing nerve growth factor release from urothelium or smooth muscle; and (4) reducing expression of TRPV1 or P2X3 receptors on sensory nerve terminals. NGF, nerve growth factor.

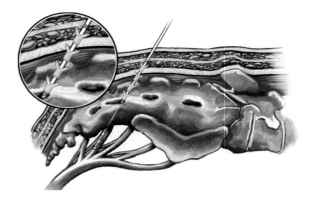

Figure 25.4 The quadripolar electrode in position in the S$_3$ foramen. The lead is secured in position by the tines at the level of the lumbodorsal fascia (inset). (Reprinted with the permission of Medtronic, Inc. © 2006)

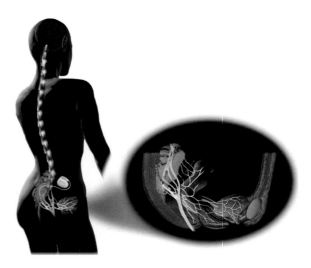

Figure 25.6 Sacral neuromodulation influences both the central and peripheral nervous systems through a variety of pathways. (Reprinted with the permission of Medtronic, Inc. © 2006)

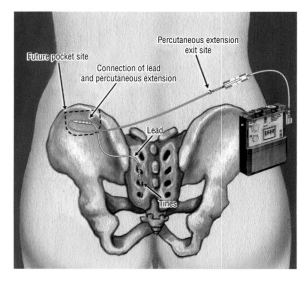

Figure 26.5 Test stimulation with chronic lead. (Reprinted with the permission of Medtronic, Inc. © 2006)

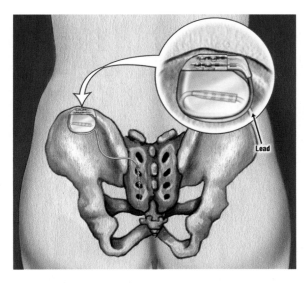

Figure 26.6 Implanted lead, extension connector, and implantable pulse generator (IPG). (Reprinted with the permission of Medtronic, Inc. © 2006)

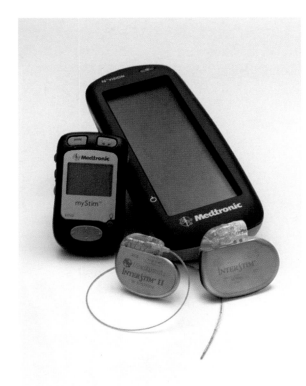

Figure 26.7 Patient programmer with control magnet. Physician programmer also viewed. (Reprinted with the permission of Medtronic, Inc. © 2006)

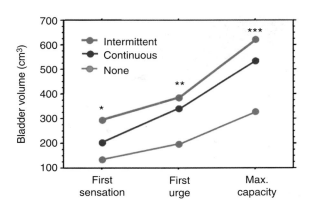

Figure 27.2 Percutaneous stimulation trial data. $*p = 0.005; **p = 0.01; ***p = 0.01$ (Kruskal–Wallis).

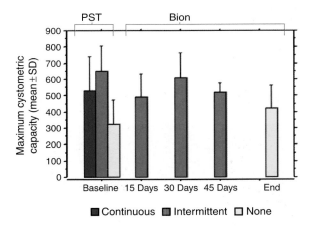

Figure 27.3 RF-Bion™ microstimulator data. PST, percutaneous stimulation trial.

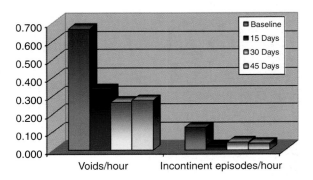

Figure 27.4 RF-Bion™ microstimulator stimulation only data: mean voiding diaries, stimulation for 8–12 hours daily.

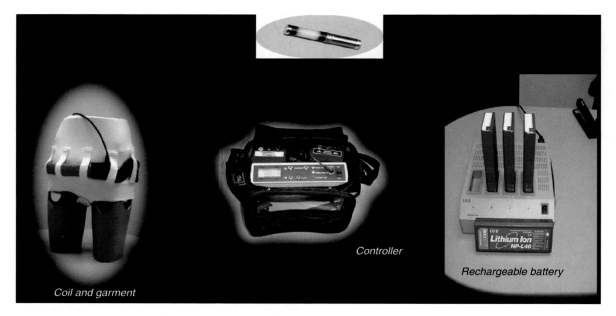

Figure 27.5 RF-Bion™ microstimulator system.

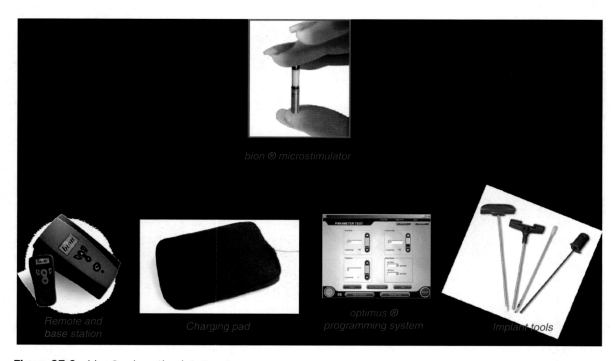

Figure 27.6 bion® microstimulator system.

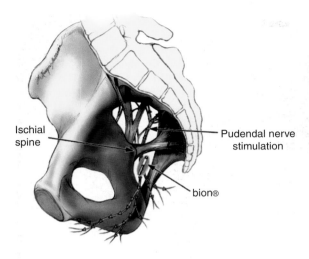

Figure 27.11 Implanted bion® microstimulator.

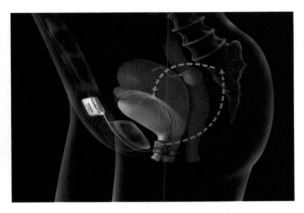

Figure 28.2 Schematic drawing of the implanted Miniaturo™-I system showing the electrode in a paraurethral position and indicating the inhibitory effect of stimulated external urethral sphincter contraction on the detrusor vesicae muscle.

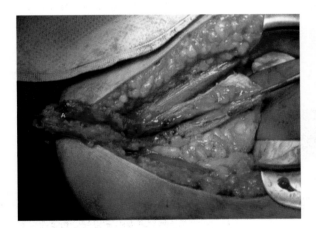

Figure 31.1 Lateral view of open bladder. Bladder split coronally: "clam". A, anterior; P, posterior.

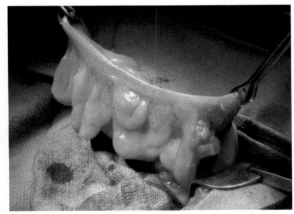

Figure 31.2 Segment of sigmoid colon isolated on mesentery.

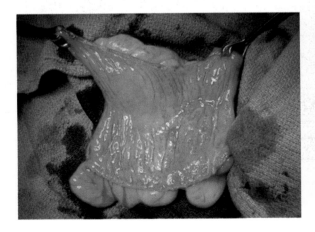

Figure 31.3 Bowel opened on antimesenteric border.

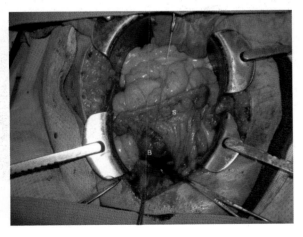

Figure 31.4 Open segment of sigmoid (S) sutured to posterior wing of clammed bladder (B).

Introduction

1

Nomenclature

Jerry G Blaivas

Introduction • Lower urinary tract symptoms

INTRODUCTION

There are two basic methods by which the meanings of words are defined – by common usage and by standardizing committee. Usage is the method that was employed in the compilation of the first edition of the *Oxford English Dictionary*. The brainchild of a passionate and indefatiguable Scotsman named James Murray who devoted nearly his entire adult life to it, the *Oxford English Dictionary* was completed in 1928 after an incredible 49 years of research.[1] The scientific methodology employed to develop this dictionary is worth considering. Thousands of volunteer readers were assigned individual words to research. In a systematic way, each reader searched out his word in contemporary and ancient writings. Each time a word was identified in a text, a citation was generated which consisted of the word and the complete sentence in which it was used. Murray and his associates meticulously read each citation and compiled all of the possible definitions for each word, based on the way the words were actually used.

Another approach to defining the meaning of words is to assign a single, very specific, unique definition to each word. In theory, this serves the interest of science so that there can be no ambiguity in experimental observations, studies, and reports. However, contextual differences and subtleties may not be completely captured when definitions are so specific.

The International Continence Society (ICS) has used the latter approach in defining overactive bladder (OAB) and many other terms.[2,3]

According to the ICS, lower urinary tract dysfunction is comprised of symptoms, signs, urodynamic observations, and conditions.[3,4] *Signs* are observed by the physician by simple means (e.g. observation of the loss of urine with a cough), or by the use of diaries, pad tests, symptom scores, and validated quality of life instruments. *Urodynamic observations* are made during urodynamic studies and reflect the definitive pathophysiological *condition* that is causing the symptom (e.g. detrusor overactivity or sphincter weakness causing incontinence). When a condition cannot be documented by urodynamic observation, it may be "presumed" by clinical documentation.[4] All definitions cited conform to ICS standards except when specifically stated to be otherwise.

LOWER URINARY TRACT SYMPTOMS

Lower urinary tract symptoms are composed of three groups: storage, voiding, and postmicturition. *Storage symptoms* include *increased daytime frequency, dysuria* (pollakisuria), *nocturia* (waking one or more times to void at night), *urgency* (a sudden compelling desire to pass urine, which is difficult to defer), and *urinary incontinence* (the involuntary leakage of urine).

Urinary incontinence is further subdivided into the following eight categories:

1. *Stress incontinence*: involuntary leakage on effort or exertion, or on sneezing or coughing. The sign of stress incontinence is the

observation of urine loss from the urethra during coughing or straining. There are two conditions that may cause stress incontinence – sphincteric weakness and stress hyperreflexia. *Stress hyperreflexia* is a term abandoned by the ICS that describes incontinence due to an involuntary detrusor contraction precipitated by a sudden increase in abdominal pressure. *Urodynamic stress incontinence,* as defined by the ICS, is the involuntary leakage of urine during increased abdominal pressure, in the absence of a detrusor contraction. However, we believe the terms *stress hyperreflexia* and *urodynamic sphincteric incontinence* are more appropriate. There are various urodynamic measurements of sphincteric function (see Chapter 6), but the condition stress incontinence can be diagnosed on physical examination alone.

2. *Urge incontinence*: involuntary leakage accompanied by or immediately preceded by urgency.
3. *Mixed urinary incontinence*: involuntary leakage associated with urgency and also with exertion, effort, sneezing, or coughing.
4. *Enuresis*: synonymous with incontinence.
5. *Nocturnal enuresis*: loss of urine occurring during sleep.
6. *Continuous urinary incontinence*: continuous leakage.
7. *Unconscious (unaware) incontinence* is a term not addressed by the ICS, but is the involuntary loss of urine that is unaccompanied by either urge or stress. The patient has no awareness of the actual moment of urinary loss, but rather just finds himself wet.[4]
8. *Overflow incontinence* is not a symptom or condition, but rather a term used to describe leakage of urine associated with urinary retention.

Voiding symptoms include the following six symptoms:

- slow stream
- splitting or spraying of the urine stream
- intermittent stream (intermittency)
- hesitancy: difficulty in initiating micturition resulting in a delay in the onset of voiding after the individual is ready to pass urine
- straining to void.

- terminal dribble is the term used when an individual describes a prolonged final part of micturition, when the flow has slowed to a trickle/dribble.

Post-micturition symptoms are self-explanatory and include (1) feeling of incomplete emptying; and (2) post-micturition dribble.

Bladder sensation can be defined, during history taking, by five categories:

1. *Normal*: the individual is aware of bladder filling and increasing sensation up to a strong desire to void.
2. *Increased*: the individual feels an early and persistent desire to void.
3. *Reduced*: the individual is aware of bladder filling but does not feel a definite desire to void.
4. *Absent*: the individual reports no sensation of bladder filling or desire to void.
5. *Non-specific*: the individual reports no specific bladder sensation, but may perceive bladder filling as abdominal fullness, vegetative symptoms, or spasticity.

Overactive bladder (OAB) is defined by the ICS as "urgency, with or without urge incontinence, usually with frequency and nocturia . . . if there is no proven infection or other etiology." More specifically, the ICS refers to this constellation of symptoms as the "overactive bladder syndrome . . . These symptom combinations are suggestive of urodynamically demonstrable detrusor overactivity, but can be due to other forms of urethrovesical dysfunction. These terms can be used if there is no proven infection or other obvious pathology. Urge syndrome or urgency–frequency syndrome are described as synonyms of OAB."[3]

Since urgency (a sudden compelling desire to pass urine, which is difficult to defer) is the sine qua non for a diagnosis of OAB, we shall begin our discussion with its definition. In a position paper, Chapple et al.[5] specifically stated that, "it is important to differentiate between 'urge' which is a normal physiologic sensation, and urgency which we consider pathological. Central to this distinction is the debate over whether urgency is merely an extreme form of 'urge.' If this was a continuum, then normal people could experience urgency, but in the model we propose, urgency is always abnormal." This distinction between urge and urgency, though, is based on the authors educated opinion, and alternative explanations may also be operational. First, as defined, urgency is an all or none phenomenon; there can be no gradations of "a sudden compelling desire to void". In contradistinction, others believe that there are gradations of urgency and, to this end, a proposed grading system has evolved,[6] the Urge Perception Scale (UPS), which is based on the original work of DeWachter and Wyndaele.[7] The UPS (Table 1.1) describes the reason why a person voids. Grade 4 urgency is identical to the ICS definition, but grade 3 may also be considered under the rubric of urgency and, in some circumstances, grade 2 might also be considered as such. The UPS may be used in a number of ways – to grade the degree of urge that a person usually experiences prior to voiding, as a method of grading each micturition (as part of a bladder diary), or as a nomenclature for describing symptoms, e.g. the patient experiences type 3 urgency. The UPS implies that the sensations that lead to micturition are, in fact, a continuum, and that once the urge to void is felt, if one waits too long, one will experience the same sensation (except for the sudden onset) that is perceived as urgency according to the ICS definition.

Even the ICS standardization document itself recognizes that urgency may be graded. In the discussion of the bladder diary, it states that the "bladder diary . . . records the times of micturitions and voided volumes . . . and other information such as . . . the degree of urgency . . ." At the present time, the only other validated instrument that is designed to grade urgency is the Urgency Severity Score (USS).[8,9] The USS grades urgency, per toilet void, as none, mild, moderate, or severe, and, by implication, supports the contention that the sensations describing the urge to void are a continuum.

These proposed scales may prove to be more clinically useful than the simple yes/no ICS definition of urgency as "a sudden compelling desire to void", whether or not urgency is on a continuum with the normal desire to void. For example, if a person experiences the gradual onset of a strong desire to void over the course of 1 hour after his last micturition, and the volume of urine in his bladder is 60 ml, it might seem reasonable to propose that that sensation is pathologic and should be considered a severe symptom, yet it does not conform to the current definition of urgency (and there is no other word that conveys this meaning).

The definition of OAB requires that there is "no proven infection or other pathology". This implies that if there is an underlying pathology that causes the symptoms, the condition is not OAB. For example, the majority of men with prostatic obstruction have exactly the same symptoms as described for OAB, but since there is "other pathology", the term OAB does not apply. This is much more than a semantic argument; it has important medical implications. If one considers OAB a syndrome, it presupposes that there is no underlying pathology and no differential diagnosis to consider until such time as empiric treatment has proved ineffective. But there is a differential diagnosis for these symptoms and we believe that a proper evaluation should be undertaken to discover them in a timely fashion. Most algorithms for overactive bladder recommend a basic evaluation to consist of a focused history and examination, bladder diary, and urinalysis. A more detailed diagnostic evaluation is only recommended after treatment failure or if there is microhematuria or an obviously elevated residual urine.[10,11]

Consider the following scenario. A patient presents with OAB and has a normal urinalysis. He or she could be empirically treated with behavior modification for 4–6 weeks followed by each of the six commercially available antimuscarinics for 4–6 weeks each for a total of 7 months of unsuccessful treatment before being considered a treatment failure. Only then would a proper

Table 1.1 The Urge Perception Scale
What is the reason you usually urinate?
Grade 0: Out of convenience? (no urge)
Grade 1: Mild urge (can hold > 1 hour)
Grade 2: Moderate urge (can hold > 10–60 min)
Grade 3: Severe urge (can hold < 10 min)
Grade 4: Desperate urge (must go immediately)

evaluation be done and a differential diagnosis be considered. There is, in fact, a well known differential diagnosis for OAB symptoms, the most important of which is bladder cancer (even without hematuria) and, in our judgment, 7 months is simply too long to wait to diagnose bladder cancer. For this reason, we believe that OAB should be considered a symptom complex (with a differential diagnosis) and not a syndrome.

The OAB symptom complex can be caused by one or more of the following conditions: detrusor overactivity, sensory urgency, and low bladder compliance. *Sensory urgency* is a term abandoned by the ICS that refers to an uncomfortable need to void that is unassociated with detrusor overactivity (see below). Conditions causing and/or associated with OAB are diverse, as depicted in Table 1.2.[12–21] In patients with OAB, diagnostic evaluation should be directed at early detection of these conditions, because in many instances the symptoms are reversible if the underlying etiology is successfully treated.

Detrusor overactivity is a generic term that refers to the presence of involuntary detrusor contractions during cystometry, which may be spontaneous or provoked. The ICS further describes two patterns of detrusor overactivity: terminal and phasic. *Terminal detrusor overactivity* is defined as a single involuntary detrusor contraction occurring at cystometric capacity, which cannot be suppressed, and results in incontinence, usually resulting in bladder emptying (Figure 1.1). *Phasic detrusor overactivity* is defined by a characteristic waveform, and may or may not lead to urinary incontinence (Figure 1.2). Involuntary detrusor contractions are not always accompanied by sensation. Some patients have no symptoms at all. Others void uncontrollably without any awareness. Still others may detect them as a first sensation of bladder filling, or a normal desire to void. The ICS classifies detrusor overactivity as either *idiopathic* or *neurogenic*. In the prior ICS standardization report these were referred to as *detrusor instability and detrusor hyperreflexia* respectively. Further, according to the previous ICS terminology, a bladder that did not exhibit involuntary detrusor contractions could be described as a *stable bladder*. The new terminology offers no word to replace a stable bladder other than "bladder without detrusor

Table 1.2   Causes of detrusor overactivity
I   *Idiopathic detrusor overactivity*

II   *Neurogenic detrusor overactivity*
 Supraspinal neurological lesions
    stroke
    Parkinson's disease
    hydrocephalus
    brain tumor
    traumatic brain injury
    multiple sclerosis
 Suprasacral spinal lesions
    spinal cord injury
    spinal cord tumor
    multiple sclerosis
    myelodysplasia
    transverse myelitis
 Diabetes mellitus

III *Non-neurogenic detrusor overactivity*
 Bladder infection
 Bladder outlet obstruction
    men – prostatic and bladder neck,
      stricture
    women – pelvic organ prolapse,
      post-surgical, urethral, diverticulum,
      primary bladder neck, stricture
 Bladder tumor
 Bladder stones
 Foreign body
 Aging

overactivity", and therefore this term may still have clinical utility.

By definition, neurogenic and idiopathic detrusor overactivity are distinguished not by specific symptoms or urodynamic characteristics, but rather by the presence or absence of an identified or previously diagnosed neurological lesion or disorder. For example, a spinal cord injury patient with involuntary bladder contractions is said to have neurogenic detrusor overactivity (detrusor hyperreflexia), whereas an elderly male with such a finding associated with prostatic obstruction is said to have idiopathic detrusor overactivity (detrusor instability). While in some cases the origin of the involuntary detrusor contractions is unknown, in other cases they are caused by, or at least associated with, a variety

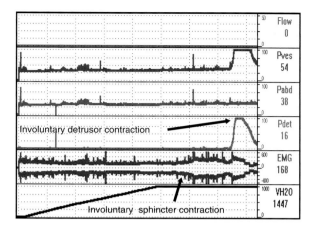

Figure 1.1 Terminal detrusor overactivity in a man with type 1 detrusor external sphincter dyssynergia (EMG relaxes after onset of detrusor contraction). During this examination he was incontinent and voided to completion, but the examination was performed in the supine position, so uroflow was not measured. Flow, uroflow; Pves, vesical pressure; Pabd, abdominal pressure; Pdet, detrusor pressure; EMG, sphincter electromyography; VH20, infused bladder volume. (See also color plate section).

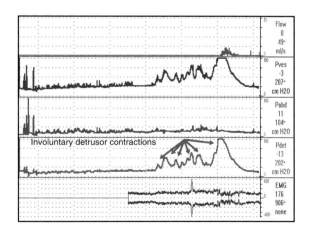

Figure 1.2 Phasic detrusor overactivity in a 53-year-old man with prostatic obstruction. Flow, uroflow; Pves, vesical pressure; Pabd, abdominal pressure; Pdet, detrusor pressure; EMG, sphincter electromyography. (See also color plate section).

of non-neurogenic clinical conditions, the same as listed above for overactive bladder.

A *urodynamic OAB classification* based on the presence of detrusor overactivity, patient awareness, and ability to abort the involuntary contraction

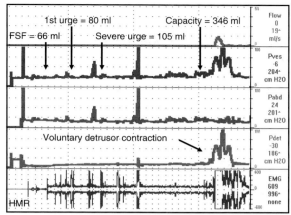

Figure 1.3 Type 1 overactive bladder (OAB). This is a 54-year-old woman with mild exacerbating–remitting multiple sclerosis who complains of urinary frequency, urgency and urge incontinence. *Urodynamic tracing:* first sensation of bladder filling (FSF) = 66 ml, 1st urge = 80 ml; severe urge = 105 ml; bladder capacity = 346 ml. Although she complains of urge incontinence, there are no involuntary detrusor contractions and she had a voluntary detrusor contraction at 346 ml. The apparent increase in EMG activity during the detrusor contraction is artifact. Unintubated maximum uroflow (Q_{max}) = 20 ml/s. Flow, uroflow; Pves, vesical pressure; Pabd, abdominal pressure; Pdet, detrusor pressure; EMG, sphincter electromyography. (See also color plate section).

was recently proposed.[22] The authors defined four types of OAB. In type 1, the patient complains of OAB symptoms, but no involuntary detrusor contractions are demonstrated (Figure 1.3). In type 2, there are involuntary detrusor contractions, but the patient is aware of them and can voluntarily contract his or her sphincter, prevent incontinence, and abort the detrusor contraction (Figure 1.4). In type 3, there are involuntary detrusor contractions, the patient is aware of them and can voluntarily contract his or her sphincter and momentarily prevent incontinence, but is unable to abort the detrusor contraction, and once the sphincter fatigues, incontinence ensues (Figure 1.5). In type 4, there are involuntary detrusor contractions, but the patient is neither able to voluntarily contract the sphincter nor abort the detrusor contraction and simply voids involuntarily (Figure 1.6). This classification system serves two purposes. First, it is a shorthand method of describing the urodynamic

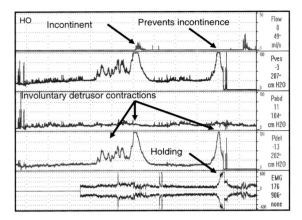

Figure 1.4 Type 2 overative bladder (OAB) and prostatic obstruction in a 53-year-old man with a 20-year history of refractory urgency, urge incontinence, and enuresis. *Urodynamic tracing*. During bladder filling he is instructed to neither void nor prevent micturition and to report his sensations to the examiner. There are a series of poorly sustained involuntary detrusor contractions (arrows) that he perceives as a severe urge to void and then there is a sustained voiding contraction whence he relaxes his sphincter and is incontinent. The bladder is filled again and there is another involuntary detrusor contraction. This time he is instructed to try to hold. He contracts his sphincter, obstructing the urethra, the detrusor contraction subsides, and he is not incontinent. Flow, uroflow; Pves, vesical pressure; Pabd, abdominal pressure; Pdet, detrusor pressure; EMG, sphincter electromyography. (See also color plate section).

characteristics of the OAB patient. Second, it provides a substrate for therapeutic decision making. For example, a patient with type 1 and 2 OAB exhibits normal neural control mechanisms and, at least theoretically, is an excellent candidate for behavioral therapy. It is likely that over time (with or without treatment), an individual patient can change from one type to another. Further, this classification only relates to the storage stage and can coexist with normal voiding, bladder outlet obstruction, and/or impaired detrusor contractility.

Low bladder compliance denotes an abnormal volume–pressure relationship, in which there is a high incremental rise in detrusor pressure during bladder filling. It can only be diagnosed by cystometry.

In conclusion, "words are the building blocks of language and the principal means by which

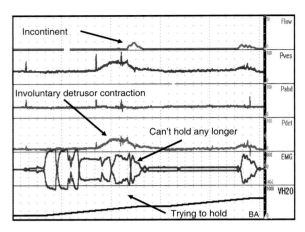

Figure 1.5 Type 3 overactive bladder (OAB) in a 42-year-old woman with refractory urge incontinence. *Urodynamic study*. A strong urge is felt at a bladder volume of 50 ml and she contracts her sphincter to prevent incontinence. At a volume of 275 ml, she develops an involuntary detrusor contraction and is able to continue contracting her sphincter, preventing incontinence. At 350 ml, she can no longer hold and she voids involuntarily. Flow, uroflow; Pves, vesical pressure; Pabd, abdominal pressure; Pdet, detrusor pressure; EMG, sphincter electromyography; VH20, infused bladder volume. (See also color plate section).

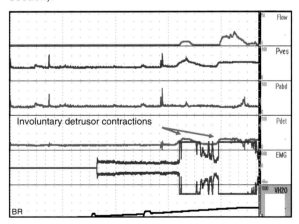

Figure 1.6 Type 4 overactive bladder (OAB) in an otherwise normal woman with refractory urge incontinence. *Urodynamic tracing*. There are two involuntary detrusor contractions; each time she voids involuntarily without control. The apparent increase in EMG activity is artifact, likely due to poor contact of the EMG electrodes, possibly due to urine leakage. Flow, uroflow; Pves, vesical pressure; Pabd, abdominal pressure; Pdet, detrusor pressure; EMG, sphincter electromyography; VH20, infused bladder volume. (See also color plate section).

we communicate with one another. Some words convey their meaning with uniform precision and understanding; others lead to confusion and controversy."[23] Choose the words that best fit your needs.

REFERENCES

1. Winchester S. The Professor and the Madman. New York: Harper Collins, 1998.
2. Abrams P, Blaivas JG, Stanton SL, Andersen JT. Standardisation of terminology of lower urinary tract function. Neurourol Urodyn 1988; 7: 403–26.
3. Abrams P, Cardozo L, Fall M et al. The standardisation of terminology of lower urinary tract function: report from the Standardisation Sub-committee of the International Continence Society. Neurourol Urodyn 2002; 21: 167–78.
4. Blaivas JG, Appell RA, Fantl JA et al. Standards of efficacy for evaluation of treatment outcomes in urinary incontinence: recommendations of the Urodynamic Society. Neurourol Urodyn 1997; 16: 145–7.
5. Chapple CR, Artibani W, Cardoza LD et al. The role of urinary urgency and its measurement in the overactive bladder symptom syndrome: current concepts and future prospects. BJU Int 2005; 95: 335–40.
6. Blaivas JG, Panagopoulos G, Weiss JP, Somaroo C, Chaikin DC. The urgency perception score: validation and test re-test. J Urol 2007; 177: 199–202.
7. DeWachter S, Wyndaele JJ. Frequency-volume charts: a tool to evaluate bladder sensation. Neurourol Urodyn 2003; 22: 638–43.
8. Nixon A, Colman S, Sabounjian L et al. A validated patient reported measure of urinary urgency severity in overactive bladder for use in clinical trials. J Urol 2005; 174: 604–07.
9. Zinner N, Harnett M, Sabounjian L et al. The overactive bladder-symptom composite score: a composite symptom score of toilet voids, urgency severity and urge urinary incontinence in patients with overactive bladder. J Urol 2005; 173: 1639–43.
10. Abrams P, Andersson K, Brubaker T et al. Evaluation and treatment of urinary incontinence, pelvic organ prolapse, and faecal incontinence. In: Abrams P, Cardozo L, Khoury S, Wein A. Incontinence. Plymouth, UK: Health Publication Ltd, 2005: 1589–631.
11. Agency for Health Care Policy and Research Urinary Incontinence Guideline Panel. Urinary Incontinence in Adults: Clinical Practice Guidelines (AHCPR publication #92-0038). Rockville, MD: US Department of Health and Human Services, 1992.
12. Awad SA, McGinnis RH. Factors that influence the incidence of detrusor instability in women. J Urol 1983; 130: 114–15.
13. Blaivas JG. The neurophysiology of micturition. J Urol 1982; 127: 958–63.
14. Kaplan SA, Chancellor MB, Blaivas JG. Bladder and sphincter behavior in patients with spinal cord injuries. J Urol 1991; 146: 113–17.
15. Chou ECL, Flisser AJ, Panagopoulos G, Blaivas JG. Effective treatment for mixed incontinence with a pubovaginal sling. J Urol 2003; 170: 494–7.
16. Fusco F, Groutz A, Blaivas JG, Chaikin DC, Weiss JP. Videourodynamic studies in men with lower urinary tract symptoms: a comparison of community based versus referral urological practices. J Urol 2001; 166: 910–13.
17. Groutz A, Blaivas JG, Chaikin DC. Bladder outlet obstruction in women: definition, prevalence and characteristics. Neurourol Urodyn 2000; 19: 213–20.
18. Groutz A, Blaivas JG, Sassone AM. Detrusor pressure – uroflow studies in women: effect of a 7f transurethral catheter. J Urol 2000; 164: 109–14.
19. Hebjorn S, Andersen JT, Walter S, Dam AM. Detrusor hyperreflexia: a survey on its etiology and treatment. Scand J Urol Nephrol 1976; 10: 103–9.
20. Resnick NM, Yalla SV, Laurino E. The pathophysiology of urinary incontinence among institutionalized elderly persons. N Engl J Med 1989; 320: 1–7.
21. Romanzi LJ, Groutz A, Heritz DM, Blaivas JG. Involuntary detrusor contractions: correlation of urodynamic data to clinical categories. Neurourol Urodyn 2001; 20: 249–57.
22. Flisser AJ, Wamsley K, Blaivas JG. Urodynamic classification of patients with symptoms of overactive bladder. J Urol 2003; 169: 529–33.
23. Blaivas JG. Detrusor instability and other "words" [Editorial]. Neurourol Urodyn 1982; 2: 125.

2

The neurophysiology of lower urinary tract function

William C de Groat

Introduction • Innervation of the lower urinary tract • Urothelium • Anatomy of central nervous
pathways controlling the lower urinary tract • Reflex control of the lower urinary tract
• Neurotransmitters in central micturition reflex pathways • Conclusions

INTRODUCTION

The functions of the lower urinary tract to store and periodically release urine are dependent upon neural circuitry in the brain and spinal cord. This dependence on central nervous control distinguishes the lower urinary tract from many other visceral organs that maintain a certain level of activity even after the elimination of extrinsic neural input. The lower urinary tract is also unusual in regard to the complexity of its neural regulation. For example, micturition depends on the integration of autonomic and somatic efferent mechanisms within the lumbosacral spinal cord. This is necessary to coordinate the activity of visceral organs (the bladder and urethra) with that of urethral striated muscles. In addition, micturition is under voluntary control and depends upon learned behavior that develops during maturation of the nervous system, whereas many other visceral functions are regulated involuntarily. This chapter will review the peripheral and central neural mechanisms controlling the lower urinary tract.

INNERVATION OF THE LOWER URINARY TRACT

The storage and elimination of urine are dependent upon the coordinated activity of two functional units in the lower urinary tract: (1) a reservoir (the urinary bladder) and (2) an outlet, consisting of bladder neck, urethra, and striated muscles of the urethral sphincter.[1,2] These structures are, in turn, controlled by three sets of peripheral nerves: sacral parasympathetic (pelvic nerves), thoracolumbar sympathetic (hypogastric nerves and sympathetic chain), and sacral somatic nerves (pudendal nerves) (Figure 2.1).

Sacral parasympathetic pathways

The sacral parasympathetic outflow provides the major excitatory input to the urinary bladder. Cholinergic preganglionic neurons located in the intermediolateral region of the sacral spinal cord send axons via the pelvic nerves to ganglion cells in the pelvic plexus and in the wall of the bladder. Transmission in bladder ganglia is mediated by a nicotinic, cholinergic mechanism, which can be modulated by the activation of various receptors including muscarinic, adrenergic, purinergic, and peptidergic (Table 2.1).[3] The ganglion cells in turn excite bladder smooth muscle via the release of cholinergic (acetylcholine) and non-adrenergic, non-cholinergic transmitters. Cholinergic excitatory transmission in the bladder is mediated by muscarinic receptors,[4–6] whereas non-cholinergic excitatory transmission is mediated by adenosine triphosphate (ATP), acting on P2X purinergic

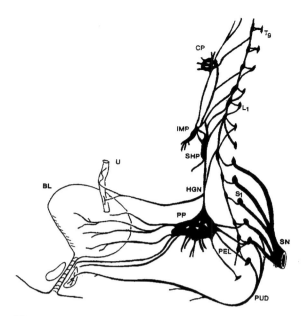

Figure 2.1 Diagram showing the innervation of the female lower urinary tract. BL, urinary bladder; CP, celiac plexus; HGN, hypogastric nerve; IMP, inferior mesenteric plexus; L_1, first lumbar root; PEL, pelvic nerves; PP, pelvic plexus; PUD, pudendal nerve; S_1, first sacral root; SN, sciatic nerve; SHP, superior hypogastric plexus; T_9, ninth thoracic root; U, ureter.

receptors (Table 2.1).[5,7] Inhibitory input to the urethral smooth muscle is mediated by nitric oxide released by parasympathetic nerves.[2] Both M_2 and M_3 muscarinic receptor subtypes are expressed in bladder smooth muscle; however, the M_3 subtype is the principal receptor involved in excitatory transmission. Muscarinic receptors are also present prejunctionally on parasympathetic nerve terminals.[8] Activation of these receptors by acetylcholine can enhance (M_1 receptors) or suppress (M_4 receptors) transmitter release, depending upon the intensity of neural firing. Postganglionic neurons innervating the bladder also contain neuropeptides, such as vasoactive intestinal polypeptide (VIP) and neuropeptide Y (NPY). These substances are coreleased with acetylcholine or ATP and may function as modulators of neuroeffector transmission.

Thoracolumbar sympathetic and sacral somatic efferent pathways

Sympathetic pathways to the lower urinary tract that originate in the lumbosacral sympathetic

chain ganglia as well as in the prevertebral inferior mesenteric ganglia pass to the bladder via the hypogastric and pelvic nerves. Sympathetic efferent pathways elicit various effects including: (1) inhibition of detrusor muscle via β-adrenergic receptors; (2) excitation of the bladder base and urethra via α_1-adrenergic receptors; and (3) inhibition and facilitation in bladder parasympathetic ganglia via α_2- and α_1-adrenergic receptors, respectively (Table 2.1).[2,3,5]

The efferent innervation of the urethral striated muscles in various species originates from cells in a circumscribed region of the lateral ventral horn that is termed Onuf's nucleus.[9] Sphincter motoneurons send their axons into the pudendal nerve and excite sphincter muscles via the release of acetylcholine which stimulates postjunctional nicotinic receptors.

Afferent pathways

Afferent axons innervating the urinary tract originate in the lumbosacral dorsal root ganglia and pass through the three sets of peripheral nerves.[2] The most important afferents for initiating micturition are those passing in the pelvic nerve to the sacral spinal cord. Two types of bladder afferents have been identified: small myelinated (Aδ) and unmyelinated (C) fibers. Aδ bladder afferents in the cat respond in a graded manner to passive distention as well as active contraction of the bladder, and exhibit pressure thresholds in the range of 5–15 mmHg, which are similar to those pressures at which humans report the first sensation of bladder filling.[2] These fibers also code for noxious stimuli in the bladder. On the other hand, C-fiber bladder afferents in the cat have very high thresholds and commonly do not respond to even high levels of intravesical pressure. However, activity in some of these afferents is unmasked or enhanced by chemical irritation of the bladder mucosa. Thus, C-fiber afferents seem to have specialized functions, such as the signaling of inflammatory or noxious events in the lower urinary tract. A large percentage of bladder afferent neurons contain neuropeptides, raising the possibility that these substances may be transmitters in the afferent pathways from the lower urinary tract.[2,10,11] C-fiber afferents are sensitive to the neurotoxins capsaicin and resiniferatoxin as well as to other substances

Table 2.1 Receptors for putative transmitters in the lower urinary tract			
Tissue	*Cholinergic*	*Adrenergic*	*Other*
Bladder body	+ (M_2) + (M_3)	− (β_2) − (β_3)	+ Purinergic (P2X$_1$) − VIP + Substance P (NK$_2$)
Bladder base	+ (M_2) + (M_3)	+ (α_1)	− VIP + Substance P (NK$_2$) + Purinergic (P2X)
Urothelium	+ (M_2) + (M_3)	+ (α) + (β)	+ TRPV1 + TRPM8 + (P2X) + (P2Y) + Substance P + Bradykinin (B2)
Urethra	+ (M)	+ (α_1) + (α_2) − (β)	+ Purinergic (P2X) − VIP − Nitric oxide
Sphincter striated muscle	+ (N)		
Adrenergic nerve terminals	− (M_4) + (M_1)	− (α_2)	− NPY
Cholinergic nerve terminals	− (M_4) + (M_1)	+ (α_1)	− NPY
Afferent nerve terminals			+ Purinergic (P2X$_{2/3}$) + TRPV1
Ganglia	+ (N) + (M_1)	+ (α_1) − (α_2) + (β)	− Enkephalinergic (δ) − Purinergic (P$_1$) + Substance P

VIP, vasoactive intestinal polypeptide; NPY, neuropeptide Y; TRP, transient receptor potential. Letters in parentheses indicate receptor type, e.g. M (muscarinic) and N (nicotinic). Plus and minus signs indicate excitatory and inhibitory effects.

(tachykinins, nitric oxide, ATP, prostaglandins, and neurotrophic factors) released in the bladder.[10–12] These substances can sensitize the afferent nerves and change their response to mechanical stimuli. Intravesical administration of ATP en-hances the firing of bladder afferent nerves by acting on P2X$_3$ or P2X$_{2/3}$ receptors on afferent terminals within or adjacent to the urothelium.[13,14]

The properties of lumbosacral dorsal root ganglion cells innervating the bladder, urethra, and external urethral sphincter in the rat have been studied with patch clamp recording techniques.[15,16] Based on responsiveness to capsaicin it is estimated that approximately 70% of bladder afferent neurons in the rat are of the C-fiber type. Approximately 90% of the bladder C-fiber afferent neurons are also excited by ATP.[2]

C-fiber bladder afferent neurons also express a slowly decaying A-type K$^+$ current that controls spike threshold and firing frequency.[15] Suppression of this K$^+$ current by drugs or chronic bladder inflammation induces hyperexcitability of the afferent neurons.[15]

UROTHELIUM

The urothelium, which has been traditionally viewed as a passive barrier, also has specialized sensory and signaling properties that allow it to respond to chemical and mechanical stimuli and to engage in reciprocal chemical communication with neighboring nerves in the bladder wall (Figure 2.2).[1,2,17–20] These properties include: (1) expression of nicotinic, muscarinic, tachykinin, adrenergic, and capsaicin (TRPV1) receptors;

(2) responsiveness to transmitters released from sensory nerves; (3) close physical association with afferent nerves; and (4) the ability to release chemical mediators such as ATP and nitric oxide that can regulate the activity of adjacent nerves and thereby trigger local vascular changes and/or reflex bladder contractions.[13,17–22]

The role of ATP in urothelial-afferent communication has attracted considerable attention because bladder distention releases ATP from the urothelium[19] and intravesical administration of ATP induces bladder hyperactivity, an effect blocked by administration of P2X purinergic receptor antagonists that suppress the excitatory action of ATP on bladder afferent neurons.[2] Mice in which the P2X$_3$ receptor was knocked out exhibited hypoactive bladder activity and inefficient voiding, suggesting that activation of P2X$_3$ receptors on bladder afferent nerves by ATP released from the urothelium is essential for normal bladder function.[13] In humans and cats with interstitial cystitis, a painful bladder condition, ATP release from urothelial cells is enhanced.[17] Higher levels of ATP may induce abnormal afferent nerve firing and pain.

Transmitter release mechanisms in the urothelium may also be a target for botulinum toxin A (BTX-A), which is injected into the bladder wall to treat patients with various types of detrusor overactivity. BTX-A can act at multiple sites in the bladder, because it reduces the release of ATP into the bladder lumen in rats with cyclophosphamide-induced cystitis or spinal cord injury and suppresses the release of acetylcholine and norepinephrine from autonomic nerves.[23] BTX-A also blocks the stretch-evoked release of ATP from cultured urothelial cells. Thus, the clinical efficacy of BTX-A in the treatment of bladder dysfunction may be related to its action on urothelial sensory mechanisms as well as to its effects on neurotransmitter release from efferent nerves.

NO release from the urothelium has been implicated in an inhibitory modulatory mechanism.[10,23] Exogenous NO inhibits Ca^{2+} channels in dissociated lumbosacral dorsal ganglion neurons, innervating the urinary bladder. In addition, the intravesical administration of NO donors suppresses bladder hyperactivity in cyclophosphamide-induced cystitis. The intravesical administration of oxyhemoglobin, an NO

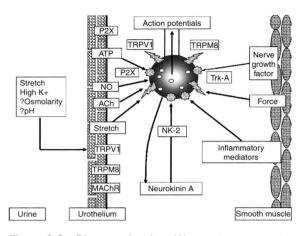

Figure 2.2 Diagram showing: (1) receptors present in the urothelium and in sensory nerve endings in the bladder mucosa and (2) putative chemical mediators that are released by the urothelium, nerves, or smooth muscle that can modulate the excitability of sensory nerves. Urothelial cells and sensory nerves express common receptors (P2X, TRPV1, and TRPM8). Distention of the bladder activates stretch receptors and triggers the release of urothelial transmitters such as ATP, ACh, and NO that may interact with adjacent nerves. Receptors in afferent nerves or the urothelium can respond to changes in pH, osmolality, high K$^+$ concentration, chemicals in the urine, or inflammatory mediators released in the bladder wall. Neuropeptides (neurokinin A) released from sensory nerves in response to distention or chemical stimulation can act on NK-2 autoreceptors to sensitize the mechanosensitive nerve endings. The smooth muscle can generate force which may influence some mucosal endings. Nerve growth factor released from muscle or urothelium can exert an acute and chronic influence on the excitability of sensory nerves via an action on Trk-A receptors. ATP, adenosine triphosphate; ACh, acetylcholine; MAChR, muscarinic acetylcholine receptor; TRPV1, transient receptor potential vanilloid receptor 1 sensitive to capsaicin; TRPM8, menthol/cold receptor; NO, nitric oxide, Trk-A, tyrosine kinase A receptor.

scavenger, produces bladder hyperactivity in normal rats. These data indicate that NO released from the urothelium can suppress the excitability of adjacent afferent nerves.[23]

The presence of muscarinic and nicotinic receptors in the urothelium has focused attention on the role of acetylcholine as a chemical mediator of neural–urothelial interactions.[17,18,23] Urothelial cells express the various proteins necessary for the synthesis and storage of acetylcholine, including the plasma membrane choline transporter, choline acetyltransferase, and the vesicle acetycholine transporter as well as the enzyme responsible for the metabolism of acetylcholine (acetylcholinesterase). In addition it has been reported that acetylcholine is released from the bladder urothelium in rats and humans by other chemical or mechanical stimuli.[23] Reverse transcriptase polymerase chain reaction (RTPCR) experiments revealed the expression of multiple subtypes of nicotinic (α_7, α_3, β_4, and β_5) and muscarinic receptors (M_1–M_5) in rat urothelial cells. In addition, exogenous cholinergic muscarinic and nicotinic agonists applied to cultured urothelial cells can elicit an increase in intracellular Ca^{2+} concentration and evoke the release of NO and ATP.[17,18,22] In bladder strips or whole bladder preparations, muscarinic agonists also stimulate the release of a smooth muscle inhibitory factor from the urothelium.[5]

The function of cholinergic receptors in the urothelium has also been evaluated by testing the effects of intravesically administered cholinergic agonists and antagonists on voiding function in cats and rats. The intravesical application of nicotine in the rat elicits two effects: a decrease in the frequency of reflex micturition in low concentrations and an increase in frequency in high concentrations.[22] The inhibitory effect was blocked by methyllycaconitine, an antagonist of α_7 nicotinic receptors, whereas the facilitatory effect was blocked by hexamethonium, an antagonist of α_3 type nicotinic receptors. Methyllycaconitine alone did not alter reflex bladder activity, whereas hexamethonium alone decreased reflex bladder activity, suggesting the existence of a tonically active nicotinic facilitatory mechanism.

In chronic spinal cord injured cats, intravesical infusion of oxotremorine methiodide, a quaternary ammonium muscarinic agonist that should have a relatively low ability to penetrate the urothelial barrier, or carbachol, a muscarinic–nicotinic agonist, decreased bladder capacity and enhanced the number of premicturition contractions during cystometrograms, but did not alter the amplitude of micturition contractions.[23] These effects were blocked by the intravesical administration of atropine methyl nitrate, indicating that activation of muscarinic receptors in the urothelium or in urothelial afferent nerves facilitates the spinal micturition reflex mediated by C-fiber afferent nerves. Intravesical administration of muscarinic agonists and antagonists elicits similar responses in the rat. Thus, the clinical effect of antimuscarinic agents to decrease sensory symptoms in overactive bladder may be related to the block of muscarinic receptors in the urothelium or afferent nerves.

ANATOMY OF CENTRAL NERVOUS PATHWAYS CONTROLLING THE LOWER URINARY TRACT

The reflex circuitry controlling micturition consists of four basic components: primary afferent neurons, spinal efferent neurons, spinal interneurons, and neurons in the brain that modulate spinal reflex pathways.

Pathways in the spinal cord

Afferent projections in the spinal cord

Afferent pathways from the bladder project into Lissauer's tract at the apex of the dorsal horn and then send collaterals laterally and medially around the dorsal horn into laminae V–VII and X at the base of the dorsal horn (Figure 2.3a).[24] The lateral pathway terminates in the region of the sacral parasympathetic nucleus and also sends some axons to the dorsal commissure (Figure 2.3a). Pudendal afferent pathways from the urethra and urethral sphincter exhibit a similar pattern of termination in the sacral spinal cord.

Efferent neurons

Parasympathetic preganglionic neurons are located in the intermediolateral gray matter (laminae V–VII) in the sacral segments of the spinal cord whereas sympathetic preganglionic neurons are located in medial (lamina X) and lateral sites (laminae V–VII) in the rostral lumbar spinal cord.[25] External urethral sphincter (EUS) motoneurons are located in lamina IX in Onuf's nucleus.[9]

Spinal interneurons

As shown in Figure 2.3c, interneurons retrogradely labeled by the injection of pseudorabies

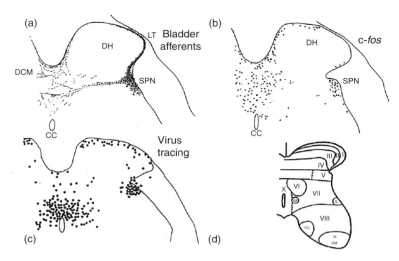

Figure 2.3 Comparison of the distribution of bladder afferent projections to the L$_6$ spinal cord of the rat (a) with the distribution of c-*fos* positive cells in the L$_6$ spinal segment following chemical irritation of the lower urinary tract of the rat (b) and the distribution of interneurons in the L$_6$ spinal cord labeled by transneuronal transport of pseudorabies virus injected into the urinary bladder (c). Afferents are labeled by wheat germ agglutinin-horseradish peroxidase (WGA-HRP) injected into the urinary bladder. c-*fos* immunoreactivity is present in the nuclei of cells. DH, dorsal horn; SPN, sacral parasympathetic nucleus; CC central canal. (d) This drawing shows the laminar organization of the cat spinal cord.

virus (PRV) into the urinary bladder or urethra of the rat are located in regions of the spinal cord receiving afferent input from the bladder.[26,27] Large populations of interneurons are located just dorsal and medial to the preganglionic neurons as well as in the dorsal commissure and lamina I.

The spinal neurons involved in processing afferent input from the lower urinary tract have been identified by the expression of the immediate early gene, c-*fos* (Figure 2.3b).[28] In the rat, chemical or mechanical stimulation of the bladder and urethra increases the levels of Fos protein primarily in the dorsal commissure, the superficial dorsal horn, and the area of the sacral parasympathetic nucleus (Figure 2.3b). Some of these interneurons make local connections in the spinal cord and participate in segmental spinal reflexes,[29] whereas others send long projections to supraspinal centers, such as the periaqueductal gray (PAG) and nucleus gracilis that are involved in the supraspinal control of micturition.

Pathways in the brain

In the rat, transneuronal virus tracing methods have identified many populations of neurons

in the brain that are involved in control of the bladder, urethra, and the urethral sphincter, including Barrington's nucleus (the pontine micturition center, PMC); medullary raphe nuclei, which contain serotonergic neurons; the locus coeruleus, which contains noradrenergic neurons; periaqueductal gray; and the A5 noradrenergic cell group (Figure 2.4).[26,27] Several regions in the hypothalamus and the cerebral cortex also exhibited virus-infected cells. Neurons in the cortex were located primarily in the medial frontal cortex.

Other anatomical studies in which anterograde tracer substances were injected into brain areas and then identified in terminals in the spinal cord (Figure 2.5) are consistent with the virus tracing data. Tracer injected into the paraventricular nucleus of the hypothalamus labeled terminals in the sacral parasympathetic nucleus as well as the sphincter motor nucleus. On the other hand, neurons in the anterior hypothalamus project to the PMC. Neurons in the PMC in turn project primarily to the sacral parasympathetic nucleus and the lateral edge of the dorsal horn and the dorsal commissure, areas containing dendritic projections from preganglionic neurons, sphincter motoneurons, and afferent inputs from the

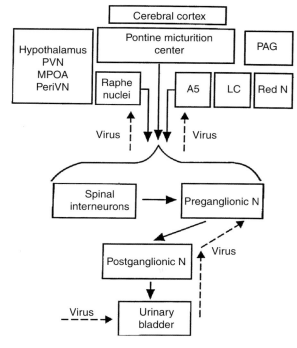

Figure 2.4 Structures in the brain and spinal cord of the adult and neonatal rat labeled after injection of pseudorabies virus into the urinary bladder or the urethra. Virus is transported transneuronally in a retrograde direction (dashed arrows). Normal synaptic connections are indicated by solid arrows. At long survival times the virus can be detected in neurons at specific sites in the spinal cord and brain, extending to the pontine micturition center in the pons (i.e. Barrington's nucleus) and to the cerebral cortex. Other sites in the brain labeled by the virus are: (1) the paraventricular nucleus (PVN), medial preoptic area (MPOA), and periventricular nucleus (PeriVN) of the hypothalamus; (2) periaqueductal gray (PAG); (3) locus coeruleus (LC) and subcoeruleus; (4) red nucleus (Red N); (5) medullary raphe nuclei; and (6) the noradrenergic cell group designated as A5.

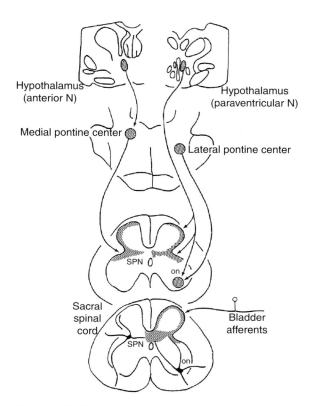

Figure 2.5 Neural connections between the brain and the sacral spinal cord that may be involved in the regulation of the lower urinary tract in the cat. Lower section of spinal cord shows the location and morphology of a preganglionic neuron in the sacral parasympathetic nucleus (SPN), a sphincter motoneuron in Onuf's nucleus (ON), and the sites of central termination of afferent projections from the urinary bladder. Upper section of the spinal cord shows the sites of termination of descending pathways arising in the medial pontine micturition center (PMC), the lateral pontine sphincter or urine storage center, and the paraventricular nuclei of the hypothalamus. Section through the pons shows the projection from the anterior hypothalamic nuclei to the pontine micturition center.

bladder (Figure 2.5).[2] Conversely, projections from neurons in the lateral pons, an area implicated in the control of urethral sphincter function, terminate rather selectively in the sphincter motor nucleus. Thus, the sites of termination of descending projections from the pontine micturition center are optimally located to regulate reflex mechanisms at the spinal level.

REFLEX CONTROL OF THE LOWER URINARY TRACT

The neural pathways controlling lower urinary tract function are organized as simple on–off switching circuits (Figures 2.6 and 2.7) that maintain a reciprocal relationship between the urinary bladder and urethral outlet. Intravesical pressure measurements during bladder filling in both humans and animals reveal low and relatively constant bladder pressures when bladder volume is below the threshold for inducing voiding (Figure 2.6). The accommodation of the bladder to increasing volumes of urine is primarily a passive phenomenon dependent upon the intrinsic properties of the vesical smooth muscle and quiescence of the parasympathetic efferent pathway. In addition, in some species urine storage is also facilitated by sympathetic reflexes that mediate an inhibition of bladder activity, closure of the bladder neck, and contraction of the proximal urethra (Table 2.2, Figure 2.7). During bladder filling the activity of the sphincter electromyogram (EMG) also increases (Figure 2.6), reflecting an increase in efferent firing in the pudendal nerve and an increase in outlet resistance that contributes to the maintenance of urinary continence.

The storage phase of the urinary bladder can be switched to the voiding phase either involuntarily (Figure 2.6a) or voluntarily (Figure 2.6b). The former is readily demonstrated in the human infant (Figure 2.6a) when the volume of urine exceeds the micturition threshold. At this point, increased afferent firing from tension receptors in the bladder produces firing in the sacral parasympathetic pathways and an inhibition of sympathetic and somatic pathways. The expulsion phase consists of an initial relaxation of the urethral sphincter (Figure 2.6a) followed by a contraction of the bladder, an increase in bladder pressure, and flow of urine. Relaxation of the urethral outlet is mediated by the activation of a parasympathetic reflex pathway to the urethra (Table 2.2) that triggers the release of nitric oxide, an inhibitory transmitter, as well as by removal of adrenergic and somatic excitatory inputs to the urethra.

Organization of urine storage reflexes

Sympathetic storage reflex

Although the integrity of the sympathetic input to the lower urinary tract is not essential for the performance of micturition, it does contribute to the storage function of the bladder. Surgical interruption or pharmacological blockade of the sympathetic innervation can reduce urethral outflow resistance, reduce bladder capacity, and increase

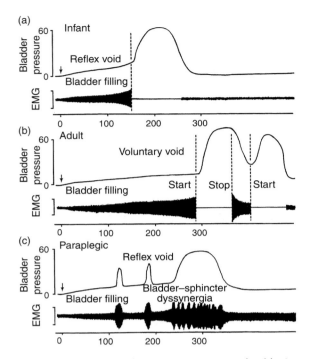

Figure 2.6 Combined cystometrograms and sphincter electromyograms (EMG) comparing reflex voiding responses in an infant (a) and in a paraplegic patient (c) with a voluntary voiding response in an adult (b). The abscissa in all records represents bladder volume in milliliters and the ordinates represent bladder pressure in cmH₂O and electrical activity of the EMG recording. On the left side of each trace the arrows indicate the start of a slow infusion of fluid into the bladder (bladder filling). Vertical dashed lines indicate the start of sphincter relaxation which precedes by a few seconds the bladder contraction in (a) and (b). In (b) note that a voluntary cessation of voiding (stop) is associated with an initial increase in sphincter EMG followed by a reciprocal relaxation of the bladder. A resumption of voiding is again associated with sphincter relaxation and a delayed increase in bladder pressure. On the other hand, in the paraplegic patient (c) the reciprocal relationship between bladder and sphincter is abolished. During bladder filling, transient uninhibited bladder contractions occur in association with sphincter activity. Further filling leads to more prolonged and simultaneous contractions of the bladder and sphincter (bladder–sphincter dyssynergia). Loss of the reciprocal relationship between bladder and sphincter in paraplegic patients interferes with bladder emptying.

the frequency and amplitude of bladder contractions recorded under constant volume conditions.

Sympathetic reflex activity is elicited by a sacrolumbar intersegmental spinal reflex pathway

Table 2.2 Reflexes to the lower urinary tract

Afferent pathway	Efferent pathway	Central pathway
Urine storage		
Low level vesical afferent activity (pelvic nerve)	1. External sphincter contraction (somatic nerves)	Spinal reflexes
	2. Internal sphincter contraction (sympathetic nerves)	
	3. Detrusor inhibition (sympathetic nerves)	
	4. Ganglionic inhibition (sympathetic nerves)	
	5. Sacral parasympathetic outflow inactive	
Afferent activity from the external urethral sphincter	6. Inhibition of parasympathetic outflow	Spinal reflex
Micturition		
High level vesical afferent activity (pelvic nerve)	1. Inhibition of external sphincter activity	Spinobulbospinal reflexes
	2. Inhibition of sympathetic outflow	
	3. Activation of parasympathetic outflow to the bladder	
	4. Activation of parasympathetic outflow to the urethra	Spinal reflex

that is triggered by vesical afferent activity in the pelvic nerves (Figure 2.7a).[2] The reflex pathway is inhibited when the bladder pressure is raised to the threshold for producing micturition (Figure 2.7b). This inhibitory response is abolished by transection of the spinal cord at the lower thoracic level, indicating that it originates at a supraspinal site, possibly the pontine micturition center. Thus, the vesicosympathetic reflex represents a negative feedback mechanism (Figure 2.7a) that allows the bladder to accommodate larger volumes during bladder filling but is turned off during voiding to allow the bladder to empty completely.

Urethral sphincter storage reflex

Motoneurons innervating the striated muscles of the urethral sphincter exhibit a tonic discharge that increases during bladder filling. This activity is mediated in part by low-level afferent input from the bladder (Figure 2.7a). During micturition the firing of sphincter motoneurons is inhibited. This inhibition is dependent in part

on supraspinal mechanisms, since it is less prominent in chronic spinal animals.

Sphincter-to-bladder reflexes may also contribute to urine storage, because afferent activity arising in the striated sphincter muscles during contractions can suppress reflex bladder activity and in turn increase bladder capacity.[9] Studies in cats and monkeys revealed that direct electrical stimulation of the sphincter muscles or electrical stimulation of motor pathways to induce a contraction of the sphincters suppresses reflex bladder activity. Similar inhibitory responses are elicited by electrical stimulation of afferent axons in the pudendal nerve, some of which must arise in the sphincter muscles.

Organization of voiding reflexes

Spinobulbospinal micturition reflex pathway

Micturition is mediated by activation of the sacral parasympathetic efferent pathway to the bladder and the urethra as well as reciprocal inhibition of the somatic pathway to the urethral sphincter (Table 2.2) (Figure 2.7b). Studies in cats

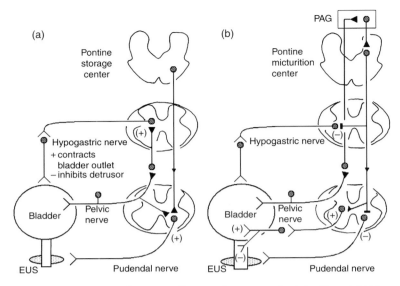

Figure 2.7 Diagram showing neural circuits controlling continence and micturition. (a) Urine storage reflexes. During the storage of urine, distention of the bladder produces low level vesical afferent firing, which in turn stimulates (1) the sympathetic outflow to the bladder outlet (base and urethra) and (2) pudendal outflow to the external urethral sphincter (EUS). These responses occur by spinal reflex pathways and represent guarding reflexes, which promote continence. Sympathetic firing also inhibits detrusor muscle and modulates transmission in bladder ganglia. A region in the rostral pons (the pontine storage center) increases external urethral sphincter activity. (b) Voiding reflexes. During elimination of urine, intense bladder afferent firing activates spinobulbospinal reflex pathways passing through the pontine micturition center, which stimulate the parasympathetic outflow to the bladder and internal sphincter smooth muscle and inhibit the sympathetic and pudendal outflow to the urethral outlet. Ascending afferent input from the spinal cord may pass through relay neurons in the periaqueductal gray (PAG) before reaching the pontine micturition center.

using brain-lesioning and electrophysiological techniques revealed that the micturition reflex is mediated by a spinobulbospinal pathway that passes through the pontine micturition center in the rostral brain stem (Figures 2.5 and 2.7b).[30] In the cat, afferent input from the bladder reaches the pontine micturition center after passing through a relay station in the periaqueductal gray (PAG).[31] The micturition reflex pathway functions as an "on–off" switch that is activated by a critical level of afferent activity arising from tension receptors in the bladder and is, in turn, modulated by inhibitory and excitatory influences from areas of the brain rostral to the pons (e.g. diencephalon and cerebral cortex) (Figures 2.8 and 2.9).

Suprapontine control of micturition

Lesion and electrical stimulation studies indicate that voluntary control of micturition depends on connections between the frontal cortex, hypothalamus, and other forebrain structures such as the anterior cingulate gyrus, amygdala, bed nucleus of the stria terminalis, and septal nuclei, where electrical stimulation elicits excitatory bladder effects. Damage to the cerebral cortex due to tumors, aneurysms, or cerebrovascular disease appears to remove inhibitory control of the pontine micturition center resulting in bladder overactivity.[32]

Human brain imaging studies (Figure 2.8) using single photon emission computed tomography (SPECT), positron emission tomography (PET), and functional magnetic resonance imaging (fMRI) have examined the areas of the brain involved in the control of micturition.[32] Some studies evaluated the brain areas responsible for the perception of bladder fullness and the sensation of the desire to void during bladder filling, whereas others examined brain activity during micturition, and voluntary contractions of the

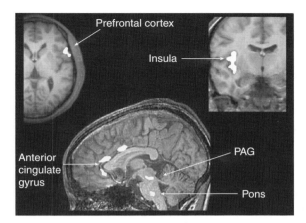

Figure 2.8 Regions of the human brain identified in positron emission tomography (PET) imaging studies that exhibit differences in activity based on whether the bladder is full or empty. PAG, periaqueductal gray.

Micturition reflex pathways

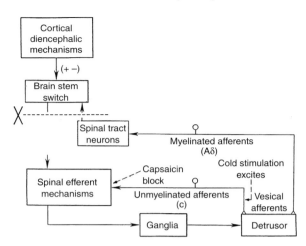

Figure 2.9 Diagram showing the organization of the parasympathetic excitatory reflex pathway to the detrusor muscle. Scheme is based on electrophysiologic studies in cats. In animals with an intact spinal cord, micturition is initiated by a supraspinal reflex pathway passing through a center in the brain stem. The pathway is triggered by myelinated afferents (Aδ fibers), which are connected to the tension receptors in the bladder wall. Injury to the spinal cord above the sacral segments interrupts the connections between the brain and spinal autonomic centers and initially blocks micturition. However, over a period of several weeks following cord injury, a spinal reflex mechanism emerges, which is triggered by unmyelinated vesical afferents (C fibers); the A-fiber afferent inputs are ineffective. The C-fiber reflex pathway is usually weak or undetectable in animals with an intact nervous system. Stimulation of the C-fiber bladder afferents by instillation of ice water into the bladder (cold stimulation) activates voiding responses in patients with spinal cord injury. Capsaicin (20–30 mg, subcutaneously) blocks the C-fiber reflex in chronic spinal cats, but does not block micturition reflexes in intact cats. Intravesical capsaicin also suppresses detrusor hyperreflexia and cold-evoked reflexes in patients with neurogenic bladder dysfunction.

pelvic floor during urine withholding or during cold stimulation of the bladder. PET scan studies revealed that two cortical areas (dorsolateral prefrontal cortex and the anterior cingulate gyrus) were active (i.e. exhibited increased blood flow) during voiding.[32,33] The hypothalamus, including the preoptic area as well as the pons and the PAG, also showed activity in concert with voluntary micturition. Other PET studies that examined the changes in brain activity during filling of the bladder revealed that increased activity occurred in the PAG, the midline pons, the mid-cingulate gyrus, and bilaterally in the frontal lobes. The results were consistent with the notion that the PAG receives information about bladder fullness and then relays this information to other brain areas involved in the control of bladder storage.

It has been speculated that the role of the prefrontal cortex, which is thought to be the seat of planning of complex behaviors, is to make a decision as to whether or not micturition should take place at a particular time or place.[33] On the other hand, the anterior cingulate, which is a part of the limbic system and which is thought to be involved in cognitive processes involving attention and executive control, may be involved in the integration of afferent input with the control of autonomic efferent outflow to the lower urinary tract. SPECT scanning of patients with urgency incontinence revealed hypoperfusion of the anterior cingulate gyrus as well as other frontal lobe regions such as the prefrontal cortex.

Spinal micturition reflex pathway

Spinal cord injury rostral to the lumbosacral level eliminates voluntary and supraspinal control of voiding, leading initially to an areflexic bladder and complete urinary retention followed by a slow development of automatic micturition and bladder hyperactivity (Figure 2.6c) mediated by spinal reflex pathways.[2,30] However, voiding is commonly inefficient due to simultaneous contractions of the bladder and urethral sphincter (bladder–sphincter dyssynergia) (Figure 2.6c). Electrophysiologic studies in animals have shown that the micturition reflex pathway changes after spinal cord injury. For example, the afferent limb of the micturition reflex in cats with chronic spinal transection above the lumbar level consists of unmyelinated (C-fiber) axons (Figure 2.9), whereas in cats with an intact spinal cord, myelinated (Aδ) afferents activate the micturition reflex (Figure 2.9).[12,30] In normal cats, capsaicin did not block reflex contractions of the bladder or the Aδ-fiber-evoked bladder reflex. However, in cats with chronic spinal injury, capsaicin, a neurotoxin known to disrupt the function of C-fiber afferents, completely blocked C-fiber-evoked bladder reflexes.[12,30] Evidence of the contribution of C-fiber bladder afferents to bladder hyperactivity and involuntary voiding in humans has been obtained in studies in which capsaicin or resiniferatoxin, another C-fiber afferent neurotoxin, was administered intravesically to patients with neurogenic detrusor overactivity due to multiple sclerosis or spinal cord injuries. In these patients the toxins increased bladder capacity and reduced the frequency of incontinence.[30]

The emergence of C-fiber bladder reflexes seems to be mediated by several mechanisms, including changes in central synaptic connections and alterations in the properties of the peripheral afferent receptors that lead to sensitization of the "silent" C fibers and the unmasking of responses to mechanical stimuli.[2] In rats it has been shown that bladder afferent neurons undergo both morphologic (neuronal hypertrophy) and physiologic changes (upregulation of tetrodotoxin (TTX)-sensitive Na^+ channels and downregulation of TTX-resistant Na^+ channels) following spinal cord injury.[11,16,30] It has been speculated that this neuroplasticity is mediated by the actions of neurotrophic factors such as nerve growth factor (NGF) released within the spinal cord or the urinary bladder. The production of neurotrophic factors including NGF

increases in the bladder after spinal cord injury, whereas chronic administration of NGF into the bladder of rats induces bladder hyperactivity and increases the firing frequency of dissociated bladder afferent neurons.[11,30] On the other hand, intrathecal application of NGF antibodies to neutralize NGF in the spinal cord suppresses detrusor hyperreflexia and detrusor–sphincter dyssynergia in spinal cord injured rats.

NEUROTRANSMITTERS IN CENTRAL MICTURITION REFLEX PATHWAYS

Excitatory neurotransmitters

Excitatory transmission in the central pathways to the lower urinary tract depends on several types of neurotransmitters, including: glutamic acid, neuropeptides, nitric oxide, and ATP.[2,10] Pharmacological experiments in rats have revealed that glutamic acid is an essential transmitter in the ascending, pontine, and descending limbs of the spinobulbospinal micturition reflex pathway and in spinal reflex pathways controlling the bladder and external urethral sphincter.[34] N-methyl-D-aspartate (NMDA) and non-NMDA glutamatergic synaptic mechanisms appear to interact synergistically to mediate transmission in these pathways.

Inhibitory neurotransmitters

Several types of inhibitory transmitters, including inhibitory amino acids (γ-aminobutyric acid (GABA), glycine) and opioid peptides (enkephalins) can suppress the micturition reflex when applied to the central nervous system. Experimental evidence in anesthetized animals indicates that GABA and enkephalins exert a tonic inhibitory control in the PMC and regulate bladder capacity. These substances also have inhibitory actions in the spinal cord.[10,35]

Transmitters with mixed excitatory and inhibitory actions

Some transmitters (dopamine, 5-hydroxytryptamine, norepinephrine, acetylcholine, and non-opioid peptides including vasoactive intestinal polypeptide and corticotropin-releasing factor) have both inhibitory and excitatory effects on reflex bladder activity. In some instances different effects are mediated by different types of receptors. For example, the inhibitory effects of dopamine are mediated by D_1-like (D_1 and D_5) and the facilitatory effects are mediated by D_2-like (D_2, D_3, and D_4) receptor subtypes. Loss of forebrain dopaminergic mechanisms in patients with idiopathic Parkinson's disease is associated with bladder hyperactivity.

Interest in the role of 5-hydroxytryptamine in the central control of micturition has increased following the introduction of duloxetine, a serotonin–norepinephrine reuptake inhibitor, for the treatment of stress urinary incontinence. 5-Hydroxytryptamine (5-HT) has complex effects on the lower urinary tract which vary in different species.[36–40] In the cat, activation of central 5-HT_{1A} receptors inhibits reflex bladder activity,[38] whereas activation of 5-HT_2 receptors enhances urethral sphincter activity.[40] On the other hand, activation of central 5-HT_{1A} receptors in the rat enhances bladder and sphincter reflexes.[39] The similarities in the effects of duloxetine in the cat and the human indicate that micturition in the cat may be a useful model for developing centrally acting serotonergic agents for the treatment of lower urinary tract dysfunction.

CONCLUSIONS

The functions of the lower urinary tract to store and periodically eliminate urine are regulated by a complex neural control system that performs like a simple switching circuit to maintain a reciprocal relationship between the bladder and urethral outlet. The switching circuit is modulated by several neurotransmitter systems and is therefore sensitive to a variety of drugs and neurologic diseases. A more complete understanding of the neural mechanisms involved in bladder and urethral control will no doubt facilitate the development of new diagnostic methods and therapies for lower urinary tract dysfunction.

REFERENCES

1. Fry CH, Brading AF, Hussain M et al. Cell biology. In: Abrams P, Cardozo L, Khoury S, Wein A, eds. Incontinence. Plymouth, UK: Health Publication Ltd, 2005: 363–432.
2. Morrison J, Birder L, Craggs M et al. Neural control. In: Abrams P, Cardozo L, Khoury S, Wein A, eds. Incontinence. Plymouth, UK: Health Publication Ltd, 2005: 363–432.
3. de Groat WC, Booth AM. Synaptic transmission in pelvic ganglia. In: Maggi CA, ed. The Autonomic Nervous System, Vol. 3, Nervous Control of the Urogenital System. London: Harwood Academic Publisher, 1993: 291–347.
4. Matsui M, Motomura D, Karasawa H et al. Multiple functional defects in peripheral autonomic organs in mice lacking muscarinic acetylcholine receptor gene for the M3 subtype. Proc Natl Acad Sci USA 2000; 97: 9579–84.
5. Andersson KE, Arner A. Urinary bladder contraction and relaxation: physiology and pathophysiology. Physiol Rev 2004; 84: 935–86.
6. Hegde SS. Muscarinic receptors in the bladder: from basic research to therapeutics. Br J Pharmacol 2006; 147 (Suppl 2): S80–7.
7. Burnstock G. Purinergic signaling in the lower urinary tract. In: Abbracchio MP, Williams M, eds. Handbook of Experimental Pharmacology. Berlin: Springer Verlag, 2001: 423–515.
8. Somogyi GT, Tanowitz M, Zernova G, de Groat WC. M1 muscarinic receptor-induced facilitation of ACh and noradrenaline release in the rat bladder is mediated by protein kinase. C. J Physiol 1996; 496: 245–54.
9. de Groat WC, Fraser MO, Yoshiyama M et al. Neural control of the urethra. Scand J Urol Nephrol Suppl 2001; 207: 35–43.
10. de Groat WC, Yoshimura N. Pharmacology of the lower urinary tract. Ann Rev Pharmacol Toxicol 2001; 41: 691–721.
11. Vizzard MA. Neurochemical plasticity and the role of neurotrophic factors in bladder reflex pathways after spinal cord injury. Prog Brain Res 2006; 152: 97–115.
12. Cheng CL, Liu JC, Chang SY, Ma CP, de Groat WC. Effect of capsaicin on the micturition reflex in normal and chronic spinal cord-injured cats. Am J Physiol 1999; 277: R786–94.
13. Cockayne DA, Hamilton SG, Zhu QM et al. Urinary bladder hyporeflexia and reduced pain-related behaviour in P2X3-deficient mice. Nature 2000; 407: 1011–15.
14. Rong W, Spyer KM, Burnstock G. Activation and sensitisation of low and high threshold afferent fibres mediated by P2X receptors in the mouse urinary bladder. J Physiol 2002; 541: 591–600.

15. Yoshimura N, de Groat WC. Increased excitability of afferent neurons innervating rat urinary bladder after chronic bladder inflammation. J Neurosci 1999; 19: 4644–53.

16. Yoshimura N, de Groat WC. Plasticity of Na$^+$ channels in afferent neurones innervating rat urinary bladder following spinal cord injury. J Physiol 1997; 503: 269–76.

17. Birder LA. More than just a barrier: urothelium as a drug target for urinary bladder pain. Am J Physiol Renal Physiol 2005; 289: F489–95.

18. de Groat WC. The urothelium in overactive bladder: passive bystander or active participant? Urology 2004; 64: 7–11.

19. Ferguson DR, Kennedy I, Burton TJ. ATP is released from rabbit urinary bladder epithelial cells by hydrostatic pressure changes—a possible sensory mechanism? J Physiol 1997; 505: 503–11.

20. Birder LA, Apodaca G, de Groat WC, Kanai AJ. Adrenergic- and capsaicin-evoked nitric oxide release from urothelium and afferent nerves in urinary bladder. Am J Physiol 1998; 275: F226–9.

21. Birder LA, Nakamura Y, Kiss S et al. Altered urinary bladder function in mice lacking the vanilloid receptor TRPV1. Nat Neurosci 2002; 5: 856–60.

22. Beckel JM, Kanai A, Lee SJ, de Groat WC, Birder LA. Expression of functional nicotinic acetylcholine receptors in rat urinary bladder epithelial cells. Am J Physiol Renal Physiol 2006; 290: F103–10.

23. de Groat WC. Integrative control of the lower urinary tract: preclinical perspective. Br J Pharmacol 2006; 147 (Suppl 2): S25–40.

24. Steers WD, Ciambotti J, Etzel B, Erdman S, de Groat WC. Alterations in afferent pathways from the urinary bladder of the rat in response to partial urethral obstruction. J Comp Neurol 1991; 310: 401–10.

25. Morgan CW, de Groat WC, Felkins LA, Zhang SJ. Intracellular injection of neurobiotin or horseradish peroxidase reveals separate types of preganglionic neurons in the sacral parasympathetic nucleus of the cat. J Comp Neurol 1993; 331: 161–82.

26. Nadelhaft I, Vera PL, Card JP, Miselis RR. Central nervous system neurons labelled following the injection of pseudorabies virus into the rat urinary bladder. Neurosci Lett 1992; 143: 271–4.

27. Vizzard MA, Erickson VL, Card JP, Roppolo JR, de Groat WC. Transneuronal labeling of neurons in the adult rat brainstem and spinal cord after injection of pseudorabies virus into the urethra. J Comp Neurol 1995; 355: 629–40.

28. Birder LA, de Groat WC. Induction of c-fos expression in spinal neurons by nociceptive and non-nociceptive stimulation of LUT. Am J Physiol 1993; 265: R326–33.

29. Araki I, de Groat WC. Unitary excitatory synaptic currents in preganglionic neurons mediated by two distinct groups of interneurons in neonatal rat sacral parasympathetic nucleus. J Neurophysiol 1996; 76: 215–26.

30. de Groat WC, Yoshimura N. Mechanisms underlying the recovery of lower urinary tract function following spinal cord injury. Prog Brain Res 2006; 152: 59–84.

31. Blok BF, De Weerd H, Holstege G. Ultrastructural evidence for a paucity of projections from the lumbosacral cord to the pontine micturition center or M-region in the cat: a new concept for the organization of the micturition reflex with the periaqueductal gray as central relay. J Comp Neurol 1995; 359: 300–9.

32. Fowler CJ. Integrated control of lower urinary tract – clinical perspective. Br J Pharmacol 2006; 147 (Suppl 2): S14–24.

33. Kavia RB, Dasgupta R, Fowler CJ. Functional imaging and the central control of the bladder. J Comp Neurol 2005; 493: 27–32.

34. Yoshiyama M, de Groat WC. Supraspinal and spinal alpha-amino-3-hydroxy-5-methylisoxazole-4-propionic acid and N-methyl-D-aspartate glutamatergic control of the micturition reflex in the urethane-anesthetized rat. Neuroscience 2005; 132: 1017–26.

35. Mallory BS, Roppolo JR, de Groat WC. Pharmacological modulation of the pontine micturition center. Brain Res 1991; 546: 310–20.

36. de Groat WC. Influence of central serotonergic mechanisms on lower urinary tract function. Urology 2002; 59: 30–6.

37. Ramage AG. The role of central 5-hydroxytryptamine (5-HT, serotonin) receptors in the control of micturition. Br J Pharmacol 2006; 147 (Suppl 2): S120–31.

38. Tai C, Miscik CL, Ungerer TD, Roppolo JR, de Groat WC. Suppression of bladder reflex activity in chronic spinal cord injured cats by activation of serotonin 5-HT(1A) receptors. Exp Neurol 2006; 199: 427–37.

39. Chang HY, Cheng CL, Chen JJ, de Groat WC. Roles of glutamatergic and serotonergic mechanisms in reflex control of the external urethral sphincter in urethane-anesthetized female rats. Am J Physiol Regul Integr Comp Physiol 2006; 291: R224–34.

40. Thor KB. Serotonin and norepinephrine involvement in efferent pathways to the urethral rhabdosphincter: implications for treating stress urinary incontinence. Urology 2003; 62 (4 Suppl 1): 3–9.

3

Diagnosis of overactive bladder

Eric S Rovner and Melissa Walls

**History • Physical examination • Urine analysis • Post-void residual urine measurement
• Urodynamics • Cystourethroscopy • Imaging • Other laboratory tests • Conclusions**

Overactive bladder (OAB) is a highly prevalent disorder impacting on millions of people's lives throughout the world.[1,2] Despite its high prevalence, many sufferers do not seek medical attention and are not aware that OAB is treatable. Over the past few years, several changes in terminology and advances in therapy for this condition have occurred. Because of these developments, considerable confusion exists within and outside the medical community with respect to the diagnosis of this burdensome condition. In order to optimize the identification and subsequent diagnosis of individuals who may suffer from OAB, it is important to fully understand the current definition of the term.

The exact origin of the term "overactive bladder" is unknown, but nevertheless, it became widely utilized and popularized in the medical lexicon in the latter half of the 1990s. It is interesting that, although much controversy was engendered by the use of the phrase "overactive bladder", this exact term was never actually defined or described by the International Continence Society (ICS) in prior terminology reports until 2001. The term overactive detrusor function (generally shortened to overactive detrusor) does appear[3] in the lexicon as a finding on urodynamic testing. This term is defined by the occurrence of involuntary detrusor contractions during the filling phase of cystometry, which may be spontaneous or provoked.

Thus, overactive detrusor function and the terms which, correctly or incorrectly, have been used as substitutes (overactive detrusor, detrusor overactivity, and, eventually, overactive bladder) were all urodynamic terms, and were utilized to describe abnormalities of detrusor function during filling cystometry. Thus, a urodynamic study was required to describe the finding of detrusor overactivity, which in turn then provided the patient with a de facto diagnosis of overactive bladder despite the fact that the term did not yet exist in the urologic literature. The limitations of this model were recognized by several authors.[4,5] It was apparent that the requirement of urodynamics in making the diagnosis placed an undue burden on the practicing physician, the patient, and the healthcare system in general. In addition, the term overactive bladder would need to be formally defined.

Several important ICS reports with substantial clinical and research implications were subsequently published, including a report on 'The standardisation of terminology of lower urinary tract function'.[3] The definitions and descriptions were meant to restate or update those presented in previous ICS standardization of terminology reports.[6] Among other important changes and updates, this report addressed the definition and use of the term "overactive bladder" and classified it as a type of syndrome. According to this document, syndromes "describe constellations or varying combinations of symptoms but cannot be used for precise diagnosis ... [syndromes] are functional abnormalities for which a precise cause has not been defined."[3] Overactive bladder syndrome, urge syndrome, or urgency–frequency syndrome is thus defined as "urgency with or without urge incontinence, usually with frequency and nocturia". Although the document indicates that these symptoms are suggestive of detrusor overactivity (a term later defined in this document as the observation of involuntary detrusor contractions during the filling phase of cystometry), a urodynamic demonstration of detrusor overactivity is not necessary, nor evident, in all cases. Furthermore, the definition allows that a variety of other conditions of urethrovesical dysfunction may result in a similar symptom complex.

Within the framework of this definition of OAB, it is important to emphasize that the use of the term overactive bladder is necessarily restricted to those situations in which local pathology such as infection and malignancy have been excluded. A large number of clinical conditions, both commonly encountered and rarely seen, can present with symptoms suggestive of OAB (Table 3.1).

Table 3.1 Differential diagnosis of overactive bladder (OAB)

Excessive fluid intake
Urinary retention (overflow)
Bacterial cystitis
Prostatitis
Radiation cystitis
Sexually transmitted disease (GC, *Chlamydia*, etc.)
Interstitial cystitis, sensory urgency syndromes
Bladder cancer
Bladder stones
Pelvic mass (GI, GU, GYN, vascular aneurysm, etc.)
Gynecological problem
  vaginitis, endometriosis, malignancy, etc.
  postmenopausal atrophic vaginitis
  vaginal prolapse: cystocele, rectocele, etc.
  severe stress urinary incontinence
Medical illnesses producing fluid shifts:
  CHF, cirrhosis, etc.
Drugs (e.g. diuretics)
Other

GC, *Neisseria gonorrhoeae*; GI, gastrointestinal; GU, genitourinary; GYN, gynecological; CHF, congestive heart failure.

The goal of the practitioner in the evaluation of OAB should be to assess the individual for the presence of symptoms suggestive of OAB, and then be able to comfortably, confidently, and accurately exclude the coexistence of most of these conditions. Fortunately, a well done and complete medical history consistent with OAB, a normal physical examination, and an unremarkable urine analysis will usually be adequate to exclude many of these conditions and arrive at the proper diagnosis. The diagnosis of OAB is usually not difficult; however, in appropriate cases, the use of additional selected, adjunctive studies may be helpful.

In this chapter, we will discuss the usual diagnostic evaluation of the patient with suspected OAB and briefly review some of the adjunctive studies that may be indicated in selected cases. The evaluation of an individual with suspected OAB should be simple, rapid, and accurate, in order to initiate effective therapy and alleviate the symptoms associated with the condition.

HISTORY

Symptom assessment

As noted in the definition discussed above, OAB is a symptomatic diagnosis. Therefore, a proper symptom assessment, both qualitatively and quantitively, is of paramount importance. Typical symptoms of the overactive bladder include an increased number of micturitions (urinary frequency, usually greater than 8×/day), a strong and sudden desire to void which is difficult to defer (urinary urgency), and, if the urgency cannot be suppressed, urinary urge incontinence.[7] People suffering from bladder overactivity typically have to empty their bladders frequently, and when they experience a sensation of urgency, they may leak urine if they are unable to reach the toilet quickly. The amount of urine lost may be large, as the bladder may empty completely and involuntarily. Sleep may be disturbed, as the need to void may awaken the patient. Nighttime frequency and nocturnal enuresis (bedwetting) is often particularly disruptive. Urinary incontinence occurring shortly after, or in concert with, the sensation of impending leakage is called urge incontinence. Urinary incontinence of any kind may not be present in up to two-thirds of individuals with OAB.[2] In 2001,

Milsom et al. reported on the OAB symptom prevalence in a cohort of over 16 000 patients across six countries in Europe; of the 16.6% of individuals reporting OAB related symptomatology, frequency was the most commonly reported symptom (85%) followed by urgency (54%) and urge incontinence (36%).[8]

Frequency and nocturia can be assessed by patient report or voiding diaries (discussed below). Patient self-report of voiding frequency is quite variable, subject to considerable recall bias, and thus not generally considered highly reliable. Normative values for 24-hour urinary frequency are not universally agreed upon. Urinary frequency is obviously dependent on a number of variables including, but not limited to, volume intake (total fluid intake, etc.), insensible losses due to sweating and respiration, and climate factors (ambient humidity, etc.,) as well as the functional bladder capacity. Generally, urinary frequency of > 8 episodes/24 hours is considered consistent with a diagnosis of OAB and represents the threshold for inclusion into many OAB pharmacotherapy studies. The ICS conveniently quantified nocturia in defining the term: awakening from sleep one or more times in order to void.[9] Urgency is the cardinal symptom of OAB. Urinary urgency is defined as the compelling sensation to void which is difficult to defer.[3] Given its inherently subjective nature, this symptom is indeed difficult to quantify or qualify. It is unclear whether the severity or magnitude of each episode of urgency is important or whether the total number of episodes of urgency is important. Urgency episodes can be quantified by patient report or by voiding diaries, and are thus subject to the same limitations as quantifying frequency. Various urgency severity scales have been developed and validated.[10–12] Their role in assisting with the diagnosis of OAB is unknown, although they may assist in quantifying the magnitude of symptom bother related to this specific symptom of OAB.

In addition to assessing symptoms, a detailed past medical, gynecological, and surgical history should be obtained, specifically looking for possible causes of the patient's symptoms. The patient should be asked whether they have a history of sexually transmitted diseases, or vaginal or urethral discharge. The patient's menstrual history and bowel habits should be reviewed.

The patient's medications, both prescription and over the counter, should be assessed as potential causes for their symptoms as many classes of medications can have wide ranging and well documented collateral effects on lower urinary tract function.[13] The review of systems should concentrate on factors potentially related to etiology (neurologic, metabolic, medication(s), for example) or related diagnoses. A history of diabetes, neurologic disease, excess fluid intake, and prior pelvic/abdominal surgery are just some of the factors that should be specifically queried. As noted previously, a number of conditions may contribute to, or simulate, the overactive bladder, and a careful history will allow the practitioner to begin to differentiate between the possibilities.

Symptoms may not be completely diagnostic of the underlying problem, however. For example, OAB and stress incontinence are widespread problems in the general population and affect all age groups. Differentiating between the two, as well as recognizing increased frequency of micturition and urgency, is vital prior to selecting appropriate treatment. Patients with stress incontinence may void frequently in an attempt to avoid leakage ("defensive voiding"), as this condition is generally worse when the bladder is full. A careful history of the condition, with special emphasis on onset, progression/regression, and response/non-response to treatments, is valuable. The use of a diagnostic aid is sometimes helpful, in order to distinguish between the symptoms of OAB and stress incontinence (Table 3.2). However, it is important to realize that these two conditions often coexist (Figure 3.1).

Questionnaires

When assessing patients' symptoms, it is important to remember that the spectrum of overactive bladder and its effect on quality of life are quite broad. The degree by which the patient is affected by their symptoms may direct treatment planning. There exists a wide variety of validated questionnaires for the study of voiding dysfunction. Questionnaires employed for OAB have many utilities, both clinically and in the research arena, including screening, symptom assessment, and disease impact, or as a measure of health-related quality of life. The majority of

Table 3.2   Differentiating overactive bladder (OAB) from stress incontinence[14]

Symptoms	OAB	Stress incontinence
Urgency (strong, sudden desire to void)	Yes	No
Frequency with urgency	Yes	Rarely
Leaking during physical activity, e.g. coughing, sneezing, lifting, etc.	No	Yes
Amount of urinary leakage with each episode of incontinence	Large if present	Usually small
Ability to reach the toilet in time following an urge to void	No or just barely	Yes
Nocturnal incontinence (presence of wet pads or undergarments in bed)	Yes	Rare
Nocturia (waking to pass urine at night)	Usually	Seldom

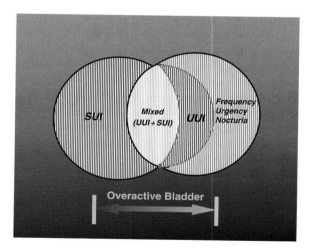

Figure 3.1   Spectrum of overactive bladder (OAB). OAB and stress incontinence may coexist. In addition, the OAB symptom complex includes those patients with irritative voiding symptoms such as urinary frequency, urgency, and nocturia, as well those with urgency incontinence and mixed (stress and urgency) incontinence. UUI, urgency incontinence; SUI, stress incontinence. (See also color plate section).

instruments are currently utilized as research tools, are not OAB specific, and are not generally used for diagnostic purposes. The specific details of each questionnaire are beyond the scope of this chapter (Table 3.3).

Voiding diaries

As noted previously, urinary frequency and urgency can be assessed by patient recall at the time of interview, or by self-monitoring using frequency–volume charts or voiding diaries. Urinary incontinence episodes can be captured in a likewise fashion. Although useful for quantifying symptoms, voiding diaries are not usually utilized as an initial diagnostic tool for OAB as the symptoms of OAB may be due to a variety of causes. However, voiding diaries are extremely useful in numerically assessing patient symptoms and evaluating patient outcomes before and after the initiation of treatment regimens. In short, voiding diaries are simple and inexpensive ways to obtain reasonably objective information on voiding behavior in the patient's usual environment. It should be noted that, although self-monitoring techniques may in themselves modify the behavior they are measuring, reported micturition frequency and number of incontinence episodes as recorded on a voiding diary have been found to be highly reproducible on a test–retest analysis.

Multiple studies have been performed in assessing the reliability, reproducibility, and accuracy of voiding diaries as a tool in the evaluation of lower urinary tract symptoms. Voiding diary parameters, specifically urinary frequency and incontinent episodes, have often been utilized as primary and secondary outcome measures in efficacy studies of various agents for the treatment of OAB.[23–30] Most voiding diaries will include intake volume, voided volumes, and incontinent and urgency episodes, as well as types of activities being performed during these episodes. Although 72-hour micturition

Table 3.3 Examples of questionnaires utilized in the evaluation of individuals with lower urinary tract symptoms

Questionnaire	Acronym	Item
Incontinence Impact Questionnaire[15,16]	IIQ-7	QoL
Urge Incontinence Impact Questionnaire[17]	Urge-IIQ	QoL
King's Health Questionnaire[18]	ICIQ-KHQ	QoL
Bristol Female Lower Urinary Tract Symptoms Questionnaire[19]	BFLUTS	QoL, symptoms, sexual function
Urinary Incontinence Quality of Life Instrument[20]	I-QoL	QoL
Overactive Bladder Questionnaire[21,22]	OAB-q	QoL, symptoms

QoL, quality of life.

diaries have shown excellent reliability, 24-hour micturition diaries are more convenient for the patient and seem to provide valid data.[31–33]

Pad tests

If incontinence is present in the setting of OAB, there are a variety of pad tests available to quantitate the amount of urine loss. However, urinary incontinence is not necessary for the diagnosis of OAB and may only be present in a minority of such patients.[2] Thus, they have limited diagnostic utility. Nevertheless, they can be extremely helpful and serve as a baseline for outcome assessments under certain conditions.[3]

PHYSICAL EXAMINATION

A directed physical examination is important in every patient presenting with lower urinary tract symptoms suggestive of OAB. There are no signs or findings on physical examination which are specific to OAB, and therefore the goal of the abdominal, pelvic, rectal, and neurological examinations are to help the clinician to exclude many of the differential diagnostic possibilities.

The abdomen is examined for wounds suggestive of prior surgery, skin abnormalities (e.g. rashes), hernias, and masses. Percussion or palpation may be performed to evaluate for a distended bladder, suggesting poor bladder emptying and chronic urinary retention as a cause of the patient's symptoms. The lower back is also examined for scars reflecting prior lower back surgery, as well as a dimple or hair tuft

suggestive of spina bifida occulta. A directed neurological assessment should be performed. The presence of motor or sensory deficits of the patient's lower extremities or perineum should be identified. Knee and ankle reflexes are assessed and the patient's gait is observed. A rectal examination should be performed in men and women specifically for the assessment of rectal tone and integrity of the sacral reflex arc (anal wink, bulbocavernosal reflex). Objective neurological abnormalities found on physical examination may prompt a referral to a neurologist and/or appropriate imaging of the central nervous system. During the assessment of rectal tone, the patient's ability to perform pelvic floor exercises properly (Kegel's exercises) can be determined.

In men, the prostate should be evaluated for size, texture, symmetry, nodules and tenderness. The male genital examination should specifically look for evidence of meatal stenosis, phimosis, urethral discharge, testicular abnormalities, and genital lesions.

Female pelvic examinations include an evaluation for pelvic organ prolapse (cystocele, vault prolapse, enterocele, rectocele, and perineal laxity), urethral hypermobility, vaginal mucosal atrophy, vaginal dryness, and rugation. The vaginal walls and surrounding perineal skin are examined for lesions, excessive vaginal discharge, or evidence of maceration or ulceration, implying chronic urinary incontinence. In some cases, urethral diverticula may be diagnosed by careful palpation of the anterior vaginal wall and digital stripping of the urethra. A cough stress test is performed to evaluate for the presence of stress urinary incontinence. A careful bimanual pelvic examination is performed for the evaluation of adnexal, uterine, or other pelvic masses.

URINE ANALYSIS

An integral part of the evaluation of the patient with OAB is a urine analysis. Patients should be asked to provide a clean-catch midstream urine specimen. A screening dipstick can be performed, specifically looking for hematuria, proteinuria, glucosuria, and the presence of nitrates and leukocytes. Altered bladder sensation during urinary tract infections can cause symptoms similar to those of OAB. Urine microscopy and culture are the diagnostic gold standard, but reagent strip testing of urine is a sensitive and cheaper screening method. Tumors of the lower urinary tract may likewise cause urgency, frequency, and urge incontinence. Hematuria mandates urologic referral and further urologic investigation. OAB symptoms should not be treated empirically in the setting of hematuria without a proper evaluation of the hematuria. Irritative symptoms may prompt a voided urine sent for cytology which, if positive for tumor or dysplastic cells, should likewise mandate further urologic evaluation. Significant glucosuria or proteinuria should prompt further medical or nephrologic evaluation.

POST-VOID RESIDUAL URINE MEASUREMENT

It remains a point of contention whether all patients presenting with symptoms of OAB require a post-void residual measurement prior to the initiation of treatment. Patients with incomplete bladder emptying (chronic urinary retention) may present with symptoms indistinguishable from OAB, including urinary frequency, urgency, or nocturia, with or without urinary incontinence. A low post-void residual urine determination excludes chronic urinary retention as a cause of lower urinary tract symptoms. In thin female patients a bimanual pelvic examination is a simple method of examining for a distended or incompletely emptied bladder. Males and obese females are more challenging. Pelvic ultrasound or urethral catheterization may be used to measure the volume of urine remaining in the bladder after voiding, with distinct advantages to each method. It is desirable to measure post-void residual urine in some groups of patients, particularly the elderly with voiding symptoms and/or recurrent or persistent urinary tract infections; in those with complicated neurological disease and voiding dysfunction; and in all those with symptoms which suggest poor bladder emptying.

URODYNAMICS

Urodynamics assesses the activity of the bladder and bladder outlet during filling/storage and emptying phases of micturition.[34] When combined with fluoroscopy (i.e. videourodynamics) this study evaluates both the anatomy and the function of the lower urinary tract simultaneously. However, the role of urodynamics in the diagnosis of OAB is, for the most part, quite limited. As noted previously, OAB is a symptomatic diagnosis which does not require urodynamic confirmation of detrusor overactivity. It is important to emphasize that OAB and detrusor overactivity are not synonymous, although it is widely believed that involuntary bladder contractions are the primary underlying pathophysiology of OAB in such patients. The sine qua non of a well done diagnostic urodynamic study is reproducing the patient's symptoms during the study. The absence of detrusor overactivity on urodynamics does not exclude OAB, and the finding of detrusor overactivity in an otherwise asymptomatic individual does not make the diagnosis. Furthermore, urodynamics is invasive (requiring urethral or suprapubic catheterization of the bladder), can be associated with significant morbidity, is relatively expensive, and is not widely available outside the industrialized world.

Nevertheless, urodynamics may have a role in the evaluation of lower urinary tract symptoms in selected patients, including those who have failed previous therapy for OAB, or those who have OAB symptoms in the setting of neurological disease, vaginal prolapse, suspected bladder outlet obstruction, prior lower urinary tract surgery, prior pelvic radiotherapy, radical pelvic surgery, or a number of other complicated clinical scenarios. Flisser and Blaivas have suggested that urodynamics may have a role in defining the exact pathophysiology of OAB in some individuals such that an accurate diagnosis can be confirmed and appropriate therapy directed.[35]

These investigators have also suggested that urodynamics, specifically cystometry, may have a central role in the classification of OAB, which in turn permits the application of optimal therapy in individual patients.[36] Nevertheless, most authors and clinicians would argue that urodynamics in the setting of an uncomplicated, untreated individual with symptoms, physical examination findings, and a urine analysis consistent with the diagnosis of OAB is unnecessary. These uncomplicated patients probably do not require urodynamics in order to initiate therapy, which is planned to be completely reversible, inexpensive, and non-invasive, such as behavioral modification with or without pharmacotherapy.

Urodynamics is covered in more detail in Chapter 6.

CYSTOURETHROSCOPY

Cystourethroscopy has a limited role in the evaluation of uncomplicated lower urinary tract symptoms as well as in the diagnosis of OAB. There are no endoscopic findings diagnostic of OAB, although bladder trabeculation may be suggestive of long-term detrusor overactivity in some patients. In the presence of a normal urine analysis and physical examination, endoscopic examination probably provides little additional diagnostic information for the patient with OAB. Cystoscopy is typically performed in patients with hematuria or sterile pyuria, and patients with refractory urgency, frequency, and/or urge incontinence (i.e. following failure of initial therapy). Cystoscopy can also be helpful in the diagnosis or evaluation of urethral diverticulum, ureteroceles, ureteral ectopia, radiation cystitis, interstitial cystitis, bladder stones, urethral strictures, bladder outlet obstruction, and bladder trabeculation.

IMAGING

Similar to urodynamic and endoscopic examination of the lower urinary tract in patients with OAB, the role of radiographic imaging is limited. No radiographic findings are specific to OAB. The role of imaging in the evaluation of OAB primarily involves excluding other conditions such as urethral diverticulum or vaginal prolapse. The limitations of static imaging are obvious when evaluating a dynamic condition

such as OAB. Videourodynamics may provide some advantages in this setting by combining the static images during cystourethrography with the dynamic information obtained during pressure–flow urodynamics. As mentioned previously, imaging of the central nervous system may be indicated in some individuals with suspected relevant neurological conditions.

OTHER LABORATORY TESTS

There are no specific serum studies necessary in the evaluation of overactive bladder. Diabetes and thyroid disorders can cause symptoms mimicking OAB, and thus the use of serum chemistry, thyroid stimulating hormone (TSH), or hemoglobin A1c (HgbA1c) could be useful. Prostate-specific antigen (PSA) is often checked as well, as a screening test for prostate cancer.

CONCLUSIONS

An *initial evaluation* of the patient with OAB should include, at a minimum: (1) an assessment of the patient's symptoms; (2) a physical examination; and (3) urinalysis. A sequential, organized approach should be employed, in which confounding conditions are identified and addressed. Once urinary tract infection has been excluded, it is possible in most cases to establish a working diagnosis based on the patient's description of symptoms (Figure 3.2).

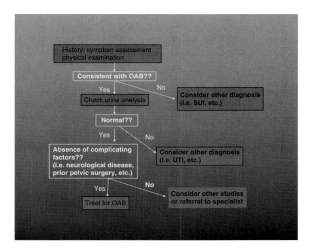

Figure 3.2 Algorithm for evaluation of overactive bladder (OAB). SUI, stress incontinence; UTI, urinary tract infection. (See also color plate section).

In some patients being evaluated for OAB it may be desirable to measure post-void residual urine by catheterization or ultrasound. In cases where there is uncertainty regarding the diagnosis, more advanced investigations such as urodynamic assessment and/or cystoscopy may be carried out, usually by the specialist.

REFERENCES

1. Milsom I, Stewart W, Thuroff J. The prevalence of overactive bladder. Am J Manag Care 2000; 6 (11 Suppl): S565–73.
2. Stewart W, Van Rooyen JB, Cundiff G et al. Prevalence and burden of overactive bladder in the United States. World J Urol 2003; 20: 327–36.
3. Abrams P, Cardozo L, Fall M et al. The standardisation of terminology of lower urinary tract function: report from the Standardisation Subcommittee of the International Continence Society. Neurourol Urodyn 2002; 21: 167–78.
4. Abrams P, Wein AJ. The overactive bladder: from basic science to clinical management. Urology 1997; 150: 1–3.
5. Abrams P, Wein AJ. The overactive bladder and incontinence: definitions and a plea for discussion. Neurourol Urodyn 1999; 18: 413–16.
6. Abrams P, Blaivas JG, Stanton SL, Andersen JT. The standardisation of terminology of lower urinary tract function. The International Continence Society Committee on Standardisation of Terminology. Scand J Urol Nephrol Suppl 1988; 114: 5–19.
7. Rovner ES, Wein AJ. Overactive bladder and urge incontinence: establishing the diagnosis. Womens Health Prim Care 2000; 3: 117–26.
8. Milsom I, Abrams P, Cardozo L et al. How widespread are the symptoms of an overactive bladder and how are they managed? A population-based prevalence study. BJU Int 2001; 87: 760–6.
9. Van Kerrebroeck P, Abrams P, Chaikin D et al. The standardization of terminology in nocturia: report from the standardization subcommittee of the International Continence Society. BJU Int 2002; 90 (Suppl 3): 11–15.
10. Cardozo L, Coyne KS, Versi E. Validation of the urgency perception scale. BJU Int 2005; 95: 591–6.
11. Freeman R, Hill S, Millard R et al. Reduced perception of urgency in treatment of overactive bladder with extended-release tolterodine. Obstet Gynecol 2003; 102: 605–11.
12. Zinner N, Harnett M, Sabounjian L et al. The overactive bladder-symptom composite score: a composite symptom score of toilet voids, urgency severity and urge urinary incontinence in patients with overactive bladder. J Urol 2005; 173: 1639–43.
13. Thomas A, Woodward C, Rovner ES, Wein AJ. Urologic complications of non-urologic medications. Urol Clin North Am 2003; 30: 123–32.
14. Rovner ES, Wein AJ. Today's treatment of overactive bladder and urge incontinence. Womens Health Prim Care 2000; 3: 179–92.
15. Uebersax JS, Wyman JF, Shumaker SA, McClish DK, Fantl JA. Short forms to assess life quality and symptom distress for urinary incontinence in women: the Incontinence Impact Questionnaire and the Urogenital Distress Inventory. Continence Program for Women Research Group. Neurourol Urodyn 1995; 14: 131–9.
16. Harvey YMA, Kristjansson B, Griffith D, Versi E. The Incontinence Impact Questionnaire and the Urogenital Distress Inventory: a revisit of their validity in women without a urodynamic diagnosis. Am J Obstet Gynecol 2001; 185: 25–31.
17. Brown JS, Posner SF, Stewart AL. Urge incontinence: new health-related quality of life measures. J Am Geriatr Soc 1999; 47: 980–8.
18. Reese PR, Pleil AM, Okano GJ, Kelleher CJ. Multinational study of reliability and validity of the King's Health Questionnaire in patients with overactive bladder. Qual Life Res 2003; 12: 427–42.
19. Brookes ST, Donovan JL, Wright M, Jackson S, Abrams P. A scored form of the Bristol Female Lower Urinary Tract Symptoms questionnaire: data from a randomized controlled trial of surgery for women with stress incontinence. Am J Obstet Gynecol 2004; 191: 73–82.
20. Wagner TH, Patrick DL, Bavendam TG, Martin ML, Buesching DP. Quality of life of persons with urinary incontinence: development of a new measure. Urology 1996; 47: 67–72.
21. Coyne K, Revicki D, Hunt T et al. Psychometric validation of an overactive bladder symptom and health-related quality of life questionnaire: the OAB-q. Qual Life Res 2002; 11: 563–74.
22. Coyne K, Matza LS, Thompson CL. The responsiveness of the Overactive Bladder Questionnaire (OAB-q). Qual Life Res 2005; 14: 849–55.
23. Appell RA, Sand P, Dmochowski R et al. Prospective randomized controlled trial of extended-release oxybutynin chloride and tolterodine tartrate

in the treatment of overactive bladder: results of the OBJECT Study [Comment]. Mayo Clin Proc 2001; 76: 358–63.

24. Burgio KL. Influence of behavior modification on overactive bladder. Urology 2002; 60 (5 Suppl 1): 72–6.

25. Chapple CR, Rechberger T, Al Shukri S et al. Randomized, double-blind placebo- and tolterodine-controlled trial of the once-daily antimuscarinic agent solifenacin in patients with symptomatic overactive bladder. BJU Int 2004; 93: 303–10.

26. Diokno AC, Appell RA, Sand PK et al. Prospective, randomized, double-blind study of the efficacy and tolerability of the extended-release formulations of oxybutynin and tolterodine for overactive bladder: results of the OPERA trial. Mayo Clin Proc 2003; 78: 687–95.

27. Dmochowski RR, Sand PK, Zinner NR et al. Comparative efficacy and safety of transdermal oxybutynin and oral tolterodine versus placebo in previously treated patients with urge and mixed urinary incontinence. Urology 2003; 62: 237–42.

28. Haab F, Stewart L, Dwyer P. Darifenacin, an M3 selective receptor antagonist, is an effective and well tolerated once-daily treatment for overactive bladder. Eur Urol 2004; 45: 420–9.

29. Van Kerrebroeck P, Kreder K, Jonas U, Zinner N, Wein A, Tolterodine Study Group. Tolterodine once-daily: superior efficacy and tolerability in the treatment of the overactive bladder. Urology 2001; 57: 414–21.

30. Zinner N, Gittelman M, Harris R et al. Trospium chloride improves overactive bladder symptoms: a multicenter phase III trial. J Urol 2004; 171: 2311–15.

31. Mazurick CA, Landis JR. Evaluation of repeat daily voiding measures in the National Interstitial Cystitis Data Base Study. J Urol 2000; 163: 1208–11.

32. Brown JS, McNaughton KS, Wyman JF et al. Measurement characteristics of a voiding diary for use by men and women with overactive bladder. Urology 2003; 61: 802–9.

33. Fitzgerald MP, Brubaker L. Variability of 24-hour voiding diary variables among asymptomatic women. J Urol 2003; 169: 207–9.

34. Homma Y, Batista J, Bauer S et al. Urodynamics. In: Abrams P, Cardozo L, Khoury S, Wein A, eds. Incontinence. Plymouth, UK: Plymbridge Distributors Ltd, 2002: 317–72.

35. Flisser AJ, Blaivas JG. Role of cystometry in evaluating patients with overactive bladder. Urology 2002; 60 (5 Suppl 1): 33–42.

36. Flisser AJ, Walmsley K, Blaivas JG. Urodynamic classification of patients with symptoms of overactive bladder. J Urol 2003; 169: 529–33.

4

Measuring overactive bladder syndrome symptoms

Rufus Cartwright and Linda Cardozo

Introduction • Frequency–volume charts • Urgency measures • Overactive bladder symptom questionnaires • Conclusions

INTRODUCTION

The defining symptoms of overactive bladder syndrome (OAB) are urinary urgency, with or without urge incontinence, frequency, and nocturia.[1] These symptoms may be described by the individual or caregiver, or elicited through history taking. An accurate urological history helps describe incontinence, and guides investigation and treatment. However "the bladder is an unreliable witness",[2] and symptoms alone cannot make a definitive diagnosis.

The symptoms of OAB each have objective correlates, but nonetheless are subjective to varying degrees. The magnitude of symptoms has an unpredictable relationship to their bothersomeness. Based on history alone, doctors tend to underestimate the impact of symptoms upon their patients.[3] Lower urinary tract symptoms are considerably stigmatizing, which may enhance this effect. Patient-completed methods of assessing OAB are thus essential to overcome this bias, in both clinical and research settings.

Simple objective measures should be used to verify and quantify the symptoms. Validated disease-specific quality of life questionnaires should be employed in order to accurately assess the level of bother.

A wide range of tools has been developed for use in a variety of populations and clinical settings. This chapter will focus on frequency–volume charts, in their many varieties, as well as the self-completion questionnaires available for capturing the more subjective aspects of the patient experience.

FREQUENCY–VOLUME CHARTS

Frequency–volume charts (FVCs) are employed both in clinical practice, and for recording outcome measure data in trials of OAB medications. In clinical practice at least, they have a two-fold function. Not only are they a non-invasive method of assessing voiding and drinking patterns, but they may also have a therapeutic role.[4] Completion of the FVC can provide unexpected insight into a dysfunctional voiding pattern for the patient herself, acting as a form of behavioral feedback.

Types of frequency–volume chart

No standardization of these charts exists, either for the instructions given to patients, or for the types of data collected. The International Continence Society (ICS) classifies FVCs into three varieties, according to sophistication.[5] A micturition time chart records only the timing of intentional voids. A frequency–volume chart records both the timing of each void and the volume passed at each void. A bladder diary records this information, as well as a selection of other factors, potentially including: volume, type, and timing of fluid intake; severity, type, and timing of incontinence episodes; severity and timing of urgency; and pad usage. The choice of type of chart should be determined by the information required, and the capabilities of the patient or caregiver to complete the chart (Figures 4.1–4.3).

Various lengths of time have been advocated for completion of FVCs, ranging from 1 day to 2 weeks; 24 hours is clearly the minimum if we wish to distinguish nocturia from nocturnal polyuria. Patient compliance with chart completion is reduced if the time period is too long.[6] A 3-day chart may be optimal for diagnostic accuracy.[7]

Interpretation of frequency–volume charts

There is a range of problems that may be subjectively reported in history, and which may also be objectively recorded in a FVC. The analysis of these measures from FVCs forms the basis for interpretation of the charts. This can be done either by hand, or with the aid of an automated

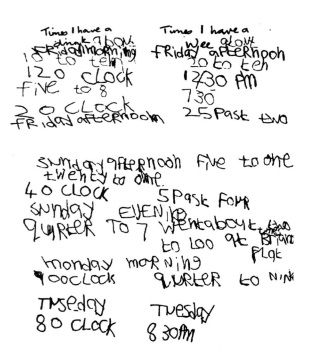

Figure 4.2 Poorly completed chart.

KINGS COLLEGE HOSPITAL
FREQUENCY–VOLUME CHART

Time	Day 1 In	Day 1 Out	W	Day 2 In	Day 2 Out	W	Day 3 In	Day 3 Out	W	Day 4 In	Day 4 Out	W	Day 5 In	Day 5 Out
6 am		75		180	50		180	125					240	300
7 am	180									125	225	w		
8 am	180	150	✓	360	125		360	125			100		360	125
9 am		100					180	350	✓	320	100			100
10 am	360	75		180	250	✓					100 75	w		125
11 am							180	200	✓	180	50		180	100
12	180	225	✓	110	325	✓		100						
1 pm		100		180			180	75		180	300 75	w	180	125
2 pm	100	50			100						200			
3 pm		75 75		180	75 75		220	220	✓	360	100	w	240	
4 pm	240	100	✓				75	90		75			180	320
5 pm				220	200	✓					100			100
6 pm	180	220	w	220	50		100	125		120			180	100
7 pm	180				50			200			100	w		
8 pm		225					200			240				75
9 pm				180	100		150		✓				360	
10 pm	180	100		180	75		180	100		180	225	✓		180
11 pm								75		180	150		180	200
12	240	100		180	150	✓	240	25			100		180	225
1 am							100		✓					
2 am				180	125	✓				180	100			350
3 am	180	300	w				180						220	
4 am					300	w		225	✓	180	100			100
5 am														180

Figure 4.1 Well completed chart.

Figure 4.3 Computerized frequency–volume chart.

scanner and computer. None of the calculations and corrections is so complicated as to require a computer, and in fact "eyeballing" the chart may provide salient information that would be overlooked during automated interpretation.

Daytime frequency

This comprises the mean daily voids between, and inclusive of, the first void after waking and rising, and the last void before sleeping. Frequency is defined as the subjective impression of needing to void too often. A cut-off of eight voids per day is often employed in research, but may not be clinically relevant.[8]

Night-time frequency *(see also 'Nocturia' below)*

This includes the mean number of voids between the time of going to bed with the intention of sleeping, and the time of waking with the intention of rising. There is some overlap between sleep disorders and overactive bladder, and for this reason nocturia may be a more helpful measure.

24-Hour frequency

This is the mean total number of voids per 24-hour period, both daytime and night-time.

Nocturia

This is defined as the mean number of voids recorded between the onset of sleep on going to bed, and the end of the last period of sleep before rising. Nocturia becomes more common with increasing age, so no single cut-off for normality can be given.[9] However, rising twice or more per night is usually felt to be abnormal for those under 60 years.

24-Hour production

This is the mean total volume of urine produced per 24-hour period. It is conventional to commence the collection after the first void of the day, and complete the collection with the first void of the subsequent day. Polyuria is defined as passing more than 2.8 liters per 24-hour period. Although this may be a reflection of an underlying medical condition, more commonly it is due to idiopathic polydipsia.

Dividing 24-hour production by 24-hour frequency gives the mean voided volume. This is the average volume of urine passed per void: one measure of the bladder capacity.

Nocturnal urine volume

This is defined as the volume of urine passed between the time of going to bed with the intention of sleeping, and the end of the last void after rising. It is possible to further "correct" this measure, to exclude the volume of urine passed from the kidneys between the time of rising and first voiding.[10] The rate of urine production is assumed to be constant between the last void during or before sleep, and the first void of the morning. The clinical significance of such a correction is uncertain.

Nocturnal urine production increases as a percentage of 24-hour production with age. Thus, in a young person nocturnal polyuria is present when greater than 20% of urine production occurs at night, whereas in a 65-year-old, it is only present if greater than 33% of the total occurs at night.

Incontinence episode frequency

This is the mean number of accidental episodes of urine leakage occurring per 24-hour period. Depending on the instruction given, patients may also be able to classify these episodes as stress related, urge related, or unconscious. They may also rate the episodes for severity of leakage (a few drops, wet pad, soaked), giving a useful indication of bother or inconvenience.

Pad usage

Pad usage is a more objective way of quantifying accidental leakage. Although it relies on self-reporting, it may be more informative than a formal pad test (performed as part of urodynamics), because measurement occurs during normal daily life. However, behavior and hygiene variations limit the usefulness of this particular variable.

Urgency

Urgency is the most subjective of lower urinary tract symptoms. There are many ways of recording or measuring its presence, not all of which are based on FVCs. They are described fully below in the section on 'Urgency measures'. FVCs can be used to record either the timing or the severity of urgency episodes.

Maximum voided volume

This is the largest volume passed at a single void, indicating the maximum functional capacity of the bladder.

Although these concepts are useful when communicating with other healthcare professionals, it is important to remember that they may have little significance in themselves for patients. The impact of the same symptom may be entirely different for two patients, depending on their lifestyles and expectations. This idea is explored more in the section on 'Overactive bladder symptom questionnaires'.

URGENCY MEASURES

Urgency is the cardinal symptom in OAB. Except in those patients with absent bladder sensation, urgency leads to frequency, nocturia, and incontinence.[11] The experience of urgency has a greater negative effect on quality of life than any of the other components of OAB.[12]

However, because of its subjective nature, it is difficult in a clinical or research setting to distinguish urgency from urge. Urge is a normal physiological sensation, synonymous with the desire to void. Urgency, as currently defined, is a pathological sensation: "a sudden compelling desire to pass urine which is difficult to defer."[1] It is unclear whether urge and urgency lie on a continuum. Equally we cannot be sure that urgency is always abnormal.

During filling cystometry, urgency may be accompanied by its objective correlate of uninhibited detrusor contraction, but this is not invariably the case. In assessing the frequency, severity, and impact of urgency we are therefore forced to rely on a variety of subjective measures.

The intensity of urgency

It is good practice during filling cystometry to check that the symptom of urgency is being reproduced.[13] Due to anxiety during the test, this typically requires some prompting from the clinician. Oliver et al.[14] attempted to measure sensation during bladder filling more objectively. Patients undergoing urodynamics were asked to continuously grade their sensation of urge and urgency on a discrete 0–4 scale, using a keypad device. During a pseudo-random cycle of filling and emptying, scores were found to correlate reliably with bladder volumes. The method was further validated through test–retesting, and through demonstration that scores were reduced during non-invasive neuromodulation. Although this is a potentially useful adjunct to filling cystometry,[15] it has not been established whether increased bladder sensation, defined as "an early and persistent desire to void",[1] is necessarily associated with urgency. Furthermore, even in healthy volunteers there is a wide variation in the volumes at which first sensation, first desire to void, and strong desire to void occur.[16]

OAB symptom questionnaires will be considered more fully in the next section. However the Leicester Urinary Symptoms Questionnaire[17] (LUSQ) serves as a good example of the controversies in designing a question to grade the severity of urgency. The LUSQ has a variety of items validated for abnormal storage symptoms. The question for urgency asks directly about intensity of sensation: "When you first feel the need to pass urine how strong is the urge to go usually? Is it overwhelming, very strong, strong, normal, weak, or do you have no sensation?"

Chapple et al.[11] have argued that urgency is by definition a "maximal" sensation, and that it is unnecessary to measure its severity in this way. It would seem that in the LUSQ, only the first response (overwhelming) corresponds to the ICS definition of urgency as a "compelling" desire. Although the LUSQ may not assess severity of urgency, it is an effective screening question for the presence of urgency.

The timing of urgency

It has been said that urgency demands both attention and action. The Urgency Perception Scale (UPS)[18] focuses on the action demanded by urgency. It asks patients to agree with one of three responses:

1. "I am usually not able to hold urine."

2. "I am usually able to hold urine until I reach the toilet if I go immediately."
3. "I am usually able to finish what I am doing before going to the toilet."

Again urge and urgency are placed on a continuum, with response 3 above corresponding to normal urge. The psychometric variables have been validated during the use of the UPS in three clinical trials of tolterodine. The UPS score correlates moderately well with incontinence episodes and pad usage. However, the correlation with frequency and symptomatic urgency is poor. This may be because the scale cannot discriminate between dry patients. A patient who gives response 3, "I am usually able to finish what I am doing before going to the toilet", at baseline, cannot improve their score despite treatment.

There is a further concern with the UPS, as no timescale is provided. Some patients involved in the studies noted that the scale would be more descriptive if it included an item such as, "I am usually able to hold urine for 5, 10, 15 minutes".

Warning time is a new concept that attempts to more accurately assess the temporal characteristics of urgency. Warning time is defined as the time from the "first sensation of urgency to voluntary micturition or incontinence". It may be a clinically relevant measure,[19] because it corresponds to the time available to find a toilet. An increased warning time should allow more patients to achieve or maintain continence.

Warning time has been used as a primary outcome measure in a proof of concept randomized control trial[20] comparing darifenacin and placebo. In the study, women with at least 6 months of urgency, and more than four episodes of urgency daily, on bladder diary, were randomized to darifenacin 30 mg daily or placebo. At the start and end of the study, warning time was measured by the women themselves, using electronic event recorders. Data were collected across three urge void cycles, or 6 hours, whichever was shorter.

Women in the darifenacin group showed significant improvements in both median (1.8 minutes) and minimum (1.1 minutes) warning time, compared with placebo (−1.0 and −0.1 minutes respectively). Despite this, the frequency of urgency was unchanged. The data regarding severity of urgency were equivocal, with improvements only being noted during clinic visits, but not on home diaries.

Although it seems probable that an increase in warning time of over 1 minute would be clinically meaningful, it has yet to be validated as a clinical tool. It is of particular concern that the range of warning times both for individuals and for the population is quite wide. The population 75th centiles were 13.8 and 14.7 minutes (for darifenacin and placebo groups respectively). It has been suggested[21] that these long times are inconsistent with the definition of urgency.

Further evidence that warning time fails to measure urgency has been presented by Wagg and Woo.[22] In their, as yet, unpublished study they asked asymptomatic men to measure their "urge time", a delay between first desire to void, and micturition. In this study many younger men (aged 18–30) were able to delay voiding for over 1 hour. However, the median "urge time" for this same group was 5 minutes. This compares closely to the median warning times in the earlier darifenacin[20] study of 4.7 and 9.3 minutes for each group. Minimum warning time may more accurately reflect urgency rather than urge. Further studies to validate this concept are ongoing.

The frequency of urgency

Two large clinical trials have asked subjects to complete frequency–volume charts that include episodes of urgency.[23,24] Both these trials used "reduction in number of urgency episodes" as an outcome measure. However, it is unclear from the reports of these trials how subjects were asked to identify or classify episodes of urgency. No validation of this measure has been undertaken.

Measuring the severity and frequency of urgency

De Wachter and Wyndaele[25] have employed modified frequency–volume charts that allow patients to record the intensity of urge or urgency each time they void or leak. Subjects were asked to grade sensation of bladder fullness as:

- no desire to void
- normal desire to void

- strong desire to void
- urgent desire to void.

Desire to void was strongly correlated with voided volume, and as in the earlier keypad study,[14] also correlated with subsequently assessed cystometric volumes. In normal volunteers they found that 65% of voids were made without desire to void. Furthermore, no voids were associated with urgent desire, except when subjects were asked to voluntarily postpone micturition as long as possible. This scale would appear to make a strong distinction between normal urge and urgency, with relevant clinical associations. Combining it with a frequency–volume chart gives a practical measure of the amount of urgency occurring with each void or leak. No attempt was made to measure urgency that might have occurred without leakage or voiding.

Brown et al.[26] further validated a similar modified frequency–volume chart in a population of patients with urge incontinence (or mixed incontinence with urge as the primary component). Subjects completed 7-day "voiding diaries", and again graded episodes of urgency associated with each void. Their scale makes little distinction between urge and urgency, but they found it had excellent test–retest reliability.

The Indevus Urgency Severity Scale (IUSS)[27] again asks patients to assess the severity of "urgency" at each void. The scale employs the following wording:

> Degree of urgency is meant to describe your urge to urinate. Sometimes you may feel a very strong urge to urinate, and at other times, you may feel a milder urge prior to the onset of a toilet void. Rate this feeling by circling 0, 1, 2, or 3, defined as:
>
> 0: None – no urgency
> 1: Mild – awareness of urgency, but it is easily tolerated and you can continue with your usual activity or tasks
> 2: Moderate – enough urgency discomfort that it interferes with or shortens your usual activity or tasks
> 3: Severe – extreme urgency discomfort that abruptly stops all activity or tasks.

Responses 0 and 1 correspond to normal desire to void, while responses 2 and 3 correspond to two levels of urgency. An argument could be made for combining responses 0 and 1, so that the scale measures urgency alone. In all analyses so far performed, the average score per void has been studied.

This questionnaire has been validated for use in OAB[28] in a 12-week double-blind placebo controlled trial of trospium. It shows moderate correlations with the number of incontinence episodes, and Incontinence Impact Questionnaire scores. This is to be expected, as these are multifactorial, situation dependent variables. The IUSS is highly responsive to change in frequency, and change in urge incontinence frequency. It also shows good temporal stability. At present the IUSS is perhaps the best validated tool for measuring urgency. There are many possible ways to improve it further. It has already been used as the basis of a unified measure of urgency and frequency severity.[29] In common with other urgency frequency measures, it is a notable omission that it does not assess urgency that occurs without voiding or leakage.

OVERACTIVE BLADDER SYMPTOM QUESTIONNAIRES

We have already briefly discussed the LUSQ and UPS, but there is a range of other questionnaires that assess OAB symptoms. To an extent these questionnaires have overlapping functions, although they are designed for use in different populations. Some have been modified or revalidated for other populations (Table 4.1).

The 3rd International Consultation on Incontinence gave eight questionnaires for OAB symptoms a grade A recommendation: DANpss, OAB-q, BFLUTS/BFLUTS-SF, ICSmale/ICSmaleSF, KHQ, and UDI/UDI6. In addition we will consider one newly validated questionnaire, the OAB-V8.

The King's Health Questionnaire

The King's Health Questionnaire (KHQ) was developed at King's College Hospital, London for the assessment of incontinence-related quality of life in women.[31] It remains primarily a quality of life tool, but contains a symptom questionnaire section. The symptom section has

Table 4.1   Properties of recommended questionnaires[30]

Questionnaire	Men	Women	UUI	UI	OAB
ICIQ	✓	✓	✓	✓	
IqOL	✓	✓		✓	
SEAPI-QMM	✓	✓		✓	
BFLUTS-SF		✓		✓	✓
ICSmaleSF	✓		✓	✓	✓
KHQ		✓		✓	✓
UDI/UDI6		✓	✓		✓
IIQ/IIQ-7		✓		✓	
ISI		✓		✓	
SUIQQ		✓	✓	✓	
UISS		✓		✓	
CONTILIFE		✓		✓	
OAB-q	✓	✓		✓	✓
BFLUTS		✓	✓	✓	✓
DAN-PSS	✓		✓		✓
ICSmale	✓		✓		✓

UUI, Urge urinary incontinence; UI, Urinary incontinence.

How much do they affect you?

FREQUENCY: going to the toilet very often
1. A little   2. Moderately   3. A lot
   ○   ○   ○

NOCTURIA: getting up at night to pass urine
1. A little   2. Moderately   3. A lot
   ○   ○   ○

URGENCY: a strong and difficult to control desire to pass urine
1. A little   2. Moderately   3. A lot
   ○   ○   ○

URGE INCONTINENCE: urinary leakage associated with a strong desire to pass urine
1. A little   2. Moderately   3. A lot
   ○   ○   ○

Box 4.1   Sample questions from the symptom domain of the KHQ.

11 items asking about bother associated with urinary symptoms (Box 4.1).

The KHQ is one of the most widely validated questionnaires available. It has been translated into 26 languages, adapted for use in men, and used in a large number of observational and interventional trials to demonstrate sensitivity to change. The minimal important difference in quality of life measured with the KHQ has also been calculated.[32]

The KHQ is being revalidated as part of the International Consultation on Incontinence Questionnaire (ICIQ) project,[33] in order to make it a standard disease-specific quality of life instrument. It will then be known as the ICIQ-LUTSqol.

Urogenital Distress Inventory

The Urogenital Distress Inventory (UDI/UDI6) was developed in the United States specifically to assess the degree of bother associated with incontinence symptoms in women. The full questionnaire has 19 items relating to different lower urinary tract symptoms. The short form has just six items (Box 4.2).

The UDI has been used in a range of populations and interventional trials to demonstrate sensitivity to change. A version adapted for use in men has received some limited validation.

ICSmale

The ICSmale,[34] sometimes called ICSmaleLF, in common with the UDI asks both about the frequency of symptoms and about their bother

(Box 4.3). There are 22 items, and the first four specifically address the key tetrad of symptoms of OAB: frequency, nocturia, urgency, and urgency incontinence.

ICSmaleSF

The ICSmaleSF is a simplified version, with 14 items, of which 13 ask directly about the frequency of different symptoms. There is only one quality of life item. The questionnaire is designed to differentiate men with bladder outlet obstruction from those with other causes of lower urinary tract symptoms (LUTS). For this reason the questions about frequency and nocturia are not

1. Do you experience frequent urination?

1 YES	0 NO—skip to 2

1a. If yes, how much does it bother you?

1 Not at all	2 Slightly	3 Moderately	4 Greatly	

2. Do you experience a strong feeling of urgency to empty your bladder?

1 YES	0 NO—skip to 3

2a. If yes, how much does it bother you?

1 Not at all	2 Slightly	3 Moderately	4 Greatly	

Box 4.2 Sample questions from the UDI6.

2	During the night, how many times do you have to get up to urinate, on average?			
		none		0
		one		1
		two		2
		three		3
		four or more		4
	How much of a problem is this for you?	not a problem		1
		a bit of a problem		2
		quite a problem		3
		a serious problem		4

Box 4.3 A sample question from the ICSmale.

11	Do you have to rush to the toilet to urinate?		
		never	0
		occasionally	1
		sometimes	2
		most of the time	3
		all of the time	4

Box 4.4 A sample question from the ICSmaleSF.

14a. During the night, how many times do you have to get up to urinate, on average?

none	0
one	1
two	2
three	3
four or more	4

14b. How much does this bother you?
   Please ring a number between 0 (not at all) and 10 (a great deal)

0   1   2   3   4   5   6   7   8   9   10
not at all   a great deal

Box 4.5 A sample question from the ICIQ-MLUTS.

included in the scoring system. They are added only to give a rounded picture of all LUTS as part of clinical screening (Box 4.4).

ICIQ-MLUTS

Both these questionnaires are currently being superseded by the ICIQ-MLUTS (International Consultation on Incontinence Questionnaire – Male Lower Urinary Tract Symptoms).[33] This questionnaire again has short and long forms. It aims to be fully validated in a wide range of populations, such that it can become a standard tool in both clinical and research settings. Instead of asking patients to rate bother as "not a problem", "a bit of a problem", "quite a problem", or "a serious problem", it uses a 10-point scale, as shown in Box 4.5. Only three of the questions, all pertinent to voiding difficulties, do not follow this format. One (Figure 4.4) asks: "Would you say that the strength of your urinary stream is . . . (please ring one number)?"

15. Would you say that the strength of your urinary stream is...
(please ring one number)

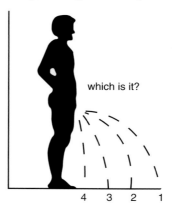

which is it?

4   3   2   1

Figure 4.4 Strength of urinary stream on the ICIQ-MLUTS. (From reference 35, with permission)

Overactive bladder screener

The overactive bladder screener (OAB-V8) is an eight-item questionnaire designed to allow primary care physicians to confidently diagnose OAB.[36] It asks about bother associated with different LUTS. Compared to the other questionnaires described here, it has received very limited validation. Although it has been employed in several large trials, validity, reliability, and responsiveness have not been established. Nor indeed have data from this questionnaire been compared with urodynamic diagnoses. Compared to the other questionnaires, the question set appears to have some redundancy. There are too many items asking about urgency, with just slightly varied wording.

Overactive bladder symptom and health-related quality of life

As the name implies, the overactive bladder symptom and health-related quality of life questionnaire (OAB-q) contains both symptom questions and quality of life questions. The questionnaire was the first to be developed specifically for OAB.[37] Its original format contained 13 symptom questions (from 62 total items). This has been modified down to eight items (from 33 total) (Box 4.6). The remaining items concern health-related and general quality of life. Although the questionnaire has received less wide ranging validation than those so far discussed, its specific focus on OAB makes it very promising. Sensitivity to change with antimuscarinic treatment has been demonstrated,[38] and the questionnaire also distinguishes between OAB-dry and OAB-wet patients.

Danish-prostate symptom score

Uniquely among these recommended questionnaires, the Danish-prostate symptom score (DAN-pss)[39] has not originally been developed and validated in the English language. It again asks about LUTS and their bothersomeness. It has paper and computerized versions, both of which can be completed by patients. It has no specificity for OAB, but functions similarly to the ICSmale.

Bristol Female Lower Urinary Tract Symptoms

As with ICSmale and ICIQ-MLUTS, the Bristol Female Lower Urinary Tract Symptoms (BFLUTS) and BFLUTS-SF questionnaires are being

During the past 4 weeks, how bothered were you by...	Not at all	A little bit	Some-what	Quite a bit	A great deal	A very great deal
1. Frequent urination during the daytime hours	1	2	3	4	5	6
2. An uncomfortable urge to urinate	1	2	3	4	5	6
3. A sudden urge to urinate with little or no warning	1	2	3	4	5	6
4. Accidental loss of small amounts of urine	1	2	3	4	5	6
5. Nighttime urination	1	2	3	4	5	6
6. Waking up at night because you had to urinate	1	2	3	4	5	6
7. An uncontrollable urge to urinate	1	2	3	4	5	6
8. Urine loss associated with a strong desire to urinate	1	2	3	4	5	6

Box 4.6   The OAB-q questionnaire.

17a. Do you have a burning feeling when you urinate?

never ☐

occasionally ☐

sometimes ☐

most of the time ☐

all of the time ☐

17b. How much does this bother you?

Please ring a number between 0 (not at all) and 10 (a great deal)

0 1 2 3 4 5 6 7 8 9 10

not at all   a great deal

Box 4.7 A sample question from the ICIQ-FLUTS.

superseded by the ICIQ-FLUTS.[33] The BFLUTS itself is a well validated questionnaire,[40] with clear evidence of reliability, consistency, and responsiveness. It has been widely used in epidemiological research.

ICIQ-FLUTS

The ICIQ-FLUTS is closely based on the BFLUTS. They both follow similar formats to their male versions, but with a modified question set. BFLUTS uses the same grading system for bother as the ICSmale, whereas ICIQ-FLUTS uses a 10-point scale like ICIQ-MLUTS. The ICIQ-MLUTS and ICIQ-FLUTS are the most detailed of all the available symptom questionnaires. They include potentially important items to sufferers of OAB, which have been overlooked by other questionnaires. This includes an item about dysuria (Box 4.7).

At the time of writing, validation has yet to occur for the ICIQ-FLUTS. However, region-specific versions are in preparation, to enable it to become a standard tool worldwide. It follows the format of the BFLUTS closely, and there is every reason to expect that it will perform as well as that questionnaire. A subset of these items, specific only to OAB, is also being validated, and will be known as the ICIQ-OAB.[33]

Implementation of symptom questionnaires

In clinical practice, where possible, a symptom questionnaire should be completed before diagnosis and after treatment has been established.

This can be useful for the clinician in guiding history taking, and directing therapy. Repeating the same questionnaire over a period of time forms a useful record of progress, in treating what is usually a chronic disease. Questionnaires should not form a substitute for a full history. Accurate history taking remains the mainstay of diagnosis. However, history taking tends to underestimate the impact of LUTS. Patients may be reluctant to reveal potentially stigmatizing symptoms in person.[41] We should therefore encourage patients to fill out questionnaires themselves. Many studies have compared telephone administration with postal administration of questionnaires, with inconsistent results. The optimal method of administration may thus depend on the clinical or research setting.

All trials in OAB should aim to include both subjective and objective outcomes. Much of the symptom data obtained from standard questionnaires can also be obtained, in a more objective way, from sophisticated bladder diaries. However, for the moment, standardization of symptom questionnaires is more advanced than for bladder diaries. There is emerging evidence that reporting of frequency and nocturia may be significantly different, depending on whether FVCs or symptom questionnaires are employed.[6] Both methods are thus complementary.

CONCLUSIONS

OAB is primarily considered a quality-of-life disorder.[42] Objective outcomes such as urodynamic parameters have only modest correlations with magnitude of symptoms.[43] Both bladder diaries and symptom questionnaires are thus essential methods of objectifying the individual experience. They both provide reproducible ways of monitoring disease progress or treatment success.

Urgency is the most subjective of the OAB symptoms. Assessment of urgency is more difficult than assessment of nocturia, frequency, or episodes of leakage. The experience of urgency is highly individualized, making it difficult for patients to communicate. As yet no ideal tool exists for measuring urgency.

Increasing standardization of all these instruments should enable a more accurate comparison between different clinical populations, and between different research efforts.

REFERENCES

1. Abrams P, Cardozo L, Fall M et al. The standardisation of terminology of lower urinary tract function: report from the Standardisation Subcommittee of the International Continence Society. Neurourol Urodyn 2002; 21: 167–78.
2. Blaivas JG. The bladder is an unreliable witness. Neurourol Urodyn 1996; 15: 443–5.
3. Litwin MS, Lubeck DP, Henning JM, Carroll PR. Differences in urologist and patient assessments of health related quality of life in men with prostate cancer: results of the CaPSURE database. J Urol 1998; 159: 1988–92.
4. Burgio KL, Locher JL, Goode PS et al. Behavioral vs drug treatment for urge urinary incontinence in older women: a randomized controlled trial. JAMA 1998; 280: 1995–2000.
5. Staskin D, Hilton P, Emmanuel A et al. Initial assessment of incontinence. In: Abrams P, Cardozo L, Khoury S, Wein A, eds. Incontinence. Plymouth, UK: Health Publication Ltd, 2005: 485–518.
6. Kenton K, FitzGerald MP, Brubaker L. What's a clinician to do? Believe the patient or her urinary diary? Abstract presented at ICS Scientific Meeting, Montreal, 2005.
7. Dmochowski RR, Sanders SW, Appell RA, Nitti VW, Davila GW. Bladder-health diaries: an assessment of 3-day vs 7-day entries. BJU Int 2005; 96: 1049–54.
8. Fitzgerald MP, Brubaker L. Variability of 24-hour voiding diary variables among asymptomatic women. J Urol 2003; 169: 207–9.
9. Fitzgerald MP, Stablein U, Brubaker L. Urinary habits among asymptomatic women. Am J Obstet Gynecol 2002; 187: 1384–8.
10. Parsons M, Tissot W, Cardozo L, Amundsen C, Diokno A. Is computer correction of a frequency-volume chart more accurate? Abstract presented at ICS (UK) Annual Scientific Meeting, Glasgow, 2005.
11. Chapple C, Wein A. The urgency of the problem and the problem of urgency in the overactive bladder. BJU Int 2005; 95: 274–5.
12. Coyne KS, Payne C, Bhattacharyya SK et al. The impact of urinary urgency and frequency on health-related quality of life in overactive bladder: results from a national community survey. Value Health 2004; 7: 455–63.
13. Schafer W, Abrams P, Liao L et al. Good urodynamic practice: uroflowmetry, filling cystometry, and pressure flow studies. Neurourol Urodyn 2002; 21: 261–74.
14. Oliver S, Fowler C, Mundy A et al. Measuring the sensations of urge and bladder filling during cystometry in urge incontinence and the effect of neuromodulation. Neurourol Urodyn 2003; 22: 7–16.
15. Freeman R. How urgent is urgency? A review of current methods of assessment. Int Urogynaecol J 2005; 16: 93–5.
16. Wyndaele J, De Wachter S. Cystometrical sensory data from a normal population: comparison of two groups of young healthy volunteers examined with 5 years interval. Eur Urol 2002; 42: 34–48.
17. Shaw C, Matthews RJ, Perry SI et al. Validity and reliability of an interviewer-administered questionnaire to measure the severity of lower urinary tract symptoms of storage abnormality: the Leicester Urinary Symptom Questionnaire. BJU Int 2002; 90: 205–15.
18. Cardozo L, Coyne KS, Versi E. Validation of the Urgency Perception Scale. BJU Int 2005; 95: 591–6.
19. Chalifoux P. Recognizing warning time: a critical step towards continence. Geriatr Nurs 1980; 1: 254–5.
20. Cardozo L, Dixon A. Increased warning time with Darifenacin: a new concept in the management of urinary urgency. J Urol 2005; 173: 1214–18.
21. Chapple C, Artibani W, Cardozo L et al. The role of urinary urgency and its measurement in the overactive bladder symptom syndrome: current

concepts and future prospects. BJU Int 2005; 95: 335–40.

22. Woo W, Wagg A. Urge time in younger versus older asymptomatic men: normal characteristics. Abstract presented at ICS (UK) Annual Scientific Meeting, Glasgow, 2005.

23. Halaska M, Ralph G, Wiedmann A et al. Controlled double-blind multicentre clinical trial to investigate long-term tolerability and efficacy of trospium chloride in patients with detrusor instability. World J Urol 2003; 20: 392–9.

24. Chapple C, Rechberger T, Al-Shukri S et al. Randomized, double-blind placebo- and Tolterodine-controlled trial of the once-daily antimuscarinic agent solifenacin in patients with symptomatic overactive bladder. BJU Int 2004; 93: 303–10.

25. De Wachter S, Wyndaele J. Frequency-volume charts: a tool to evaluate bladder sensation. Neurourol Urodyn 2003; 22: 638–42.

26. Brown J, McNaughton K, Wyman et al. Measurement characteristics of a voiding diary for use by men and women with overactive bladder. Urology 2003; 61: 802–9.

27. Dmochowski R, Heit M, Sand P. The effect of anticholinergic therapy on urgency severity in patients with overactive bladder: clinical assessment of a newly validated tool. Neurourol Urodyn 2003; 22: 411–12.

28. Nixon N, Colman S, Sabounjian L et al. A validated patient reported measure of urinary urgency severity in overactive bladder for use in clinical trials. J Urol 2005; 174: 604–7.

29. Zinner N, Harnett M, Sabounjian L et al. The overactive bladder-symptom composite score: a composite symptom score of toilet voids, urgency severity and urge urinary incontinence in patients with overactive bladder. J Urol 2005; 173: 1639–43.

30. Donovan J, Bosch R, Gotoh M et al. Symptom and quality of life assessment. In: Abrams P, Cardozo L, Khoury S, Wein A, eds. Incontinence. Plymouth, UK: Health Publication Ltd; 2005: 519–84.

31. Kelleher CJ, Cardozo LD, Khullar V, Salvatore S. A new questionnaire to assess the quality of life in urinary incontinent women. BJOG 1997; 104: 1374–9.

32. Kelleher CJ, Pleil AM, Reese PR, Burgess SM, Brodish PH. How much is enough and who says so? BJOG 2004; 111: 605–12.

33. Abrams P, Avery K, Gardener N, Donovan J. The International Consultation on Incontinence Modular Questionnaire: www.iciq.net. J Urol 2006; 175: 1063–6.

34. Donovan JL, Abrams P, Peters TJ et al. The ICS-'BPH' Study: the psychometric validity and reliability of the ICSmale questionnaire. Br J Urol 1996; 78: 964.

35. Peeling WB. Diagnostic assessment of benign prostatic hyperplasia. Prostate Suppl 1989; 2: 51–68.

36. Coyne KS, Zyczynski T, Margolis MK, Elinoff V, Roberts RG. Validation of an overactive bladder awareness tool for use in primary care settings. Adv Ther 2005; 22: 381–94.

37. Coyne K, Revicki D, Hunt T et al. Psychometric validation of an overactive bladder symptom and health-related quality of life questionnaire: the OAB-q. Qual Life Res 2002; 11: 563–74.

38. Coyne KS, Matza LS, Thompson CL. The responsiveness of the Overactive Bladder Questionnaire (OAB-q). Qual Life Res 2005; 14: 849–55.

39. Meyhoff HH, Hald T, Nordling J et al. A new patient weighted symptom score system (DAN-PSS-1). Clinical assessment of indications and outcomes of transurethral prostatectomy for uncomplicated benign prostatic hyperplasia. Scand J Urol Nephrol 1993; 27: 493–9.

40. Jackson S, Donovan J, Brookes S et al. The Bristol Female Lower Urinary Tract Symptoms questionnaire: development and psychometric testing. Br J Urol 1996; 77: 805–12.

41. Khan MS, Chaliha C, Leskova L, Khullar V. A randomized crossover trial to examine administration techniques related to the Bristol female lower urinary tract symptom (BFLUTS) questionnaire. Neurourol Urodyn 2005; 24: 211–14.

42. Gray M. Overactive bladder: an overview. J Wound Ostomy Continence Nurs 2005; 32 (3 Suppl 1): S1–5.

43. Hashim H, Abrams P. Is the bladder a reliable witness for predicting detrusor overactivity? J Urol 2006; 175: 191–4.

5

Nocturia

Jeffrey P Weiss and Jerry G Blaivas

Diminished nocturnal bladder capacity • **Nocturnal polyuria** • **Polyuria, disorders of thirst, and diabetes insipidus** • **Nocturia and aging** • **Mixed causes for nocturia** • **Nocturia case study**

One of the most common reasons for interrupted sleep in the general adult population is nocturia – waking during the night to urinate.[1] Many individuals with nocturia suffer from other lower urinary tract symptoms (LUTS) such as urinary frequency, weak stream, urgency, incontinence, etc. In women, these symptoms are often considered to result from aging, or as a consequence of childbirth. In men, the symptoms are most often attributed to benign prostatic hypertrophy (BPH). In fact, recent literature suggests that the majority of men prior to transurethral prostatectomy (TURP) have nocturia >2 times, whereas over 90% of the same men arise less than twice to void following TURP.[2] So, why not just perform a TURP on all men with nocturia? We herein describe an approach to nocturia in the ensuing paragraphs which will provide an adequate answer to this question.

The majority of elderly patients with nocturia are likely to be exposed to serious health risks, since nocturia causes fatigue due to sleep deprivation, which increases the chance of traumatic injury through falling.[3] In one study comparing night-time falls in elderly people, those with nocturia were at a significantly greater risk of falling, their risk increasing from 10% to 21% with two or more micturitions per night.[4] Epidemiologic data point toward the high prevalence of nocturia in both men (65% of 400 healthy males) and women (63% of 479 healthy females).[5]

The International Continence Society's definition of nocturia is the condition of waking up to void one or more times during the night.[6] A stricter definition would be voiding during intended sleep time that is preceded and followed by sleep. This is an important distinction, because many in the general population are shift workers who sleep during the day. Nocturia is not necessarily troublesome; voiding <2 times per night is often considered to be normal. The underlying pathophysiology which accounts for nocturia in all of these conditions falls into four broad categories: (1) nocturnal polyuria (NP), (2) low nocturnal bladder capacity (NBC), (3) mixed (a combination of NP and low NBC), and (4) global polyuria. These categories are derived from the 24-hour voiding diary in which is tabulated each voided volume and its corresponding time.

In general, nocturia may be associated with medical causes, originating outside the lower urinary tract, and/or urologic causes. The former generally will be related to nocturnal urine overproduction (defined as nocturnal polyuria) or global polyuria. These are usually best evaluated and treated by a primary care physician (PCP) or internist. The latter includes conditions requiring treatment by a urologist; these conditions are generally associated with diminished nocturnal bladder capacity. An algorithm for analysis of nocturia is presented in Figure 5.1.

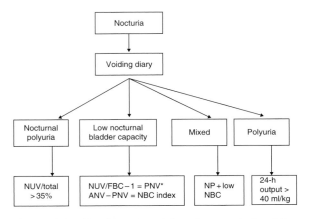

Figure 5.1 Algorithm for voiding diary analysis of the etiology of nocturia. NUV, nocturnal urine volume; ANV, actual number of nightly voids; NBC, nocturnal bladder capacity; FBC, functional bladder capacity; PNV, predicted number of nightly voids; NP, nocturnal polyuria. *Round up to nearest integer if not already an integer.

DIMINISHED NOCTURNAL BLADDER CAPACITY

Nocturia due to diminished nocturnal bladder capacity is of two general types – decreased functional bladder capacity (FBC) and decreased nocturnal bladder capacity. FBC is the maximum voided volume recorded on a bladder diary. In both conditions, nocturnal urinary volume exceeds bladder capacity and the patient is awakened by the need to void because the bladder does not hold enough. If the FBC is less than the nocturnal urine volume (NUV), nocturia ensues.[7]

In order to quantify NBC, several terms need to be defined – the *nocturia index* (Ni) and the *NBC index* (NBCi). The Ni is NUV/FBC, remembering to include the first morning void in the NUV. The Ni minus 1 (rounded up to the nearest integer) equals the predicted number of nightly voids (PNV). The NBCi is defined as the difference between the PNV and the actual nightly voids (ANV). The significance of this is that the greater is the NBCi, the more that nocturia may be attributed to diminished NBC and sensory urge disorders. For example, if the NUV is 750 ml and the FBC is 250 ml, the Ni is 750/250 = 3. This patient would have a PNV = 2 (Ni – 1 = 2) and would be expected to void twice per night – the first 500 ml during sleep hours in two voids – and then awaken and void the remaining 250 ml. For the illustration above, if the patient actually arose seven times to void the same 750 ml, he or she would have a NBCi of 5 [7 (ANV) – 2 (PNV)]. This patient, for whatever reason, has significantly diminished bladder capacity during sleep hours. Thus, the higher is the NBCi the lower is the nocturnal bladder capacity (compared to the functional bladder capacity).[8] The causes of decreased NBC are listed in Table 5.1.

Treatment of diminished nocturnal bladder capacity

An overview of Table 5.1 indicates that low NBC is primarily a urologic as opposed to a medical diagnosis. Thus, infravesical obstruction, infection, and cancer may all require specific treatment by a urologist as opposed to, for example, diabetes mellitus or obstructive sleep apnea which may cause nocturia/nocturnal polyuria and require treatment by their respective medical specialists. Interestingly, low NBC is not related to detrusor instability, at least not that which can be diagnosed through awake urodynamic studies.[9] BPH with obstruction has recently been studied as a cause for low NBC. In the VA Cooperative Study Program Trial, there were 1078 men with BPH, aged 45–80 years, whose baseline nocturnal voids averaged 2.5. Nocturia decreased to 1.8, 2.1, 2.0, and 2.1 as a result of treatment with terazosin, finasteride, combination, and placebo, respectively. While nocturia reduction with terazosin and combination therapy was statistically significantly different from that resulting from placebo, the minimal absolute differences support the observation that placebo was nearly as good as drug in the treatment of nocturia. Thus, medical treatment of the prostate is an inefficient way to treat nocturia, most likely because of confounding factors such as nocturnal urine overproduction in its many causes (see below).[10]

The role of antimuscarinics in the treatment of nocturia in patients with overactive bladder (OAB) is currently being investigated. Episodes of nocturia were statistically significantly decreased in patients treated with solifenacin 10 mg (−0.71, −38.5%) versus placebo (−0.52, −16.4%; $p = 0.036$).[11] Tolterodine extended release caused a

Table 5.1 Common causes of low nocturnal bladder capacity
Infravesical obstruction (prostate, pelvic organ prolapse, post-surgical)
Idiopathic nocturnal detrusor overactivity
Neurogenic bladder
Cystitis: bacterial, interstitial, tuberculous, radiation
Cancer of bladder, prostate, urethra
Acquired voiding dysfunction
Anxiety disorders
Pharmacologic: xanthines (theophylline, caffeine); beta-blockers
Bladder calculi
Ureteral calculi

Table 5.2 Causes of nocturnal polyuria	
Category	Causes
Nocturnal polyuria	Congestive heart failure
	Diabetes mellitus
	Obstructive sleep apnea
	Peripheral edema
	Excessive night-time fluid intake
	Loss in circadian rhythmicity of arginine vasopressin secretion

59% median reduction in OAB-specific nocturnal voids compared with 43% reduction by placebo ($p = 0.02$), although overall benefit for all types of nocturic micturitions was not seen.[12]

NOCTURNAL POLYURIA

The increased production of urine at night experienced in NP is offset by lowered daytime urine production, such that the 24-hour urine volume remains normal.[13] Nocturnal urine volume is defined as the total urinary output during the hours of sleep to which is added the volume of the first morning void within 30 minutes of arising. It is assumed that the patient voids just prior to retiring, so that all urine voided during sleep time plus the first morning void belongs with the tally of NUV. There are several definitions of nocturnal polyuria, including nocturnal urine volume (NUV) >6.4 ml/kg; nocturnal diuresis >0.9 ml/minute; NUV/24-hour urine volume >35%.[14] We favor the last definition. Data supporting the last definition include a study of over 200 age-matched elderly (>70 years) men and women in whom NUV/24-hour volume was 45% in nocturics as compared with 31% in non-nocturics.[15] In the same study, nocturics excreted a greater NUV than non-nocturics (700 ml and 417 ml, respectively) and had smaller functional bladder capacities (325 vs. 400 ml). The most dramatic parametric distinction between nocturics and non-nocturics, however, lies in analysis of the nocturia index (Ni = NUV/FBC), where Ni = 2.1 for nocturics and 1.0 for non-nocturics, implying that the most significant reason for nocturia in the elderly is a mismatch between the volume of urine excreted and the bladder's capacity to hold adequate urine volumes during the hours of sleep.[15]

The etiology of NP is manifold, and includes congestive heart failure, diabetes mellitus, sleep apnea, diabetes insipidus, cerebrovascular accident (via an effect on the hypothalamic–pituitary axis and resultant loss in circadian rhythmicity of arginine vasopressin secretion)[16] third-space fluid resorption (venous stasis, nephrotic syndrome, hepatic failure) and late evening diuretic/fluid intake (Table 5.2).

Abnormalities of arginine vasopressin secretion

Urine production assumes a standard circadian pattern which is age-dependent: in young people (<25 years), mean NUV = 14% as compared with those over the age of 65 whose mean NUV = 34%.[17] This circadian pattern appears to be closely related to a corresponding increase in secretion of antidiuretic hormone (ADH) during the hours of sleep, a change in which may cause nocturnal polyuria in the elderly.[14] One reason for this diurnal change is thought to be a disruption of the diurnal variation in secretion of ADH, otherwise known as arginine vasopressin (AVP). Antidiuretic hormone is synthesized in the supraoptic and paraventricular nuclei of the hypothalamus and is released by the posterior pituitary in response to various stimuli such as increased plasma osmolality.[14] AVP, normally secreted in a diurnal pattern, is partly responsible for the regulation of urine production.[18] Since AVP increases the resorption of water from the renal tubule, higher concentrations of AVP occurring at night result in the production of lower volumes of concentrated urine. Plasma AVP levels are often undetectable during the night in elderly subjects with nocturia, thus implying a cause and effect relationship between AVP secretion and NP.[19]

In the renal inner medullary collecting duct, AVP regulates two key transporters: aquaporin-2 (AQP2) and vasopressin-regulated urea transporter (VRUT). Aquaporin-2 is present in intracellular vesicles as well as the apical plasma membrane. Short-term regulation of AQP2 (but not VRUT) occurs by vasopressin-induced trafficking of AQP2-containing vesicles to the apical plasma membrane.[20] Long-term regulation is such that a prolonged (>24 h) increase in circulating vasopressin in turn leads to increased AQP2 production.[21] Reduced secretion of vasopressin and absorptive hypercalciuria are independently associated with decreases in nocturnal urinary AQP2 and resulting nocturnal polyuria.[21] AVP causes water reabsorption in the collecting duct via the "V2 receptor", which promotes a cascade of events leading to the activation of "G-protein" which then causes adenylate cyclase to convert adenosine triphosphate (ATP) to cyclic adenosine monophosphate (cAMP).[22] Cyclic AMP then activates "protein kinase A" which stimulates intracellular vesicles containing aquaporin-2 water channels. The latter translocate to the apical membrane by exocytosis of intracellular vesicles, leading to water transport from urine into the circulation. When AVP levels are low, water permeability is decreased by a shift of AQP2 channels back into the intracellular vesicles.[20] Vasopressin "escape" is associated with relative vasopressin resistance of the collecting duct cells manifested by decreased intracellular cAMP levels.[23] Decreased cAMP levels contribute to a decrease in collecting duct water permeability in two ways: by causing a decrease in aquaporin-2 expression and by limiting the acute action of vasopressin to increase collecting duct water permeability.

Nocturia in a large proportion of elderly men with LUTS is caused by NP and natriuresis.[14] Interestingly, a positive correlation has been observed between NUV and daytime mean arterial blood pressure. While significant negative correlation has been found between NUV and plasma angiotensin II, NP is associated with decreased plasma AVP levels.[14] A possible explanation for NP and natriuresis in these patients is that pressure-induced lesions in the renal medulla and distal tubular system may be caused by long-lasting urinary tract obstruction. This may interfere with normal circadian renal handling of sodium by decreasing daytime sodium excretion.[14]

Obstructive sleep apnea

Sleep apnea, a form of sleep-disordered breathing, is defined as sudden cessation of respiration due to airway obstruction during sleep. Respiratory diseases associated with increased airway resistance such as obstructive sleep apnea (OSA) are associated with increased renal sodium and water excretion mediated by plasma atrial natriuretic peptide (ANP) levels.[14,24] The prevalence of OSA is about 2% in women and 4% in adult men.[25] The mechanism for elevated ANP release associated with OSA has been demonstrated as being due to increased right atrial transmural pressure resulting from hypoxia-induced pulmonary vasoconstriction.[24] Hence, a population of patients with nocturia may result from OSA and secondary nocturnal polyuria.[26] Polysomnographic sleep studies including measurement of plasma oxygen saturation and respiratory patterns are therefore recommended in patients with nocturia having a suspected relation to OSA. Patient selection is based upon increased risk as follows: patients with nocturnal polyuria, morbid obesity, acromegaly, asthma, hypertension, adult onset diabetes mellitus, and craniofacial abnormalities may be submitted for sleep studies owing to their 30–40% chances of having OSA.[25,26] Treatment of OSA includes nasal continuous positive airway pressure during sleep and uvulectomy/tonsillectomy when these structures are causing obstruction.

Treatment of nocturnal polyuria

Remediable medical causes of NP should be identified and treated, but in some instances nocturia persists, and in most patients clearly identifiable remediable conditions are not found. Empiric treatment options include evening fluid restriction (a form of behavior modification), timed diuretics,[27,28] afternoon naps and/or elevation of the legs, application of compressive stockings in patients with edema or varicosities, and antidiuretic hormone administration.[29,30] The latter should be avoided or used judiciously at best in patients with congestive heart failure.

In the elderly, simple fluid restriction is rarely effective in reducing NP which is due to the mobilization of gravitational-induced third spacing of interstitial fluid residing in the lower extremities upon achieving the recumbent position during the hours of sleep. Compressive devices may prevent this fluid accumulation and help to diminish nocturnal urinary output. In addition, late afternoon naps with elevation of the legs simulate sleep hours during the day and may diminish the burden of fluid excretion otherwise inevitable during normal sleep time. If edema is present either in the legs or presacral area, diuretics may be helpful to diminish this third spacing. Virtually all diuretics act within 2 hours of administration and, therefore, may be given in mid- to late afternoon or early evening, as they are least needed just after arising and may exacerbate NP if given later in the evening. Bumetanide has been shown to reduce the number of weekly night-time voids by 4 in patients without obstructive symptoms.[28] In addition, furosemide has been shown to be effective at reducing both nocturia and NP.[27] Doses of the diuretic taken 6 hours before bedtime were shown to reduce the number of night-time voids by 0.5, and to lower the percentage night-time voided volume by 18%. Recent evidence has been presented for the treatment of nocturnal polyuria with imipramine.[31] The mechanism for such an antidiuretic effect is thought to result from imipramine-mediated α-adrenergic stimulation in the proximal nephron along with increased urea and water reabsorption in the distal nephron. Non-steroidal antiinflammatories have been proposed as treatment for nocturnal polyuria mediated by inhibition of prostaglandin E_2-mediated diuresis.[32]

Exogenous administration of antidiuretic treatment is effective in preventing NP. Desmopressin (1-deamino-8-D-arginine-vasopressin; dDAVP) is an AVP analog that has been proven effective and well tolerated in the treatment of neurogenic diabetes insipidus[33] and enuresis, both in children[34] and in adults.[35] Desmopressin has also been shown to reduce or eliminate nocturnal voiding in patients with autonomic dysfunction and Parkinson's disease.[36] Patients with nocturia due to multiple sclerosis have been successfully treated with desmopressin, experiencing a decrease in the number of voids per night and a corresponding increase in nights free from voiding and hours of uninterrupted sleep.[37] In addition, patients previously diagnosed with BPH were found to have a reduced number of voids when treated with desmopressin, particularly those with a high nocturnal urine output.[38]

Our protocol involves beginning with 10 μg of intranasally or 0.1 mg orally administered desmopressin increased by increments of 10 μg or 0.1 mg, respectively, every third night until the desired effect is reached, to a maximum dose of 40 μg or 0.4 mg, respectively, each bedtime. The patient is seen again 7 days after the first dose, because if electrolyte abnormalities or fluid overload occurs, it is most likely to commence during this initial time interval. After each dose increment the patient should be questioned about headache, nausea, vomiting, light-headedness, etc. If any of these symptoms occur, the medication should be discontinued until electrolyte values are known. The patient or a caregiver should be taught to monitor the legs and presacral area for edema and do daily weights for early identification of excess fluid retention induced by desmopressin in susceptible patients. Significant weight increases, new onset or worsening of edema, or symptoms of hyponatremia such as headache or visual disturbance should be reported immediately to the physician and the medication discontinued. The above protocol may be prescribed to appropriately selected patients with nocturia owing to nocturnal urine overproduction having reached the age of 21 years.

In the opinion of the authors, claims of lack of side effects from antidiuretic treatment apply to pediatric patients with enuresis and cannot be expected in the elderly, especially those with a history of congestive heart failure. It is important to remind patients receiving desmopressin that they should sharply curtail their evening water intake in order to minimize the occurrence of fluid retention. Recent work suggests that there is a relationship between gender, plasma level of desmopressin, and the incidence of adverse events. Specifically, women seem to have a significantly higher plasma desmopressin concentration and more adverse events than do men.[39]

Mannucci was the first to demonstrate the therapeutic value of desmopressin in the treatment and prevention of bleeding complications in patients with mild forms of hemophilia A and von Willebrand's disease.[40] However, the doses of desmopressin used in the treatment of coagulation disorders are about 10 times higher than those recommended for antidiuretic therapy. Thus, it is unlikely that dosage levels of desmopressin used in the treatment of NP would be associated with thrombotic complications.

The efficacy of any combination of the above treatment methods for NP may be easily determined using repeated voiding diaries.

POLYURIA, DISORDERS OF THIRST, AND DIABETES INSIPIDUS

Polyuria (defined as 24-hour urine output in excess of 40 ml/kg/24 hours) is related to increased intake, so that polyuria and polydipsia (at least in the steady state) are closely related.[17] Polyuria thus results in both day and night urinary frequency due to global urine overproduction in excess of bladder capacity. Causes of polyuria include diabetes mellitus and insipidus and primary thirst disorders (Table 5.3). While polyuria causes increased nocturnal urine volume similar to the situation for nocturnal polyuria, treatment is directed at reduction in both water intake and its resultant output through specific measures such as insulin replacement, voluntary restriction of water intake, or supplementary administration of vasopressin analogs where appropriate.

The causes of diabetes insipidus (DI) are generally classified into two categories: central (neurogenic) and renal (nephrogenic); polydipsia (either dipsogenic or psychogenic) may cause polyuria but is not considered a form of DI. In central DI, there is a lack of production of vasopressin (AVP; antidiuretic hormone, ADH) from the posterior pituitary, for example due to loss of neurosecretory neurons in the hypothalamus as a result of surgery, infection (tuberculosis, meningitis), primary (craniopharyngioma), or metastatic (lung, breast) tumor or head trauma. Infiltrative disease such as sarcoid or Wegener's granulomatosis, plus idiopathic conditions, account for the remainder of cases of central DI. Renal

Table 5.3 Causes of polyuria

Category	Causes
Global polyuria	Diabetes mellitus Diabetes insipidus Primary polydipsia (dipsogenic, psychogenic)

(nephrogenic) DI is caused by defective renal responsiveness to adequate circulating levels of ADH so that the renal tubules are incapable of water reabsorption, leading to dehydration and excessive thirst with secondary polydipsia. Etiologies of nephrogenic DI include hypercalcemia, hypokalemia, lithium, tetracyclines, and abnormal secretion of atrial natriuretic peptide. Psychogenic polydipsia presents as DI due to compulsive water drinking. There may be an associated secondary nephrogenic component to DI in these patients owing to washout of the countercurrent multiplier gradient responsible for renal concentration of urine. This defect may reverse with psychiatric treatment of the underlying compulsion to drink excessive volumes of water. Patients with primary thirst disorders (dipsogenic polydipsia) may present with global polyuria and secondary NP.[41] Dipsogenic polydipsia usually occurs in the setting of central neurologic disorders related to brain tumors, trauma, or radiation injury.

The differential diagnosis of diabetes insipidus may be made by careful diary evaluation of urinary output in addition to use of both the overnight dehydration test and the renal concentrating capacity test (RCCT). Overnight dehydration normally results in transformation of initially dilute urine to urine concentrated to an osmolality of over 600 mOsm/kg. A normal overnight dehydration test assures that both central production of and peripheral renal responsiveness to AVP is normal, thus excluding all forms of diabetes insipidus. These patients with polyuria have a primary thirst disorder, either psychogenic or dipsogenic. Patients with psychogenic polydipsia usually have low to low-normal serum sodium levels. If polyuric patients continue to have dilute urine after overnight dehydration, a test of renal responsiveness to desmopressin is in order. In adults, 40 μg desmopressin is administered intranasally owing to greater reliability of absorption as compared with the enteric route of administration. The bladder is emptied and a urine sample for osmolality obtained 3–5 hours later. Water intake is restricted for the first 12 hours after drug administration (so as to avoid hyponatremia from desmopressin in patients with polydipsia). The reference level for normal urine osmolality after desmopressin administration is 800 mOsm/kg, though polyurics rarely attain this degree of urine concentration; a more realistic target is >600 mOsm/kg. Post-desmopressin administration urine osmolality under 550 mOsm/kg suggests nephrogenic (or chronic central) diabetes insipidus, whereas urine osmolality 600–800 mOsm/kg is consistent with psychogenic or dipsogenic polydipsia. However, after several days of desmopressin administration, patients with central diabetes insipidus develop normal concentrating capacity.

Treatment of polyuria is in accordance with etiologic diagnosis: reduced water intake for those without DI; specific treatment of diabetes mellitus; vasopressin analogs for central DI; and psychotherapy for compulsive water drinkers.

NOCTURIA AND AGING

In a study of 850 patients with symptoms of OAB, younger men and women were more likely to have diminished nocturnal bladder capacity (higher NBCi) and older men and women were more likely to have nocturnal urine overproduction.[42] In a cohort of aged men patients, nocturics had significantly greater nocturnal urine output (mean 700 ml) and diminished nocturnal bladder capacity (mean 325 ml) than their counterparts without nocturia (417 ml and 400 ml, respectively). The combination of increased output and decreased bladder capacity at night appears to account for the increasing incidence of nocturia which accompanies aging.[15]

MIXED CAUSES FOR NOCTURIA

Many patients with nocturia are found to have a combination of NP and low NBC ("mixed" etiology of nocturia). We recently reviewed 194 patients with nocturia and found that 13 (7%) had pure nocturnal polyuria, 111 (57%) had diminished nocturnal bladder capacity, and 70 (36%) a combination of the two. Of these 194, 45 (23%) additionally had global polyuria.[43] Specific treatment of these patients should be directed at both disorders.

NOCTURIA CASE STUDY

Patient: 62-year-old G1 P1 (one pregnancy, one delivery) woman
History: Chief complaint post-void suprapubic cramping; nocturia × 3
Past medical history: Crohn's disease treated with purinethol, azulfidine, minocycline. Recent body computed tomography (CT) scan unremarkable
Examination: Mild cystocele. No peripheral edema. Neurourologic: Normal
Urinalysis/culture: Normal
PVR = 0 ml
Uroflow: Peak flow (Q_{max}) = 35 ml/s (Figure 5.2)
Cystoscopy: Unremarkable
Stress test: No stress incontinence noted
Voiding diary:
  24-hour urinary volume = 5190 ml
  Usual voided volume = 300 ml
  Functional bladder capacity = 1220 ml
  Awake hours: number of voids = 14
  Sleep hours: number of voids = 3
  Nocturnal urine volume (NUV) = 1530 ml
  Nocturia index (NUV/FBC) = 1.2
  NUV/total (NPi) = 29%
  NBC index = 2
Urodynamic studies (done to determine whether underlying vesicourethral function was normal in view of the cramping symptoms): Revealed large capacity bladder, normal vesicourethral function, cystocele (Figures 5.3 and 5.4).

Comment: Mrs PD has nocturia and suprapubic cramping associated with polyuria (>40 ml/kg/24 hours) and no relevant endoscopic or urodynamic abnormalities. In our view the global polyuria accounted for her LUTS. Thus, testing was directed at identifying the cause for her polyuria.

An overnight dehydration test revealed the results given in Table 5.4.

The patient was unable to fully concentrate her urine overnight, although this is a common problem in patients who are chronically overhydrated. A fasting serum antidiuretic hormone level was normal, excluding central diabetes insipidus.

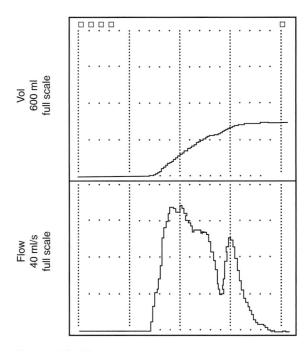

Figure 5.2 Flow–volume chart.

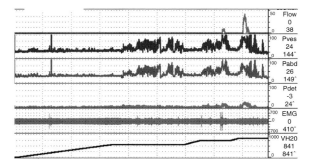

Figure 5.3 Urodynamic tracing. Pves, vesical pressure; Pabd, abdominal pressure; Pdet, detrusor pressure. No leakage with cough or valsalva; capacity 990 ml; peak uroflow (Q_{max}) = 38 ml/s; $PdetQ_{max}$ = 18 cmH$_2$O.

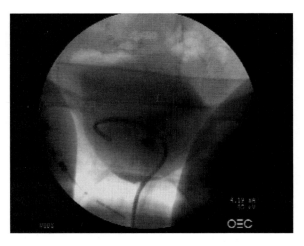

Figure 5.4 Cystogram demonstrating mild cystocele.

Therefore, a renal concentrating capacity test (RCCT) was subsequently carried out, comparing baseline serum and urine osmolality with the same parameters obtained 4 hours following administration of desmopressin 40 μg intranasally (Table 5.5). Her baseline serum sodium was 140 mmol/l.

Comment: Her baseline urine osmolalities were low, but the RCCT excluded nephrogenic DI as the cause (post-desmopressin urine osmolality <500 mOsm/kg is necessary for a diagnosis of nephrogenic DI). This left psychogenic versus dipsogenic polydipsia in the differential diagnosis. Magnetic resonance imaging (MRI) scanning of the head done to exclude a pituitary tumor was normal.

Comment: As the patient denied water drinking to result from abnormal thirst and in view of the lack of a history of head trauma, surgery, or

Table 5.4 Results of overnight dehydration test		
	Baseline	*NPO after full night sleep*
Serum osmolality (mOsm/kg)	286	288
Urine osmolality (mOsm/kg)	203	497

Non par os (fasting.)

Table 5.5   Results of renal concentrating capacity test

	Baseline	After DDAVP 40 μg IN
Serum osmolality (mOsm/kg)	288	287
Urine osmolality (mOsm/kg)	197	676

DDAVP. desmopressin; IN, intranasally.

radiation (along with a normal brain MRI), we established the diagnosis of psychogenic polydipsia. She was thus treated using behavior modification with the following outcome.

Subsequent voiding diary after behavior modification for psychogenic polydipsia:
24-hour urinary volume = 2490 ml
Usual voided volume = 350 ml
Functional bladder capacity = 950 ml
Awake hours: number of voids = 8
Sleep hours: number of voids = 0
Nocturnal urine volume (NUV) = 730 ml
Nocturia index (NUV/FBC) = 0.77
NUV/total = 29%
NBC index = 0

Comment: Symptoms of both nocturia and suprapubic cramping have now resolved with near-resolution of her polyuria. Her serum sodium levels have remained normal throughout treatment. If she had evidence of central DI, we would expect AVP replacement therapy with desmopressin to have equally beneficial results. While it is our routine to perform urodynamic studies in most patients with voiding dysfunction, in retrospect Mrs PD could have been managed without them.[44,45]

REFERENCES

1. Van Kerrebroeck P, Weiss J. Classification of Nocturia. BJU Int 1999; 84 (Suppl 1): 1–4.
2. Bruskewitz RC, Larsen EH, Madsen PO et al. 3-year follow-up of urinary symptoms after transuretheral resection of the prostate. J Urol 1986; 136: 613–15.
3. Barker JC, Mitteness LS. Nocturia in the elderly. Gerontologist 1988; 28: 99–104.
4. Stewart RB, Moore MT, May FE et al. Nocturia: a risk factor for falls in the elderly. J Am Geriatr Soc 1992; 40: 1217–20.
5. Fultz NH, Herzog AR. Epidemiology of urinary symptoms in the geriatric population. Urol Clin North Am 1996; 23: 1–10.
6. Abrams P, Cardozo L, Fall M et al. The standardisation of terminology in lower urinary tract function: report from the standardisation sub-committee of the International Continence Society. Urology 2003; 61: 37–49.
7. Abrams P, Blaivas JG, Stanton S et al. The standardisation of terminology of lower urinary tract function. International Continence Society Committee on standardisation of terminology. Scand J Urol Nephrol Suppl 1988; 114: 5–19.
8. Weiss JP, Stember DS, Chaikin DC, Blaivas JG. Evaluation of the etiology of nocturia in men: the nocturia and nocturnal bladder capacity indices. Neurourol Urodyn 1999; 18: 559–65.
9. Blaivas JG, Stember DS, Weiss JP. Etiology of voiding symptoms in men: correlation of individual AUA symptom scores with urodynamic and diary parameters. Neurourol Urodyn 1998; 17: 398–9.
10. Johnson TM, Jones K, Williford WO et al. Changes in nocturia from medical treatment of benign prostatic hyperplasia: secondary analysis of the department of Veterans Affairs Cooperative Study Trial. J Urol 2003; 170: 145–8.
11. Cardozo L, Lisee M, Millard R et al. Randomized, double-blind placebo-controlled trial of the once-daily antimuscarinic agent solifenacin succinate in patients with overactive bladder. J Urol 2004; 172: 1919–24.
12. Rackley R, Weiss JP, Rovner ES, Wang JT, Guan Z. Nighttime dosing of tolterodine extended release reduces overactive bladder-related nocturnal

frequency in patients with overactive bladder and nocturia. Urology 2006; 67: 731–6.

13. Asplund R. The nocturnal polyuria syndrome (NPS). Gen Pharmac 1995; 26: 1203–9.

14. Matthiesen TB, Rittig S, Norgaard JP et al. Nocturnal polyuria and natriuresis in male patients with nocturia and lower urinary tract symptoms. J Urol 1996; 156: 1292–9.

15. Rembratt A, Weiss J, Robertson G. Pathogenesis of nocturia in the elderly: relationship of functional bladder capacity to nocturnal urine output. J Urol 2001; 165 (Suppl): 250.

16. Ozawa T, Oyanagi K, Tanaka H et al. Suprachiasmatic nucleus in a patient with multiple system atrophy with abnormal circadian rhythm of arginine-vasopressin secretion into plasma. J Neurol Sci 1998; 154: 116–21.

17. Kirkland JL, Lye M, Levy DW, Banerjee AK. Patterns of urine flow and electrolyte excretion in healthy elderly people. Br Med J 1983; 287: 1665–7.

18. Baylis PH. Osmoregulation and control of vasopressin secretion in healthy humans. Am J Physiol 1987; 235: R671–8.

19. Asplund R, Åberg H. Diurnal variation in the levels of antidiuretic hormone in elderly subjects with nocturia. J Intern Med 1991; 229: 131–4.

20. Inoue T, Terris J, Ecelbarger CA et al. Vasopressin regulates apical targeting of aquaporin-2 but not of UT1 urea transporter in renal collecting duct. Am J Physiol 1999; 276: F559–66.

21. Valenti G, Laera A, Pace G et al. Urinary aquaporin 2 and calciuria correlate with the severity of enuresis in children. J Am Soc Nephrol 2000; 1: 1873.

22. Nishimoto G, Zelenina M, Li D et al. Arginine vasopressin stimulates phosphorylation of aquaporin-2 in rat renal tissue. Am J Physiol 1999; 276: F254–9.

23. Ecelbarger CA, Chou CL, Lee AJ et al. Escape from vasopressin-induced antidiuresis: role of vasopressin resistance of the collecting duct. Am J Physiol 1998; 274: F1161–6.

24. Yalkut D, Lee LY, Grider J et al. Mechanism of atrial natriuretic peptide release with increased inspiratory resistance. J Lab Clin Med 1996; 128: 322–8.

25. Partinen M. Epidemiology of obstructive sleep apnea syndrome. Curr Opin Pulm Med 1995; 1: 482–7.

26. Krieger J, Petian C, Sforza E et al. Nocturnal pollakiuria is a symptom of obstructive sleep apnea. Urol Int 1993; 50: 93–7.

27. Reynard JM, Cannon A, Yang Q, Abrams P. A novel therapy for nocturnal polyuria: a double-blind randomized trial of furosemide against placebo. Br J Urol 1998; 81: 215–8.

28. Pedersen PA, Johansen PB. Prophylactic treatment of adult nocturia with bumetanide. Br J Urol 1988; 62: 145–7.

29. Asplund R. The nocturnal polyuria syndrome. Gen Pharmac 1995; 26: 1203–9.

30. Donahue JL, Lowenthal DT. Nocturnal polyuria in the elderly person. Am J Med Sci 1997; 314: 232–8.

31. Hunsballe J, Rittig S, Pederson E, Oleson O, Djurhuus L. Single dose imipramine reduces nocturnal urine output in patients with nocturnal enuresis and nocturnal polyuria. J Urol 1997; 158: 830–6.

32. Al-Waili NS. Increased urinary nitrite excretion in primary enuresis: effects of indomethacin treatment on urinary and serum osmolality and electrolytes, urinary volumes and nitrite excretion. BJU Int 2002; 90: 294–301.

33. Robinson AG. DDAVP in the treatment of diabetes insipidus. N Engl J Med 1976; 294: 507–11.

34. Klauber GT. Clinical efficacy and safety of desmopressin in the treatment of nocturnal enuresis. J Pediatr 1989; 114: 719–22.

35. Belmaker RH. The use of desmopressin in adult enuresis. Mil Med 1986; 151: 660–2.

36. Suchowersky O, Furtado S, Rohs G. Beneficial effect of desmopressin for nocturnal polyuria in Parkinson's disease. Mov Disord 1995; 10: 337–40.

37. Valiquette G, Herbert J, Meade-D'Alisera P. Desmopressin in the management of nocturia in patients with multiple sclerosis. Arch Neurol 1996; 53: 1270–5.

38. Månsson W, Sundin T, Gullberg B. Evaluation of synthetic vasopressin analogue for treatment of nocturia in benign prostatic hypertrophy. Scand J Urol Nephrol 1980; 14: 139–41.

39. Hvistendahl GM, Riis A, Norgaard JP, Djurhuus JC. The pharmacokinetics of 400 microg of oral desmopressin in elderly patients with nocturia, and the correlation between the absorption of desmopressin and clinical effect. BJU Int 2005; 95: 804–9.

40. Mannucci PM. Desmopressin: a nontransfusional form of treatment for congenital and acquired bleeding disorders. Blood 1988; 72: 1449–55.

41. Britton JP, Dowell AC, Whelan P. Prevalence of urinary symptoms in men aged over 60. Br J Urol 1990; 66: 175–6.

42. Weiss JP, Blaivas JG, Guan Z, Wang JT. Age-related pathogenesis of nocturia in patients with overactive bladder. J Urol 2005; 173 (Suppl 4): 307.

43. Weiss JP, Blaivas JG, Stember DS, Brooks MM. Nocturia in adults: etiology and classification. Neurourol Urodyn 1998; 17: 467–72.

44. Zerbe RL, Robertson GL. Osmotic and nonosmotic regulation of thirst and vasopressin secretion. In: Narins RG, ed. Clinical Disorders of Fluid and Electrolyte Metabolism, 5th edn. New York: McGraw-Hill, 1994: 81–100.

45. Reddi AS. Essentials of Renal Physiology. E Hanover, NJ: College Book Publishers, 1999.

6

Urodynamics

Melissa C Fischer and Victor W Nitti

Introduction • **Indications for urodynamics** • **Urodynamic testing** • **Summary**

INTRODUCTION

The lower urinary tract is responsible for the storage and evacuation of urine. Storage should occur at low pressure in order to assure continence and protection of the kidneys, and evacuation should be voluntary. However, a variety of problems may arise which interfere with these two basic functions. Urodynamics (UDS) is the dynamic study of the transport, storage, and evacuation of urine by the urinary tract. It comprises a number of tests which individually or collectively can be used to gain invaluable information about lower urinary tract function. The term "urodynamics" was first described by Davis in 1953, but the study of bladder pressure began in earnest in the late 19th century.[1,2]

Components of UDS include from simple, non-invasive tests such as uroflowmetry, to more sophisticated, invasive multichannel pressure–flow studies with sphincter electromyography and video-fluoroscopy (videourodynamics). The following is a review of UDS with an emphasis on the diagnostic evaluation of detrusor overactivity and related conditions. The terminology used conforms to the standards recommended by the International Continence Society (ICS), except where specifically noted, and is intended to provide an effective means of communication between clinicians.[3]

INDICATIONS FOR URODYNAMICS

The initial evaluation of any patient includes a thorough history, physical examination, and formulation of a differential diagnosis. While there have been many technological advances in the field of UDS, clinical expertise in deciding when, why, and how to perform the study is critical to the accurate interpretation and ultimate utility of the test. In general, UDS is indicated when the information and diagnosis provided will guide patient treatment. Examples of indications for urodynamics in the patient with overactive bladder (OAB) include: an inconclusive diagnosis after simpler tests, associated poor bladder emptying (elevated post-void residual), a poor response to empiric therapy (e.g. anticholinergic medication), suspected bladder outlet obstruction or other voiding phase abnormality, presence of a condition with known deleterious effects, particularly OAB associated with neurological disease or pelvic radiation, mixed stress and urge incontinence (particularly when the predominate component is not obvious by history), prior surgical procedures on the lower urinary tract, or when a proposed treatment has significant risks.

UDS is just one tool that can be used to assist in the diagnosis of genitourinary abnormalities and is best utilized when the clinician has specific questions to be answered. UDS is an interactive test between the clinician and the patient, and should attempt to reproduce the patient's symptoms. Often the objective data obtained are influenced by the circumstances and conditions of the test. Therefore, the ultimate interpretation of the data is subjective, requiring experience and an understanding of the patient's history. Three general principles should always be remembered: (1) a study which does not reproduce the patient's symptoms is non-diagnostic; (2) failure to record an abnormality does not rule out its existence; and (3) not all abnormalities are clinically significant.[4]

A basic understanding of the physiology of urine storage and voiding and the pathophysiology of voiding dysfunction is required to formulate appropriate questions to be answered by a urodynamic study. One should always focus on the possible urodynamic findings in a given case and how each of the findings may ultimately affect treatment. The functional classification system described by Wein is a useful framework with which to conceptualize voiding dysfunction and characterize it based on urodynamic findings.[5] Of equal importance is that treatment options can be guided by this system. The Functional Classification system is based on the simple concept that the lower urinary tract (comprising the bladder and the bladder outlet) must store and empty urine. For normal storage and emptying to occur, the bladder and bladder outlet must function in a proper and coordinated fashion. Hence, lower urinary tract dysfunction can be classified under the following rubrics: "failure to store", "failure to empty", or a combination of both. Urodynamic abnormalities may result from bladder dysfunction, bladder outlet dysfunction, or a combination of both.

URODYNAMIC TESTING

Uroflowmetry

Uroflowmetry is a non-invasive means of quantifying the general effectiveness of voiding. The information may be used as an initial screening test or for comparison to monitor therapy, but is not diagnostic as a single tool. Uroflowmetry is simple, non-invasive, and inexpensive. The test relies on physiologic bladder filling to normal capacity, until the patient is comfortably full and has a normal desire to void. The patient is encouraged to sit and void as usual in a private setting. Prior to interpretation the patient should be asked whether the void was typical.

The flow rate is directly related to the intravesical volume. The ideal volume for uroflowmetry is dependent upon the individual, but generally the volume should be greater than 150 ml for accurate interpretation.[6] While we agree with the statement that a voided volume of $\geq$ 150 ml is optimal, we also realize that some patients cannot hold such a volume, and in these cases, the knowledge that the study was "typical" is important. This is particularly true for patients with severe OAB. Low volume voids can be correlated with voiding diaries.

The urinary flow pattern is the result of the expulsion pressure, both detrusor and abdominal, and the outlet resistance. The following parameters can be measured during a noninvasive uroflow:

1. Flow rate: the volume of urine expelled via the urethra per unit time (ml/s);
2. Voided volume: total volume expelled via the urethra (ml);
3. Maximum flow rate (Q_{max}): the maximum measured flow rate after correction for artifact (ml/s);
4. Voiding time: the total duration of micturition, including interruptions (s);
5. Flow time: the time over which measurable flow actually occurs (s);
6. Average flow rate (Q_{ave}): voided volume divided by flow time (ml/s);
7. Time to maximum flow: elapsed time from onset of flow to maximum flow (s);
8. Post-void residual volume (PVR) may be determined after uroflowmetry to assess how well the patient emptied her bladder. PVR may be measured by a bladder ultrasound or catheterization.

When interpreting a uroflow tracing it is important to look at not only the objective parameters listed above, but also the shape of the flow curve, which can give insight into the way the patient voids. The pattern of flow can be described as continuous or intermittent, smooth or fluctuating.[3] A typical flow is a continuous, smooth, bell-shaped curve with high amplitude. A decreased detrusor contraction and/or increased outlet resistance will result in a lower flow rate and a smooth flat curve.[7]

How can uroflowmetry be applied to clinical practice? If a patient with significant voiding symptoms has a completely normal uroflow (rate and pattern) and a low PVR, then more invasive urodynamic testing may initially be deferred. Conversely, an abnormal uroflow might prompt further testing. An abnormal uroflow indicates that emptying is altered, but is not diagnostic of etiology. Emptying abnormalities that affect uroflowmetry include impaired contractility and increased outlet resistance (obstruction).[8] UDS with a formal pressure–flow study is necessary to distinguish between the two. Uroflowmetry is particularly useful to evaluate a patient after an intervention which can affect emptying, such as anticholinergic therapy, medical or surgical therapy for an enlarged prostate, anti-incontinence procedures, etc.

Cystometry

A cystometrogram (CMG) is a measure of the bladder's response to being filled. It allows the clinician to determine the pressure–volume relationship within the bladder during bladder filling and storage of urine. A function of the bladder is to store increasing volumes of urine at low pressure. In addition, with the cooperation of the patient, it provides a subjective measure of bladder sensation. CMG provides correlation of the patient's symptoms with objective measures. Cystometry can be performed as a single channel study where the bladder pressure (Pves) is measured and recorded during filling and storage, or as a multichannel study where abdominal pressure (Pabd) is subtracted from Pves to give the detrusor pressure (Pdet). We believe that cystometry whether conducted alone, or as part of a pressure–flow study, is ideally done by monitoring both Pves and Pabd (Figure 6.1).[9]

It is beyond the scope of this chapter to describe all of the technical nuisances of performing proper cystometry and UDS. The reader is referred elsewhere for more detail.[7] However, it is important to remember several basic principles. First, the patient should be adequately prepared, with an understanding of what to except, before the study is started. Intravesical catheters (usually 6–8 French) should be double- or triple-lumen to allow for both filling and simultaneous measurement (bladder and urethra if desired). Abdominal pressure can be measured by placing a catheter in the rectum, vagina, or an abdominal stoma. Subtracted Pdet (Pves − Pabd) is usually calculated automatically by the UDS software. The transducers should be at the level of the pubic symphysis then zeroed to atmospheric pressure. If the transducers are not at the level of the pubic symphysis then the baseline readings

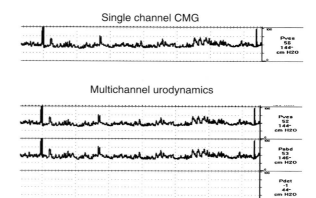

Figure 6.1 Adding intraabdominal pressure monitoring gives a better representation of the true detrusor pressure. The top tracing is a single channel cystometrogram (CMG) with measurement of only total vesical pressure (Pves). Note the multiple spikes and rises in pressure. Without having simultaneous monitoring of intraabdominal pressure, it is impossible to know whether these pressure spikes are due to a rise in detrusor or abdominal pressure. The lower tracing depicts the same CMG with intraabdominal pressure (Pabd) monitoring added. The changes in Pves were due to the changes in abdominal pressure. The subtracted detrusor pressure (Pdet) curve is noted to be flat and without any rises in pressure, i.e. a stable and compliant bladder. (From reference 9, with permission)

should be adjusted accordingly. At the beginning of the test the patient is asked to cough, to assess accurate transmission of pressure in both Pabd and Pves. If there is unequal transmission, then the catheters need to be adjusted or recalibrated prior to initiating the study. Typically, medium fill is recommended (10–100 ml/min), and we usually fill between 30 and 50 ml/min with normal saline or radiographic contrast for videourodynamics.

Several parameters may be evaluated during cystometry, including: filling pressure, sensation, presence of involuntary or unstable contractions, compliance, capacity, and control over micturition.

Filling pressure

Normally, as the bladder fills it maintains a relatively constant and low pressure. Detrusor pressure usually does not exceed 5–10 cmH$_2$O due to the vesicoelastic properties of the bladder; Pdet remains low until the voluntary voiding phase. Rises in Pdet may be caused by involuntary detrusor contractions (IDCs) or impaired compliance.

Sensation

Sensation is the part of cystometry that is truly subjective, and therefore requires both an alert and attentive patient and clinician. Bladder sensation can be described in many ways. The ICS recommends judging bladder sensation by three defined points: first sensation of bladder filling, first desire to void (the feeling that would lead the patient to pass urine at the next convenient moment, but voiding can be delayed if necessary), and strong desire to void (persistent desire to void without the fear of leakage).[3] Patients can further be described as having normal, increased, reduced, or absent bladder sensation. Also, the ICS has provided terms to describe non-specific bladder sensations, bladder pain, and urgency (a sudden compelling desire to void). If any of these sensations are experienced, the examiner should ask whether they correlate with any of the patient's symptoms. Also, these sensations can be correlated to voiding dairies. Many patients with OAB will only demonstrate a heightened sensation to filling without other measurable urodynamic abnormalities. In the past some have referred to this as sensory urgency, but that term is no longer recommended.

Capacity

Cystometric capacity is the bladder volume at the end of the filling cystometrogram. The end point should be specified, e.g. the patient had a normal desire to void, a void was precipitated by detrusor overactivity, or the study was terminated for another reason. Maximum cystometric capacity (MCC) is the volume at which a patient feels she can no longer delay micturition because of a strong desire to void.[3] If during the study there is a question as to the bladder volume, the recorded instilled volume can be verified by adding the measured voided volume to the residual, which can be estimated by fluoroscopy or measured with an ultrasound or catheter.

MCC can also be correlated with voiding dairies to determine its correlation to a "real life" setting.

Compliance

Bladder compliance is the change in bladder volume over a change in bladder pressure expressed in ml/cmH$_2$O. Compliance is generally calculated by subtracting the baseline Pdet from the premicturition pressure (Pdet just prior to the initial isovolumetric contraction, also termed end-filling pressure) divided by the change in volume. Compliance is a reflection of the viscoelastic properties of the bladder, which normally allow storage of increasing volumes of urine at low pressures (Figure 6.1).[9] Abnormal or decreased compliance (increased pressure for a given volume) usually occurs in patients with underlying neurological conditions, chronic catheterization or certain inflammatory states. Decreased compliance is generally accepted to be less than 20 ml/cmH$_2$O, which implies a poorly accommodating bladder.[10] The absolute value of compliance is probably less important than premicturition pressure. Typically the Pdet at the end of filling should not exceed 6–10 cmH$_2$O.[11] Clinically, it is most important to decide whether the bladder is storing urine at elevated pressures for prolonged periods of time. An example of impaired compliance is shown in Figure 6.2.

Detrusor contractions

The urodynamic observation of involuntary detrusor contractions (IDCs) during the filling or storage phase is termed detrusor overactivity (DO) (Figure 6.3).[12] Detrusor overactivity may be phasic or terminal (occurring at MCC). DO is usually, but not always, associated with an urge to void, and may be associated with urgency or incontinence. If incontinence occurs with an IDC, it is known as DO incontinence. DO incontinence is a urodynamic observation, as opposed to "urgency incontinence" which is a symptom. If an IDC is present, then the following should be noted: the volume at which the IDC occurred, the amplitude of the contraction, and whether there was an associated leak. Furthermore, DO and DO incontinence are urodynamic observations and the clinician must

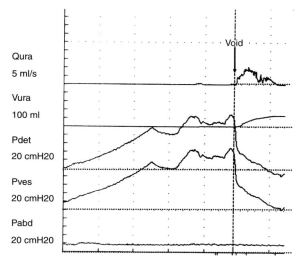

Figure 6.2 An example of severely impaired compliance in a woman with incontinence, hydronephrosis, and renal insufficiency after high dose radiation for a pelvic malignancy. Baseline detrusor pressure (Pdet) is zero; however, with slow filling there is a steady rise in Pdet to over 100 cmH_2O. When the patient is allowed to void, there is an immediate drop in pressure with the voluntary release of outlet resistance. This represents a dangerous situation and impaired compliance is responsible for hydronephrosis and renal insufficiency. Qura, flow rate (mL/s); Vura, voided volume (mL); Pves, vesical pressure; Pabd, abdominal pressure.

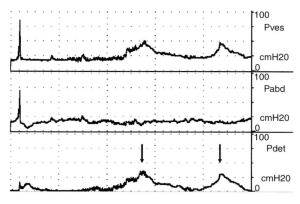

Figure 6.3 Detrusor overactivity. Note the rises in vesical pressure (Pves) and detrusor pressure (Pdet) (arrows) with no rise in abdominal pressure (Pabd). (From reference 12, with permission)

interpret the significance of these findings within the clinical context. Unequal transmission of Pabd and Pves or rectal contractions may falsely suggest an IDC. Careful attention to the

tracings, patient activity, and associated rise in Pabd should help delineate the situation.

According to the ICS, DO may also be described according to cause: neurogenic DO when there is a relevant neurological condition and idiopathic DO when there is no defined cause.[3] The term idiopathic is a bit of a misnomer, in that the cause of detrusor overactivity in a non-neurogenic patient may be readily apparent (e.g. bladder outlet obstruction or inflammatory process) versus truly "unknown". Thus, from a practical standpoint, the terms neurogenic and non-neurogenic DO may be used.

Urodynamic stress incontinence

Urodynamic stress incontinence is defined as the involuntary leakage of urine during UDS with increased abdominal pressure, in the absence of a detrusor contraction.[3] There are various urodynamic measurements of sphincteric function (e.g. abdominal leak point pressure, maximal urethral closure pressure) but the diagnosis of urodynamic stress incontinence, per se, can be made without any such measurements. During cystometry, filling can be stopped and the patient is asked to increase abdominal pressure by progressive valsalva maneuvers or coughing. The demonstration of leakage with such maneuvers, in the absence of a detrusor contraction, confirms the diagnosis of urodynamic stress incontinence. Many patients with OAB will have the symptom and urodynamic finding of stress incontinence. Urodynamic stress incontinence can be present in the OAB patient with urge incontinence (mixed incontinence) or without urge incontinence (OAB with stress incontinence).

Abdominal pressure monitoring will also allow for the identification of IDCs brought on by changes in abdominal pressure. This is particularly useful in the evaluation and management of stress incontinence. Symptomatically it may seem as if incontinence is being caused by a cough or other stressful maneuver, but it is actually being caused by an IDC that is provoked by a preceding increase in abdominal pressure. This phenomenon of stress induced DO is defined as an increase in detrusor pressure triggered by an increase in intraabdominal pressure (Figure 6.4).[9] In this scenario, if there is associated incontinence, then it is the detrusor

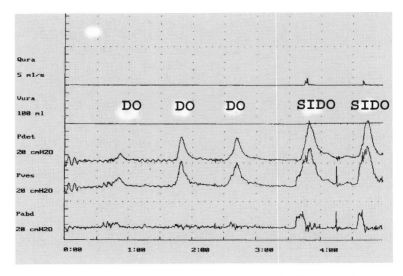

Figure 6.4 Stress induced detrusor overactivity. Urodynamic tracing of a 52-year-old woman complaining of combined stress and urge incontinence. Loss of urine with straining was clearly demonstrated on physical examination. There are three episodes of detrusor overactivity (DO) preceding two episodes of stress induced DO (SIDO). In the case of SIDO, note that as abdominal pressure (Pabd) increases so does vesical pressure (Pves). Shortly *after* this, detrusor pressure (Pdet) rises and continues long after Pabd returns to baseline. With both episodes of stress induced instability, incontinence occurred, as can be seen on the flow rate (Qura) curve. Vura, voided volume (mL). (From reference 9, with permission)

contraction and not the increase in abdominal pressure that is the cause of the incontinence.

Leak point pressures

There are two distinct types of leak point pressures that can be measured in the incontinent patient. The two are independent of each other and represent completely different pathologic conditions. The abdominal leak point pressure (ALPP) is a measure of sphincter strength (its ability to resist changes in abdominal pressure).[13] ALPP is defined as the intravesical pressure at which urine leakage occurs due to increased abdominal pressure in the absence of a detrusor contraction (Figure 6.5).[3,12] This measure of intrinsic urethral function is applicable to patients with stress urinary incontinence (SUI). ALPP cannot be determined if the patient does not demonstrate urodynamic stress incontinence. Conceptually, the lower is the ALPP, the weaker is the sphincter. There is no normal ALPP as patients without SUI will not leak at any physiologic abdominal pressure. In cases of pelvic organ prolapse, ALPP can be measured after reduction of the prolapse to simulate surgical

repair. Furthermore, UDS may be beneficial in women who report pure SUI prior to surgical intervention, as only 51% had pure urodynamic SUI on UDS.[14] The term Valsalva leak point pressure (VLPP) has also been used to describe the ALPP.

The second type of leak point pressure is detrusor leak point pressure (DLPP), which is a measure of detrusor pressure in the setting of decreased bladder compliance. It is defined as the lowest detrusor pressure at which urine leakage occurs in the absence of either a detrusor contraction or increased abdominal pressure (Figure 6.6).[3] The higher is the DLPP, the higher is the urethral resistance. From a clinical perspective, DLPP is most useful in patients with lower motor neuron disease affecting the bladder (e.g. spina bifida, spinal cord tumors, or after radical pelvic surgery) and in non-neurogenic patients with low bladder compliance (e.g. multiple bladder surgeries, or radiation or tuberculous cystitis). The higher is the DLPP, the more likely that upper tract damage can occur as intravesical pressure is transmitted to the kidneys. McGuire et al. documented the deleterious effects that a high leak point pressure has on the

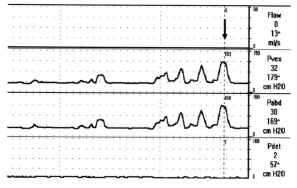

Figure 6.5 Abdominal leak point pressure (ALPP). At a fixed volume (usually 150–200 ml) the patient is asked to perform progressive valsalva maneuvers until leakage is demonstrated. In this case leakage occurs at the arrow and the vesical pressure (Pves) at that point is 109 cmH$_2$O, which is the ALPP. Note the equal rise in abdominal pressure (Pabd) and Pves. If there is no leakage demonstrated at the fixed volume the patient can be retested at 50-ml increments until leakage is demonstrated. If leakage does not occur with a slow valsalva, then the patient may be asked to cough. It is often necessary to perform ALPP testing in the standing position. If incontinence is not demonstrated with a urethral catheter in place in patients in whom stress urinary incontinence (SUI) is suspected, stress maneuvers should be repeated without the catheter in place and the ALPP can be determined from the Pabd curve. (From reference 12, with permission)

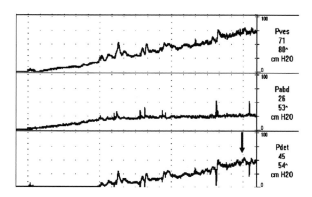

Figure 6.6 Detrusor leak point pressure (DLPP). Urodynamic tracing of an incontinent patient with neurogenic bladder secondary to myelomeningocele. There is impaired compliance (steady rise in detrusor pressure (pdet)) and incontinence is demonstrated at the arrow where Pdet is 45 cmH$_2$O, which is the DLPP. Note that there is no rise in abdominal pressure (Pabd). Pves, vesical pressure.

upper urinary tract: leak point pressures greater than 40 cmH$_2$O result in hydronephrosis or vesicoureteral reflux in 85% of myelodysplastic patients.[15]

Voiding pressure–flow studies

Multichannel invasive assessment of pressure–flow during the voiding phase of micturition can precisely define voiding dynamics and evaluate for abnormalities in contractility and/or outlet resistance (e.g. obstruction). Normal voiding starts by voluntary relaxation of the striated urethral sphincter followed by a detrusor contraction, opening of the bladder neck, and initiation of urine flow. Urodynamics allows investigation of each of these phases. During the voiding phase the parameters which were described for uroflowmetry are measured (Q_{max}, Q_{ave}, voided volume, etc.), as well as Pdet at Q_{max} (PdetQ_{max}) and maximum detrusor pressure (Pdet$_{max}$). Voiding phase abnormalities occur when there are problems with detrusor contractility, increased outlet resistance, or abnormal coordination between the detrusor and sphincters. It is well known that abnormalities of storage are associated with abnormalities of emptying (e.g. association of detrusor overactivity with outlet obstruction or the association of incontinence with incomplete emptying). Patients should be carefully questioned about voiding symptoms, especially when such symptoms are not the primary presenting symptom.

The ICS defines normal detrusor function as a voluntarily initiated continuous contraction that leads to complete bladder emptying within a normal time span.[3] The degree of amplitude and duration of the contraction is dependent upon outlet resistance. The greater is the outlet resistance, the greater is the detrusor pressure required to empty the bladder. A contraction that is of reduced strength and/or duration is termed detrusor underactivity. It is important to note that in some cases, especially in women, when outlet resistance is low, a low pressure detrusor contraction can result in normal voiding and emptying, and should not be considered a detrusor of reduced strength (Figure 6.7).[16] An acontractile detrusor is one that does not demonstrate any contractility during urodynamics. An examiner should be careful not to

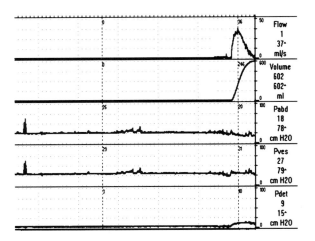

Figure 6.7 Multichannel UDS tracing of a 72-year-old woman with stress incontinence and low pressure voiding. Note the minimal rise in detrusor pressure (Pdet) (most of which is actually a fall in abdominal pressure (Pabd)) with very little rise, about 2 cmH$_2$O, in vesical pressure (Pves) associated with a "super-flow" rate of > 35 ml/s and complete bladder emptying. Although this patient voids with a low detrusor pressure, she does not have impaired contractility. (From reference 16, with permission)

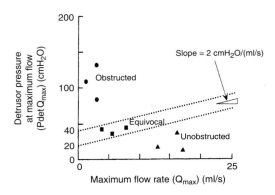

Figure 6.8 International Continence Society (ICS) nomogram: see text for details. (From reference 18, with permission)

$$BOOI = PdetQ_{max} - 2(Q_{max})$$
$$BOOI > 40 = obstructed;$$
$$BOOI < 20 = unobstructed;$$
$$BOOI\ 20–40 = equivocal\ obstruction$$

erroneously diagnose detrusor acontractility. For example, if a patient does not void during the study, but does void in daily life, then the diagnosis should not be made, because the UDS was not representative of the clinical situation. This often happens when patients are inhibited in the clinical setting and are unable to relax the striated sphincter and initiate the micturition reflex. In our experience, approximately 24% of women are unable to void characteristically during urodynamic testing.[17]

Bladder outlet obstruction (BOO) is a generic term for obstruction during voiding, and is classically diagnosed by synchronous comparison of Pdet and flow rate.[3] In men there are numerous nomograms which express the pressure–flow dynamic and allow for the diagnosis of obstruction and/or impaired contractility.[18–20] An example of a universally accepted nomogram in the evaluation of male pressure–flow studies is the ICS nomogram (Figure 6.8).[18] Currently this is the most widely used tool to diagnose BOO in men. The bladder outlet obstruction index (BOOI), derived from the ICS nomogram, is a simple formula that can be used to categorize BOO in most men:[20]

The etiology of BOO in men may be anatomic (i.e. benign prostatic enlargement, bladder neck contracture, etc.) or functional (i.e. primary bladder neck obstruction, dysfunctional voiding, etc.). Men who present with predominantly OAB symptoms should be evaluated for DO and BOO. DO can often coexist with BOO and may have developed as a result of the BOO (Figure 6.9). More than 50% of men with benign prostatic hyperplasia and associated LUTS will have DO, but the presence of DO does not correlate with BOO.[21–23] Therefore urodynamics are essential if a specific diagnosis is required.

In men, the model of BOO secondary to benign prostatic enlargement provides a highly prevalent condition with predictable outcomes after treatment. BOO in women is far less common then in men, but is probably more prevalent than previously suspected. Furthermore, nomograms derived for men cannot be applied to women as voiding dynamics differ. In addition, anatomic differences allow many women to empty their bladders by simply relaxing the pelvic floor, and some will augment voiding by abdominal straining. Minor elevations in detrusor pressure or decreases in flow rate, which might be considered insignificant in the male population, might signify obstruction in women. Accordingly, clinicians must have a high index

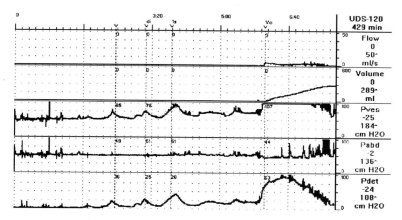

Figure 6.9 Detrusor overactivity (DO) and bladder outlet obstruction (BOO) in a male. Urodynamic tracing of a 64-year-old man with lower urinary tract symptoms (LUTS) including urgency, frequency, and decreased force of stream. Urodynamics shows DO with three separate involuntary detrusor contractions (IDCs) and voluntary voiding with high pressure–low flow voiding dynamics. Maximum detrusor pressure (Pdet) is near 100 cmH$_2$O. (BOO index (BOOI) is 63 − 2(3) = 57). Pves, vesical pressure; Pabd, abdominal pressure.

of suspicion based on lower urinary tract symptoms, incomplete emptying, persistent urinary tract infections, and a history of anti-incontinence surgery, prolapse, or other conditions.

There are a variety of causes of BOO in women including anatomic and functional etiologies.[24] Anatomic causes (i.e. urethral stricture, cystocele, iatrogenic obstruction after anti-incontinence procedures) are more obvious than functional causes and are often suspected prior to urodynamics. Functional causes (i.e. primary bladder neck obstruction) require urodynamics (and often videourodynamics in women) to make a precise diagnosis. Figure 6.10 shows an example of a woman with primary bladder neck obstruction and associated DO. Recent interest in female BOO has resulted in the publication of several diagnostic urodynamic criteria.[25–28] Each of these proposals has merit, and none is perfect in diagnosing obstruction. We believe that a combination of clinical parameters and urodynamic findings is currently the best way to diagnose obstruction in women.

Sphincter coordination and electromyography

Coordination refers to the bladder–urethral sphincter mechanism relationship during voiding. Normally, during voiding the urethra is open, and is continually relaxed to allow for effective emptying. Sphincteric electromyography (EMG)

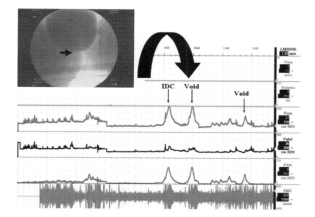

Figure 6.10 Primary bladder neck obstruction. Videourodynamic tracing of a healthy 37-year-old woman with urinary retention. The filling phase shows detrusor overactivity (IDC), and attempts to void show adequate pressure, but no flow. With attempts to void, simultaneous fluoroscopic imaging shows no opening of the bladder neck (horizontal arrow). There is some increase in electromyogram (EMG) activity, but failure of the bladder neck to open in the face of a sustained detrusor contraction is diagnostic of primary bladder neck obstruction. The patient subsequently underwent a transurethral incision of the bladder neck and now voids and empties normally.

studies the bioelectric potentials of the external urethral sphincter complex (EUS). Surface or needle electrodes may be used. Surface electrodes are placed on the skin overlying the muscle of interest and detect potentials for a group of muscles in the area. The electrodes should be placed near the periurethral or perianal area. Needle electrodes are more precise, measuring the potential of one motor unit, but are invasive. Generally, surface electrodes are accurate in providing the necessary information.[29] The EMG tracing should be assessed at various points during filling to ensure proper lead placement and recording prior to the voiding phase. At the beginning of the study, the patient should be asked to contract and relax the sphincter. Also, during the initial cough test and subsequent stress maneuvers there are often increases in the EMG recording. Furthermore, a normal response to bladder filling is a gradual and sustained rise in the EMG potential. During the voiding phase, the first action is relaxation of the EUS, measured as silence of the EMG.[29] The EUS should remain relaxed until voiding is completed.

EMG is useful in patients with suspected pelvic floor dysfunction or neurogenic voiding dysfunction. The goal of EMG during UDS is to determine whether the EUS is coordinated or discoordinated with the bladder during voiding.[11] If an abnormality is present, the examiner will observe a failure of the sphincter to appropriately relax during voiding. If the patient has a known neurological condition, the phenomenon is termed detrusor–external sphincter dyssynergia (DESD); usually, the disease affects the suprasacral spinal cord (Figure 6.11).[12] If there is no known neurological abnormality, the discoordination is likely a learned behavior and the term dysfunctional voiding should be applied.[30]

Imaging of the bladder outlet during voiding allows for assessment of the bladder neck/internal sphincter coordination (see below). Failure of the bladder neck to open in the face of a sustained detrusor contraction is abnormal. In cases of neurogenic voiding dysfunction, especially with lesions above the lower thoracic cord, true internal sphincter dyssynergia can occur. Primary bladder neck obstruction has a similar radiographic appearance to internal sphincter dyssynergia and is the diagnosis if there is no known neurological disease.

Videourodynamics

Videourodynamics involves simultaneous fluoroscopy images of the lower urinary tract and

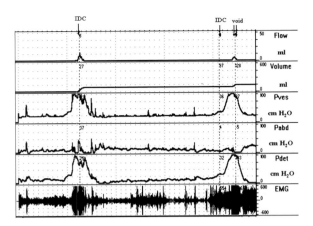

Figure 6.11 Detrusor overactivity with detrusor–external sphincter dyssynergia (DESD). Urodynamic tracing of an 18-year-old woman with frequency, urgency, and urge incontinence, who was diagnosed with a tethered cord. Note the involuntary detrusor contraction (IDC, arrow) associated with high volume urine loss as registered in the flow meter. There is increased sphincter activity as demonstrated by increased electromyogram (EMG) activity consistent with DESD. On the second fill there is again an IDC, but this time the patient is instructed to void (double arrow). Note that there is increased EMG activity throughout the IDC and "voluntary void". Detrusor pressures (Pdet) with IDCs are quite high because of the resistance of the contracting striated sphincter. Pves, vesical pressure; Pabd, abdominal pressure. (From reference 12, with permission)

urodynamic studies. The filling solution contains radiographic contrast which allows visualization of the lower urinary tract during storage and voiding. Most systems allow for imaging and urodynamic recordings on one monitor, as well as recording of the image with the simultaneous urodynamic tracing. Images may be obtained with the patient supine, seated, or standing. Often in clinical practice, office videourodynamics is not practical and not necessary for an accurate diagnosis in many patients. Furthermore, images of the lower urinary tract may be obtained separate from UDS, but there are several situations in which simultaneous imaging and urodynamics is crucial. Videourodynamics provides the clinician with the essential ability to correlate anatomy with function at a specific moment in time.

Imaging can assist with the diagnosis of complex incontinence cases by demonstrating involuntary loss of urine with an IDC or with stress maneuvers.[29] Fluoroscopy greatly improves the accuracy of determining ALPP as it is often easier to visualize the flow of contrast on video rather than on examination.[11] Video also allows the assessment of urethral hypermobility and degree of cystocele. In patients who demonstrate bladder outlet obstruction on pressure–flow studies, imaging allows determination of the level of obstruction. Videourodynamics is critical to make the diagnosis of bladder neck obstruction or detrusor internal sphincter dyssynergia and is especially helpful when high pressure–low flow voiding is not demonstrated.[25] Cases of complex voiding dysfunction may be less common, but it is precisely in those patients in whom videourodynamics is invaluable. Simultaneous fluoroscopy can also identify vesicoureteral reflux, prominent bladder diverticula, or urinary fistulae.

SUMMARY

UDS can be an invaluable part of the diagnosis and management of the overactive bladder and associated voiding abnormalities. Prior to termination of the study, the clinician must assess whether all posed questions have been adequately answered.[7] If the study is inconclusive with regard to pivotal issues, then every effort should be made to better elucidate the pathology. This may require adjustments, repetition, and creativity. Current technology provides accurate and precise information detailing the storage and emptying dynamics of the lower urinary tract that can be used to guide therapy and properly counsel patients. The relevance of the study is dependent upon appropriate patient selection, proper technique, and experienced interpretation.

REFERENCES

1. Davis DM. The Mechanism of Urology Diseases. Philadelphia: WB Saunders, 1953.
2. Kraklau DM, Bloom DA. The cystometrogram at 70 years. J Urol 1998; 160: 316–19.
3. Abrams P, Cardozo L, Fall M et al. The standardisation of terminology in the lower urinary tract function: report from the standardisation subcommittee of the International Continence Society. Urology 2003; 61: 37–49.
4. Nitti VW, Coombs AJ. Urodynamics: when, why and how. In: Nitti VW, ed. Practical Urodynamics. Philadelphia: WB Saunders, 1998: 15–26.
5. Wein AJ. Classification of neurogenic voiding dysfunction. J Urol 1981; 125: 605–9.
6. Golomb J. Uroflometry. In: Raz S, ed. Female Urology, 2nd edn. Philadelphia: WB Saunders, 1996: 97–105.
7. Shafer W, Abrams P, Liao L et al. Good urodynamic practices: uroflowmetry, filling cystometry, and pressure-flow studies. Neurourol Urodyn 2002; 21: 261–74.
8. Chancellor MB, Blaivas JG, Kaplan SA, Alexrod S. Bladder outlet obstruction versus impaired detrusor contractility: the role of outflow. J Urol 1991; 145: 810–12.
9. Nitti VW. Cystometry and abdominal pressure monitoring. In: Nitti VW, ed. Practical Urodynamics. Philadelphia: WB Saunders, 1998: 38–51.
10. Stohrer M, Goepel M, Kondo A et al. The standardization of terminology in neurogenic lower urinary tract dysfunction with suggestions for diagnostic procedures. Neurourol Urodyn 1999; 18: 139–58.
11. Webster GD, Guralnick ML. The neurourologic evaluation. In: Walsh PC, Retik, AB, Vaughan ED, Wein AJ, eds. Campbell's Urology, 8th edn. Philadelphia: WB Saunders, 2002: 905–28.
12. Kelly CE, Nitti VW. Evaluation of neurogenic bladder dysfunction: basic urodynamics. In: Corcos J, Schick E, eds. Textbook of the Neurogenic Bladder. London: Martin Dunitz, 2004: 415–23.
13. McGuire EJ, Fitzpatrick CC, Wan J et al. Clinical assessment of urethral sphincter function. J Urol 1993; 150: 1452–4.
14. Weidner AC, Myers ER, Visco AG, Cundiff GW, Bump RC. Which women with stress incontinence require urodynamic evaluation prior to intervention? Am J Obstet Gynecol 2001; 184: 20–7.
15. McGuire EJ, Woodside JR, Borden TA, Weiss RM. Prognostic value of urodynamic testing in myelodysplastic patients. J Urol 1981; 126: 205–9.
16. Nitti VW. Bladder outlet obstruction in women. In: Nitti VW, ed. Practical Urodynamics. Philadelphia: WB Saunders, 1998: 197–210.
17. Carlson KV, Fiske J, Nitti VW. Value of routine evaluation of the voiding phase when performing urodynamic testing on women with lower urinary tract symptoms. J Urol 2000; 164: 1614–17.
18. Griffiths D, Hofner K, van Mastrigt R et al. Standardization of terminology of lower urinary tract function: pressure-flow studies of voiding, urethral resistance, and urethral obstruction. International Continence Society Subcommittee

on standardization of terminology of pressure-flow studies. Neurourol Urodyn 1997; 16: 1–18.

19. Schafer W. Analysis of bladder outlet function with the linearized passive urethral resistance, linPURR, and a disease-specific approach for grading obstruction from complex to simple. World J Urol 1995; 13: 47–58.

20. Abrams P. Bladder outlet obstruction index, bladder contractility index and bladder voiding efficiency: three simple indices to define bladder voiding function. BJU Int 1999; 84: 14–15.

21. Abrams P. In support of pressure-flow studies for evaluating men with lower urinary tract symptoms. Urology 1994; 44: 153–5.

22. Blaivas JG. Pathophysiology and differential diagnosis of benign prostatic hypertrophy. Urology 1988; 32: 5–11.

23. Andersen JT. Prostatism: clinical. Radiologic and urodynamic aspects. Neurourol Urodyn 1982; 1: 241–93.

24. Nitti VW, Raz S. Urinary retention. In: Raz S, ed. Female Urology, 2nd edn. Philadelphia: WB Saunders, 1996: 197–213.

25. Nitti VW, Tu LM, Gitlin J. Diagnosing bladder outlet obstruction in women. J Urol 1999; 161: 1535–40.

26. Chassange S, Bernier PA, Haab F et al. Proposed cutoff values to define bladder outlet obstruction in women. Urology 1998; 51: 408–11.

27. Lemack GE, Zimmern PE. Refinement and application of cut-off values for bladder outlet obstruction in women. J Urol 2000; 163: 1823–8

28. Blaivas JG, Groutz A. Bladder outlet obstruction nomogram for women with lower urinary tract symptomatology. Neurourol Urodyn 2000; 19: 553–64.

29. Rovner ES, Wein AJ. Practical urodynamics. AUA Update Series 2002; XXI: Lessons 19–20.

30. Carlson KV, Rome S, Nitti VW. Dysfunctional voiding in adult females. J Urol 2001; 165: 143–7.

7

Urgency–frequency syndrome and pelvic pain, and interstitial cystitis

Harris E Foster Jr

Introduction • **Etiology of interstitial cystitis** • **Diagnosis of interstitial cystitis** • **Treatment of interstitial cystitis** • **Conclusion**

INTRODUCTION

Managing patients with urgency frequency and pelvic pain syndrome/interstitial cystitis is one of the greatest challenges facing physicians and other healthcare providers who treat those with this disorder. The symptoms of urgency, frequency, dysuria, and chronic pelvic pain characterize interstitial cystitis (IC), but it is often the debilitating pelvic pain associated with interstitial cystitis that is the most difficult to control. The pathophysiology of IC is poorly understood, but is thought to be a complex entity involving inflammatory and immunologic components. Currently there are no single universally effective therapies available; however, oral treatments frequently used include antimuscarinics, nonsteroidal anti-inflammatory drugs (NSAIDs), tricyclic antidepressants, gabapentin, and pentosan polysulfate, all of which have varying degrees of efficacy. The recognition that the pain of IC is multifactorial, probably with a neuropathic component, has led to the effective use of some of these agents that have previously been prescribed for various neurologic conditions associated with chronic pain. Intravesical and surgical options are also available, which expands the armamentarium for those who treat patients with this perplexing disease. Treating IC requires managing all of the symptoms of this disease.

Interstitial cystitis (IC) treatment primarily involves managing a patient's symptoms in order to improve their quality of life. This difficult disease process, with an etiology as yet undefined, is a benign disorder that can result in devastating effects on a patient's physical and mental health. Although frequency and urgency (both symptoms of overactive bladder) are problematic for the patient, pain remains the hallmark of this disease and can be difficult to manage, which is typically frustrating to both the patient and the treating physician.

ETIOLOGY OF INTERSTITIAL CYSTITIS

Interstitial cystitis is a chronic, probably, although not established, inflammatory, non-infectious disorder of the urinary bladder that primarily affects women (approximately 90% of cases are female).[1] The disease can also affect men and possibly children; however, these groups of patients have been studied or characterized to a lesser extent than women. It is believed that IC prevalence ranges from 1/100 000 to 510/100 000 of the general population, and by definition includes some component of pain, usually chronic pelvic pain (CPP).[2,3] Some feel that the diagnosis of non-bacterial chronic prostatitis (CP) in men may actually represent IC.[4] IC symptoms include urinary frequency and urgency, dyspareunia, and, most commonly, debilitating pelvic pain. It is believed that the symptoms associated with IC can be progressive if left untreated.

Severe decreases in quality of life can occur in patients with IC, leading to symptoms such as depression, social isolation, and, in rare instances, suicidal ideations.[5]

IC is a diagnosis based primarily on clinical criteria without disease-specific pathological or physiological findings. Many of the symptoms and signs are shared with various disease processes of an infectious or inflammatory nature. Although many promising theories exist, a unifying etiology has been elusive. Some of the more popular potential etiologies include infectious (bacterial, viral, or fungal), autoimmune, lymphovascular obstruction, neurologic overactivity, deficient mucosal barrier, and excretion of toxic substances in the urine (Table 7.1). An infectious cause for IC has been proposed for many years, particularly because of the similarity in symptoms to its bacterial counterpart. Furthermore, the temporal association of urinary tract infection with the onset of interstitial cystitis symptoms in many patients makes this theory more reasonable. Unfortunately, no studies exist which clearly establish a link between bacterial infection and IC; however, some have suggested that non-traditional uropathogens such as mycoplasmas may explain why cultures are always negative.[6] Nevertheless, the majority of patients have been treated with multiple courses of antibiotics to no avail, shedding much doubt on this potential pathophysiologic mechanism.

IC shares some clinical characteristics with systemic lupus prompting some investigators to conclude that it also has an autoimmune origin.[7] In addition, several studies have demonstrated the presence of antinuclear antibodies, bladder specific antibodies, and antibodies to Tamm–Horsfall protein in certain patients with IC.[8–10] The presence of vascular and lymphatic dilatation in bladder biopsies has led some to propose lymphovascular obstruction as a potential etiology; however, this is a non-specific finding, and has not received much support. Reflex sympathetic dystrophy (RSD) exists as the most popular neurologic theory for the development of IC. Patients with RSD develop symptoms related to an exaggerated sympathetic discharge, resulting in increased vasomotor tone and ischemia.[11] Reasons that suggest similar etiologies between IC and RSD include the demographics of the affected patient population and the associated pain. Likewise, many treatment modalities that have been successful in RSD have also been shown to be effective in IC, such as tricyclic antidepressants and transcutaneous electrical nerve stimulation.[12,13]

Another theory for the development of IC is a defect in the bladder's mucosal barrier, thereby allowing absorption of noxious substances. The principle barrier felt responsible for protecting the underlying urothelium is the glycosaminoglycan (GAG) layer, which is composed of hyaluronic acid, and the sulfates heparan, chondroitin, dermatan, and keratan.[14] This layer protects against invasion of the urothelium by bacteria, toxic metabolites, or certain electrolytes (primarily potassium) in the urine which ultimately either directly injure the underlying detrusor muscle or induce an inflammatory reaction with similar results. The protective effect of the GAG layer primarily results from it being highly negatively charged and hydrophilic.[15] This layer is thought to be relatively impermeable, thereby preventing urine solutes from diffusing into the subepithelial components of the bladder. IC may affect this layer by increasing solute permeability, possibly resulting in subsequent irritation, inflammation, and sensory nerve hypersensitivity in the bladder. Potassium may be the main offending substance (although its continuous presence in urine calls this supposition into question), and its diffusion across the permeable transitional epithelium may be the primary irritant, hence the evolution of the potassium sensitivity test for the diagnosis of IC. Medications designed to facilitate regeneration such as intravesical heparin and oral pentosanpolysulfate have shown only moderate success, although the latter is presently

---

Table 7.1 Proposed etiologies for interstitial cystitis

Infectious (bacterial, viral, fungal)
Autoimmune
Lymphovascular obstruction
Neurologic overactivity (reflex sympathetic dystrophy)
Deficient mucosal barrier
Excretion of toxic substances in urine

the only Food and Drug Administration (FDA) approved oral treatment for IC.[16,17] Parsons et al. have suggested the possibility that a toxic substance excreted in the urine of patients with interstitial cystitis may be a potential mechanism by which the epithelial protective layer is injured.[18] In elaborate studies by Keay and associates, increased levels of antiproliferative factor (APF), a frizzled-8 protein which inhibits transitional epithelial growth, has been found in the urine of patients with IC.[19,20]

Unfortunately, no one theory can encompass all the patients who present with what is now called IC. Future research may ultimately reveal that IC will fail to subscribe to a single etiology, and is more likely multifactorial, for which specific treatments hopefully can be developed. At present, however, our incomplete understanding of its true etiology clearly hampers efforts to improve our diagnostic capabilities, but more importantly, efforts to develop better treatments. Ideally, elucidation of the underlying pathophysiology will further enhance our ability to make the above goals achievable. Until more progress is made in this area, our inadequate understanding of this disease process will continue to result in relatively non-specific and poorly successful treatments.

DIAGNOSIS OF INTERSTITIAL CYSTITIS

Because of the similarities in symptomatology between IC and other infectious, inflammatory, and neoplastic diseases, the diagnosis can often be difficult. A high index of suspicion is therefore necessary in addition to a thorough understanding of the criteria needed to confirm the presence of IC. All patients require a careful medical history, physical examination, and pertinent laboratory testing to exclude other treatable diagnoses. The introduction of the potassium sensitivity test (PST) and questionnaires, such as the O'Leary–Sant, and Pelvic Pain and Urinary Frequency Questionnaire (PUF), have provided other tools to assist in the assessment of IC.[21,22] It is critical, however, that a thorough evaluation elicits any reversible causes of patient symptoms, including infection, cancer, urolithiasis, obstruction, neurologic disease, or gynecologic disorders such as endometriosis. Once other causes are ruled out and a diagnosis of IC is confirmed,

therapy should be aimed at controlling symptoms, particularly pelvic pain, which can often be debilitating. The diagnosis of IC requires the presence of irritative voiding symptoms (mainly urgency, frequency, and nocturia), pelvic and/or bladder pain, which worsens with bladder filling, in the absence of other known bladder disease. Initial evaluation should include a urine analysis and culture and cytology, to assist in ruling out urinary tract infection and neoplasia, respectively. Cystoscopic examination is generally normal if performed in the office under local anesthesia. It is for this reason that a normal cystoscopy performed in this situation should not be used to rule out IC. Correct diagnosis of interstitial cystitis, according to many clinicians, requires cystoscopy and hydrodistention under anesthesia. The hydrodistention should be performed under a pressure of 80–100 cmH$_2$O for several minutes, and often should be repeated at the same sitting.[23] Following hydrodistention, the terminal effluent is generally bloody, and the bladder demonstrates the characteristic submucosal hemorrhages, termed "glomerulations", which are representative of petechial submucosal hemorrhage. These glomerulations should be widely distributed, occupying at least three quadrants of the bladder. Although glomerulations are required to diagnose IC following hydrodistention, they are not specific for this disease, occurring in a variety of other processes in which bladder inflammation exists and also in patients without symptoms. These can include diseases such as tuberculous, radiation, and cyclophosphamide induced cystitis, carcinoma in situ, and distention of a defunctionalized bladder.[24] This is further complicated by the fact that cystoscopic findings consistent with interstitial cystitis have been noted in normal women undergoing tubal ligation, following hydrodistention.[25] The classic Hunner's ulcer can also be used to make the cystoscopic diagnosis; however, it occurs infrequently and is not necessary for diagnosis. The need for routine bladder biopsy in the diagnosis of IC has not been entirely established. Certain well defined treatable bladder disorders such as eosinophilic and tuberculous cystitis, and carcinoma in situ, can be easily diagnosed by bladder biopsy. The pathologic changes seen in IC are generally diffuse, and do not reflect the severity of the cystoscopic or clinical findings.

Typical findings include a non-specific chronic inflammatory infiltrate, edema, and vasodilatation in the submucosa and detrusor layers of the bladder wall.[24] Perineural inflammation, eosinophilic leukocyte infiltrates, and detrusor fibrosis are other patterns that can be identified pathologically.[26] Increased numbers of nerve fibers within the submucosa and detrusor muscle have been demonstrated, along with fibrosis around the nerve fibers and perineural inflammatory cell infiltrates, possibly explaining the bladder hypersensitivity seen in these patients.[27] Alterations in collagen distribution have been demonstrated in some patients with IC, consistent with the chronic inflammatory process known to exist in this condition. The collagen deposition can occur between the muscle fasicles (interfascicular) and, as a special feature in some with IC, also within the muscle fascicles (intrafascicular).[28] The underlying detrusor muscle cells are generally unaltered. Mast cell infiltrates have been found in the submucosa and detrusor musculature of many patients with IC, although its presence is still non-specific.[29] Mast cells are known to contain secretory granules with many vasoactive substances such as histamine and prostaglandins that are potentially injurious to the bladder. Paradoxically, the release of these substances actually facilitates the recruitment of more mast cells to the area, setting a vicious cycle into progress. There is some evidence to suggest that the autonomic nervous system may also play a role in mast cell activation, possibly explaining the proliferation of autonomic nerve fibers in this population.[27, 30]

Urodynamic studies are not typically required in patients with IC; however, when performed, they demonstrate decreased functional bladder capacity, pain during filling, and sensory instability.[24] As mentioned previously, there is an increase in pain and urgency in response to intravesical instillation of potassium chloride (40 ml; 400 mEq/l).

Intravesical potassium has also been suggested as a potential diagnostic test that obviates the need for a procedure requiring anesthesia.[22] It is not necessary to perform radiographic evaluation of the upper or lower urinary tract unless indicated by other findings such as hematuria. Serum studies are also of no benefit at this time. Assays for urinary substances such as eosinophilic cationic protein, histamine metabolites, epidermal and heparin binding growth factors, and components of the glycosaminoglycan layer remain purely investigational. Studies by Keay et al. from the University of Maryland indicating an increased level of antiproliferative factor (APF) and heparin binding epidermal growth factor (HB-EGF), in addition to decreased levels of epidermal growth factor (EGF), in patients with IC have generated excitement that potential biomarkers for this disease exist and can be measured easily.[19]

In an attempt to more uniformly characterize the diagnosis of IC, the National Institutes of Health-National Institute of Arthritis, Diabetes, Digestive, and Kidney Diseases (NIH-IDDK) has compiled a list of inclusion and exclusion criteria.[31] At least 10–15% of patients with known IC will fail to satisfy one or more of these inclusion criteria, potentially leading to a significant underestimation of its prevalence if adhered to strictly.[23] These criteria should mainly serve as a mechanism to identify a homogeneous group of patients with IC, for entrance into clinical trials, to allow adequate scientific assessment of this disease. It should not be used routinely in clinical practice to exclude the diagnosis. The validated O'Leary–Sant symptom and problem index questionnaire can be a helpful adjunct in the diagnosis and assessment of treatment response in patients with IC (Table 7.2).[21]

TREATMENT OF INTERSTITIAL CYSTITIS

The most successful approaches to treating patients with IC have included multimodal therapies incorporating psychological interventions, physical therapy, pharmacotherapy, and periodically procedural treatments, such as cystoscopy

---

Table 7.2 Evaluation of patient suspected of having interstitial cystitis

History (O'Leary–Sant symptom score?)
Physical examination
Urinalysis/culture/cytology
Cystoscopy (with or without hydrodistention)
Potassium chloride test (?)

with hydrodistention and sacral neuromodulation. It should be noted that there are few well performed placebo-controlled randomized trials investigating various IC treatments, and those that are will be highlighted when mentioned. Historically, for a variety of reasons (i.e. chronic pain syndrome, low incidence of disease), it has been difficult to enroll IC patients in randomized studies, particularly those that involve the use of a placebo. Since there is no universally agreed successful therapy, randomized clinical trials for IC should include a placebo arm whenever possible. It has been suggested that limiting the length of treatment and follow-up, allowing open-label treatment at completion, and/or providing appropriate, reasonable compensation can help ameliorate the disadvantages to being potentially randomized to the placebo arm.[32]

Oral treatments (Table 7.3)

Antihistamines

Since the number of mast cells has been shown to be increased in bladder biopsies from some IC patients, reducing mast cell activity may therefore decrease bladder inflammation and improve symptoms.[33] As histamine, released in many instances by mast cells, has been implicated in the pathophysiology of IC, antihistamines have been utilized with varying efficacy for the treatment of this disease. The most commonly used antihistamine for IC has been hydroxyzine.[34,35] It acts by blocking both mast cell secretion and the H_1 receptor. An additional neurogenic mechanism of mast cell release has been the involvement of substance P.[36] Studies in animal models have demonstrated that the release of substance P is inhibited by hydroxyzine.[37] Inhibition of histamine

---

Table 7.3   Oral treatment of interstitial cystitis

Antihistamines (i.e. hydroxyzine)
Pentosan polysulfate
Amitriptyline
Gabapentin (?)
Immunosuppressants (?)
   cyclosporine
   prednisone

---

and substance P release can presumably lessen the ensuing hyperemia that is associated with both of these substances, and the fibrosis associated with substance P. In an open-label study, the use of hydroxyzine was shown to improve symptom scores by 40% from baseline.[34] Drowsiness, however, is a common adverse effect associated with antihistamines, but may abate after chronic use. A recent randomized trial comparing hydroxyzine to pentosan polysulfate either alone or in combination, however, failed to show a significant advantage over placebo.[35]

Pentosan polysulfate

Pentosan polysulfate sodium (PPS; Elmiron®; Ortho-McNeil Pharmaceuticals, Inc., Raritan, NJ) remains the only FDA-approved oral agent for the treatment of IC. An oral heparinoid, PPS is purported to augment the glycosaminoglycan layer of the bladder, thereby repairing deficiencies in this layer which may lead to IC. PPS was demonstrated to be effective in the treatment of IC in a randomized trial in which significant improvement (> 25%) was seen in 28% of affected patients compared to 13% in the control group.[38] A 2005 randomized control trial investigating three different doses of PPS (300–900 mg/day) to treat IC revealed overall response rates ranging from 45% to 50%, with no significant improvement seen with higher doses.[39] Ultimately, the duration of dose appears to be more important than the actual dosage. The severity of symptoms does not appear to affect responses to pentosan polysulfate. Modest improvements in symptoms have been described at 4 weeks into therapy with continued steady improvements over time.[39] Interestingly, on closer inspection of the 2005 study, this agent appears to improve urinary symptoms more than pain. Adverse effects associated with PPS have generally been modest and resolve without intervention or long-term sequelae. The most common adverse effects have included gastrointestinal disorders, headache, and alopecia. The risk of coagulation disorder associated with this agent remains undetermined.

Amitriptyline

Hanno and Wein in 1987 first described the use of amitriptyline for the treatment of IC.[40]

Its anecdotal efficacy has led to its rise as one of the most frequently prescribed oral agents for IC.[41] It was not, however, until recently that amitriptyline was shown to be effective in a randomized, placebo-controlled, double-blind study.[42] In this report, 63% of patients reported satisfaction with therapy as compared to 4% in the placebo group. Specifically, mean pain intensity, as measured by a visual analog scale, revealed statistically significant improvements in the amitriptyline group but not in those who received placebo. The exact mechanism of how amitriptyline treatment achieves pain relief is still not completely understood. Its effects on frequency symptoms and bladder capacity are more readily explained by its concomitant anticholinergic properties.

Amitriptyline also has serotonergic effects via its inhibition of 5-hydroxytryptamine (5-HT) reuptake. This mechanism of action is thought to occur within the spinal and supraspinal neuronal pathways that coordinate bladder function.[43] Current data indicate that 5-HT receptor activation induced by amitriptyline affects the neuromodulation of afferent and efferent pathways that signal pain and urgency sensation within the bladder. In addition, amitriptyline may improve IC symptoms through its antihistamine properties. Amitriptyline is a potent tricyclic antidepressant, blocking H_1-specific receptors, including those on mast cells. A beneficial side effect of this drug is its sedative properties that can help in enhancing restorative sleep. This can vastly improve the quality of life of IC patients, although these sedative effects can also limit the dose that can be tolerated. Adverse effects associated with amitriptyline's anticholinergic properties are present in over 90% of patients, and have proved to be an important limitation in the use of this drug.[42] Nonetheless, this tricyclic antidepressant represents a powerful, safe, and apparently effective tool in the treatment of IC pain.

Gabapentin

The use of the anticonvulsant agent gabapentin for treating IC is aimed at harvesting the drug's well documented efficacy in chronic pain conditions. The mechanism of action of gabapentin is not fully understood, but the agent has been shown to be effective for neuropathic pain in conditions such as diabetic neuropathy, reflex sympathetic dystrophy, and postherpetic neuralgia.[44] It could be considered an ideal drug, because it does not require monitoring of blood levels as in the case of other anticonvulsants such as carbamazepine. Additionally, gabapentin is not metabolized by the liver but is excreted unchanged in the urine.

Gabapentin is structurally related to the neurotranmsitter γ-aminobutyric acid (GABA); however, it is not known to bind to GABA receptors or have any effect on the activity or metabolism of GABA. It is believed to modulate calcium channels, specifically at the $\alpha_2\delta$ subunit, which are thought to be specifically involved in neuropathic pain.[45] There is also evidence that gabapentin might exert some activity against the N-methyl-D-aspartate (NMDA) receptor.[46] Gabapentin may exhibit an indirect action on the NMDA receptor, thereby improving pain symptoms in addition to reducing sympathetic tone in the bladder. Furthermore, it is known that gabapentin enhances endogenous opioid release in the limbic system, subsequently increasing pain control.[46]

Over the past decade, the use of gabapentin for IC pain has increased anecdotally, but no clinical trials have tested its efficacy in a randomized, prospective, double-blind setting. Most descriptions of its use in the literature are case reports and open-label studies. A single institution clinical trial by Sasaki et al. in 2001 reported the efficacy of gabapentin on refractory genitourinary tract pain.[47] There was a reduction in pain observed in nearly 50% of the 21 patients treated with gabapentin. Additionally, Hansen reported significant improvements in IC pain in two patients in a case report.[48] Given its minimal adverse effect profile and overall safety, gabapentin can be used effectively and safely when treating pain secondary to IC. Dosing starts at 100 mg daily and can be titrated up to 3600 mg. A multicenter randomized clinical trial will need to be performed to truly establish its efficacy in the treatment of this disease.

Immunosuppressive drugs

Efforts to use immunosuppressive drugs such as prednisone or cyclosporine have shown some success in treating the symptoms associated with IC. Immunosuppressive agents are thought to reduce the inflammatory response in the bladder and empirically treat autoimmune processes that are thought to be associated with IC. In a small, Canadian study, 14 patients with the ulcerative form of IC were treated with 25 mg of prednisone daily.[49] A significant decrease in the O'Leary symptom and problem index and pain was reported in 22% and 69% of patients respectively. Although the results of this study are thought-provoking, it was small, and only targeted patients with confirmed Hunner's ulcers; this limits its applicability to the approximately 90% of patients who do not have the ulcerative form of the disease. Another factor that could limit the use of immunosuppressants is that diabetic control was compromised with the use of steroids in some of the patients in the study.

The use of low dose cyclosporine for the treatment of IC has also been investigated by a group in Finland.[50,51] In their original report, 11 patients with IC were initially treated with 2.5–5.0 mg/kg of cyclosporine daily, which was then reduced to 1.5–3.0 mg/kg/day maintenance for 3–6 months. Bladder pain either decreased or disappeared in 10 patients, in addition to significant increases in mean and maximum voided volumes and reduction in voiding frequency. A more recent study from the same group reporting on the effects of long-term treatment (greater than 1 year) with cyclosporine (initially 3 mg/kg/day gradually decreasing to as low as 1 mg/kg/day) demonstrated that 20 out of 23 patients were relieved of their bladder pain.[51] Furthermore, mean 24-hour urinary frequency decreased from 20.8 ± 6.3 to 10.2 ± 3.8, mean maximal bladder capacity increased from 161.8 ± 74.6 to 360.7 ± 99.3 ml, and mean voided volume increased from 101.4 ± 42.7 to 246.4 ± 97.9 ml, all of which were highly statistically significant. It should be noted that symptoms recurred in all patients, nine in the study, who stopped cyclosporine. No renal toxicity occurred; however, seven patients developed side effects such as hypertension, gingival hyperplasia, and increased hair growth. There is concern about the development of skin malignancies after long-term use of cyclosporine, and one patient did develop a basalioma after 5 years of treatment. In a randomized study from the same group, cyclosporine treatment was compared with pentosan polysulfate.[52] Cyclosporine was superior to pentosan polysulfate in all clinical outcome parameters measured at 6 months. Clinical response as measured by the global response assessment was 75% and 19% in the cyclosporine and pentosan polysulfate groups, respectively. Furthermore, 24-hour voids decreased by 6.7 (mean) in those treated with cyclosporine, compared to only 2.0 in those who received pentosan polysulfate. While immunosuppressive drugs, particularly prednisone and cyclosporine, have shown some early promise, it is clear that larger, prospective randomized trials are still needed to demonstrate therapeutic improvement in IC symptoms before their widespread use can be advocated.

Invasive treatments (Table 7.4)

Hydrodistention

Cystoscopy combined with hydrodistention under anesthesia is often the first diagnostic and therapeutic choice for IC in many urological practices. The efficacy of hydrodistention has proved to be variable.[53] Hanno and Wein have described response rates ranging from 12% to 26%.[54] A more recent study from Japan reported a 70% improvement in symptoms in patients whose bladder capacity is greater than 100 ml, following hydrodistention under anesthesia.[55] The mechanism of action behind this treatment is believed to be a mechanical stretch of the bladder mucosa and damage to the submucosal neuronal plexus, thereby decreasing afferent pain transmission. Although the efficacy may range

Table 7.4   Invasive treatments of interstitial cystitis

Hydrodistention
Intravesical agents
  DMSO
Combination therapies (e.g.)
  DMSO
  methylprednisolone
  heparin
  bupivicaine
  sodium bicarbonate
Sacral neuromodulation

DMSO, dimethylsulfoxide.

from 12 to 70%, the effects of therapy have been reported to be brief, lasting at most 3–6 months, although prolonged response can occur.

Dimethylsulfoxide

With the exception of PPS, dimethylsulfoxide (DMSO), delivered intravesically, is the only other FDA-approved drug for the treatment of IC. The exact mechanism of action is not entirely clear, but DMSO is known to deplete substance P from the bladder and to stimulate mast cell degranulation.[56] Originally popularized by Stewart et al. in 1967, overall improvement in IC symptoms (not specifically pain) was reported in up to 75% of patients.[57] In a 1988 study, Perez-Marrero et al. showed improvements in pain symptoms in 93% of patients versus 35% improvement in the saline placebo group.[58] Unfortunately, the same study revealed that 59% of the patients relapsed in 4 weeks. The same group later showed that the beneficial effects of DMSO instillation can be moderately prolonged with the use of heparin.[59] In a European study of 28 patients, a modest response to DMSO instillations was also noted.[60] More importantly, the study showed that the adverse effects associated with DMSO therapy could be well tolerated, so that a 6-week course of treatment could generally be completed. Urethral irritation was evident in nearly 50% of patients, but was reported as tolerable. Although certainly not a durable treatment for the pain and other symptoms associated with IC, instillation of DMSO offers another useful tool in the clinician's armamentarium.

Bacillus Calmette–Guérin and resiniferatoxin

The use of intravesical bacillus Calmette–Guérin (BCG) for the treatment of IC is based on the proposed role of an immune dysregulation in the etiology of IC, specifically an imbalance of the Th1 and Th2 T-helper cells. First reported in an open-label study by Zeidman et al., in which improvement was seen in all categories of IC symptoms, BCG treatment appeared promising.[61] In fact, Peters et al. performed a small randomized, placebo-controlled study and reported that 67% of patients treated with BCG noticed an improvement in IC symptoms compared to 33% in the placebo group.[62] With respect to pelvic pain,

53% of BCG-treated and 33% of placebo-treated patients had a subjective improvement in symptoms. When followed for at least 2 years, 81% of initial BCG responders continued to experience a reduction in pelvic pain.[63] In contrast, a recently published large-scale study conducted by the Interstitial Cystitis Clinical Trials Group demonstrated little benefit of this therapy when compared to placebo: 21% versus 12% who reported moderate or marked improvement in their IC symptoms on global response assessment, respectively ($p = 0.06$).[64] Similarly, resiniferatoxin held theoretical promise as an intravesical agent to help control pain in patients with IC. It is a vanilloid receptor agonist that desensitizes C fibers that transmit pain within the bladder. In a randomized, double-blind, placebo-controlled trial published in 2005, no statistically significant benefit was seen with the use of this agent.[65] Based on currently available evidence, both BCG and resiniferatoxin should still be considered investigational interventions for the management of IC symptoms.

Sacral neuromodulation

The use of sacral nerve-root stimulation for the treatment of bladder dysfunction has been well described since Schmidt, Bruschini, and Tanagho reported on this technique in 1979.[66] Most studies have evaluated the effects of sacral neuromodulation on urinary frequency, urgency, incontinence, and non-obstructive urinary retention.[67,68] An implantable neuroprosthetic transforaminal sacral nerve stimulating device (InterStim®; Medtronic Inc., Minneapolis, MN) has been FDA approved for these symptoms. There is a paucity of information available on the effects of sacral neuromodulation on chronic pain.

Studies have suggested that pelvic pain can be ameliorated in some instances by the use of this device.[69,70] In a study of just 10 patients, Siegel et al. demonstrated that nine of the 10 received some level of pain relief with sacral nerve stimulation.[69] Similarly, a more recent study revealed that nearly two-thirds of IC patients treated with sacral nerve stimulation had improved pain following implantation.[70] Peters and Konstandt reported a 36% decrease in narcotic use, as defined by morphine dose equivalents, after implantation of the InterStim device, with four out of 18 patients completely stopping narcotics.[71] These data are preliminary and involve small numbers of patients, and it is clear that this mode of therapy needs further investigation. Sacral neuromodulation may, however, offer a promising option for the treatment of IC (at least the symptoms of urgerncy and frequency) in the future.

CONCLUSION

Interstitial cystitis continues to be a frustrating clinical problem for any physician treating this disorder, particularly the debilitating pain associated with IC. The pathophysiology of this disease remains poorly understood, but current knowledge has spurred the investigation of novel therapies. A number of oral agents are currently available for the treatment of IC including amitriptyline, gabapentin, and PPS, which have demonstrated an ability to improve symptoms although not necessarily all in randomized controlled studies. While intravesical therapy has not been shown to be particularly successful, some instillations may help to temporarily alleviate symptoms, particularly management of chronic pain and acute flairs. There are also a limited number of surgical options available that could potentially treat the pain caused by IC. A multimodal approach is likely necessary to obtain the most successful outcomes when treating patients afflicted by this perplexing disease.

REFERENCES

1. Nordling J. Interstitial cystitis: how should we diagnose it and treat it in 2004? Curr Opin Urol 2004; 14: 323–7.
2. Hanno P, Keay S, Moldwin R, Van Ophoven A. International consultation on IC – Rome, September 2004/Forging an International Concensus: progress in painful bladder syndrome/ interstitial cystitis. Int Urogynecol J Pelvic Floor Dysfunct 2005; 16: S2–34.
3. Jones CA, Nyberg L. Epidemiology of interstitial cystitis. Urology 1997; 49: 2–9.
4. Parsons CL. Prostatitis, interstitial cystitis, chronic pelvic pain, and urethral syndrome share a common pathophysiology: lower urinary dysfunctional epithelium and potassium recycling. Urology 2003; 62: 976–82.
5. Foster HE. Urologic causes of pelvic pain. Infertil Reprod Med Clin North Am 1999; 10: 701–15.
6. Wilkins EG, Payne SR, Pead PJ, Moss ST, Maskell RM. Interstitital cystitis and the urethral syndrome: a possible answer. Br J Urol 1989; 64: 39–44.
7. Peeker R, Atanasiu L, Logadottir Y. Intercurrent autoimmune conditions in classic and non-ulcer interstitial cystitis. Scand J Urol Nephrol 2003; 37: 60–3.
8. Neal DE, Dilworth JP, Kaack MB. Tamm-Horsfall autoantibodies in interstitial cystitis. J Urol 1991; 145: 37–9.
9. Oravisto K, Alfthan O, Jolinen E. Interstitial cystitis: clinical and immunological findings. Scand J Urol Nephrol 1970; 4: 37–40.
10. Silk M. Bladder autoantibodies in interstitial cystitis. J Urol 1970; 103: 307–9.
11. Galloway NT, Gabale DR, Irwin PP. Interstitial cystitis or reflex sympathetic dystrophy of the bladder? Semin Urol 1991; 9: 148–53.
12. Fall M. Transcutaneous electrical nerve stimulation in interstitial cystitis: update on clinical experience. Urology 1987; 29 (Suppl): 40–2.
13. Ratliff TL, Klutke CG, McDougall EM. The etiology of interstitial cystitis. Urol Clin North Am 1994; 21: 21–30.
14. Parsons CL. Bladder surface glycosaminoglycan: efficient mechanism of environmental adaptation. Urology 1990; 171: 9–14.
15. Parsons CL, Boychuk D, Jones S, Hurst R, Callahan H. Bladder surface glycosaminoglycans: an epithelial permeability barrier. J Urol 1990; 143: 139–42.
16. Holm-Bentzen M, Jacobsen F, Nerstrom B et al. A prospective double-blind clinically controlled multicenter trial of sodium pentosanpolysulfate in the treatment of interstitial cystitis and related painful bladder disease. J Urol 1987; 138: 503–7.
17. Parsons CL, Housley T, Schmidt JD, Lebow D. Treatment of interstitial cystitis with intravesical heparin. Br J Urol 1994; 73: 504–7.
18. Parsons CL, Bautista SL, Stein PC, Zupkas P. Cyto-injury factors in urine: a possible mechanism for the development of interstitital cystitis. J Urol 2000; 164: 1381–4.
19. Keay S, Zhang CO, Hise MK et al. A diagnostic in vitro urine assay for interstitial cystitis. Urology 1998; 52: 974–8.
20. Keay S, Szekely Z, Conrad TP et al. An antiproliferative factor from interstitial cystitis patients is a frizzled 8 protein-related sialoglycopeptide. Proc Natl Acad Sci USA 2004; 101: 11803–8.

21. O'Leary MP, Sant GR, Fowler FJ Jr, Whitmore KE, Spolarich-Kroll J. The interstitial cystitis symptom index and problem index. Urology 1997; 49 (5A Suppl): 58–63.

22. Parsons CL, Dell J, Stanford EJ et al. Increased prevalence of interstitial cystitis: previously unrecognized urologic and gynecologic cases identified using a new symptom questionnaire and intravesical potassium sensitivity. Urology 2002; 60: 573–8.

23. Batra AK, Wein AJ, Hanno PM. Interstitial cystitis. AUA Update Series 1993; 12: Lesson 8.

24. Sant GR. Interstitial cystitis. Monogr Urol 1991; 12: 37.

25. Waxman JA, Sulak PJ, Kuehl TJ. Cystoscopic findings consistent with interstitial cystitis in normal women undergoing tubal ligation. J Urol 1998; 160: 1663–7.

26. Christmas TJ, Smith GL, Rode J. Detrusor myopathy: an accurate predictor of bladder hypocompliance and contracture in interstitial cystitis. Br J Urol 1996; 78: 862–5.

27. Christmas TJ, Rode J, Chapple CR, Milroy EJ, Turner-Warwick RT. Nerve fibre proliferation in interstitial cystitis. Virchows Arch A Pathol Anat Histopathol 1990; 416: 447–51.

28. Holm-Bentzen M, Lose G. Pathology and pathogenesis of interstitial cystitis. Urology 1987; 29 (4 Suppl): 8–13.

29. Lynes WL, Flynn SD, Shortliffe LD, Stamey TA. The histology of interstitial cystitis. Am J Surg Pathol 1990; 14: 969–76.

30. Christmas TJ, Rode J. Characteristics of mast cells in normal bladder, bacterial cystitis and IC. Br J Urol 1991; 68: 473–8.

31. Gillenwater JY, Wein AJ. Summary of the National Institute of Arthritis, Diabetes, Digestive, and Kidney Diseases workshop on interstitial cystitis. J Urol 1988; 140: 203–6.

32. Propert KJ, Payne C, Kusek JW, Nyberg LM. Pitfalls in the design of clinical trials for interstitial cystitis. Urology 2002; 60: 742–8.

33. Lynes WL, Flynn SD, Shortliffe LD et al. Mast cell involvement in interstitial cystitis. J Urol 1987; 138: 746–2.

34. Theoharides TC, Sant GR. Hydroxyzine therapy for interstitial cystitis. Urology 1997; 49 (Suppl 5A): 108–10.

35. Sant GR, Propert KJ, Hanno PM et al. A pilot clinical trial of oral pentosan polysulfate and oral hydroxyzine in patients with interstitial cystitis. J Urol 2003; 170: 810–15.

36. Sant GR, Theoharides TC. The role of mast cell in interstitial cystitis. Urol Clin North Am 1994; 21: 41–53.

37. Minogiannis P, El-Mansoury M, Betnaces JA, Sant GR, Theoharides TC. Hydroxyzine inhibits neurogenic bladder mast cell activation. Int J Immunopharmacol 1998; 20: 553–63.

38. Mulholland SG, Hanno P, Parsons CL, Sant GR, Staskin DR. Pentosan polysulfate sodium for the therapy of interstitial cystitis – a double blind placebo controlled clinical study. Urology 1990; 35: 552–8.

39. Nickel JC, Barkin J, Forrest J et al. Randomized, double blind, dose ranging study of pentosan polysulfate sodium for interstitial cystitis. Urology 2005; 65: 654–8.

40. Hanno PM, Wein AJ. Medical treatment of interstitial cystitis (other than Rimso-50/Elmiron). Urology 1987; 29 (Suppl): 22–6.

41. Rovner E, Propert KJ, Brensinger C et al. Treatments used in women with interstitial cystitis: the interstitial cystitis data base (ICDB) study experience. The Interstitial Cystitis Data Base Study Group, Urology 2000; 56: 940–5.

42. van Ophoven A, Pokupic S, Heinecke D, Hertle L. A prospective, randomized, placebo controlled, double-blind study of amitriptyline for the treatment of interstitial cystitis. J Urol 2004; 172: 533–6.

43. Pilowsky I, Hallett EC, Bassett DL, Thomas PG, Penhall RK. A controlled study of amitriptyline in the treatment of chronic pain. Pain 1982; 14: 169–79.

44. Backonga M, Glanzman RL. Gabapentin dosing for neuropathic pain: evidence from randomized, placebo-controlled clinical trials. Clin Ther 2003; 25: 81–104.

45. Gee NS, Brown JP, Dissanayake VU et al. The novel anticonvulsant drug, gabapentin, binds to the alpha2delta subunit of a calcium channel. J Biol Chem 1996; 271: 5768–76.

46. Nicholson B. Gabapentin use in neuropathic pain syndromes. Acta Neurol Scand 2000; 101: 359–71.

47. Sasaki K, Smith CP, Chuang YC et al. Oral gabapentin treatment for refractory genitourinary tract pain. Tech Urol 2001; 7: 47–9.

48. Hansen H. Interstitial cystitis and the potential role of gabapentin. Southern Med J 2000; 93: 238–42.

49. Soucy F, Gregoire M. Efficacy of prednisone for severe refractory ulcerative interstitial cystitis. J Urol 2005; 173: 841–3.

50. Forsell T, Ruutu M, Isoniemi H, Ahonen J, Alfthan O. Cyclosporine in severe interstitial cystitis. J Urol 1996; 155: 1591–3.

51. Sairanen J, Forsell J, Ruutu M. Long term outcome of patients with interstitial cystitis treated with low dose cyclosporine A. J Urol 2004; 171: 2138–41.

52. Sairanen J, Tammela TL, Leppilanhti M et al. Cyclosporine A and pentosan polysulfate sodium for the treatment of interstitial cystitis: a randomized comparative study. J Urol 2005; 174: 2235–8.

53. Turner K, Stewart H. How do you stretch a bladder? A survey of UK practice, literature review, and a recommendation of a standard approach. Neurourol Urodyn 2005; 24: 74–6.

54. Hanno P, Wein A. Conservative therapy for interstitial cystitis. Semin Urol 1991; 9: 143–7.

55. Yamada T, Murayama T, Andoh M. Adjuvant hydrodistension under epidural anesthesia for interstitial cystitis. Int J Urol 2003; 10: 463–8.

56. Moldwin R, Sant GR. Interstitial cystitis: a pathophysiology and treatment update. Clin Obstet Gynecol 2002; 45: 259–72.

57. Stewart BH, Persky L, Kiser WS. The use of dimethyl sulfoxide (DMSO) in the treatment of interstitial cystitis. J Urol 1967; 98: 671–2.

58. Perez-Marrero R, Emerson LE, Feltis JT. A controlled study of dimethyl sulfoxide in interstitial cystitis. J Urol 1988; 140: 36–9.

59. Perez-Marrero R, Emerson LE, Maharajh DO, Juma S. Prolongation of response to DMSO by heparin maintenance. Urology 2003; 41(1 Suppl): 64–6.

60. Rossberger J, Fall M, Peeker R. Critical appraisal of dimethyl sulfoxide treatment for interstitial cystitis: discomfort, side effects and treatment outcome. Scand J Urol Nephrol 2005; 39: 73–7.

61. Zeidman EJ, Helfrick B, Pollard C, Thompson IM. Bacillus-Calmette-Guérin immunotherapy for refractory interstitial cystitis. Urology 1994; 43: 121–4.

62. Peters D, Diokno A, Steinert B et al. The efficacy of intravesical Tice strain BCG in the treatment of interstitial cystitis: a double blind, prospective, placebo controlled trial. J Urol 1997; 157: 2090–4.

63. Peters KM, Diokno AC, Steinert BW, Gonzales JA. The efficacy of intravesical BCG in the treatment of interstitial cystitis: long term follow up. J Urol 1998; 159: 1483–6.

64. Mayer R, Propert KJ, Peters KM et al. A randomized controlled trial of intravesical bacillus Calmette-Guérin for the treatment of refractory interstitial cystitis. J Urol 2005; 173: 1186–91.

65. Payne CK, Mosbaugh PG, Forrest JB et al. Intravesical resiniferatoxin for the treatment of interstitial cystitis: a randomized, double blind, placebo controlled trial. J Urol 2005; 173: 1590–4.

66. Schmidt RA, Bruschini H, Tanagho EA. Urinary bladder and sphincter responses to stimulation of dorsal and ventral sacral roots. Invest Urol 1979; 16: 300–4.

67. Hassouna MM, Siegel SW, Nyeholt AA et al. Sacral neuromodulation in the treatment of urgency-frequency symptoms: a multicenter study of efficacy and safety. J Urol 2000; 163: 1849–54.

68. Abrams P, Blaivas JG, Fowler CJ et al. The role of neuromodulation in the management of urinary urge incontinence. BJU Int 2003; 91: 355–9.

69. Siegel S, Paszkiewicz E, Kirkpatrick C, Hinkel B, Oleson K. Sacral nerve stimulation in patients with intractable pelvic pain. J Urol 2001; 166: 1742–5.

70. Peters KM, Carey JM, Konstandt DB. Sacral neuromodulation for the treatment of refractory interstitial cystitis: outcomes based on technique. Int Urogynecol J Pelvic Floor Dysfunct 2003; 14: 223–8.

71. Peters KM, Konstandt D. Sacral neuromodulation decreases narcotic requirements in refractory interstitial cystitis. BJU Int 2004; 93: 777–9.

8

Pelvic floor muscle exercises and behavioral therapy

Kathryn L Burgio and Diane F Borello-France

Changing bladder habits • **Behavioral training and the role of the pelvic floor** • **Changing behavior: changing attitudes** • **Nocturia** • **Behavioral lifestyle changes** • **Conclusion**

Behavioral interventions are a group of treatments that have been used for several decades to restore bladder control by improving bladder habits and teaching skills for inhibiting bladder overactivity. Cortical control of the micturition reflex is learned in childhood. The skills we learn as children allow us to empty the bladder when conditions are suitable or to delay voiding to a time when conditions are more appropriate. These skills include the ability to inhibit or disinhibit bladder contraction and to contract or relax pelvic floor muscles. When control over the micturition reflex is lost, symptoms of overactive bladder (OAB), including urgency, frequency, urge incontinence, and/or nocturia manifest. While pharmacological agents can inhibit the bladder directly, it is optimal to have volitional control over bladder activity.

The primary behavioral interventions for overactive bladder are bladder training and behavioral training, which utilizes pelvic floor muscle exercise. In clinical practice, the best behavioral programs are those that tailor multiple components to the needs of the individual patient. Components of behavioral treatment can include biofeedback, bladder inhibition training, urge suppression techniques (urge strategies), urethral occlusion, voiding schedules, self-monitoring with a bladder diary, and fluid and diet management.

CHANGING BLADDER HABITS

Patients who experience frequent urges to urinate often respond with frequent voiding. This behavioral response relieves the immediate sensation of urge, but sets the stage for more frequent episodes of urgency. Once frequent voiding becomes a habit, it can be difficult to break and may lead to reduced functional bladder capacity, diminished ability to control urges, and detrusor overactivity (Figure 8.1). In turn, the detrusor overactivity further promotes urgency and can lead to the more disabling condition of urge incontinence. One way to break this cycle is to place the patient on a voiding schedule using bladder training.

Bladder training

Bladder training is a behavioral intervention developed originally for the treatment of urge urinary incontinence. The goal of bladder training is to break the cycle of urgency and frequency using consistent, incremental voiding schedules. First known as bladder drill, the intervention was intensive and, therefore, was often conducted in an inpatient setting. Patients, mostly women, were placed on a strict expanded voiding schedule for 7–10 days to establish a normal voiding pattern.[2,3] Bladder training is a sequel to this

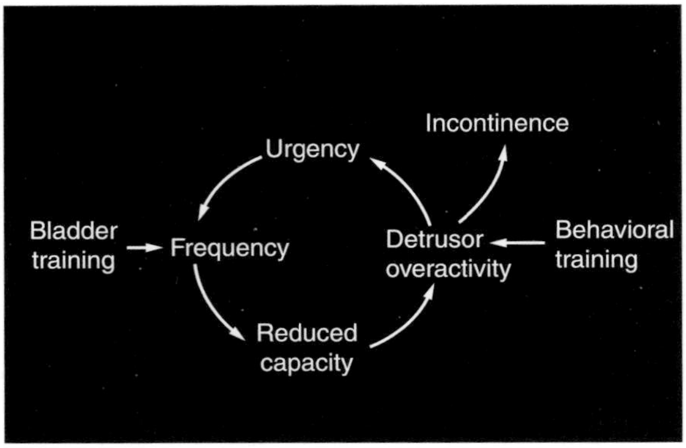

Figure 8.1 Cycle of urgency and frequency, depicting the two points where bladder training and behavioral training are thought to break the cycle.
(From reference 1, with permission)

procedure that increases the voiding interval more gradually, over a longer period of time, and is conducted in the outpatient setting.[4–12]

In bladder training the patient completes a voiding diary, which shows the clinician when and how often the patient is voiding. Using data from the bladder diary, the clinician and patient agree to a baseline voiding interval that maximizes the time between voids, but that is comfortable and reasonable for the patient. Patients are instructed to void first thing in the morning, then every time the interval passes, and finally before going to bed at night. Over time, the voiding interval is gradually increased. To follow a voiding schedule, patients must resist the sensation of urgency and postpone urination. This is believed to increase bladder capacity, decrease overactivity, and result in improved bladder control. Guidelines for conducting bladder training appear in Table 8.1.

Several clinical series studies have demonstrated the efficacy of outpatient bladder training or a mixture of inpatient and outpatient intervention.[4–10,12] The most definitive study is a randomized clinical trial that demonstrated a mean 57% reduction in frequency of incontinence in older women.[11] In this trial, bladder training also reduced incontinence associated with sphincter insufficiency, possibly because patients acquired a greater awareness of bladder function or because the exercise of postponing urination increased the use of pelvic floor muscles.

One positive feature of bladder training is that it dissociates voiding from urgency. Voiding by the clock, not in response to an urge sensation, weakens the urge–void response.

Delayed voiding

Delayed voiding is another approach to teaching patients bladder control without implementing a voiding schedule. Initially, whenever an urge strikes, patients are encouraged to wait 5 minutes before they void. For patients who have experienced incontinence, the smallest sensation to void can trigger anxiety or tension and result in a learned disuse of previously established bladder control skills. Even these most urgent patients can usually be convinced to try a 5-minute delay as a way to practice or reestablish bladder control skills. Many patients are surprised to find that after a brief wait, the urge subsides or disappears altogether, and they gradually recognize that they have improved control of their bladder. Once patients experience some success, they can extend the delay in voiding over a longer period. Longer intervals build confidence and enhance this new sense of control.

Urge control techniques

To be successful with bladder training or delayed voiding, most patients also need to learn strategies for coping with the urge while they wait to void. The traditional approach to urge control has been to suggest various techniques for relaxation or distraction to another activity. Patients are encouraged to divert attention away from their bladder by engaging in a task that requires mental but not physical effort. Examples include reading, balancing a checkbook, or making a to-do list. Taking the focus off the bladder can reduce anxiety and allows time for the urge to subside. Also used are affirming self-statements such as, "I am in control, not my bladder", or "I can wait".

More recently, clinicians have enhanced traditional bladder training by incorporating techniques from behavioral training to improve treatment outcomes. One very useful behavioral training method is to employ repeated pelvic floor muscle contractions as a mechanism to suppress urgency and bladder contractions.

Table 8.1 Instructions for bladder training

Step 1: Review voiding diary with the patient. Note the voiding intervals and their variability.

Step 2: With the patient, select the longest voiding interval that he/she finds comfortable.

Step 3: Instruct the patient:

　　　　　Empty your bladder...
- first thing in the morning
- every time your voiding interval passes during the day
- just before you go to bed

Step 4: Teach patient techniques for coping with urge to void that occurs before the interval has passed:
- distraction to another task that is mentally but not physically engaging (e.g. reading, writing a letter, balancing a checkbook)
- deep breathing and relaxation
- self-statements (e.g. "I can wait until it is time to go")
- urge suppression strategy: using pelvic floor muscle contraction to keep bladder relaxed

Step 5: Gradually increase the voiding interval...
- when the patient is comfortable on the voiding schedule for at least 3 days
- by 30-minute intervals, more or less, as determined by the patient's confidence and clinical judgment

---

BEHAVIORAL TRAINING AND THE ROLE OF THE PELVIC FLOOR

Behavioral training is an intervention that combines exercise science, motor learning, motor control, and behavior therapy principles into an increasingly accepted, conservative treatment for urge incontinence and OAB. The goal of behavioral training is to improve bladder control by teaching the patient to voluntarily suppress detrusor contractions. This involves a new response to urgency through learned use of pelvic floor muscle (PFM) contractions to control urgency and inhibit detrusor contractions. Historically, PFM exercises have been regarded primarily as a treatment for stress incontinence, but it is increasingly recognized that pelvic floor muscles play a role in OAB and urge urinary incontinence in women as well as in men.

Pelvic floor muscle training

PFM training is now a central element of behavioral training. The science behind using PFM training to treat OAB stems from observations that electrical stimulation of the pudendal nerve or PFMs results in bladder muscle inhibition.[13,14] It has also been shown that bladder distention

during urine storage stimulates both sympathetic and pudendal nerve activity, leading to an increase in external urethral sphincter and PFM activity. This "guarding reflex", mediated by spinal pathways, helps to promote continence.[15] Finally, clinical studies have shown that most patients can learn the skill of using a voluntary PFM contraction to inhibit or abort detrusor contractions, leading to a significant reduction of incontinence.[16]

The first step in behavioral training is for the patient to learn the skill of contracting and relaxing their muscles without increasing pressure on the bladder or pelvic floor. Several techniques can be used to help patients learn to exercise correctly, including biofeedback,[17] verbal feedback using vaginal or anal palpation,[16] or electrical stimulation.[13] Confirming that patients have identified the correct muscles is an essential and often overlooked step. Failure to identify the correct muscles or to exercise them properly is a key cause of treatment failure. Providing patients with a pamphlet or brief verbal instructions on how to exercise are insufficient teaching methods that do not ensure that patients will know how to proceed with exercise once they return home. It is unrealistic to expect patients to adhere to exercises when they are uncertain whether they are performing them correctly.

Once patients demonstrate the ability to properly contract their PFMs in the clinic, they can be sent home with written instructions for daily progressive exercises. Table 8.2 presents general guidelines for proper PFM exercise. Although there are several published reports on the effectiveness of PFM exercise to reduce urinary incontinence, there is great variability between studies regarding specific exercise methods. In many studies, women with stress, urge, or mixed incontinence were included and few studies reported results by diagnosis.[18,19] Therefore, strong evidence for an "optimal exercise prescription" for OAB does not yet exist. The degree to which the PFM exercise program should emphasize building muscle strength versus muscle endurance and/or coordination is unknown.[20,21] However, a program requiring the patient to perform 45–50 muscle contractions per day, sustaining each contraction for 10 seconds, has been shown to yield good results.[17,22]

Given this recommendation, we believe it is also prudent that the PFM exercise program be individualized to the patient's specific needs. The patient may need to perform fewer or more than the recommended 45–50 contractions, gradually progress to the 10-second contraction duration, or contract their PFMs with maximal versus submaximal force to achieve their continence goals. In this context, the focus on strength, endurance, and/or coordination will vary according to the patient's initial muscle function and functional complaints. A patient who cannot prevent urine loss in the event of a sudden, very strong urge may benefit from exercise that increases muscle strength and the timing of muscle force. In this case, the patient may be instructed to contract their muscles as fast as possible and with maximal force.[23] The maximal force requirement may prevent the patient from contracting their muscles for the full 10 seconds. If the patient's functional limitation is the inability to suppress several, small urges in order to get to a distant bathroom, then the exercise program should focus more on enhancing muscle endurance. In this scenario, the patient should be encouraged to sustain a submaximal muscle contraction for the full 10 seconds.[23] In most cases, patients will need to work on improving both strength and endurance.

In addition to improving muscle strength and endurance, the PFM exercise program should aim to improve muscle coordination, or the ability to use muscle strength in a functional context. Contracting the PFMs to suppress urges while walking to the bathroom requires the patient's nervous and muscular systems to control two simultaneous tasks, locomotion and prevention of a bladder accident. Without functional or task-specific PFM training, the patient may gain improved muscle strength or endurance, but most likely will have difficulty reaching their continence goal. To become continent, the patient will need to control their PFMs during a variety

---

Table 8.2 General instructions for pelvic muscle exercise

1. The muscles you want to exercise are the same muscles that you use if you are trying to prevent the passage of gas or stool from the rectum. As you squeeze these muscles you should feel a tightening around your vagina and anus.
2. As you get better with exercise, think about drawing the pelvic floor (the area around your vagina and anus) upwards and inwards toward your pubic bone.
3. Never strain or bear down when doing your exercises. This will cause strain on your pelvic floor.
4. Never hold your breath when doing your exercises.
5. Always relax the muscles completely after each contraction. This is important to restore oxygen to the muscles and prevent them from getting sore.
6. Try to relax your buttocks and thigh muscles during exercise. Your bottom should not lift off the exercise surface, nor should you notice much movement of your thighs when you are exercising correctly.

of tasks and situations throughout the day. Varied practice is essential in the development of skill. Skill is evidenced when the patient is able to use their PFM effortlessly, consistently, and in response to a variety of continence demands. For example, a patient who can stop or prevent an urge when reaching into the freezer at the grocery store, when putting the key in the door, and when taking a shower has developed skill.

Other important exercise prescription considerations include preventing muscle fatigue and enhancing exercise adherence. To avoid muscle fatigue, it is recommended that patients space the exercises across the day. If the exercise prescription calls for 45 contractions per day, the patient is advised to perform three separate exercise sessions of 15 PFM contractions each. It is also important to advise total relaxation between muscle contractions. In general, a 1 : 2 (for weak muscles) or a 1 : 1 (for stronger muscles) muscle contraction/relaxation ratio is recommended to allow muscles to restore energy and oxygen and to prevent exercise-induced muscle soreness.[23]

Exercise position is another variable that may impact on fatigue, exercise adherence, and the development of skill. Typically, patients are told to perform exercises while in the lying position first. As the patient becomes stronger, it is important to progress the exercise position to sitting, and eventually standing to promote skill. It is also more convenient to exercise in upright postures, therefore potentially reducing exercise burden. However, some patients find exercise in the standing position to be more difficult and fatiguing, which may negatively impact on adherence. Such differences in ability reinforce the notion that "one exercise program does not fit all". Instead clinicians need to be flexible and innovative in their approach to exercise prescription in order to maximize the patient's exercise adherence and, subsequently, their continence skills.

In addition to the scheduled exercises, patients with urge incontinence can often benefit from practice in interrupting or slowing the urinary stream during voiding once per day. Not only does this provide practice in occluding the urethra and interrupting detrusor contraction, it does so in the presence of the urge sensation, when patients with OAB need the skill most. Some clinicians have expressed concerns that repeated interruption of the stream could lead to incomplete

bladder emptying in certain groups of patients. Therefore, caution should be used when recommending this technique for patients who may be susceptible to voiding dysfunction.

Behavioral training: a new response to urge

The other essential component of behavioral training is teaching patients a new way to respond to urgency: the urge suppression strategy.[24] Usually, patients with OAB feel compelled to rush to the nearest bathroom when they feel the urge to void. In behavioral training, they are told how this natural response is actually counterproductive and can increase the probability of incontinence. Not only does rushing add physical pressure on the bladder, it enhances the sensation of fullness, exacerbates urgency, and triggers detrusor contraction. Further, when the patient reaches the vicinity of the toilet, he/she is exposed to visual cues that can trigger incontinence. Although the new response is counterintuitive at first, patients can learn instead to stop what they are doing, sit down if possible, and contract the PFM repeatedly to diminish urgency and suppress the detrusor contraction and prevent urine loss. They concentrate on voluntarily inhibiting the urge sensation and wait for the urge to subside before they walk at a normal pace to the toilet. See Table 8.3 for patient instructions for using the urge suppression strategy.

Table 8.3 Patient instructions for the urge suppression strategy

When you experience a strong urge to urinate. . .

Step 1: Stop and stay still. Sit down if you can.

Step 2: Squeeze your pelvic floor muscles quickly 3–5 times and repeat as needed.

Step 3: Relax the rest of your body. Take several deep breaths.

Step 4: Concentrate on suppressing the urge feeling.

Step 5: Wait until the urge subsides.

Step 6: Walk to the bathroom at a normal pace.

The effectiveness of behavioral training has been established in several studies.[16,17,25,26] In the first randomized controlled trial, behavioral training reduced incontinence episodes significantly more than drug treatment, and patient perceptions of improvement and satisfaction with their progress were higher with behavioral training.[26] A subsequent study demonstrated that the results of behavioral training using biofeedback versus verbal feedback based on vaginal palpation did not differ significantly,[16] indicating that careful training with either method can achieve good results.

CHANGING BEHAVIOR: CHANGING ATTITUDES

Many patients hold beliefs about toileting that can postpone or interfere with their goal of gaining bladder control. For instance, most patients are firm in the attitude that, "When you gotta go, you gotta go". To fully commit to a delayed voiding program or to become skillful in using the urge strategy, patients must suspend these beliefs. If the patient is skeptical about trying the urge strategy, the clinician can encourage them to try this new behavior in the safest possible environment and with absorbent protection to avoid embarrassment. Any positive results including partial success should be highlighted by the clinician as evidence of progress in order to encourage the persistence that will lead to further skill development. Once the patient enjoys some success in controlling their urge, that experience can be used to debunk the "gotta go" attitude. "When you gotta go, you *don't* gotta go", is a useful mantra the patient can use in the face of urgency. Whether the problem is incontinence or frequency, the patient must learn to stay away from the toilet until the urge subsides.

NOCTURIA

Nocturia is a multidimensional problem that requires differential diagnosis. When it is truly due to OAB, behavioral strategies can be helpful. While getting up once per night is widely regarded as normal, getting up two or more times can be very bothersome when it results in sleep disruption or daytime fatigue, or increases the risk of falls. One practical approach to reducing nocturia is to restrict fluid intake for 3–4 hours prior to bedtime. In patients who retain fluid during the day and have nocturia due to fluid mobilization at night, interventions focus on managing daytime accumulation of fluid. This can be facilitated by wearing support stockings, elevating the lower extremities in the late afternoon, or using a diuretic. For patients who are already taking a diuretic, nocturia can often be improved by altering the timing of the diuretic (so that most of the effect has occurred prior to bedtime) or by changing the prescription to a long-acting diuretic.

In addition to the medical management of nocturia, behavioral training for daytime urge incontinence has also been shown to reduce nocturia in older women.[27] Patients are instructed to use the urge suppression strategy when they wake up at night. If the technique is successful and the urge subsides, they are encouraged to go back to sleep. If after a minute or two the urge to void has not remitted, they may get up and void so as not to interfere unnecessarily with their sleep.

BEHAVIORAL LIFESTYLE CHANGES

Fluid management

Changes in the type or volume of fluids are recommended by many clinicians either as a primary or as an adjunctive strategy to optimize outcomes. Many patients with OAB attempt to manage their symptoms by restricting fluid intake overall, or at particular times of day when they anticipate limited restroom access or they believe they are at risk of having an incontinence episode. In some cases, their fluid restriction places them at risk of dehydration. Though it may seem counterintuitive, it is usually good advice to encourage the patient to consume at least six glasses of fluid each day. This will prevent the urine from becoming too concentrated, making it less irritating to the bladder.

When patients consume an abnormally high volume of fluid (e.g. > 2100 ml of output per 24 hours), fluid restriction is often an appropriate measure and can be helpful for reducing urine loss. Some people increase their fluid intake deliberately in an effort to "flush" their kidneys, lose weight, or avoid dehydration. In others it is simply a habit. In these cases, reducing excess fluids can relieve problems with sudden bladder fullness and help to reduce urgency, frequency, and urge incontinence.

Caffeine, in addition to being a diuretic, has also been shown to be a bladder irritant for many people. Many patients are reluctant initially to forgo their caffeinated beverages, but they may be convinced to try it for a short period of time, such as 3–5 days. If they experience relief from their symptoms, they are often more willing to reduce or eliminate caffeinated beverages from their diet. To avoid problems with caffeine withdrawal, it is recommended that caffeine reduction be approached gradually, and may include mixing caffeinated and decaffeinated beverages. Though there are few data on the role of sugar substitutes in incontinence, there are clinical cases in which these substances appear to aggravate incontinence, and reduction has provided clinical improvement.

Weight loss

Obesity is a common health problem that is now an established risk factor for urinary incontinence. Women with a high body mass index are more likely to develop incontinence, and they tend to have more severe incontinence than women with a lower body mass index.[28] A small body of literature now exists showing significant improvement in continence status with a weight loss of 45–50 kg after bariatric surgery,[29] and with as little as 5% weight reduction with conventional weight loss programs.[30] Because this small percentage weight loss is achievable for many overweight women, it is reasonable to recommend weight loss as a component in a behavioral program for incontinence in overweight women.

Bowel management

Fecal impaction and constipation have been recognized as factors contributing to urinary incontinence, particularly in nursing home populations.[31] In severe cases, fecal impaction can be an irritating factor in overactive bladder, or obstruct normal voiding, causing incomplete bladder emptying and overflow incontinence. Some patients experience immediate relief with disimpaction, but a bowel management program is often needed to avoid recurrence. Normal fluid intake and dietary fiber (or supplements)

are important in maintaining normal stool consistency and regular bowel movements. When hydration and fiber are not enough, bowel management may include enemas to stimulate a regular daily bowel movement, preferably after a regular meal such as breakfast to take advantage of postprandial motility.

CONCLUSION

Behavioral interventions are safe and without the risks and side effects of some other therapies. However, they require the active participation of a motivated patient and usually take some time and persistence to reach maximum benefit. Behavioral interventions are widely used and have an abundance of evidence demonstrating their efficacy. Although the majority of patients are not cured with these approaches, most can achieve significant improvement in continence status. This makes behavioral intervention a very reasonable first line approach to the care of men and women with overactive bladder.

Further, there is now evidence that combining behavioral interventions with drug therapy can improve outcomes over those achieved with either treatment alone. Studies of both bladder training and behavioral training indicate that for some patients, combined therapy will be the best way to optimize the treatment of overactive bladder.[32,33]

REFERENCES

1. Burgio KL. Current perspectives on management of urgency using bladder and behavioural training. Journal of the American Academy of Nurse Practitioners 2004; 16: 4–7.
2. Frewen WK. Role of bladder training in the treatment of the unstable bladder in the female. Urol Clin North Am 1979; 6: 273–7.
3. Frewen WK. A reassessment of bladder training in detrusor dysfunction in the female. Br J Urol 1982; 54: 372–3.
4. Elder DD, Stephenson TP. An assessment of the Frewen regime in the treatment of detrusor dysfunction in females. Br J Urol 1980; 52: 467–71.
5. Jarvis GJ, Millar DR. Controlled trial of bladder drill for detrusor instability. Br Med J 1980; 281: 1322–3.

6. Jarvis GJ. A controlled trial of bladder drill and drug therapy in the management of detrusor instability. J Urol 1981; 53: 565–6.

7. Jarvis GJ. The management of urinary incontinence due to primary vesical sensory urgency by bladder drill. Br J Urol 1982; 54: 374–6.

8. Pengelly AW, Booth CM. A prospective trial of bladder training as treatment for detrusor instability. Br J Urol 1980; 52: 463–6.

9. Svigos JM, Matthews CD. Assessment and treatment of female urinary incontinence by cystometrogram and bladder retraining programs. Obstet Gynecol 1977; 50: 9–12.

10. Jeffcoate TNA, Francis WJ. Urgency incontinence in the female. Am J Obstet Gynecol 1966; 94: 604–18.

11. Fantl JA, Wyman JF, McClish DK et al. Efficacy of bladder training in older women with urinary incontinence. JAMA 1991; 265: 609–13.

12. Colombo M, Zanetta G, Scalambrino S, Milani R. Oxybutynin and bladder training in the management of female urinary urge incontinence: a randomized study. Int Urogynecol J 1995; 6: 63–7.

13. Godec C, Cass A, Ayala G. Bladder inhibition with functional electrical stimulation. Urology 1975; 6: 663–6.

14. Ohlsson BL, Fall M, Frankenberg-Sommar S. Effects of external and direct pudendal nerve maximal stimulation in the treatment of the uninhibited overactive bladder. Br J Urol 1989; 64: 374–89.

15. DeGroat W. A neurologic basis for the overactive bladder. Urology 1997; 50 (Suppl 6A): 36–52.

16. Burgio KL, Goode PS, Locher JL et al. Behavioral training with and without biofeedback in the treatment of urge incontinence in older women: a randomized, controlled trial. JAMA 2002; 288: 2293–9.

17. Burgio KL, Whitehead WE, Engel BT. Urinary incontinence in the elderly. Bladder-sphincter biofeedback and toileting skills training. Ann Intern Med 1985; 103: 507–15.

18. Hay-Smith EJC, Bo K, Berghmans LCM et al. Pelvic floor muscle training for urinary incontinence in women. Cochrane Database Syst Rev 2001; (1): CD001407.

19. Hay-Smith EJC, Dumoulin C. Pelvic floor muscle training versus no treatment, or inactive control treatments for urinary incontinence in women. Cochrane Database Syst Rev 2006; (1): CD005654.

20. Bo K, Berghmans LCM. Nonpharmacologic treatments for overactive bladder-pelvic floor exercises. Urology 2000; 55 (5A Suppl): 7–11.

21. Bo K, Talseth T, Holm I. Single blind, randomized trial of pelvic floor muscle exercises, electrical stimulation, vaginal cones, and no treatment in management of genuine stress incontinence in women. BMJ 1999; 318: 487–93.

22. Goode PS, Burgio KL, Locher JL et al. Effect of behavioral training with or without pelvic floor electrical stimulation on stress incontinence in women: A randomized controlled trial. JAMA 2003; 290: 345–52.

23. Kisner C, Colby LA. Therapeutic Exercise. Foundations and Techniques, 4th edn. Philadelphia: FA Davis, 2003.

24. Burgio KL, Pearce KL, Lucco A. Staying Dry: A Practical Guide to Bladder Control. Baltimore: The Johns Hopkins University Press, 1989.

25. Burton JR, Pearce KL, Burgio KL et al. Behavioral training for urinary incontinence in elderly ambulatory patients. J Am Geriatr Soc 1988; 36: 693–8.

26. Burgio KL, Locher JL, Goode PS et al. Behavioral vs. drug treatment for urge urinary incontinence in older women: a randomized controlled trial. JAMA 1998; 280: 1995–2000.

27. Johnson TM, Burgio KL, Goode PS et al. Effects of behavioral and drug therapy on nocturia in older incontinent women. J Am Geriatr Soc 2005; 53: 846–50.

28. Brown J, Grady D, Ouslander J et al. Prevalence of urinary incontinence and associated risk factors in postmenopausal women. Heart & Estrogen/Progestin Replacement Study (HERS) Research Group. Obstet Gynecol 1999; 94: 66–70.

29. Bump RC, Sugerman HJ, Fantl JA, McClish DK. Obesity and lower urinary tract function in women: effect of surgically induced weight loss. Am J Obstet Gynecol 1992; 167: 392–7.

30. Subak LL, Johnson C, Whitcomb E et al. Does weight loss improve incontinence in moderately obese women? Int Urogynecol J Pelvic Floor Dysfunct 2002; 13: 40–3.

31. Ouslander JG, Schnelle JF. Incontinence in the nursing home. Ann Intern Med 1995; 122: 438–9.

32. Mattiasson AJ, Blaakaer J, Hoye K, Wein AJ; Tolterodine Scandinavian Study Group. Simplified bladder training augments the effectiveness of tolterodine in patient with an overactive bladder. BJU Int 2003; 91: 54-60.

33. Burgio KL, Locher JL, Goode PS. Combined behavioral and drug therapy for urge incontinence in older women. J Am Geriatr Soc 2000; 48: 370–4.

Pharmacology

9

Overactive bladder: basic pharmacology

Karl-Erik Andersson

Introduction • Activation of the bladder and peripheral targets for micturition control • Targets for pharmacologic intervention • Conclusion • Acknowledgment

INTRODUCTION

Several drugs with different modes and sites of action have been tried for the treatment of urodynamically demonstrated detrusor overactivity (DO), and the overactive bladder (OAB) syndrome.[1,2] Antimuscarinic drugs are still first line pharmacotherapy, but have well known limitations.[2] To be able to optimize treatment with current drug alternatives and to find new pharmacological treatment targets, further knowledge about the mechanisms of micturition is necessary.

The lower urinary tract is controlled by a complex interplay between the central and peripheral nervous systems and local regulatory factors.[3,4] Malfunction at various levels may result in micturition disorders, which can be classified as disturbances of storage or emptying. Failure to store urine may lead to various forms of incontinence (mainly urgency and stress incontinence). Theoretically, these disorders may be improved by agents that decrease detrusor activity and increase bladder capacity, and/or increase outlet resistance, either by acting peripherally or on the central nervous system (CNS).

A brief review is given of the basic pharmacology of the lower urinary tract, its central control, and of some therapeutic targets for drugs meant for treatment of DO/OAB.

ACTIVATION OF THE BLADDER AND PERIPHERAL TARGETS FOR MICTURITION CONTROL

Possible peripheral targets for pharmacologic intervention may be: (1) afferent neurotransmission, (2) efferent neurotransmission, and (3) the smooth muscle itself, including ion channels and intracellular second messenger systems. Although many drugs are available targeting these systems, most of them are less useful clinically due to the lack of selectivity for the lower urinary tract, which may result in intolerable or bothersome side effects. Thus, a main task is to find systems or receptors via which a selective action on the lower urinary tract (LUT) can be obtained.

Muscarinic receptors

Acetylcholine, acting on muscarinic receptors on the detrusor, is the main contractile transmitter. Muscarinic receptors comprise five subtypes, encoded by five distinct genes.[5] In the human bladder, the mRNAs for all muscarinic receptor subtypes have been demonstrated,[6] with a predominance of mRNAs encoding M_2 and M_3 receptors.[6,7] These receptors are functionally coupled to G-proteins, but the signal transduction systems vary.[8–10] Detrusor smooth muscle contains muscarinic receptors of the M_2 and M_3 subtypes.[8–10]

The M_3 receptors in the human detrusor are believed to be the most important for detrusor contraction.[3] Even in the obstructed rat bladder, M_3 receptors were found to play a predomiant role in mediating detrusor contraction.[11] Stimulation of M_3 receptors has previously been considered to cause contraction through phosphoinositide hydrolysis.[12,13] However, Jezior et al.[14] suggested that muscarinic receptor activation of detrusor muscle includes both non-selective cation channels and activation of Rho-kinase. Supporting a role of Rho-kinase in the regulation of rat detrusor contraction and tone, Wibberley et al.[15] found that in the rat, Rho-kinase inhibitors (Y-27632, HA 1077) inhibited contractions evoked by carbachol without affecting the contraction response to KCl. They also demonstrated high levels of Rho-kinase isoforms (I and II) in detrusor muscle. In line with this, Schneider et al.,[16] confirming that in the human detrusor carbachol-induced contraction is mediated via M_3 receptors, concluded that contraction largely depends on Ca^{2+} entry through nifedipine-sensitive channels and activation of the Rho-kinase pathway.

There may be species differences in the signaling pathways used by the different muscarinic receptor subtypes.[17] However, taken together, available evidence suggests that the main pathways for M_3 receptor activation of the human detrusor are *calcium influx via L-type calcium channels and inhibition of myosin light chain phosphatase through activation of Rho-kinase and protein kinase C*, leading to increased sensitivity of the contractile machinery to calcium.[16,18]

The functional role for the M_2 receptors has not been clarified, but it has been suggested that M_2 receptors may oppose sympathetically mediated smooth muscle relaxation through β-adrenoceptors.[19] M_2 receptor stimulation may also activate non-specific cation channels,[20] inhibit K_{ATP} (adenosine triphosphate (ATP)-sensitive potassium) channels through activation of protein kinase C,[21,22] and use other signaling pathways.[17] On the other hand, in certain disease states, M_2 receptors may contribute to contraction of the bladder. Thus, in the denervated rat bladder, M_2 receptors, or a combination of M_2 and M_3, mediated contractile responses.[23-26] In obstructed, hypertrophied rat bladders, there was an increase in total and M_2 receptor density, whereas there was a reduction in M_3 receptor density.[27] The functional significance of this change for voiding function has not been established, and preliminary experiments on the human detrusor[28,29] could not confirm these observations. Pontari et al.[30] analyzed bladder muscle specimens from patients with neurogenic bladder dysfunction to determine whether the muscarinic receptor subtype mediating contraction shifts from M_3 to the M_2 receptor subtype, as found in the denervated, hypertrophied rat bladder. They concluded that whereas normal detrusor contractions are mediated by the M_3 receptor subtype, in patients with neurogenic bladder dysfunction, contractions can be mediated by the M_2 receptors.

Muscarinic receptors may also be located on the presynaptic nerve terminals and participate in the regulation of transmitter release. The inhibitory prejunctional muscarinic receptors have been classified as M_2 in the rabbit[31,32] and rat,[33] and M_4 in the guinea-pig,[34] rat,[35] and human[36] bladder. Prejunctional facilitatory muscarinic receptors appear to be of the M_1 subtype in the rat and rabbit urinary bladder.[31-33] Prejunctional muscarinic facilitation has also been detected in human bladders.[37] The muscarinic facilitatory mechanism seems to be upregulated in overactive bladders from chronic spinal cord transected rats. The facilitation in these preparations is primarily mediated by M_3 muscarinic receptors.[37,38]

Muscarinic receptors have also been demonstrated on the urothelium/suburothelium,[10,39] but their functional importance has not been clarified. It has been suggested that they may be involved in the release of an unknown inhibitory factor.[10,40] Yokoyama et al.[41] investigated whether the effects of antimuscarinics depend on the suppression of C-fiber bladder afferent nerves. They gave tolterodine intravenously or intravesically to rats with cerebral infarct (and detrusor overactivity) with and without pretreatment with resiniferatoxin (to eliminate C fibers). Yokoyama et al.[41] found that at low doses tolterodine increased bladder capacity in non-resiniferatoxin-treated animals, but was ineffective in those who had received the toxin. The amplitude of contraction was not affected in any of the groups. The authors concluded that tolterodine exerted an inhibitory effect on C-fiber bladder afferent nerves, thereby improving bladder capacity. An inhibitory effect of systemically administered oxybutynin on the afferent part of the micturition reflex in rats was demonstrated by De Laet et al.,[42] recording afferent activity in the pelvic nerve. Boy et al.,[43] who studied the effect of tolterodine on sensations evoked by intravesical electrical stimulation and during bladder filling in healthy female subjects, found that the drug had a significant effect on afferent fibers, probably located in the suburothelium. These findings are in line with the clinical observations that antimuscarinics at clinically recommended doses have little effect on voiding contractions and may act mainly during the bladder storage phase, increasing bladder capacity.[44] During storage there is normally no parasympathetic outflow from the spinal cord.[45] A basal release of acetylcholine from non-neuronal (urothelial) as well as neuronal sources has been demonstrated in isolated human detrusor muscle.[46] It has been suggested that this release, which is increased by stretching the muscle and in the aging bladder, contributes to DO and OAB by eventually increasing bladder afferent activity during storage.[47] This may be because of a direct effect on suburothelial afferents, or stimulation of contraction of detrusor muscle cells, which already have an increased myogenic activity in DO.[48] In turn, enhanced myogenic contractions can generate enhanced afferent activity ("afferent noise"), contributing to urgency and/or initiation of the micturition reflex.

Adrenergic receptors

α-Adrenoceptors

α-Adrenoceptors (α-ARs) may have effects on different locations in the bladder: the detrusor smooth muscle, detrusor vasculature, afferent and efferent nerve terminals, and intramural ganglia. The importance of the α_1-ARs in the human detrusor for contraction and for generation of lower urinary tract symptoms (LUTS) has not been established. Most investigators agree that there is a low expression of these receptors in detrusor muscle.[49–51] In the human detrusor, Malloy et al.[50] found two-thirds of the α-AR mRNA expressed to be α_{1D}, there was no α_{1B}, and one-third was α_{1A}. In the rat bladder, the α_1-mRNA distribution was different: the α_{1A} was predominating, one-third was α_{1D}, and there was very little α_{1B}. The pattern was consistent in the different parts of the detrusor.[52]

A change of subtype distribution may be produced by outflow obstruction. Hampel et al.[52] reported that there was a change in the obstructed bladder from α_{1A}- to α_{1D}-mRNA predominance. In humans, as mentioned previously, there is an α_{1D}-AR predominance already in the normal detrusor, which means that a change in a similar direction as in the rat would be of minor importance provided that the number of receptors or their sensitivity did not increase. Nomiya and Yamaguchi[53] suggested that this was not the case. They confirmed the low expression of α-AR mRNA in normal human detrusor, and further demonstrated that there was no upregulation of any of the ARs with obstruction. In addition, in functional experiments they found a small response to phenylephrine at high drug concentrations with no difference between normal and obstructed bladders. This was, however, not found by Bouchelouche et al.,[54] who showed an increased contractile response to phenylephrine in detrusor of patients with bladder outlet obstruction. Even if there seems to be no evidence for α-AR upregulation or change in subtype in the obstructed human detrusor, which would make it unlikely that the α_{1D}-ARs on the detrusor muscle are responsible for DO/OAB, this does not exclude that α_{1D}-ARs located elsewhere in the bladder would be of importance. In an attempt to establish the importance of α_{1D}-ARs for control of micturition, Chen et al.[55] studied the role in micturition of α_{1D}-AR in knockout (KO) mice. They clearly showed that these mice had a larger bladder capacity and voided volumes than their wild type controls, supporting an important role for the α_{1D}-AR in the control of voiding. However, it is not possible to draw any conclusions from the presented data about the location of the α_{1D}-ARs involved in micturition control. The α_{1D}-ARs in bladder structures involved in afferent signaling, e.g. urothelium/suburothelium, or extravesical α_{1D}-ARs on afferent pathways, ganglia, and/or CNS structures may be more important for the control of bladder function. Thus, Ishihama et al.[56] demonstrated that activation of α_{1D}-ARs in the rat urothelium facilitates the micturition reflex, and they concluded that "endogenous catecholamines appear to act on α_{1D} receptors in the urothelium to facilitate mechanosensitive bladder afferent nerve activity and reflex voiding".

Sugaya et al.[57] investigated the effects of intrathecal injection of tamsulosin (acting on $\alpha_{1A/D}$-ARs) and naftopidil (acting preferentailly on α_{1D}-ARs) on isovolumetric bladder contractions in rats. Intrathecal injection of tamsulosin or naftopidil transiently abolished these contractions. The amplitude of bladder contraction was decreased by intrathecal injection of naftopidil, but not by tamsulosin. It was speculated that in addition to the antagonistic action of these agents on the α_{1A}-ARs of prostatic smooth muscle, both agents (especially naftopidil) may also act on the lumbosacral cord, and thus may improve collecting disorders in patients with benign prostatic hyperplasia. Supporting such a view, Ikemoto et al.[58] gave tamsulosin and naftopidil to 96 patients with benign prostatic hyperplasia (BPH) for 8 weeks in a crossover study. Whereas naftopidil monotherapy decreased the International Prostate Symptom Score (I-PSS) for storage symptoms, tamsulosin monotherapy decreased the I-PSS for voiding symptoms. However, these results could not be confirmed by Gotoh et al.[59] in a randomized controlled trial (RCT).

All subtypes of α-ARs can be found in different parts of the human vascular tree, and they all mediate contraction. The expression varies with vessel bed and increases with age. In the bladder, the function of the detrusor muscle is dependent on the vasculature and the perfusion. Hypoxia induced by partial outlet obstruction is believed to play a major role in both the hypertrophic and degenerative effects of partial outlet obstruction. Das et al.[60] investigated in rats whether doxazosin affected blood flow to the bladder and reduced the level of bladder dysfunction induced by partial outlet obstruction. They found that 4 weeks of treatment with doxazosin increased bladder blood flow in both control and obstructed rats. Furthermore, doxazosin treatment reduced bladder weight increase in obstructed animals, which could be one of the mechanisms contributing to a positive effect of α-AR blockade in DO.

In a pilot study comprising 11 male patients with LUTS, tamsulosin was given for 5 weeks and effects on bladder blood flow (color Doppler methodology), bladder capacity, and compliance were measured.[61] It was found that particularly in patients with a pathologic response to intravesical KCl, tamsulosin normalized blood flow and even increased it. The authors suggested that

there was a blood flow dysregulation in BPH patients. This could be normalized by α-AR antagonists and this effect may contribute to an improved bladder function.

β-Adrenoceptors

There are many pieces of evidence from studies in various animals suggesting that the sympathetic nervous system contributes to the urine storage function by inhibiting the reflex activation of the detrusor muscle during bladder filling.[62] However, the role of β-AR mediated detrusor relaxation in humans has been questioned. One argument is that β-AR blockade seems to have no effect on normal human detrusor function, another that individuals lacking dopamine β-hydroxylase, which is necessary for noradrenaline synthesis, seem to have normal bladder function.[63] Thus, the functional importance of β-ARs for normal detrusor function in humans remains to be settled. This does not exclude β-ARs from being an interesting target for drugs mediating detrusor relaxation.

In the human detrusor, it is now generally accepted that the most important β-AR for bladder relaxation is the β_3-AR.[51,64] This can partly explain why the clinical effects of selective β_2-AR agonists in DO have not been convincing.[2] The β_2-AR agonist, clenbuterol, inhibited electrically evoked contractions in human "unstable", but not normal, bladder,[65] which is in agreement with previous experiences in humans, suggesting that clenbuterol and also other β_2-AR agonists such as terbutaline may inhibit DO.[66,67]

β-AR agonists are thought to stimulate adenylyl cyclase to increase cyclic adenosine monophosphate (cAMP). In turn, cAMP activates protein kinase A (PKA) to mediate their biological effects. Nakahira et al.[68] showed in guinea pigs that isoprenaline prevented spontaneous action potential discharges and associated calcium transients through the activation of PKA. The isoprenaline-induced inhibition of intracellular Ca^{2+} largely depended on the prevention of spontaneous action potentials since the contribution of the intracellular calcium store was small. Isoprenaline hyperpolarized the cell membrane, probably by stimulating sodium pump activity. Nakahira et al.[68] also found no effect of different K^+ channel blockers on the hyperpolarization, and concluded that activation of K$^+$ channels was not involved in this effect. This is in contrast to the findings of Kobayashi et al.,[69] who reported that the isoprenaline-induced relaxation of guinea pig bladder smooth muscle was mainly mediated by facilitation of BK$_{Ca}$ (large conductance calcium- and voltage-activated potassium) channels subsequent to the activation of the cAMP/PKA pathway. In line with this, Uchida et al.[70] suggested that in addition to the cAMP-dependent pathway, BK$_{Ca}$ channels are involved in a non-cAMP-dependent β-AR agonist-induced relaxation in precontracted detrusor muscle. Hudman et al.[65] suggested that K$_{ATP}$ channel opening and the subsequent hyperpolarization of cell membranes in response to β$_2$-adrenoceptor activation (clenbuterol) is mediated by raised cAMP levels and activation of PKA.

The β$_3$-AR seems to be an interesting target for drugs aimed at treatment of DO/OAB, and selective β$_3$-AR agonists have shown relaxant effects in vitro and in animal models of DO.[71–73] However, there seem to be no published human proof of concept studies showing that this is an effective principle to treat DO/OAB.

Ion channels

In detrusor muscle, the two most thoroughly investigated classes of ion channels are Ca^{2+} and K$^+$ channels.[74]

Calcium channels

An increase in [Ca^{2+}]$_i$ is a key process required for the activation of contraction in the detrusor. However, it is still discussed whether this increase is due to influx from the extracellular space and/or release from intracellular stores.[74] Several types of Ca^{2+} channels have been demonstrated in smooth muscle.[75] For example, in many types of smooth muscle, there are at least two, and probably more, distinct store-operated channels (SOCs), which have markedly different permeabilities to Ca^{2+} ions. They can be expected to occur also in the detrusor, but whether they have any importance for detrusor contraction does not seem to have been specifically studied. For the human detrusor, information is available mainly on voltage-operated channels.[74]

A decrease of the membrane potential (depolarization) increases the open probability for

Ca^{2+} channels, thereby increasing the Ca^{2+} influx. Several studies on animal detrusor tissue have demonstrated the importance of extracellular Ca^{2+} entry through L-type (dihydropyridine-sensitive) Ca^{2+} channels and mobilization of intracellular Ca^{2+} for activation of the detrusor via the main transmitters, acetylcholine and ATP. In addition, muscarinic receptor stimulation was suggested to increase the sensitivity of the contractile machinery to Ca^{2+}.[74] The relative contribution of these mechanisms to the activation of contraction has not been established. In the human detrusor, extracellular Ca^{2+} seems to play a major role in the activation process, irrespective of the mode of activation.[76] Dihydropyridines, e.g. nifedipine, have a potent inhibitory effect on isolated detrusor muscle.[62] Inhibitory effects have also been demonstrated on experimentally induced contractions under in vivo conditions in rats,[77] and clinically in patients with DO.[78] Mice deficient in the smooth muscle Cav1.2 Ca^{2+} channel (SMACKO, smooth muscle α$_{1C}$ subunit Ca^{2+} channel KO mice) had severely reduced micturition and an increased bladder mass. Their detrusor tissue showed no spontaneous contractile activity, and membrane depolarization- and carbachol-induced contractions were reduced 10-fold.[79] The results in SMACKO mice were considered to reveal a central role for L-type Ca^{2+} channels in urinary bladder function and mark them as candidate targets for the pharmacologic manipulation of, for example, DO.[79]

If DO is caused by increased Ca^{2+} influx, one would expect changes in the functional properties or number of Ca^{2+} channels in bladders exhibiting this property. However, this could not be verified in a study using bladder tissues from children with myelodysplasia, a condition frequently associated with neurogenic DO.[80] Clinically, the use of Ca^{2+} antagonists in the treatment of DO/OAB has been disappointing,[2] and there is currently no evidence from RCTs that Ca^{2+} antagonists represent an effective treatment principle.

Potassium channels

K$^+$ channels represent another mechanism to modulate the excitability of the smooth muscle cells. Under normal conditions, the resting membrane potential in smooth muscle cells is determined predominantly by the membrane conductivity for K^+ ions. Increased K^+ conductivity will lower the membrane potential by increasing the K^+ efflux. As a consequence, this will increase the threshold for opening of voltage-operated calcium channels and initiation of contraction. Several different types of K^+ channels have been identified in myocytes isolated from detrusor muscle,[74] and at least two subtypes have been found in the human detrusor, ATP-sensitive K^+ channels (K_{ATP}) and large conductance calcium-activated K^+ channels (BK_{Ca}). Evidence for the participation of K^+ channels in detrusor myocyte function derives from molecular genetic studies on mice, such as conditional KOs of the SK3 channel.[81] Investigations into isolated mouse detrusor myocytes and strips, as well as in vivo cystometry, have clearly indicated the importance of SK3 channels to the regulation of detrusor contractility and bladder function. Activation or increased activity of SK3 channels seemed to result in decreased bladder sensation during filling,[81] which can be assumed to be of benefit for treating DO/OAB. Studies on mice lacking the α and β_1 subunits of the BK_{Ca} channel subtype have suggested an important role for the BK_{Ca} channel. Thus, cystometric recording in α-subunit KO mice revealed DO.[82,83] In isolated detrusor strips, enhanced phasic contractile activity[82] and increased sensitivity to nerve stimulation[83] could be demonstrated. Also, in detrusor muscle strips from β_1-subunit knockout mice,[84] enhanced phasic contractile responses were observed.

In vitro findings have suggested that hyperpolarization of the detrusor muscle cell membrane via selective activation of the BK_{Ca} channel with a new class of BK_{Ca} channel openers can elicit relaxation of detrusor muscle strips.[85] In line with this, intravesical injection of *hSlo* cDNA (coding for the α subunit of the human BK_{Ca} channel) in rats was shown to improve DO due to partial outflow obstruction.[86]

Taken together, available data support the assumption that alterations in K^+ channel subtype expression, regulation, or function could have very important implications for normal bladder physiology and the etiology of DO. Supporting this, studies of isolated human detrusor muscle have demonstrated that K^+ channel openers can reduce spontaneous contractions as well as contractions induced by carbachol and electrical stimulation.[74] However, the lack of bladder selectivity of K^+ channel openers currently available for clinical use (K_{ATP} openers) has thus far limited the use of these drugs. No effects of cromakalim or pinacidil on the bladder were found in studies of patients with spinal cord lesions or DO secondary to outflow obstruction.[87,88] However, new K_{ATP}-channel openers have been developed, claimed to have selectivity towards the bladder.[74] One of them, ZD6169, which activates K_{ATP} channels in human bladder cells, was shown to reduce micturition frequency in rats at doses that produced no cardiovascular effects.[89] However, an analog of ZD6169 was shown to be ineffective in an RCT in patients with idiopathic DO.[90] Thus, there is no clinical evidence suggesting that opening of K^+ channels (K_{ATP}) is an effective treatment for patients with DO/OAB. However, this does not exclude that the selective opening of, for example, BK_{Ca} channels can be effective.

Sensory nerves and vanilloid receptors

Appropriate bladder function is dependent on an intact afferent signaling from the bladder to the CNS. This signaling conveys information about bladder filling and the status of the tissue, e.g. presence of infectious agents, etc. The afferent nerves consist of small slowly conducting myelinated Aδ fibers and slowly conducting, unmyelinated C fibers. The former are excited by mechanoreceptors and convey information about bladder filling, while C fibers may primarily mediate painful sensations recognized by chemoreceptors.[91]

By means of capsaicin (CAP), a subpopulation of primary afferent neurons innervating the bladder and urethra, the "CAP-sensitive nerves", has been identified. It is believed that CAP exerts its effects by acting on specific, "vanilloid" receptors (TPVR1), on these nerves.[92] CAP has a biphasic effect: initial excitation is followed by a long-lasting blockade, which renders sensitive primary afferents (C fibers) resistant to activation by natural stimuli. In sufficiently high concentrations, CAP is believed to cause "desensitization" initially by releasing and emptying the stores of neuropeptides, and then by blocking further release.[93] Resiniferatoxin (RTX) is an analog of CAP, approximately 1000 times more potent for desensitization than CAP,[94] but only a few hundred times more potent for excitation.[95] Possibly, both CAP and RTX can have effects on Aδ fibers. It is also possible that CAP at high concentrations (mmol/l) has additional, non-specific effects.[96]

The rationale for intravesical instillations of vanilloids is based on the involvement of C fibers in the pathophysiology of conditions such as bladder hypersensitivity and neurogenic DO.[97] In the healthy human bladder, C fibers carry the response to noxious stimuli, but they are not implicated in the normal voiding reflex. After spinal cord injury major neuroplasticity appears within bladder afferents in several mammalian species, including man. C-fiber bladder afferents proliferate within the suburothelium and become sensitive to bladder distention. Those changes lead to the emergence of a new C-fiber-mediated voiding reflex, which is strongly involved in spinal neurogenic DO. Improvement of this condition by defunctionalization of C-fiber bladder afferents with intravesical vanilloids has been widely demonstrated in humans and animals.

Cystometric evidence that CAP-sensitive nerves may modulate the afferent branch of the micturition reflex in humans was originally presented by Maggi et al.,[98] who instilled CAP (0.1–10 μmol/l) intravesically in five patients with hypersensitivity disorders, with attenuation of their symptoms a few days after administration. Intravesical CAP, given in considerably higher concentrations (1–2 mmol/l) than those administered by Maggi et al.,[98] has since been used with success in neurological disorders such as multiple sclerosis, or traumatic chronic spinal lesions.[2] Side effects of intravesical CAP include discomfort and a burning sensation at the pubic/urethral level during instillation, an effect that can be overcome by prior instillation of lidocaine, which does not interfere with the beneficial effects of CAP.[99] No premalignant or malignant changes in the bladder have been found in biopsies of patients who had repeated CAP instillations for up to 5 years.[100] The beneficial effect of CAP and RTX has been demonstrated in several studies including RCTs.[2,101]

Available information (including data from randomized controlled trials) suggests that both CAP and RTX may have useful effects in the treatment of neurogenic DO. There may be beneficial effects also in non-neurogenic DO in selected cases refractory to antimuscarinic treatment. RTX is an interesting alternative to capsaicin, but the drug is currently not in clinical development owing to formulation problems.

Botulinum toxin-sensitive mechanisms

Seven immunologically distinct antigenic subtypes of botulinum toxin (BTX) have been identified: A, B, C1, D, E, F, and G. Types A and B are in clinical use in urology, but most studies have been performed with BTX type A. BTX is believed to act by inhibiting acetylcholine release from cholinergic nerve terminals interacting with the protein complex necessary for docking acetylcholine vesicles. However, the mechanism of action seems to be much more complex.[102–105] Apostolidis et al.[105] proposed that a primary peripheral effect of BTX is "the inhibition of release of acetylcholine, ATP, substance P, and reduction in the axonal expression of the capsaicin and purinergic receptors. This may be followed by central desensitization through a decrease in central uptake of substance P and neurotrophic factors. The summation of these effects is a profound and long-lasting inhibition of those afferent and efferent mechanisms that are thought to be the pathophysiological basis for DO."

BTX injection results in decreased muscle contractility and muscle atrophy at the injection site. The produced chemical denervation is a reversible process, and axons regenerate in about 3–6 months. The BTX molecule cannot cross the blood–brain barrier and therefore has no CNS effects.

The chemical denervation of the bladder induced by BTX implies an effective treatment approach.[106,107] BTX injected into the external urethral sphincter was initially used to treat spinal cord injured patients with detrusor–external sphincter dyssynergia.[102,103] The use of BTX has increased rapidly, and successful treatment of neurogenic DO by intravesical BTX injections has now been reported by several groups.[108–112] BTX may also be an alternative to surgery in children with intractable DO.[109] However, toxin injections have also been shown to be effective in refractory idiopathic DO.[110,111] Adverse effects, e.g. generalized muscle weakness, have been reported,[112] but seem to be rare.

TARGETS FOR PHARMACOLOGIC INTERVENTION

Central nervous system targets

Anatomically, several CNS regions may be involved in micturition control: supraspinal structures, such as the cortex and diencephalon, midbrain, and medulla, but also spinal structures.[45,113–117] Griffiths et al.,[115] using functional magnetic resonance imaging (fMRI) to determine brain responses to bladder filling in subjects with normal and with poor bladder control (DO), found that poor bladder control is specifically associated with inadequate activation of the orbitofrontal cortex. Clinically, it is known that frontal cortical lesions cause bladder control problems.[114]

Many transmitters, both excitatory (e.g. glutamic acid, substance P, and ATP) and inhibitory (e.g. γ-aminobutyric acid (GABA), glycine, and enkephalins), are involved in the micturition reflex pathways.[3,4,118] There is evidence from experiments in rats that glutamic acid is an essential excitatory transmitter in the ascending, pontine and descending limbs of the spinobulbospinal micturition reflex pathway and in spinal reflex pathways controlling the bladder and external urethral sphincter,[119] but several other transmitters/modulators may be involved, and thus targets for micturition control. However, few drugs with a CNS site of action have been developed.[2,120]

Opioid receptors

Endogenous opioid peptides and corresponding receptors (μ, δ, κ) are widely distributed in many regions in the CNS that are of importance for micturition control, e.g. the periaqueductal gray (PAG), the pontine micturition center (PMC), the sacral parasympathetic nucleus, and the nucleus of Onuf.[118] It has been well established that morphine, given by various routes of administration to animals and humans, can increase bladder capacity or block bladder contractions. Furthermore, given intrathecally to anesthetized rats and intravenously to humans, the μ-opioid receptor antagonist, naloxone, has been shown to stimulate micturition,[121,122] suggesting that tonic activation of μ-opioid receptors has a depressant effect on the micturition reflex. However, intrathecal naloxone was not effective in stimulating micturition in conscious rats at doses blocking the effects of intrathecal morphine.[123,124]

Morphine given intrathecally was effective in patients with DO due to spinal cord lesions.[125] However, opioid treatment is associated with well-known side effects, such as nausea, respiratory depression, constipation, and abuse. Attempts have been made to reduce these side effects by increasing selectivity towards one of the different opioid receptor types.[126] At least three different opioid receptors – μ, δ, and κ – bind stereospecifically with morphine, and have been shown to interfere with voiding mechanisms. Theoretically, selective receptor actions, or modifications of effects mediated by specific opioid receptors, may have useful therapeutic effects for micturition control.

Tramadol is a well-known analgesic drug. By itself, it is a weak μ-receptor agonist, but it is metabolized to several different compounds, some of them almost as effective as morphine at the μ-receptor. However, the drug also inhibits serotonin (5-HT) and noradrenaline reuptake.[127] This profile is of particular interest, since both μ-receptor agonism and amine reuptake inhibition may be useful principles for the treatment of DO/OAB.

The most conspicuous changes in the cystometrogram when tramadol was given to a normal, awake rat were increases in threshold pressure and bladder capacity. Naloxone more or less completely inhibited these effects.[128] In rats, morphine has a very narrow range between the doses causing inhibition of micturition and those increasing bladder capacity and evoking urinary retention. Tramadol, on the other hand, has effects over a much wider range of doses, which means that it could be therapeutically more useful for micturition control. It may be speculated that this difference between morphine and tramadol is caused by tramadol's inhibitory effects on the reuptake of 5-HT and noradrenaline.[128]

In rats, tramadol abolished experimentally induced DO caused by cerebral infarction.[129] Tramadol also inhibited DO induced by apomorphine in rats[130] – a model of bladder dysfunction in Parkinson's disease. Whether or not tramadol may have a clinically useful effect on OAB/DO remains to be studied in RCTs.

Serotonin mechanisms

It is well established that the lumbosacral autonomic as well as the somatic motor nuclei (Onuf's nuclei) receive a dense serotonergic input from the raphe nuclei.[45] Multiple 5-HT receptors have been found at sites processing afferent and efferent impulses from and to the LUT.[131] The main receptors so far implicated in the control of micturition are the $5-HT_{1A}$, $5-HT_2$, and $5-HT_7$ receptors.[132] Although, as pointed out by de Groat,[133] there is some evidence in the rat for serotonergic facilitation of voiding, the descending pathway is essentially an inhibitory circuit, with 5-HT as a key neurotransmitter. Thus, electrical stimulation of 5-HT-containing neurons in the caudal raphe nucleus causes inhibition of bladder contractions.[134,135] Most experiments in rats and cats indicate that activation of the central serotonergic system by 5-HT reuptake inhibitors, as well as by $5-HT_{1A}$ and $5-HT_2$ receptor agonists, depresses reflex bladder contractions and increases the bladder volume threshold for inducing micturition.[133] $5-HT_{1A}$ receptors are involved in multiple inhibitory mechanisms controlling the spinobulbospinal micturition reflex pathway. The regulation of the frequency of bladder reflexes is presumably mediated by a suppression of afferent input: on the C-fiber afferent limb of the spinal micturition reflex including interneuronal pathways in the spinal cord,[136] and on the micturition switching circuitry in the pons. The regulation of bladder contraction amplitude may be related to an inhibition of the output from the pons to the parasympathetic nuclei in the spinal cord. It has been speculated that both blockade and stimulation $5-HT_{1A}$ receptors might be useful in treating DO.[120,136] However, there is evidence showing that at least blockade of these receptors leads to rapid tolerance.[136]

It has been speculated that selective serotonin reuptake inhibitors (SSRIs) may be useful for treatment of DO/OAB. On the other hand, there are reports suggesting that the SSRIs in patients without incontinence can actually cause incontinence, particularly in the elderly, and one of the drugs (sertraline) seemed to be more prone to produce urinary incontinence than the others.[137] Patients exposed to serotonin uptake inhibitors had an increased risk (15 out of 1000 patients) for developing urinary incontinence. So far, there are no RCTs demonstrating the value of SSRIs in the treatment of DO/OAB.

γ-Amino butyric acid mechanisms

Both $GABA_A$ and $GABA_B$ receptors are present in the brain[138,139] and in the spinal cord, where GABA has been identified as a main inhibitory transmitter.[118] GABA functions appear to be triggered by binding of GABA to its ionotropic receptors, $GABA_A$ and $GABA_C$, which are ligand-gated chloride channels, and its metabotropic receptor, $GABA_B$.[140] Since the blockade of $GABA_A$ and $GABA_B$ receptors in the spinal cord[141,142] and brain[142,143] stimulated rat micturition, an endogenous activation of $GABA_{A+B}$ receptors may be responsible for continuous inhibition of the micturition reflex within the CNS. In the spinal cord, $GABA_A$ receptors are more numerous than $GABA_B$ receptors, except for the dorsal horn where $GABA_B$ receptors predominate.[144,145]

GABA transporters, present on neuronal and glial cells in the brain, brain stem, and spinal cord,[146] are presumed to provide an inactivation mechanism.[144] Four different GABA transporters (GATs) have been described.[138] Tiagabine is a selective inhibitor of one of these GABA transporters, GAT1,[147] is able to increase extracellular levels of GABA,[148] and has inhibitory effects on rat micturition.[149] Intravenous administration of tiagabine decreased micturition pressure and decreased voided volume. Tiagabine given intrathecally reduced micturition pressure and increased bladder capacity,[149] suggesting that increasing endogenous levels of GABA in the CNS may improve micturition control.

Experiments using conscious and anesthetized rats demonstrated that exogenous GABA, muscimol ($GABA_A$ receptor agonist), and baclofen ($GABA_B$ receptor agonist) given intravenously, intrathecally, or intracerebroventricularly inhibit micturition.[142,150] Baclofen given intrathecally attenuated oxyhemoglobin-induced DO, suggesting that the inhibitory actions of $GABA_B$ receptor agonists in the spinal cord may be useful for controlling micturition disorders caused by C-fiber activation in the urothelium and/or suburothelium.[142] In mice, where DO was produced by intravesical citric acid, baclofen given subcutaneously had an inhibitory effect which was blocked by the selective $GABA_B$ receptor antagonist, CGP55845.[151]

Stimulation of the PMC results in an immediate relaxation of the external striated sphincter and a contraction of the detrusor muscle of the bladder. Blok et al.[152] demonstrated in cats a direct pathway from the PMC to the dorsal gray commissure of the sacral cord. It was suggested that the pathway produced relaxation of the external striated sphincter during micturition via inhibitory modulation by GABA neurons of the motoneurons in the sphincter of Onuf.[152] In rats, intrathecal baclofen and muscimol ultimately produced dribbling urinary incontinence,[141,142] and this was also found in conscious mice given muscimol and diazepam subcutaneously.[151]

Thus, normal relaxation of the striated urethral sphincter is probably mediated via $GABA_A$ receptors,[142,149] $GABA_B$ receptors having a minor influence on motoneuron excitability.[153]

Gabapentin Gabapentin is widely used not only for seizures and neuropathic pain, but for many other indications, such as anxiety and sleep disorders, because of its apparent lack of toxicity. The drug was originally designed as an anticonvulsant GABA mimetic capable of crossing the blood–brain barrier.[154] Its effects, however, do not appear to be mediated through interaction with GABA receptors, and its mechanism of action remains controversial.[154] It has been suggested that it acts by binding to the $\alpha_2\delta$ unit of voltage-dependent calcium channels.[155] The specific effects of such an action on micturition mechanisms have apparently not been studied in detail.

In a pilot study, Carbone et al.[156] reported on the effect of gabapentin on neurogenic DO. These investigators found a positive effect on symptoms and a significant improvement in urodynamic parameters after treatment with gabapentin, and suggested that the effects of the drug should be explored in further controlled studies in both neurogenic and non-neurogenic DO. Kim et al.[157] studied the effects of gabapentin in patients with OAB and nocturia not responding to antimuscarinics. They found that 14 out of 31 patients improved with oral gabapentin. The drug was generally well tolerated, and the authors suggested that it can be considered in selective patients when conventional modalities have failed. It is possible that gabapentin and other $\alpha_2\delta$ ligands (e.g. pregabalin and analogs) will offer new therapeutic alternatives.

Noradrenaline mechanisms

Neurons in the locus coeruleus react to bladder filling, and noradrenergic neurons in the brain stem project to the sympathetic, parasympathetic, and somatic nuclei in the lumbosacral spinal cord. Destruction of the noradrenergic pathways with 6-OH dopamine did not change micturition in rats; however, there is ample evidence that bulbospinal noradrenergic pathways are involved in the supraspinal control of micturition.[45]

Bladder activation through these bulbospinal noradrenergic pathways may involve excitatory α_1-adrenoceptors.[158] In rats undergoing continuous cystometry, doxazosin given intrathecally decreased micturition pressure, both in normal rats and in animals with post-obstruction bladder hypertrophy.[159] The effect was much more pronounced in the animals with hypertrophied/ overactive bladders. Doxazosin given intrathecally, but not intraarterially, to spontaneously hypertensive rats exhibiting DO normalized bladder activity.[160] It was suggested that doxazosin has a site of action at the level of the spinal cord and ganglia.

A central site of action for α_1-adrenoceptor antagonists has been discussed as an explanation for the beneficial effects of these drugs in patients with LUTS (especially storage symptoms) associated with BPH.[3] However, there are no RCTs showing that α_1-adrenoceptor antagonists represent an effective treatment of DO/OAB.[2]

Dopamine mechanisms

Parkinson's disease is one of the most common neurological causes of voiding dysfunction, often resulting in DO/OAB and impairment of relaxation of the striated urethral sphincter.[161] Patients with Parkinson's disease may have neurogenic DO, possibly as a consequence of nigrostriatal dopamine depletion and failure to activate inhibitory D_1-like (D_1 and D_5) receptors.[162] However, other dopaminergic systems may activate D_2-like (D_2, D_3, D_4) receptors, facilitating the micturition reflex.

Sillén et al.[163] showed that apomorphine, which activates both D_1- and D_2-like receptors, induced DO in anesthetized rats via stimulation of central dopaminergic receptors. The effects were abolished by infracollicular transection of the brain, and by prior intraperitoneal administration of the centrally acting dopamine receptor blocker, spiroperidol. Kontani et al.[164,165] suggested that the DO induced by apomorphine in anesthetized rats resulted from synchronous stimulation of the micturition centers in the brain stem and spinal cord, and that the response was elicited by stimulation of both dopamine D_1- and D_2-like receptors. Blockade of central dopamine receptors may be expected to influence voiding; however, the therapeutic potential of drugs having this action has not been established.

Tachykinin mechanisms

Substance P (SP), neurokinin A (NKA), and neurokinin B (NKB), the main endogenous tachykinins, are believed to be important neurotransmitters or neuromodulators within the CNS. These peptides and their preferred receptors, NK_1, NK_2, and NK_3, respectively, have been demonstrated in various CNS regions, including those involved in micturition control.[166–170] Much attention has focused on both spinal and supraspinal NK receptors as therapeutic targets in different disorders, including DO. At the spinal level, tachykinin involvement via NK_1 receptors was demonstrated in the micturition reflex induced by bladder filling,[171] both in normal rats and in rats with bladder hypertrophy secondary to bladder outflow obstruction. When NK_1 receptor-expressing neurons in the spinal cord were eliminated by using saporin, a ribosome-inactivating protein, conjugated with a specific ligand of NK_1 receptors (SSP–SAP), capsaicin-induced DO was reduced.[172]

SSP–SAP treatment also decreased c-*fos* expression in the dorsal horn of the spinal cord induced by instillation of capsaicin into the bladder, and it was suggested that SSP–SAP could be effective to treat DO induced by bladder irritation without affecting normal bladder function.[172] Spinal NK_1 receptor blockade could also suppress detrusor activity induced by dopamine receptor (L-DOPA) stimulation.[173]

At the supraspinal level, NK receptor stimulation by intracerebroventricular injection of SP (NK_1 receptors), but not by selective NK_2 and NK_3 receptor agonists, was found to inhibit isovolumetric contractions in urethane anesthetized rats.[174] However, in conscious rats, intracerebroventricular SP stimulated micturition.[175] In conscious rats undergoing continuous cystometry, antagonists of both NK_1 and NK_2 receptors inhibited micturition, decreasing micturition pressure and increasing bladder capacity at low doses, and inducing dribbling incontinence at high doses. This was most conspicuous in animals with outflow obstruction.[176] Intracerebroventricular

administration of NK_1 and NK_2 receptor antagonists to awake rats suppressed detrusor activity induced by dopamine receptor (L-DOPA) stimulation.[177] It may be that the differences between the results of Palea et al.[174] and later investigators can be attributed to differences in experimental conditions (including anesthesia).

The development of non-peptide NK_1 receptor antagonists has revealed species differences in their affinity to NK receptors (rat and mouse differing from guinea pig and humans[178]). Even if functional results are available only from animal studies, it seems reasonable to assume that spinal and supraspinal NK_1 and NK_2 receptors, but probably not NK_3 receptors, are involved in micturition control also in humans.[166] Ongoing studies with selective NK receptor antagonists will reveal whether NK receptors are useful targets for drugs aiming at control of micturition disturbances.

CONCLUSION

To effectively control bladder activity, and to treat DO/OAB, the identification of suitable targets for pharmacological intervention is necessary. Such targets may be found in the CNS or peripherally. Drugs specifically directed at the control of bladder activity are under development and will hopefully lead to improved treatment of urinary incontinence.

ACKNOWLEDGMENT

This study was supported by the Swedish Medical Research Council (grant no. 6837).

REFERENCES

1. Ouslander JG. Management of overactive bladder. N Engl J Med 2004; 350: 786–99.
2. Andersson K-E, Appell R, Cardozo L et al. Pharmacological treatment of urinary incontinence. In: Abrams P, Cardozo L, Khoury S, Wein A, eds. Incontinence. Plymouth, UK: Health Publication Ltd, 2005: 811–54.
3. Andersson KE, Wein AJ. Pharmacology of the lower urinary tract: basis for current and future treatments of urinary incontinence. Pharmacol Rev 2004; 56: 581–631.

4. Morrison J, Birder L, Craggs M et al. In: Abrams P, Cardozo L, Khoury S, Wein A, eds. Incontinence. Plymouth, UK: Health Publication Ltd, 2005: 363–422.

5. Caulfield MP, Birdsall NJM. International Union of Pharmacology: XVII. Classification of muscarinic acetylcholine receptors. Pharmacol Rev 1998; 50: 279–90.

6. Sigala S, Mirabella G, Peroni A et al. Differential gene expression of cholinergic muscarinic receptor subtypes in male and female normal human urinary bladder. Urology 2002; 60: 719–25.

7. Yamaguchi O, Shishido K, Tamura K et al. Evaluation of mRNAs encoding muscarinic receptor subtypes in human detrusor muscle. J Urol 1996; 156: 1208–13.

8. Eglen RM, Hegde SS, Watson N. Muscarinic receptor subtypes and smooth muscle function. Pharmacol Rev 1996; 48: 531–65.

9. Hegde SS, Eglen RM. Muscarinic receptor subtypes modulating smooth muscle contractility in the urinary bladder. Life Sci 1999; 64: 419–28.

10. Chess-Williams R. Muscarinic receptors of the urinary bladder: detrusor, urothelial and prejunctional. Auton Autacoid Pharmacol 2002; 22: 133–45.

11. Krichevsky VP, Pagala MK, Vaydovsky I, Damer V, Wise GJ. Function of M3 muscarinic receptors in the rat urinary bladder following partial outlet obstruction. J Urol 1999; 161: 1644–50.

12. Andersson KE, Holmquist F, Fovaeus M et al. Muscarinic receptor stimulation of phosphoinositide hydrolysis in the human isolated urinary bladder. J Urol 1991; 146: 1156–9.

13. Harriss DR, Marsh KA, Birmingham AT, Hill SJ. Expression of muscarinic M3-receptors coupled to inositol phospholipid hydrolysis in human detrusor cultured smooth muscle cells. J Urol 1995; 154: 1241–5.

14. Jezior JR, Brady JD, Rosenstein DI et al. Dependency of detrusor contractions on calcium sensitization and calcium entry through LOE-908-sensitive channels. Br J Pharmacol 2001; 134: 78–87.

15. Wibberley A, Chen Z, Hu E, Hieble JP, Westfall TD. Expression and functional role of Rho-kinase in rat urinary bladder smooth muscle. Br J Pharmacol 2003; 138: 757–66.

16. Schneider T, Fetscher C, Krege S, Michel MC. Signal transduction underlying carbachol-induced contraction of human urinary bladder. J Pharmacol Exp Ther 2004; 309: 1148–53.

17. Braverman AS, Tibb AS, Ruggieri MR Sr. M2 and M3 muscarinic receptor activation of urinary bladder contractile signal transduction. I. Normal rat bladder. J Pharmacol Exp Ther 2006; 316: 869–74.

18. Takahashi R, Nishimura J, Hirano K et al. Ca^{2+} sensitization in contraction of human bladder smooth muscle. J Urol 2004; 172: 748–52.

19. Hegde SS, Choppin A, Bonhaus D et al. Functional role of M-2 and M-3 muscarinic receptors in the urinary bladder of rats in vitro and in vivo. Br J Pharmacol 1997; 120: 1409–18.

20. Kotlikoff MI, Dhulipala P, Wang YX. M2 signaling in smooth muscle cells. Life Sci 1999; 64: 437–42.

21. Bonev AD, Nelson MT. Muscarinic inhibition of ATP-sensitive K$^+$ channels by protein kinase C in urinary bladder smooth muscle. Am J Physiol 1993; 265: C1723–8.

22. Nakamura T, Kimura J, Yamaguchi O. Muscarinic M2 receptors inhibit Ca2$^+$-activated K$^+$ channels in rat bladder smooth muscle. Int J Urol 2002; 9: 689–96.

23. Braverman AS, Luthin GR, Ruggieri MR. M2 muscarinic receptor contributes to contraction of the denervated rat urinary bladder. Am J Physiol 1998; 275: R1654–60.

24. Braverman A, Legos J, Young W, Luthin G, Ruggieri M. M2 receptors in genito-urinary smooth muscle pathology. Life Sci 1999; 64: 429–36.

25. Braverman AS, Tallarida RJ, Ruggieri MR Sr. Interaction between muscarinic receptor subtype signal transduction pathways mediating bladder contraction. Am J Physiol Regul Integr Comp Physiol 2002; 283: R663–8.

26. Braverman AS, Doumanian LR, Ruggieri MR Sr. M2 and M3 muscarinic receptor activation of urinary bladder contractile signal transduction. II. Denervated rat bladder. J Pharmacol Exp Ther 2006; 316: 875–80.

27. Braverman AS, Ruggieri MR Sr. Hypertrophy changes the muscarinic receptor subtype mediating bladder contraction from M3 toward M2. Am J Physiol Regul Integr Comp Physiol 2003; 285: R701–8.

28. Stevens L, Chapple C, Tophill P, Chess-Williams R. A comparison of muscarinic receptor-mediated function in the normal and the neurogenic overactive bladder. J Urol 2004; 171: 143 (abstr 535).

29. Stevens L, Chess-Williams R, Chapple C. Muscarinic receptor function in the idiopathic overactive bladder. J Urol 2004; 171: 140–1 (abstr 527).

30. Pontari MA, Braverman AS, Ruggieri MR Sr. The M2 muscarinic receptor mediates in vitro bladder contractions from patients with neurogenic bladder dysfunction. Am J Physiol Regul Integr Comp Physiol 2004; 286: R874–80.
31. Tobin G, Sjögren C. Prejunctional facilitatory and inhibitory modulation of parasympathetic nerve transmission in the rabbit urinary bladder. J Auton Nerv Syst 1998; 68: 153–6.
32. Inadome A, Yoshida M, Takahashi W et al. Prejunctional muscarinic receptors modulating acetylcholine release in rabbit detrusor smooth muscles. Urol Int 1998; 61: 135–41.
33. Somogyi GT, de Groat WC. Evidence for inhibitory nicotinic and facilitatory muscarinic receptors in cholinergic nerve terminals of the rat urinary bladder. J Auton Nerv Syst 1992; 37: 89–98.
34. Alberts P. Classification of the presynaptic muscarinic receptor subtype that regulates 3H-acetylcholine secretion in the guinea pig urinary bladder in vitro. J Pharmacol Exp Ther 1995; 274: 458–68.
35. D'Agostino G, Barbieri A, Chiossa E, Tonini M. M4 muscarinic autoreceptor-mediated inhibition of -3H-acetylcholine release in the rat isolated urinary bladder. J Pharmacol Exp Ther 1997; 283: 750–6.
36. D'Agostino G, Bolognesi ML, Lucchelli A et al. Prejunctional muscarinic inhibitory control of acetylcholine release in the human isolated detrusor: involvement of the M4 receptor subtype. Br J Pharmacol 2000; 129: 493–500.
37. Somogyi GT, de Groat WC. Function, signal transduction mechanisms and plasticity of presynaptic muscarinic receptors in the urinary bladder. Life Sci 1999; 64: 411–18.
38. Somogyi GT, Zernova GV, Yoshiyama M et al. Change in muscarinic modulation of transmitter release in the rat urinary bladder after spinal cord injury. Neurochem Int 2003; 43: 73–7.
39. Mansfield KJ, Liu L, Mitchelson FJ et al. Muscarinic receptor subtypes in human bladder detrusor and mucosa, studied by radioligand binding and quantitative competitive RT-PCR: changes in ageing. Br J Pharmacol 2005; 144: 1089–99.
40. Hawthorn MH, Chapple CR, Cock M et al. Urothelium-derived inhibitory factor(s) influences on detrusor muscle contractility in vitro. Br J Pharmacol 2000; 129: 416–19.
41. Yokoyama O, Yusup A, Miwa Y et al. Effects of tolterodine on an overactive bladder depend on suppression of C-fiber bladder afferent activity in rats. J Urol 2005; 174: 2032–6.
42. De Wachter S, De Laet K, Wyndaele JJ. Does the cystometric filling rate affect the afferent bladder response pattern? A study on single fibre pelvic nerve afferents in the rat urinary bladder. Neurourol Urodyn 2006; 25: 162–7.
43. Boy S, Schurch B, Nehring G et al. The effect of tolterodine on sensations evoked by electrical stimulation and bladder filling sensations. Eur Urol Suppl 2006; 5: 223 (abstr 804).
44. Andersson K-E. Antimuscarinics for treatment of overactive bladder. Lancet Neurol 2004; 3: 46–53.
45. De Groat WC, Booth AM, Yoshimura N. Neurophysiology of micturition and its modification in animal models of human disease. In: Maggi CA, ed. Nervous Control of the Urogenital System. London: Harwood Academic Publishers, 1993; 227–90.
46. Yoshida M, Miyamae K, Iwashita H, Otani M, Inadome A. Management of detrusor dysfunction in the elderly: changes in acetylcholine and adenosine triphosphate release during aging. Urology 2004; 63 (3 Suppl 1): 17–23.
47. Andersson K-E, Yoshida M. Antimuscarinics and the overactive detrusor – which is the main mechanism of action? Eur Urol 2003; 43: 1–5.
48. Brading AF. A myogenic basis for the overactive bladder. Urology 1997; 50 (6A Suppl): 57–67.
49. Goepel M, Wittmann A, Rubben H, Michel MC. Comparison of adrenoceptor subtype expression in porcine and human bladder and prostate. Urol Res 1997; 25: 199–206.
50. Malloy BJ, Price DT, Price RR et al. Alpha1-adrenergic receptor subtypes in human detrusor. J Urol 1998; 160: 937–43.
51. Michel MC, Vrydag W. Alpha(1)-, alpha(2)- and beta-adrenoceptors in the urinary bladder, urethra and prostate. Br J Pharmacol 2006; 147 (Suppl 2): S88–119.
52. Hampel C, Dolber PC, Smith MP et al. Modulation of bladder alpha1-adrenergic receptor subtype expression by bladder outlet obstruction. J Urol 2002; 167: 1513–21.
53. Nomiya M, Yamaguchi O. A quantitative analysis of mRNA expression of alpha 1 and beta-adrenoceptor subtypes and their functional

roles in human normal and obstructed bladders. J Urol 2003; 170: 649–53.

54. Bouchelouche K, Andersen L, Alvarez S, Nordling J, Bouchelouche P. Increased contractile response to phenylephrine in detrusor of patients with bladder outlet obstruction: effect of the alpha1A and alpha1D-adrenergic receptor antagonist tamsulosin. J Urol 2005; 173: 657–61.

55. Chen Q, Takahashi S, Zhong S et al. Function of the lower urinary tract in mice lacking alpha1d-adrenoceptor. J Urol 2005; 174: 370–4.

56. Ishihama H, Momota Y, Yanase H et al. Activation of alpha1D adrenergic receptors in the rat urothelium facilitates the micturition reflex. J Urol 2006; 175: 358–64.

57. Sugaya K, Nishijima S, Miyazato M et al. Effects of intrathecal injection of tamsulosin and naftopidil, alpha-1A and -1D adrenergic receptor antagonists, on bladder activity in rats. Neurosci Lett 2002; 328: 74–6.

58. Ikemoto I, Kiyota H, Ohishi Y et al. Usefulness of tamsulosin hydrochloride and naftopidil in patients with urinary disturbances caused by benign prostatic hyperplasia: a comparative, randomized, two-drug crossover study. Int J Urol 2003; 10: 587–94.

59. Gotoh M, Kamihira O, Kinukawa T et al. Tokai Urological Clinical Trial Group. Comparison of tamsulosin and naftopidil for efficacy and safety in the treatment of benign prostatic hyperplasia: a randomized controlled trial. BJU Int 2005; 96: 581–6.

60. Das AK, Leggett RE, Whitbeck C, Eagen G, Levin RM. Effect of doxazosin on rat urinary bladder function after partial outlet obstruction. Neurourol Urodyn 2002; 21: 160–6.

61. Pinggera G-M, Schuster A, Pallwein L et al. Alpha-blockers increase vesical and prostatic blood flow and bladder capacity. Eur Urol Suppl 2003; 2: 159 (abstr 628).

62. Andersson K-E. Pharmacology of lower urinary tract smooth muscles and penile erectile tissues. Pharmacol Rev 1993; 45: 253–308.

63. Gary T, Robertson D. Lessons learned from dopamine β-hydroxylase deficiency in humans. News Physiol Sci 1994; 9: 35–9.

64. Yamaguchi O. Beta3-adrenoceptors in human detrusor muscle. Urology 2002; 59 (Suppl 1): 25–9.

65. Hudman D, Elliott RA, Whitaker P et al. Inhibition of the contractile responses of isolated human and rat bladders by clenbuterol. J Urol 2001; 166: 1969–73.

66. Grüneberger A. Treatment of motor urge incontinence with clenbuterol and flavoxate hydrochloride. Br J Obstet Gynaecol 1984; 91: 275–8.

67. Lindholm P, Lose G. Terbutaline (Bricanyl) in the treatment of female urge incontinence. Urol Int 1986; 41: 158–60.

68. Nakahira Y, Hashitani H, Fukuta H et al. Effects of isoproterenol on spontaneous excitations in detrusor smooth muscle cells of the guinea pig. J Urol 2001; 166: 335–40.

69. Kobayashi H, Adachi-Akahane S, Nagao T. Involvement of BK(Ca) channels in the relaxation of detrusor muscle via beta-adrenoceptors. Eur J Pharmacol 2000; 404: 231–8.

70. Uchida H, Shishido K, Nomiya M, Yamaguchi O. Involvement of cyclic AMP-dependent and -independent mechanisms in the relaxation of rat detrusor muscle via beta-adrenoceptors. Eur J Pharmacol 2005; 518: 195–202.

71. Woods M, Carson N, Norton NW, Sheldon JH, Argentieri TM. Efficacy of the beta3-adrenergic receptor agonist CL-316243 on experimental bladder hyperreflexia and detrusor instability in the rat. J Urol 2001; 166: 1142–7.

72. Kaidoh K, Igawa Y, Takeda H et al. Effects of selective beta2 and beta3-adrenoceptor agonists on detrusor hyperreflexia in conscious cerebral infarcted rats. J Urol 2002; 168: 1247–52.

73. Takeda H, Yamazaki Y, Igawa Y et al. Effects of beta(3)-adrenoceptor stimulation on prostaglandin E(2)-induced bladder hyperactivity and on the cardiovascular system in conscious rats. Neurourol Urodyn 2002; 21: 558–65.

74. Andersson KE, Arner A. Urinary bladder contraction and relaxation: physiology and pathophysiology. Physiol Rev 2004; 84: 935–86.

75. Berridge MJ, Bootman MD, Roderick HL. Calcium signalling: dynamics, homeostasis and remodelling. Nat Rev Mol Cell Biol 2003; 4: 517–29.

76. Forman A, Andersson KE, Henriksson L et al. Effects of nifedipine on the smooth muscle of the human urinary tract in vitro and in vivo. Acta Pharmacol Toxicol 1978; 43: 111–18.

77. Diederichs W, Sroka J, Graff J. Comparison of Bay K 8644, nitrendipine and atropine on spontaneous and pelvic-nerve-induced bladder contractions on rat bladder in vivo. Urol Res 1992; 20: 49–53.

78. Andersson KE. Current concepts in the treatment of disorders of micturition. Drugs 1988; 35: 477–94.

79. Wegener JW, Schulla V, Lee TS et al. An essential role of Cav1.2 L-type calcium channel for urinary bladder function. FASEB J 2004; 18: 1159–61.

80. Shapiro E, Tang R, Rosenthal E, Lepor H. The binding and functional properties of voltage dependent calcium channel receptors in pediatric normal and myelodysplastic bladders. J Urol 1991; 146: 520–3.

81. Herrera GM, Pozo MJ, Zvara P et al. Urinary bladder instability induced by selective suppression of the murine small conductance calcium-activated potassium (SK3) channel. J Physiol 2003; 551: 893–903.

82. Meredith AL, Thorneloe KS, Werner ME, Nelson MT, Aldrich RW. Overactive bladder and incontinence in the absence of the BK large conductance Ca^{2+}-activated K^+ channel. J Biol Chem 2004; 279: 36746–52.

83. Thorneloe KS, Meredith AL, Knorn AM, Aldrich RW, Nelson MT. Urodynamic properties and neurotransmitter dependence of urinary bladder contractility in the BK channel deletion model of overactive bladder. Am J Physiol Renal Physiol 2005; 289: F604–10.

84. Petkov GV, Bonev AD, Heppner TJ et al. Beta1-subunit of the Ca^{2+}-activated K^+ channel regulates contractile activity of mouse urinary bladder smooth muscle. J Physiol 2001; 537: 443–52.

85. Turner SC, Carroll WA, White TK et al. Structure-activity relationship of a novel class of naphthyl amide KATP channel openers. Bioorg Med Chem Lett 2003; 13: 1741–4.

86. Christ GJ, Day NS, Day M et al. Bladder injection of "naked" hSlo/pcDNA3 ameliorates detrusor hyperactivity in obstructed rats in vivo. Am J Physiol Regul Integr Comp Physiol 2001; 281: R1699–709.

87. Hedlund H, Mattiasson A, Andersson KE. Effects of pinacidil on detrusor instability in men with bladder outlet obstruction. J Urol 1991; 146: 1345–7.

88. Komersova K, Rogerson JW, Conway EL et al. The effect of levcromakalim (BRL 38227) on bladder function in patients with high spinal cord lesions. Br J Clin Pharmacol 1995; 39: 207–9.

89. Howe BB, Halterman TJ, Yochim CL et al. Zeneca ZD6169: a novel KATP channel opener with in vivo selectivity for urinary bladder. J Pharmacol Exp Ther 1995; 274: 884–90.

90. Chapple CR, Patroneva A, Raines RR. Effects of ZD0947, an ATP-sensitive potassium channel opener, in subjects with overactive bladder: a randomized, double-blind, placebo-controlled study (ZD0947IL/0004). Eur Urol 2006; 49: 879–86.

91. Maggi CA. The mammalian tachykinin receptors. Gen Pharmacol 1995; 26: 911–44.

92. Szallasi A. The vanilloid (capsaicin) receptor: receptor types and species differences. Gen Pharmacol 1994; 25: 223–43.

93. Maggi CA. The dual sensory and "efferent" function of the capsaicin-sensitive primary sensory neurons in the urinary bladder and urethra. In: Maggi CA, ed. Nervous Control of the Urogenital System. London: Harwood Academic Publishers, 1993: 383–422.

94. Ishizuka O, Mattiasson A, Andersson KE. Urodynamic effects of intravesical resiniferatoxin and capsaicin in conscious rats with and without outflow obstruction. J Urol 1995; 154: 611–16.

95. Szallazi A, Blumberg PM. Vanilloid receptors: new insights enhance potential as a therapeutic target. Pain 1996; 68: 195–208.

96. Kuo H-C. Inhibitory effect of capsaicin on detrusor contractility: further study in the presence of ganglionic blocker and neurokinin receptor antagonist in the rat urinary bladder. Urol Int 1997; 59: 95–101.

97. de Groat WC, Yoshimura N. Mechanisms underlying the recovery of lower urinary tract function following spinal cord injury. Prog Brain Res 2006; 152: 59–84.

98. Maggi CA, Barbanti G, Santicioli P et al. Cystometric evidence that capsaicin-sensitive nerves modulate the afferent branch of micturition reflex in humans. J Urol 1989; 142: 150–4.

99. Chandiramani VA, Peterson T, Duthie GS, Fowler CJ. Urodynamic changes during therapeutic intravesical instillations of capsaicin. Br J Urol 1996; 77: 792–7.

100. Dasgupta P, Chandiramani V, Parkinson MC, Beckett A, Fowler CJ. Treating the human bladder with capsaicin: is it safe? Eur Urol 1998; 33: 28–31.

101. Silva C, Silva J, Ribeiro MJ, Avelino A, Cruz F. Urodynamic effect of intravesical resiniferatoxin in patients with neurogenic detrusor overactivity of spinal origin: results of a double-blind randomized placebo-controlled trial. Eur Urol 2005; 48: 650–5.

102. Yokoyama T, Kumon H, Smith CP et al. Botulinum toxin treatment of urethral and bladder dysfunction. Acta Med Okayama 2002; 56: 271–7.

103. Smith CP, Franks ME, McNeil BK et al. Effect of botulinum toxin A on the autonomic nervous system of the rat lower urinary tract. J Urol 2003; 169: 1896–900.

104. Simpson LL. Identification of the major steps in botulinum toxin action. Annu Rev Pharmacol Toxicol 2004; 44: 167–93.

105. Apostolidis A, Dasgupta P, Fowler CJ. Proposed mechanism for the efficacy of injected botulinum toxin in the treatment of human detrusor overactivity. Eur Urol 2006; 49: 644–50.

106. Leippold T, Reitz A, Schurch B. Botulinum toxin as a new therapy option for voiding disorders: current state of the art. Eur Urol 2003; 44: 165–74.

107. Cruz F, Silva C. Botulinum toxin in the management of lower urinary tract dysfunction: contemporary update. Curr Opin Urol 2004; 14: 329–34.

108. Sahai A, Khan M, Fowler CJ, Dasgupta P. Botulinum toxin for the treatment of lower urinary tract symptoms: a review. Neurourol Urodyn 2005; 24: 2–12.

109. Schurch B, Corcos J. Botulinum toxin injections for paediatric incontinence. Curr Opin Urol 2005; 15: 264–7.

110. Rapp D, Lucioni A, Katz EE et al. Use of botulinum-A toxin for the treatment of refractory overactive bladder symptoms: an initial experience. Urology 2004; 63: 1071–5.

111. Kalsi V, Apostolidis A, Popat R et al. Quality of life changes in patients with neurogenic versus idiopathic detrusor overactivity after intradetrusor injections of botulinum neurotoxin type A and correlations with lower urinary tract symptoms and urodynamic changes. Eur Urol 2006; 49: 528–35.

112. De Laet K, Wyndaele JJ. Adverse events after botulinum A toxin injection for neurogenic voiding disorders. Spinal Cord 2005; 43: 397–9.

113. Shefchyk SJ. Spinal cord neural organization controlling the urinary bladder and striated sphincter. Prog Brain Res 2002; 137: 71–82.

114. Griffiths DJ. Cerebral control of bladder function. Curr Urol Rep 2004; 5: 348–52.

115. Griffiths D, Derbyshire S, Stenger A, Resnick N. Brain control of normal and overactive bladder. J Urol 2005; 174: 1862–7.

116. Holstege G. Micturition and the soul. J Comp Neurol 2005; 493: 15–20.

117. Sugaya K, Nishijima S, Miyazato M, Ogawa Y. Central nervous control of micturition and urine storage. J Smooth Muscle Res 2005; 41: 117–32.

118. de Groat WC, Yoshimura N. Pharmacology of the lower urinary tract. Annu Rev Pharmacol Toxicol 2001; 41: 691–721.

119. Yoshiyama M, de Groat WC. Supraspinal and spinal alpha-amino-3-hydroxy-5-methylisoxazole-4-propionic acid and N-methyl-D-aspartate glutamatergic control of the micturition reflex in the urethane-anesthetized rat. Neuroscience 2005; 132: 1017–26.

120. Andersson KE, Pehrson R. CNS involvement in overactive bladder: pathophysiology and opportunities for pharmacological intervention. Drugs 2003; 63: 2595–611.

121. Murray KH, Feneley RC. Endorphins—a role in lower urinary tract function? The effect of opioid blockade on the detrusor and urethral sphincter mechanisms. Br J Urol 1982; 54: 638–40.

122. Dray A, Nunan L, Wire W. Naloxonazine and opioid-induced inhibition of reflex urinary bladder contractions. Neuropharmacology 1987; 26: 67–74.

123. Igawa Y, Andersson KE, Post C, Uvelius B, Mattiasson A. A rat model for investigation of spinal mechanisms in detrusor instability associated with infravesical outflow obstruction. Urol Res 1993; 21: 239–44.

124. Igawa Y, Westerling D, Mattiasson A, Andersson KE. Effects of morphine metabolites on micturition in normal, unanaesthetized rats. Br J Pharmacol 1993; 110: 257–62.

125. Herman RM, Wainberg MC, delGiudice PF, Willscher MK. The effect of a low dose of intrathecal morphine on impaired micturition reflexes in human subjects with spinal cord lesions. Anesthesiology 1988; 69: 313–18.

126. Kieffer BL. Opioids: first lessons from knockout mice. Trends Pharmacol Sci 1999; 20: 19–26.

127. Raffa RB, Friderichs E. The basic science aspect of tramadol hydrochloride. Pain Rev 1996; 3: 249–71.

128. Pandita RK, Pehrson R, Christoph T, Friderichs E, Andersson KE. Actions of tramadol on micturition in awake, freely moving rats. Br J Pharmacol 2003; 139: 741–8.

129. Pehrson R, Stenman E, Andersson KE. Effects of tramadol on rat detrusor overactivity induced by experimental cerebral infarction. Eur Urol 2003; 44: 495–9.

130. Pehrson R, Andersson KE. Tramadol inhibits rat detrusor overactivity caused by dopamine receptor stimulation. J Urol 2003; 170: 272–5.

131. Thor KB, Nickolaus S, Helke CJ. Autoradiographic localization of 5-hydroxytryptamine1A, 5-hydroxytryptamine1B and 5-hydroxytryptamine1C/2 binding sites in the rat spinal cord. Neuroscience 1993; 55: 235–52.

132. Ramage AG. The role of central 5-hydroxytryptamine (5-HT, serotonin) receptors in the control of micturition. Br J Pharmacol 2006; 147 (Suppl 2): S120–31.

133. de Groat WC. Influence of central serotonergic mechanisms on lower urinary tract function. Urology 2002; 59 (5 Suppl 1): 30–6.

134. McMahon SB, Spillane K. Brain stem influences on the parasympathetic supply to the urinary bladder of the cat. Brain Res 1982; 234: 237–49.

135. Sugaya K, Ogawa Y, Hatano T et al. Evidence for involvement of the subcoeruleus nucleus and nucleus raphe magnus in urine storage and penile erection in decerebrate rats. J Urol 1998; 159: 2172–6.

136. Tai C, Miscik CL, Ungerer TD, Roppolo JR, de Groat WC. Suppression of bladder reflex activity in chronic spinal cord injured cats by activation of serotonin 5-HT(1A) receptors. Exp Neurol 2006; 199: 427–37.

137. Movig KL, Leufkens HG, Belitser SV, Lenderink AW, Egberts AC. Selective serotonin reuptake inhibitor-induced urinary incontinence. Pharmacoepidemiol Drug Saf 2002; 11: 271–9.

138. Bowery NG. GABA$_B$ receptor pharmacology. Annu Rev Pharmacol Toxicol 1993; 33: 109–47.

139. Rudolph U, Crestani F, Möhler H. GABA$_A$ receptor subtypes: dissecting their pharmacological functions. Trends Pharmacol Sci 2001; 22: 188–94.

140. Chebib M, Johnston GAR. The 'ABC' of GABA receptors: a brief review. Clin Exp Pharmacol Physiol 1999; 26: 937–40.

141. Igawa Y, Mattiasson A, Andersson KE. Effects of GABA-receptor stimulation and blockade on micturition in normal rats and rats with bladder outflow obstruction. J Urol 1993; 150: 537–42.

142. Pehrson R, Lehmann A, Andersson KE. Effects of gamma-aminobutyrate B receptor modulation on normal micturition and oxyhemoglobin induced detrusor overactivity in female rats. J Urol 2002; 168: 2700–5.

143. Maggi CA, Furio M, Santicioli P, Conte B, Meli A. Spinal and supraspinal components of GABAergic inhibition of the micturition reflex in rats. J Pharm Exp Ther 1987; 240: 998–1005.

144. Malcangio M, Bowery NG. GABA and its receptors in the spinal cord. Trends Pharmacol Sci 1996; 17: 457–62.

145. Coggeshall RE, Carlton SM. Receptor localization in the mammalian dorsal horn and primary afferent neurons. Brain Res Brain Res Rev 1997; 24: 28–66.

146. Jursky F, Tamura S, Tamura A et al. Structure, function and brain localization of neurotransmitter transporters. J Exp Biol 1994; 196: 283–95.

147. Borden LA, Murali Dhar TG, Smith KE et al. Tiagabine, SK&F 89976-A, CI-966, and NNC-711 are selective for the cloned GABA transporter GAT-1. Eur J Pharmacol 1994; 269: 219–24.

148. Fink-Jensen A, Suzdak PD, Swedberg MDB et al. The γ-aminobutyric acid (GABA) uptake inhibitor, tiagabine, increases extracellular brain levels of GABA in awake rats. Eur J Pharmacol 1992; 220: 197–201.

149. Pehrson R, Andersson KE. Effects of tiagabine, a gamma-aminobutyric acid re-uptake inhibitor, on normal rat bladder function. J Urol 2002; 167: 2241–6.

150. Maggi CA, Santicioli P, Giuliani S et al. The effects of baclofen on spinal and supraspinal micturition reflexes in rats. Naunyn Schmiedebergs Arch Pharmacol 1987; 336: 197–203.

151. Zhu Q-M, Hu D-Q, Tsung S, Blue DR, Ford AP. Differential effects of GABA$_A$ and GABA$_B$ receptor agonists on cystometry in conscious mice. J Urol 2002; 167 (Suppl): 39–40 (abstr 157).

152. Blok BF, de Weerd H, Holstege G. The pontine micturition center projects to sacral cord GABA immunoreactive neurons in the cat. Neurosci Lett 1997; 233: 109–12.

153. Rekling JC, Funk GD, Bayliss DA, Dong XW, Feldman JL. Synaptic control of motoneuronal excitability. Physiol Rev 2000; 80: 767–852.

154. Maneuf YP, Gonzalez MI, Sutton KS et al. Cellular and molecular action of the putative GABA-mimetic, gabapentin. Cell Mol Life Sci 2003; 60: 742–50.

155. Gee NS, Brown JP, Dissanayake VU et al. The novel anticonvulsant drug, gabapentin (Neurontin), binds to the alpha2delta subunit of a calcium channel. J Biol Chem 1996; 271: 5768–76.

156. Carbone A, Tubaro A, Morello P et al. The effect of gabapentin on neurogenic detrusor overactivity, a pilot study. Eur Urol Suppl 2003; 2: 141 (abstr 555).

157. Kim YT, Kwon DD, Kim J et al. Gabapentin for overactive bladder and nocturia after anticholinergic failure. Int Braz J Urol 2004; 30: 275–8.

158. Yoshiyama M, Yamamoto T, de Groat WC. Role of spinal alpha(1)-adrenergic mechanisms in the control of lower urinary tract in the rat. Brain Res 2000; 882: 36–44.

159. Ishizuka O, Persson K, Mattiasson A et al. Micturition in conscious rats with and without bladder outlet obstruction – role of spinal alpha(1)-adrenoceptors. Br J Pharmacol 1996; 117: 962–6.

160. Persson K, Pandita RK, Spitsbergen JM et al. Spinal and peripheral mechanisms contributing to hyperactive voiding in spontaneously hypertensive rats. Am J Physiol 1998; 275: R1366–73.

161. Andersson K-E. Mechanisms of disease: central nervous system involvement in overactive bladder syndrome. Nat Clin Pract Urol 2004; 1: 103–8.

162. Yoshimura N, Mizuta E, Kuno S et al. The dopamine D1 receptor agonist SKF 38393 suppresses detrusor hyperreflexia in the monkey with parkinsonism induced by 1-methyl-4 phenyl-1,2,3,6-tetrahydropyridine (MPTP). Neuropharmacology 1993; 32: 315–21.

163. Sillén U, Rubenson A, Hjalmas K. On the localization and mediation of the centrally induced hyperactive urinary bladder response to L-dopa in the rat. Acta Physiol Scand 1981; 112: 137–40.

164. Kontani H, Inoue T, Sakai T. Dopamine receptor subtypes that induce hyperactive urinary bladder response in anesthetized rats. Jpn J Pharmacol 1990; 54: 482–6.

165. Kontani H, Inoue T, Sakai T. Effects of apomorphine on urinary bladder motility in anesthetized rats. Jpn J Pharmacol 1990; 52: 59–67.

166. Lecci A, Maggi CA. Tachykinins as modulators of the micturition reflex in the central and peripheral nervous system. Regul Pept 2001; 101: 1–18.

167. Saffroy M, Torrens Y, Glowinski J, Beaujouan JC. Presence of NK2 binding sites in the rat brain. J Neurochem 2001; 79: 985–96.

168. Saffroy M, Torrens Y, Glowinski J, Beaujouan JC. Autoradiographic distribution of tachykinin NK2 binding sites in the rat brain: comparison with NK1 and NK3 binding sites. Neuroscience 2003; 116: 761–73.

169. Covenas R, Martin F, Belda M et al. Mapping of neurokinin-like immunoreactivity in the human brainstem. BMC Neurosci 2003; 4: 3.

170. Nagano M, Saitow F, Haneda E et al. Distribution and pharmacological characterization of primate NK-1 and NK-3 tachykinin receptors in the central nervous system of the rhesus monkey. Br J Pharmacol 2006; 147: 316–23.

171. Ishizuka O, Igawa Y, Lecci A et al. Role of intrathecal tachykinins for micturition in unanaesthetized rats with and without bladder outlet obstruction. Br J Pharmacol 1994; 113: 111–16.

172. Seki S, Erickson KA, Seki M et al. Elimination of rat spinal neurons expressing neurokinin 1 receptors reduces bladder overactivity and spinal c-fos expression induced by bladder irritation. Am J Physiol Renal Physiol 2005; 288: F466–73.

173. Ishizuka O, Mattiasson A, Andersson KE. Effects of neurokinin receptor antagonists on L-dopa induced bladder hyperactivity in normal conscious rats. J Urol 1995; 154: 1548–51.

174. Palea S, Dalforno G, Gaviraghi G et al. Further studies on the effects of selective neurokinin agonists upon the activation of micturition reflex in rats. Evidence for a dual NK-1 receptor mediated excitatory and inhibitory activity. Neuropeptides 1993; 24: 285–91.

175. Dib B, Corsi MM, Fulgenzi A, Ferrero ME, Falchi M. Intracerebroventricular injection of capsaicin or substance P provokes the micturition reflex in the rat. Int J Tissue React 1998; 20: 109–14.

176. Gu BJ, Ishizuka O, Igawa Y, Nishizawa O, Andersson KE. Role of supraspinal tachykinins for micturition in conscious rats with and without bladder outlet obstruction. Naunyn Schmiedebergs Arch Pharmacol 2000; 361: 543–8.

177. Ishizuka O, Igawa Y, Nishizawa O, Andersson KE. Role of supraspinal tachykinins for volume- and L-dopa-induced bladder activity in normal conscious rats. Neurourol Urodyn 2000; 19: 101–9.

178. Stout SC, Owens MJ, Nemeroff CB. Neurokinin(1) receptor antagonists as potential antidepressants. Annu Rev Pharmacol Toxicol 2001; 41: 877–906.

10

Drug delivery and intravesical instillation

Pradeep Tyagi and Michael B Chancellor

Introduction • **Drug delivery** • **Intravesical instillation** • **Barriers to absorption after instillation**
• **Conclusion** • **Acknowledgment**

INTRODUCTION

Overactive bladder (OAB) continues to plague millions of patients. Existing management of this serious malady involves pharmacological manipulation of the micturition reflex. The reflex comprises two arms, the afferent nerve signaling by C fibers and Aδ fibers, and the efferent branch constituted by sympathetic and parasympathetic nerves. One of the predominant treatment modalities targets the cholinergic transmission in the efferent branch of the voiding reflex with the use of anticholinergic drugs.[1] Drugs acting at the afferent branch of the micturition reflex such as vanilloids have been only partly successful in the clinic so far.[2,3] Perhaps better analogs and improved drug delivery will be able to change that scenario.

Oral administration of the anticholinergic agent oxybutynin has been the major treatment for OAB for over 30 years. It has been able to produce symptomatic improvement in the majority of patients, and controlled studies have shown advantages for oxybutynin over placebo on subjective and cystometric outcomes. However, differences exist among patients in the tolerability and adverse event profile related to oxybutynin. Consequently, nearly 40% of patients withdraw from this therapy.

Since most adverse effects are produced by drugs acting at sites other than the disease location, it is not unusual for such effects to be associated with therapy acting at efferent branch of the micturition reflex. There seem to be two major ways to reduce the incidence of side effects from therapy. One is to discover drugs with a higher affinity for the drug targets expressed exclusively in the bladder, and the second is selective delivery of the drugs only at the disease site, with lower systemic exposure via the approach of drug delivery. The issue of drug delivery has proved critical in achieving therapeutic success using drugs developed by means of biotechnology. The category of drugs comprising peptides and immunotoxins is characterized by a liability for chemical degradation and an inability to cross cellular membranes.

Regional drug delivery by instillation through the urethra exists as a novel strategy for localizing the effects of the drug inside the bladder (Figure 10.1). This approach has already been evaluated for the delivery of neurotoxic agents such as vanilloids and botulinum toxin into the bladder.[2,4] Drug delivery by instillation offers many benefits compared to alternative routes of drug delivery. The following discussion will be focused on the relative merits of different drug delivery routes with an emphasis on intravesical instillation.

DRUG DELIVERY

It is well accepted that the tolerability and safety profile of oxybutynin following oral administration can be significantly improved by changes in its temporal delivery into the plasma.[5] Being a substrate for CYP3A4, oxybutynin is metabolized into its active metabolite *N*-desethyl-oxybutynin

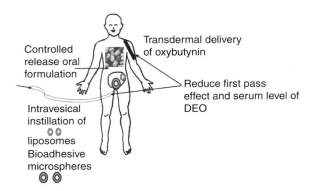

Figure 10.1 Illustration of different delivery systems for drugs in the treatment of overactive bladder: controlled release capsules and transdermal patch of oxybutynin. Oxybutynin can also be instilled as a solution or bioadhesive solution. Liposomes and microspheres are the new drug carriers for instilled drugs. DEO, N-desethyl-oxybutynin.

(DEO) in the liver. The metabolite is considered responsible for the majority of its anticholinergic side effects such as dry mouth, blurred vision, constipation, and tachycardia.[5] These side effects impair patient compliance and often result in a dose reduction or even discontinuation of therapy.

The first pass effect for oxybutynin was revealed by higher serum levels of the parent drug in patients after intravesical instillation, compared with those after oral intake.[6] This was achieved through a controlled release oral formulation of oxybutynin that uses an Oros® Push-Pull™ system. The tablet based on this system contains two layers, whereby the first layer contains the drug and osmotically active hydrophilic polymers, and the second layer (also called the "push" layer) contains a hydrophilic expansion polymer that expands to push the drug from the first layer through an orifice. The polymer expands due to osmosis driven water influx into the system.

Compared to the conventional immediate release formulation of oxybutynin, the controlled release formulation showed higher bioavailability, higher parent drug/metabolite ratio, and a significant extension in the time to achieve peak plasma concentration. The new formulation of oxybutynin not only reduced the degree of fluctuation around the average concentration, but also brought down the incidence of side effects by nearly 20%. However, the controlled release formulation failed to reduce the first pass effect and the rate of adverse effects caused by the oxybutynin metabolite. Although the toxicity of the sustained release capsule was slightly better, there was no distinct change in efficacy.

In an attempt to avoid the effects of this first pass metabolism, various alternative routes of administration have been studied in an effort to alter the spatial release profile of oxybutynin and bypass the liver. A widely acceptable method with a reduced incidence of adverse effects has been the development of a transdermal delivery system for oxybutynin.[5] Application of the transdermal system to intact skin delivers the drug over a period of 3–4 days. Delivery of oxybutynin through the skin alters its pharmacokinetics, and concentrations are maintained below the toxic range throughout the dosage interval. The peak plasma concentrations of oxybutynin and its major metabolite DEO are reached 24–48 hours after application.

Transdermal delivery of oxybutynin demonstrated clinical efficacy similar to that of oral tolterodine or oral oxybutynin, with significant reductions in incontinence episodes.[7] The reduction in plasma DEO levels improved the tolerability profile of oxybutynin, and incidences of side effects such as dry mouth were no different from those with placebo. The better tolerability of skin delivery can probably be explained by the slow and reversible binding of oxybutynin to muscarinic receptors, as demonstrated in rats. In contrast, prolonged occupation of exocrine receptors following oral delivery of oxybutynin evoked a blockade in cholinergic salivation.[7,8]

Unfortunately, the transdermal patch causes skin irritation for many patients. Not only is the patch itself irritating, but the addition of oxybutynin further aggravates the irritation. The patch without the drug showed a very low rate of dermatitis type reactions, but the dermatitis reaction rate increased to 14% after addition of the drug. Approximately 10% of patients will stop treatment due to side effects.

INTRAVESICAL INSTILLATION

Since the bladder is directly accessible from the external orifice of the urethra, diseases affecting the bladder are amenable to regional drug delivery through the intravesical route. Intravesical instillation has many advantages such as easy access via a catheter, avoiding the hepatic first pass effect, and a reduced potential of adverse effects from instillation of toxic agents into the bladder. Drug delivery by the intravesical route is usually intended for local effect and for overcoming intrinsic shortcomings of oral therapy such as variable bioavailability.

The orally administered cytoprotective drug misoprostol requires 6 months to achieve therapeutic benefit in interstitial cystitis patients.[9] The prolonged regimen needed for efficacy can be traced to low amounts of drug excreted in the urine following oral administration. The relative advantage of regional drug delivery by intravesical instillation has also been demonstrated using pharmacokinetic analysis.[10] Comparison of oxybutynin pharmacokinetics after oral and intravesical administration in children with neurogenic bladder revealed that instilled oxybutynin is systemically absorbed, with a dramatically reduced first pass effect.[11] The serum level ratio of DEO/oxybutynin was found to be much lower after instillation than after oral intake of oxybutynin.

Pharmacokinetic parameters following instillation are bound to vary with the administration of different agents. The ratio of total body clearance of a drug to its regional exchange rate is the principal determinant of therapeutic advantage. Intravesical drug delivery is characterized by its low exchange rate. Thus, the most favorable circumstances for regional delivery are with the use of drugs with high total body clearances.

The bioavailability from instillation can be influenced by numerous factors such as physicochemical attributes of the drug itself, formulation differences, or the delivery system used, such as liposomes, microspheres, or nanoparticles. These factors critically affect drug exposure in the bladder, the extent of absorption, and the pharmacokinetics of a drug or its formulation. Among chemical attributes, molecular weight seems to offer the best correlation with extent of absorption.[12] Drugs with a molecular weight of less than 200, such as thiotepa, are absorbed into the systemic circulation better than drugs with molecular weights above 400.[13]

Drugs with a large molecular weight such as bacillus Calmette–Guérin (BCG) (65 kDa) are not absorbed by normal urothelium, although minimal absorption is possible through inflamed urothelium.[14] The same is true for the botulinum toxin, whose large molecular size and weight prevents its absorption after instillation into the bladder. Therefore, cystoscopic guided injections of botulinum toxin are needed for achieving the therapeutic effect. Drug absorption is also affected by pH and pK_a factors, and drugs with a pK_a that provides a high percentage of nonionized molecules at the usual pH of urine, 6–7, are desirable for instillation. Drug absorption is more efficient when the logarithm of the partition coefficient (log P) for the drug is in the range from -0.4 to -1.2 or from -7.5 to -8.0.[12]

Instillation has proved efficacious as a second line treatment for overactive bladder. The procedure is well tolerated by the majority of patients, although the instillation of some drugs such as dimethylsulfoxide (DMSO) and capsaicin can cause bothersome irritation. Instillation is ideally suited to patients who perform intermittent catheterization. It is also suitable for patients with voiding dysfunction who are unable to tolerate orally administered anticholinergic therapy. Instillation of anticholinergic agents can achieve local cholinergic blockade and avoid systemic effects.

Patients who remain incontinent on oral anticholinergics or who cannot tolerate oral medication have frequently been instilled with oxybutynin dissolved in saline. The procedure of instilling oxybutynin twice daily for 30 minutes had a more than 90% success rate in 11 patients suffering from chronic urge incontinence.[15] Intravesical treatment with oxybutynin significantly increased the bladder capacity without eliciting any anticholinergic side effects, and a decrease in filling pressure was also noted. Subsequently reported studies confirmed these advantages of instilled oxybutynin in a different patient population.[16]

Vanilloids such as resiniferatoxin (RTX) have been instilled to successfully manage overactive bladder in patients refractory to anticholinergic agents.[17,18] Patients responding to intravesical RTX (10 nmol/l) treatment showed a decrease in adenosine triphosphate ATP-gated purinergic receptor $P2X_3$ immunoreactivity.[19] This receptor is expressed by small diameter sensory neurons, and it has been identified in bladder biopsy samples from patients and healthy subjects.

The majority of analogs for vanilloids (and similar agents such as the cannabinoids) developed so far are generally insoluble in water, which presents a major hurdle in their formulation for intravesical instillation. Numerous approaches have been tried in overcoming the aqueous insolubility of these agents for urological use. However, before we consider these recent advances in this field, it would be pertinent to consider the nature of the barriers afforded to this route of drug delivery.

BARRIERS TO ABSORPTION AFTER INSTILLATION

The major barriers to drug absorption from instillation include a limited residence time in the bladder due to regular voiding and restriction on the passage of large molecules across the urothelium. However, notwithstanding the poor permeability of the urothelium, it serves a useful purpose when instillation of toxic agents such as vanilloids is desired in the treatment of overactive bladder. The presence of a glycosaminoglycan (GAG) layer at the apical surface of umbrella cells in the urothelium serves as the main roadblock in the absorption of instilled drugs.[20] Ablation of the GAG layer improves permeability for instilled drugs.[4]

Instilled drugs can navigate the GAG layer by electrostatic, hydrophobic, or van der Waals interactions. After permeating the GAG layer, the instilled drug may cross the urothelium by either of two principal routes. First is transcellular or simple (Fickian) diffusion across the apical cell membrane. Second is paracellular transport, which involves movement through the spaces between cells and tight junctions. This pathway can be augmented by the reversible opening of tight junctions. An instilled drug may access either or both of these routes, although one is generally preferred according to the physicochemical attributes of the drug. Paracellular transport is the major route for hydrophilic drugs, whereas lipophilic drugs may prefer transcellular transport. Intravesical instillation of peptides and proteins may also offer an alternative to other parenteral routes. The bioavailability of peptides is inversely proportional to the molecular weight of the peptide. This inverse relationship suggests that the hydrophilic and globular nature of peptides and proteins may favor the paracellular mode of transport across the urothelium.

Indeed, the two most challenging issues to be addressed in intravesical instillation are undoubtedly permeability enhancement and retention of instilled drug carrier inside the bladder. Constant urine production and intermittent voiding can lead to substantial loss of drug, and hence low bioavailability. In recent years, various technological developments have taken place to increase the bioavailability from intravesical instillation that include either increasing the bladder permeability or methods to prolong the drug residence time in the bladder for both increased and sustained release.[21] These innovations are discussed below.

Drug absorption across the urothelium may be enhanced by either increasing paracellular transport or breaching the GAG layer and initiating membrane pore formation. High concentrations of heparin in the composition of the GAG layer prompted the use of protamine sulfate for reducing the barrier to drug absorption.[4] Therapy via the intravesical route can be further improved by helping drugs cross the permeability barrier of the urothelium by physical (such as iontophoresis)[22] and chemical (such as DMSO) enhancement methods.

Iontophoresis has the potential to improve the passive delivery of most compounds across epithelia. The technique generates an electrical potential gradient that facilitates the movement of solute ions across the membrane. Iontophoresis has been used with great success in the therapy of hyperhidrosis. The potential of iontophoresis for systemic delivery is being rediscovered, and the technique has been observed to be particularly effective for ionic drugs. It also enhances transdermal permeation of neutral compounds by the process of electro-osmosis.

Liposomes

Liposomes are microscopic vesicular structures having an aqueous core surrounded by membrane-like phospholipid layers (Figure 10.2). Phospholipids carry a hydrophilic head and a lipophilic tail. When dispersed in water, phospholipids arrange themselves in bilayers, which can form closed vesicles like artificial cells.

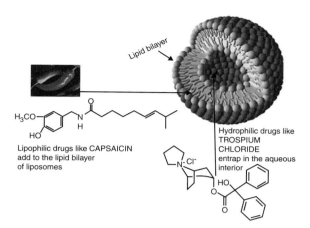

Figure 10.2 Liposomes are spherical lipid vesicles that can serve as carriers for lipophilic (in a bilayer) and hydrophilic drugs in the aqueous interior. The pungent principle of capsaicin obtained from red pepper can be entrapped in the lipid bilayer and the quaternary amine based drug trospium chloride can be entrapped in the aqueous interior.

Depending on the lipids used, the liposomes can be either neutral or anionically and cationically charged. The flexibility in their compositions makes them versatile platforms for the delivery of a variety of drugs, proteins, nucleotides, and even plasmids. Liposomes have been well tolerated from a physiological standpoint owing to their composition, which is similar to that of biological membranes. The biocompatible, biodegradable, and highly favorable toxicity profile of liposomes following parenteral administration has been well documented in decades of clinical experience.

A liposomal product in physicochemical terms can be viewed as a heterogeneous liquid: lipid vesicles suspended in a water based solution. Liposomes are better suited than micelles for use as carriers for water insoluble drugs administered into the bladder, because instillation of micelles into the bladder can have deleterious effects on the urothelium.[23] Liposomes have been used for instillation of chemotherapeutic agents with promising results, although research in this area is fairly limited. The entrapped drug is delivered inside the bladder as the lipid bilayer holding the drug eventually collapses after instillation.

Owing to their biphasic nature, liposomes have the potential to associate hydrophilic (e.g. cytarabine, $\log P = -1.25$), hydrophobic (e.g. paclitaxel, $\log P = 3.96$), and amphiphilic compounds (e.g. doxorubicin, $\log P = 0.17$; daunorubicin, $\log P = 0.73$). Amphiphilic and hydrophilic compounds are entrapped within the aqueous interior of the liposomes, while hydrophobic drugs intercalate within the hydrophobic region of the lipid bilayer. Liposomes can also be modified to impart controlled release properties. They have been able to demonstrate an improvement in aqueous solubility of hydrophobic drugs such as taxol and amphotericin.

Liposomes are ideal in the development of niche products that have a limited market, such as those used in intravesical instillation. A recent study reported from the University of Pittsburg used liposomes as a vehicle for capsaicin, and evaluated their potential as a vehicle for intravesical delivery in rats.[24] Liposomes were able to deliver capsaicin with an efficacy similar to that of ethanolic saline, but toxicity to the bladder was drastically reduced. A similar approach can prove useful in the instillation of other vanilloids such as resiniferatoxin (RTX) and water insoluble drugs.

The bioavailability of drugs improves after entrapping them in liposomes, owing to their spherical shape that increases the surface/volume ratio. Instilled liposomes can adhere to the urothelium and the drug can then freely diffuse from the lipid bilayer of liposomes to the superficial cells of the transitional epithelium. Moreover, liposomes themselves can also be absorbed into the cells, but the absorption rate of liposomal drug is slower than that of free drug owing to the larger molecular size of the liposomes. The slower diffusion of liposomes probably accounts for the longer residency time of the encapsulated drug. In addition, clearance of the absorbed liposomal drug from the urothelium is much slower than that of free drug, as the larger size of liposomes prevents them from entering the blood vessels in the urothelium.

Liposomes not only possess a benign nature but they have also been shown to be successful in promoting skin wound-healing in the absence of any drug.[25] The probable mechanism underlying this effect is the formation of a protective film on the tissue surface. The earlier encouraging reports on wound-healing properties of lipo-somes were confirmed recently in studies of non-viral gene therapy of skin wounds.[26] It seems reasonable, therefore, to hypothesize that the instillation of liposomes may be a plausible option in a rat model for palliating interstitial cystitis symptoms arising from bladder injury, because of their wound-healing properties.[27] The effect of liposomes alone in the absence of any drug was studied in a rat model of bladder hyperactivity induced by breaching the GAG layer by protamine and thereafter irritating the bladder with KCl. Liposomes were able to partially reverse the high bladder contraction frequency induced by protamine sulfate/KCl (Figure 10.3).[28] These observations suggest that liposomes might enhance the barrier properties of a dysfunctional urothelium and increase the resistance to irritant penetration.

Increased vesical residence time

Drug residence time in the urinary bladder after intravesical instillation rarely lasts beyond the first voiding of urine. Prolonged intravesical delivery of drugs can ensure uninterrupted local-ization of the drug in the bladder without the need for intermittent catheterization. It is reason-able to expect an improvement in efficacy with increased residence time of the drug inside the bladder.[29] Increased duration of residence in the bladder results in less frequent and more tolerable

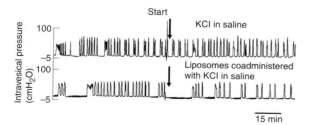

Figure 10.3 Cystometrogram tracing of injured rat bladder infused with empty liposomes. Liposomes were able to significantly decrease the bladder contraction frequency even in the presence of an irritating concentration of potassium chloride. The bladder was injured by 1 hour's infusion of protamine sulfate and then irritated with 1 hour's infusion of 500 mmol/l of KCl. Liposomes were coadministered in the bladder in the presence of 500 mmol/l of KCl.

treatment regimens that positively affect patient convenience.

A simple approach for increasing the resi-dence time of drugs inside the bladder is similar to the technique of extended intravenous infu-sion. This technique has often been applied for achieving the continuous release of drugs such as RTX inside the bladder.[30] The procedure used for treating neurogenic bladder infused RTX through a suprapubic 5Fr mono pigtail catheter for 10 days at a flow rate 25 µl per hour with the help of an infusion pump. Patients were evaluated 30 days after the end of infusion admin-istration and after 3 months. A 30% decrease in frequency, and a three-fold reduction of nocturia, with a significant reduction of symptoms of pelvic pain for at least 6 months after the end of infusion were observed.

In recent years, the development of a bio-adhesive drug delivery system intended for the urinary bladder has been the subject of intense research. Bioadhesion refers to the adherence of a drug to a biological surface through interfacial surfaces. The bioadhesive delivery system is intended to remain adhered to the bladder sur-face for a prolonged period of time and allow for complete drug absorption.[31] Adhesion between the GAG layer (mucin) and adhesive polymers is usually based on molecular attractive and repulsive forces, and, in contrast, adhesion to cell surfaces involves highly specific receptor-mediated interactions.

Bioadhesion can be understood as a two step process, in which first adsorptive contact is gov-erned by surface energy effects and a spreading process. In the latter phase, the diffusion of poly-mer chains such as that of polyethylene glycol across the polymer–mucin interface occurs to promote the final bond. Mucoadhesive materials are generally hydrophilic polymers that swell significantly in contact with water and eventu-ally undergo complete dissolution. Also called wet adhesives, these hydrophilic polymers adhere to the mucosal surface upon wetting and can be categorized into the following classes: anionic polymers such as sodium carboxymethyl cellu-lose and sodium alginate, polycationic polymers such as chitosan and dextrans, non-ionic poly-mers such as polyvinylpyrolidine, and cellu-lose derivatives such as hydroxypropylmethyl cellulose.

The strongly mucoadhesive nature of chitosan microspheres prompted their application in bioadhesive regional therapy of acyclovir via the ophthalmic route.[32] The improvement of bioadhesion was able to increase the ocular residence time and decrease the frequency of administration.[32] Similar expectations have motivated the use of bioadhesives for improving intravesical drug delivery.[33] The application of bioadhesion for instilled drugs should be able to fulfill the following criteria: they should quickly bind to the urothelium after instillation and be retained inside the bladder for at least several hours without blocking the voiding of urine. Polymers that have been tried so far for intravesical instillation in preclinical studies in rodents are carbopol, cellulose compounds, polycarbophil, and chitosan.

A cationic hydrophilic polymer that has been used as a bioadhesive in many bladder studies is chitosan. Chitosan is characterized by its high molecular weight, biodegradability, low toxicity, and ability to swell at the usual pH, 6.8, of urine. Its use for intravesical instillation has led to increased drug absorption because of its adhesive nature and its ability to alter tight junctions.[34] Isolated porcine urinary bladder was used to evaluate chitosan and polycarbophil as bioadhesive polymeric carriers for a hydrophilic drug. Drug distribution into the bladder wall was determined by sectioning the frozen bladder and extracting the drug from tissue slices for analysis.[35]

Both the intrinsic nature and molecular weight of a polymer can affect the binding ability of the polymer to the urothelium. The length of the polymer chain determines the extent of interpenetration and molecular entanglement. Other considerations for bioadhesive efficacy include the polymer concentration at the urothelium surface, and pH inside the bladder, which can alter charge potential and interactions. The hydration level of the polymer plays an important role in bioadhesion, as polymers that hydrate too soon are not ideal for intravesical instillation. Chitosan and polycarbophil can retain good adhesive qualities upon full hydration. The invading water molecules liberate polymer chains from their twisted and entangled state and, thus, expose reactive sites that can bond to macromolecules of the urothelium. Salts of the natural polymer

algin swell and form an adherent viscous layer in contact with a mucosal surface. The bioadhesive technology is capable of modulating the release and absorption characteristics of the drugs instilled using carrier particles such as microspheres, nanoparticles, liposomes, etc. These carrier particles with modified bioadhesive technology can then have more intimate contact with the urothelium, for improved efficiency of absorption.

Bioadhesion was recently evaluated clinically, and was able to achieve partial clinical success.[36] The case study involved six overactive bladder patients suffering from side effects of oxybutynin's metabolite N-desethyl-oxybutynin (DEO). Hydroxypropylcellulose (HPC) was added to the oxybutynin chloride solution (5% w/w), which lent bioadhesive characteristics to the oxybutynin.[36] The mucoadhesive solution was instilled twice daily, via the catheter used for bladder emptying, at a dosage of 0.5 mg/ml, and cystometography (CMG) was performed on the patients before starting the treatment, and at 1 week and 3 years after the first instillation of oxybutynin. A significant increase in bladder capacity was observed in four out of six patients. Intravesical delivery of oxybutynin is suitable for patients who suffer side effects from its metabolite DEO following oral administration. This intravesical oxybutynin therapy is thought to depend on three mechanisms that prevent or improve urge incontinence: a direct effect on the bladder muscle, a topical anesthetic effect, and the indirect effect of absorbed oxybutynin and its metabolite.

Formation of a drug reservoir inside the bladder may also be an alternative option to increase the drug contact time with the bladder. There are stimuli-sensitive polymers available that change their physical state on either lowering or increasing stimuli such as temperature or pH. One polymer of this class of triblock copolymers is poly(ethylene glycol-b-[DL-lactic acid-co-glycolic acid]-b-ethylene glycol) (PEG-PLGA-PEG) whose solution in water forms a free-flowing sol at room temperature but which becomes a gel at body temperature 37°C.[37] Thermosensitive hydrogel formed by PEG-PLGA-PEG has been used for in situ gel formation for a depot of hydrophobic and hydrophilic drugs following subcutaneous administration in rats.[38]

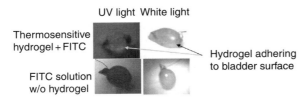

Figure 10.4 Photographs of a rat bladder instilled with thermosensitive hydrogel. Thermosensitive hydrogel was localized in the rat bladder by loading the hydrogel with a fluorescent probe that appears green in ultraviolet (UV) light 48 hours after instillation. Rat bladder instilled with a fluorescent probe without any hydrogel did not show any green color of the probe under UV light. FITC, fluorescein isothiocyanate. (See also color plate section).

Its formulation does not require organic solvent, and products from bioerosion of the biocompatible polymer are non-toxic PEG, glycolic acid, and lactic acid.

The triblock copolymer PEG-PLGA-PEG was modified for its application to intravesical instillation in order to sustain the residence time of hydrophobic drugs in the rat bladder. After its instillation as a fluid at room temperature, it formed a gel inside the bladder after coming into contact with the warm bladder surface. The thermosensitive hydrogel was entrapped with a fluorescent probe, fluorescein isothiocyanate (FITC), for studying the kinetics of drug excretion by measurement of the fluorescence in urine after instillation and for locating the hydrogel in the bladder[39] (Figure 10.4). The increased urine concentration over a period of time implies increased penetration into bladder tissue owing to the linear relationship between the two variables.[40] Therapeutic benefit of sustained delivery afforded by thermosensitive hydrogel was demonstrated by replacing FITC with misoprostol, which was able to protect against cyclophosphamide-induced cystitis and decrease the induced increase in bladder contraction frequency.

CONCLUSION

Although newer oral agents represent a significant advancement in therapy, many patients do not respond to or do not tolerate oral therapy. The paucity of side effects associated with the intravesical approach makes intravesical therapy an attractive treatment option, particularly for patients who are already using self-catheterization. Intravesical instillation provides a safe and effective method of affecting the afferent and efferent sides of the micturition reflex arc. Intravesical instillation is becoming increasingly of interest to the drug delivery community, and improvements in this field are continuing to evolve. Delivery systems for the intravesical route are usually adaptations of technologies used for other routes that may incorporate mucoadhesive polymers or particulate carriers such as liposomes. Perhaps of greater interest are more recent developments utilizing drug carriers that can offer sustained release, such as thermosensitive hydrogel. In the coming years, delivery of biomolecules such as therapeutic proteins and peptides will be of significant interest, as they may emerge as a major class of therapeutic agents. Successful delivery of such drugs in clinically efficacious amounts may be possible via intravesical instillation as it avoids the degradation observed after oral administration.

ACKNOWLEDGMENT

The authors are grateful to the Fishbein Family Foundation for financial support (Center of Urologic Research Excellence in Interstitial Cystitis (CURE-IC)) NIDDK RO1 DK 066138 R43 DK 074286.

REFERENCES

1. Andersson KE, Hedlund P. Pharmacologic perspective on the physiology of the lower urinary tract. Urology 2002; 60: 13–20; discussion 20–1.
2. Yoshimura N, Chancellor MB. Current and future pharmacological treatment for overactive bladder. J Urol 2002; 168: 1897–913.
3. Cannon TW, Chancellor MB. Pharmacotherapy of the overactive bladder and advances in drug delivery. Clin Obstet Gynecol 2002; 45: 205–17.
4. Khera M, Somogyi GT, Salas NA et al. In vivo effects of botulinum toxin A on visceral sensory function in chronic spinal cord-injured rats. Urology 2005; 66: 208–12.
5. Abramov Y, Sand PK. Oxybutynin for treatment of urge urinary incontinence and overactive bladder: an updated review. Expert Opin Pharmacother 2004; 5: 2351–9.

6. Lehtoranta K, Tainio H, Lukkari-Lax E, Hakonen T, Tammela TL. Pharmacokinetics, efficacy, and safety of intravesical formulation of oxybutynin in patients with detrusor overactivity. Scand J Urol Nephrol 2002; 36: 18–24.

7. Dmochowski RR, Nitti V, Staskin D et al. Transdermal oxybutynin in the treatment of adults with overactive bladder: combined results of two randomized clinical trials. World J Urol 2005; 23: 263–70.

8. Oki T, Toma-Okura A, Yamada S. Advantages for transdermal over oral oxybutynin to treat overactive bladder: muscarinic receptor binding, plasma drug concentration and salivary secretion. J Pharmacol Exp Ther 2005; 316: 1137–45.

9. Kelly JD, Young MR, Johnston SR, Keane PF. Clinical response to an oral prostaglandin analogue in patients with interstitial cystitis. Eur Urol 1998; 34: 53–6.

10. Highley MS, van Oosterom AT, Maes RA, De Bruijn EA. Intravesical drug delivery. Pharmacokinetic and clinical considerations. Clin Pharmacokinet 1999; 37: 59–73.

11. Buyse G, Waldeck K, Verpoorten C et al. Intravesical oxybutynin for neurogenic bladder dysfunction: less systemic side effects due to reduced first pass metabolism. J Urol 1998; 160: 892–6.

12. Mishina T, Watanabe H, Kobayashi T et al. Absorption of anticancer drugs through bladder epithelium. Urology 1986; 27: 148–57.

13. Huben RP. Intravesical chemotherapy versus immunotherapy for superficial bladder cancer. Semin Urol Oncol 1996; 14: 17–22.

14. de Boer EC, Westerhof AC, Kolk AH et al. Polymerase chain reaction based method for the detection of BCG retention after intravesical instillation in guinea pig bladders. Eur Urol 2000; 37: 488–93.

15. Brendler CB, Radebaugh LC, Mohler JL. Topical oxybutynin chloride for relaxation of dysfunctional bladders. J Urol 1989; 141: 1350–2.

16. Buyse G, Verpoorten C, Vereecken R, Casaer P. Treatment of neurogenic bladder dysfunction in infants and children with neurospinal dysraphism with clean intermittent (self)catheterisation and optimized intravesical oxybutynin hydrochloride therapy. Eur J Pediatr Surg 1995; 5 (Suppl 1): 31–4.

17. Kuo HC. Multiple intravesical instillation of low-dose resiniferatoxin is effective in the treatment of detrusor overactivity refractory to anticholinergics. BJU Int 2005; 95: 1023–7.

18. Chancellor MB, de Groat WC. Intravesical capsaicin and resiniferatoxin therapy: spicing up the ways to treat the overactive bladder. J Urol 1999; 162: 3–11.

19. Brady CM, Apostolidis A, Yiangou Y et al. P2X3-immunoreactive nerve fibres in neurogenic detrusor overactivity and the effect of intravesical resiniferatoxin. Eur Urol 2004; 46: 247–53.

20. Hurst RE, Zebrowski R. Identification of proteoglycans present at high density on bovine and human bladder luminal surface. J Urol 1994; 152: 1641–5.

21. Ueda K, Sakagami H, Masui Y, Okamura T. Single instillation of hydroxypropylcellulose-doxorubicin as treatment for superficial bladder carcinoma. Cancer Chemother Pharmacol 1994; 35 (Suppl): S81–3.

22. Riedl CR, Stephen RL, Daha LK et al. Electromotive administration of intravesical bethanechol and the clinical impact on acontractile detrusor management: introduction of a new test. J Urol 2000; 164: 2108–11.

23. Ratliff TL. Identification of pretreatment agents to enhance adenovirus infection of bladder epithelium. J Urol 2005; 173: 2198–9.

24. Tyagi P, Chancellor MB, Li Z et al. Urodynamic and immunohistochemical evaluation of intravesical capsaicin delivery using thermosensitive hydrogel and liposomes. J Urol 2004; 171: 483–9.

25. Reimer K, Fleischer W, Brogmann B et al. Povidone-iodine liposomes—an overview. Dermatology 1997; 195 (Suppl 2): 93–9.

26. Jeschke MG, Sandmann G, Finnerty CC et al. The structure and composition of liposomes can affect skin regeneration, morphology and growth factor expression in acute wounds. Gene Ther 2005; 12: 1718–24.

27. Parsons CL. A model for the function of glycosaminoglycans in the urinary tract. World J Urol 1994; 12: 38–42.

28. Fraser MO, Chuang YC, Tyagi P et al. Intravesical liposome administration—a novel treatment for hyperactive bladder in the rat. Urology 2003; 61: 656–63.

29. Frangos DN, Killion JJ, Fan D et al. The development of liposomes containing interferon alpha for the intravesical therapy of human superficial bladder cancer. J Urol 1990; 143: 1252–6.

30. Lazzeri M, Spinelli M, Beneforti P et al. Intravesical infusion of resiniferatoxin by a temporary in situ

drug delivery system to treat interstitial cystitis: a pilot study. Eur Urol 2004; 45: 98–102.

31. Ozturk E, Eroglu M, Ozdemir N, Denkbas EB. Bioadhesive drug carriers for postoperative chemotherapy in bladder cancer. Adv Exp Med Biol 2004; 553: 231–42.

32. Genta I, Conti B, Perugini P et al. Bioadhesive microspheres for ophthalmic administration of acyclovir. J Pharm Pharmacol 1997; 49: 737–42.

33. Le Visage C, Rioux-Leclercq N, Haller M et al. Efficacy of paclitaxel released from bio-adhesive polymer microspheres on model superficial bladder cancer. J Urol 2004; 171: 1324–9.

34. Smith JM, Dornish M, Wood EJ. Involvement of protein kinase C in chitosan glutamate-mediated tight junction disruption. Biomaterials 2005; 26: 3269–76.

35. Grabnar I, Bogataj M, Mrhar A. Influence of chitosan and polycarbophil on permeation of a model hydrophilic drug into the urinary bladder wall. Int J Pharmacol 2003; 256: 167–73.

36. Saito M, Watanabe T, Tabuchi F et al. Urodynamic effects and safety of modified intravesical oxybutynin chloride in patients with neurogenic detrusor overactivity: 3 years experience. Int J Urol 2004; 11: 592–6.

37. Jeong B, Bae YH, Kim SW. Drug release from biodegradable injectable thermosensitive hydrogel of PEG-PLGA-PEG triblock copolymers. J Control Release 2000; 63: 155–63.

38. Jeong B, Bae YH, Kim SW. In situ gelation of PEG-PLGA-PEG triblock copolymer aqueous solutions and degradation thereof. J Biomed Mater Res 2000; 50: 171–7.

39. Tyagi P, Li Z, Chancellor M et al. Sustained intravesical drug delivery using thermosensitive hydrogel. Pharm Res 2004; 21: 832–7.

40. Gao X, Au JL, Badalament RA, Wientjes MG. Bladder tissue uptake of mitomycin C during intravesical therapy is linear with drug concentration in urine. Clin Cancer Res 1998; 4: 139–43.

11

Pioneering agents: immediate release

Philippe E Zimmern

Introduction • **Historical background** • **Pharmacologic agents** • **Where are we now?**
• **Conclusions**

INTRODUCTION

Over the last decade much of the pharmacologic market for overactive bladder (OAB) has evolved into a spectrum of extended release medications. The newer medications have been designed with novel delivery mechanisms to prolong their efficacy and reduce their side effects. Where does that leave the "older", immediate release (IR) agents in the treatment of the overactive bladder?

Review of bladder function and physiology has been done in previous chapters. From a pharmacologic perspective, an ideal medication would act as a bladder muscle relaxant without affecting detrusor contraction, resulting in decreased frequency and urgency, and with minimal or no side effects. The goal of this chapter is to review the IR anticholinergic medications that are currently or have previously been used in the management of OAB, with emphasis placed on the most commonly used: oxybutynin and tolterodine.

HISTORICAL BACKGROUND

To understand the development and evaluation of anticholinergic agents, it is imperative to recognize the complexity of evolution that has occurred over the past 35 years in terminology, evaluation of symptoms, and designing research studies. Although these issues are beyond the scope of this chapter and extensively covered in other areas of this book, it is important to recognize three key factors in review of the past and current literature on OAB.

First, the terminology has changed. Previously we used non-specific terms such as unstable bladder and detrusor hyperreflexia to denote whether unstable contractions were of idiopathic or neurogenic etiology respectively.[1] The preferred terminology is now detrusor overactivity (DO), further subclassified as idiopathic or neurogenic origin (Table 11.1).[2]

Additionally, outcome tools in OAB trials have improved as newer agents have strived to meet the Food and Drug Administration (FDA) requirements while trying to find a niche in a very competitive market. One example is the voiding diary, which serves to objectively document frequency, urgency, nocturia, and incontinence. Not only is the optimal duration (1, 3, or 7 days) still debated,[3,4] but this is burdensome to the patients[5] and may in itself induce a placebo effect.[3] In addition, what constitutes a meaningful response to treatment in the eyes of the patient remains a debate. Fitzgerald et al. attempted to answer this question through comparison of voiding diaries from symptomatic and asymptomatic individuals.[6] They proposed that a median reduction of three voids/24 hours and an increase in mean volume voided of 70 ml may be clinically important goals for OAB treatment.

Lastly, recent randomized controlled trials have focused on urgency as a cornerstone symptom in OAB, resulting in the development of urgency

Table 11.1 Evolution of terminology for the diagnosis of overactive bladder syndrome and detrusor overactivity[1]

	Pre-1978	1980	2002
Clinical diagnosis			Overactive bladder syndrome
Urodynamic diagnosis			
general	Unstable bladder (English) Detrusor hyperreflexia (Scandinavian)		Detrusor overactivity (DO)
idiopathic		Unstable Detrusor	Idiopathic (DO)
neurogenic		Detrusor hyperreflexia	Neurogenic (DO)

scales and validated questionnaires focusing on the symptoms of OAB.[7,8]

PHARMACOLOGIC AGENTS

Available medications can be divided into categories based on their mechanism of action or drug composition (Table 11.2). There are two broad categories of anticholinergics based on the mechanism of action. Some medications act purely through the inhibition of acetylcholine binding to the muscarinic receptors of the bladder and others have a mixed action. The latter agents not only have a variable anticholinergic effect, but also may have a musculotropic effect resulting directly in smooth muscle relaxation, and/or local anesthetic effect. Besides mixed mechanism of action, there are some drugs that are composed of multiple pharmacologic agents (e.g. Prosed®), thus resulting in variable effects.

Pure anticholinergics

Atropine/hyoscyamine

A derivative of the belladonna alkaloids, atropine, is perhaps the oldest anticholinergic medication and could be considered the prototype in terms of mechanism for treatment of OAB. The reality is that the widespread application of atropine is limited by its systemic side effects and it is primarily used for resuscitation efforts and in ophthalmology as a topical agent. From a urological perspective, atropine is found as a small component

in medications such as Prosed and Urised®, although some have investigated its use as an intravesical agent.[9,10]

The active portion of atropine, hyoscyamine, has been more clinically applicable. Hyoscyamine sulfate (Levsin®) is readily absorbed from the gastrointestinal (GI) tract and is available in oral (immediate and extended release (ER)) and sublingual (SL) formulations. Used extensively for GI complaints, hyoscyamine has also been employed in the management of bladder spasms, frequency, and urgency. However, clinical evidence in the literature supporting its utility for OAB is lacking. The hyoscyamine sulfate recommended dose for IR is 0.125–0.25 mg every 4–6 hours either orally or sublingually, and for ER 0.375 mg twice daily (bid). Like atropine, hyoscyamine is also a component of Prosed.

Propantheline bromide (Pro-Banthine®)

Propantheline is different from other "older" anticholinergic medications in that it is a quaternary amine. This property limits GI absorption, which may be further reduced in the presence of food. Once in the GI tract, propantheline is metabolized to inactive metabolites and has a short half-life, with peak plasma levels in 1.3 hours. A combination of all of these factors leads to a high recommended dose with frequent intake required, 15–30 mg orally every 4–6 hours, and titration to higher doses may be required in some patients. Thuroff et al. reviewed six randomized

Table 11.2 Mechanism of pharmacologic activity of immediate release medications for the treatment of overactive bladder

Drug	Anticholinergic	Musculotropic	Local anesthetic	Combination drug
Atropine/hyoscyamine	×			
Propantheline	×			
Tolterodine	×			
Oxybutynin	×	×	×	
Dicyclomine	×	×		
Flavoxate	×	×		
Prosed®				×
Urised®				×

controlled trials and determined that there is a variable, but positive response (Table 11.3).[11]

Tolterodine tartrate (Detrol®)

Tolterodine was one of the first medications to be developed specifically for the management of OAB and created a competitive market for oxybutynin. Though not muscarinic receptor subtype specific, relative to oxybutynin, tolterodine has a similar affinity for the bladder and less affinity for salivary glands as demonstrated in in vitro and in vivo animal models.[12] Tolterodine is metabolized to an active metabolite, 5-hydroxymethyl metabolite (5-HM), and non-active N-dealkylated tolterodine through the cytochrome P450 system. The specific enzyme for metabolism is absent in approximately 7% of Caucasians;[13,14] however, it has been demonstrated that there is no difference in clinical response for these patients.[15] The recommended dose of tolterodine is 2 mg orally bid, with time to peak plasma concentrations of the IR agent from 0.5 to 2 hours. A reduction in dose may be required if significant side effects develop.

From a clinical perspective, tolterodine consistently demonstrates a mild improvement (approximately 20%) in frequency and a more significant overall improvement with urge urinary incontinence (50–70%), with a less than 10% dropout rate in clinical trials due to adverse events (Tables 11.4 and 11.5). Based on the response rates, tolerability, and the availability of IR formulations, tolterodine IR is still being utilized in the management of OAB.

Mixed action

Oxybutynin chloride (Ditropan®)

Oxybutynin is the oldest and most widely recognized OAB medication. It was initially developed in the 1960s for treatment of hypermobility of the GI tract. Not only a potent muscarinic receptor antagonist with slight M_3 and M_1 selectivity, oxybutynin has a direct antispasmodic effect on the detrusor muscle and has been identified as a surface anesthetic agent.[22]

As a tertiary amine, it is well absorbed from the GI tract but sustains a significant first pass hepatic metabolism. The principal active metabolite, N-desethyl-oxybutynin, has similar properties to those of its parent drug. Peak plasma levels are 2–5 times higher for the metabolite[23] and higher affinity for the parotid gland may contribute to the side effect of dry mouth.[12, 24] In an effort to decrease the first pass metabolism, intravesical and transdermal routes have been explored and appear to be well tolerated, safe, and with good clinical response.[25–28]

The standard dosage of the oral IR oxybutynin is 5 mg bid – four times daily (qid). The dose can be decreased to 2.5 mg if side effects are of concern. Time to peak plasma concentration is 30–60 minutes. Because oxybutynin was the principal agent available for many years, it has served as the comparator in head-to-head randomized controlled trials (RCTs) for OAB done in the recent past.

Overall subjective improvement rate has been reported to range from 61% to 100%, with mean

Table 11.3 Summary of results for review of randomized controlled trials (adapted from reference 11). Data for tolterodine and dicyclomine are limited in this paper. Not every study reviewed evaluated each parameter

	Oxybutynin	Flavoxate	Propantheline	Placebo
Studies (n)	15	7	6	25
Total patients (n)	476	153	155	800
Micturitions per 24 h (%)	−33	−6	−23	−16
Incontinence (%)	−70	−50	−2	−22
Improvements (%)	74	44	61	37
Side effects (%)	70	25	51	33

decreases in urge incontinence and 24-hour frequency at 52% and 33% respectively.[11] The persistent challenge with oxybutynin IR is the side effect profile. The side effects such as dry mouth, constipation, drowsiness, and blurred vision are not different from those of other agents. The rate of adverse events, however, may limit patient compliance (Table 11.5).

Dicyclomine hydrochloride (Bentyl®)

Dicyclomine is a mixed action medication with both antimuscarinic and musculotropic effects. Only two randomized control trials have been published, and other data through non-controlled studies are limited.[11] Despite its mixed activity it has never been widely applied to the treatment of OAB, and optimal dosing was never specifically determined but varied in the few clinical trials from 600 to 1200 mg daily.

Flavoxate hydrochloride (Urispas®)

The exact mechanism of action of flavoxate is still not entirely known. It appears to have a combination of moderate calcium antagonist properties, local anesthetic properties, and phosphodiesterase inhibition. However, the antimuscarinic activity is controversial, with conflicting results.[29,30] Flavoxate is well absorbed from the GI tract with a plasma half-life of 3.5 hours, and is metabolized to an inactive form.

Clinically, flavoxate demonstrates a lesser degree of improvement in frequency, while still achieving a 50% reduction in incontinence. Subjective clinical improvement was reported at 44% despite weak evidence for objective improvement in parameters other than incontinence.[11] Compared to other agents, flavoxate has a lower side effect profile, with GI complaints of nausea and vomiting predominating.[11]

Other agents

For completeness we will just briefly mention some of the other anticholinergics that have been either previously available in the US market or not used in the US but available in other countries. Terodiline was available in the USA in the late 1980s but was removed from the US market after 10 reported fatalities due to the ventricular arrhythmia, torsades de pointes.[11] Propiverine and emepronium bromide are two other agents with anticholinergic properties not available in the USA. Data available on these medications indicate that both can improve voiding diary parameters by 15–30%, with a subjective improvement around 77% for propiverine and 49% for emepronium bromide.[11]

Efficacy and compliance

At this time the most commonly used IR anticholinergic medications are tolterodine and oxybutynin. In consideration of any anticholinergic efficacy, the placebo effect needs to be remembered. Over the years, 30–40% placebo response has been noted consistently in RCTs. In fact, a recent meta-analysis of 32 randomized control trials enrolling 6800 participants reviewed patient perception as well as incontinence episodes and number of micturitions in 24 hours.[31]

Table 11.4 Summary of results from several studies evaluating the efficacies of oxybutynin and tolterodine. Assessment of subjective improvement varied between studies

Author	Trial design	Treatment duration	Drug	n	Frequency/ 24 h (%)	UUI/24 h (%)	VV (%)	MCC (%)	Subjective improvement (%)
Tolterodine only									
Abrams 2001[16]	Open label extension	12 months	Tolterodine 2 mg po bid	441	−20	−74	+18		69
Tolterodine vs. oxybutynin vs. placebo									
Abrams 1998[17]	Randomized, double blind	12 weeks	Placebo	57	−10.5	−19	+7		47
			Oxybutynin 5 mg po tid	118	−19.5	−71	+31		49
			Tolterodine 2 mg po bid	118	−21	−47	+27		50
Drutz 1999[18]	Randomized, double blind	12 weeks	Placebo	56	−10	−27	+8		
			Oxybutynin 5 mg po tid	112	−17	−52	+34		
			Tolterodine 2 mg po bid	109	−17	−46	+21		

Table 11.4 Continued

Author	Trial design	Treatment duration	Drug	n	Frequency/ 24 h (%)	UUI/24 h (%)	VV (%)	MCC (%)	Subjective improvement (%)
Tolterodine vs. placebo									
Rentzhog 1998[19]	Double blind	2 weeks	Placebo	13	NA	NA		−3	−7
			Tolterodine 2 mg po bid	14	−20	−46		+10	26
Millard 1999[20]	Randomized, double blind	12 weeks	Placebo	64	−12	−37	+6		38
			Tolterodine 2 mg po bid	123	−21	−47	+23		59
Oxybutynin vs. propantheline vs. placebo									
Thuroff 1991[21]	Double blind	4 weeks	Placebo	52	−0.3			+9	43
			Oxybutynin 5 mg po tid	63	−1.8			+33	58
			Propantheline 15 mg po tid	54	−0.9			+19	45

UUI, urge urinary incontinence; VV, voided volume (based on diary); MCC, maximum cystometric capacity; po, orally; bid, twice daily; tid, three times daily

Table 11.5 Reported side effects from studies evaluating the efficacy and tolerability of tolterodine and oxybutynin

Author	Treatment duration	Drug	n	Dose reduction (%)	Dropout rate (%)		Adverse events (%)				
					Total	Adverse events	Total	Dry mouth	Mod–severe dry mouth	GI	Vision
Tolterodine only											
Abrams 2001[16]	12 months	Tolterodine 2 mg po bid	441	23		15	23	41	3	6	
Tolterodine vs. oxybutynin vs. placebo											
Abrams 1998[17]	12 weeks	Placebo	57	2		12		21		16	2
		Oxybutynin 5 mg po tid	118	32		17		86		29	7
		Tolterodine 2 mg po bid	118	8		8		50		12	3
Drutz 1999[18]	12 weeks	Placebo	56	4	14	7	75	15	7	26	
		Oxybutynin 5 mg po tid	112	23	31	21	90	69	44	39	
		Tolterodine 2 mg po bid	109	7	14	6	78	30	9	21	

Table 11.5 Continued

Author	Treatment duration	Drug	n	Dose reduction (%)	Dropout rate (%) Total	Dropout rate (%) Adverse events	Adverse events (%) Total	Dry mouth	Mod-severe dry mouth	GI	Vision
Tolterodine vs. placebo											
Rentzhog 1998[19]	2 weeks	Placebo	13				46	15		None	8
		Tolterodine 2 mg po bid	14				54	38		8	8
Millard 1999[20]	12 weeks	Placebo	64		5	None	78	13			
		Tolterodine 2 mg po bid	123		7	2	73	39			
Oxybutynin vs. propantheline vs. placebo											
Thuroff 1991[21]	4 weeks	Placebo	52			None	33	12	4		
		Oxybutynin 5 mg po tid	63			3	63	48	27		
		Propantheline 15 mg po tid	54			6	44	31	19		

po, orally; bid, twice daily; tid, three times daily

The authors reported that though the results favored the anticholinergic medications overall, the clinical improvements were small, over the placebo response. Tables 11.4 and 11.6 review some of the literature available comparing efficacies of the different available IR medications for OAB.

In addition to a modest degree of clinical improvement over placebo, the relative similarity in efficacy between drugs complicates the clinician's decision. Therefore the choice of medication depends often on other factors such as the rate of side effects, cost, and long-term patient compliance.

In fact studies have evaluated reasons for treatment discontinuation. A large Veterans Affairs (VA) study reviewed the medication database over 9 months to evaluate prescription refill habits for OAB medications.[36] Of patients prescribed oxybutynin and dicyclomine, 28% and 19% were still receiving these respective medications at 12 months. What this study did not specifically address was the reason for non-compliance.

Another study based on questionnaires mailed to participants to determine long-term compliance with oxybutynin revealed similar discontinuation rates.[37] Of the respondents, two-thirds had discontinued the medication, most within the first 4 months. Among patients who had discontinued the oxybutynin, 47% received an alternative treatment (pelvic floor exercises, surgery, other medication), 43% stopped due to side effects, 5% due to no improvement, and 5% did not like tablets. These results are similar to those of the VA study.

Regarding tolterodine, one study evaluated the tolerability and efficacy in a 12-month open label extension phase. Of the participants, approximately 38% withdrew from the study, of which 15% because of adverse effects.[16]

What we can conclude from the above literature is that a significant proportion of patients discontinue therapy or decrease the dose regardless of the medication, and the reason is often variable. From a practical perspective, Salvatore et al. emphasized the important point that due to the high discontinuation rate, patients begun on anticholinergics should be reassessed at 6 months (if not sooner) in clinical practice.[37]

Cost may be significant for some patients who require anticholinergic therapy for an extended period of time and it may influence their overall compliance. As generic formulations become available, physicians and patients may be willing to tolerate more side effects for lower cost. At this time IR oxybutynin is the only "modern" anticholinergic available in generic formulation; this translates into lower costs.

Anticholinergics and the elderly

The elderly patient with OAB is challenging to treat and warrants special consideration. The underlying etiology is often complex to understand, especially when associated comorbidities such as Alzheimer's or Parkinson's disease are present. OAB and urinary incontinence can lead to increased morbidity such as skin breakdown or falls in an effort to reach the bathroom.[38]

Concern has been raised over the routine use of anticholinergic agents in the elderly population, specifically the central nervous system (CNS) effects that the medications may exert. Medications are often a cause for delirium, dementia, or cognitive impairment in the elderly. These side effects can often be attributed to an alteration in pharmacokinetics and pharmacodynamics in older patients as well as polypharmacy.

Both oxybutynin and tolterodine are tertiary amines, but due to the lower lipophilic nature of tolterodine relative to oxybutynin, tolterodine crosses the blood–brain barrier at a much lower level.[39] Studies have been performed to evaluate the CNS effect of oxybutynin and tolterodine based on quantitative electroencephalography (qEEG) brain activity, alteration of rapid eye movement (REM) sleep, and impairment in concentration and cognition.[39,40] Ultimately it appears that oxybutynin has a greater CNS effect based on qEEG activity, but both drugs may interfere with normal REM sleep. What was not clearly demonstrated in either study was how these findings translate to the elderly. It should be remembered that anticholinergic medications have been categorized among the worst offenders at inducing cognitive impairment in the elderly.[41] Thus, prescribing such medications should be done in concert with the geriatrician, patient, and family. Starting with the lowest dose is advisable, and the patient's family needs to be aware of possible changes in cognition and be able to recognize alterations.

Table 11.6 Results of studies evaluating the effectiveness of propantheline and flavoxate

Author	Trial design	Treatment duration	Drug	n	Frequency/ 24 h (%)	MCC (%)	Incontinence score (%)	Subjective improvement (%)
Flavoxate								
Stanton 1973[32]	Double blind, crossover	2 weeks	Flavoxate HCl 200 mg po tid	38	There is more overall improvement in symptoms and cystometry with flavoxate than with emepronium			
			Emepronium bromide 200 mg po tid	38				
Chapple 1990[33]	Double blind, crossover	2 weeks	Placebo	25	Failed to demonstrate significant difference in flavoxate compared to placebo using both subjective and objective criteria			
			Flavoxate HCl 200 mg po tid	25				
Propantheline vs. oxybutynin								
Holmes 1989[34]	Single blind, crossover	4 weeks	Oxybutynin 5 mg po tid	23	−20	+36	−56	+60
			Propantheline 15 mg po tid	23	−10	+17	+11	+48
Thuroff 1991[21]	Double blind	4 weeks	Placebo	52	−0.3	+9	+43	
			Oxybutynin 5 mg po tid	63	−1.8	+33	+58	
			Propantheline 15 mg po tid	54	−0.9	+19	+44	
Propantheline only								
Coombes 1996[35]	Unblinded, crossover	4 weeks	Propantheline 15 mg po tid	23		+68	0	+56

MCC, maximum cystometric capacity; po, orally; tid, three times daily

WHERE ARE WE NOW?

Oxybutynin IR was the primary agent for treatment of OAB until the development of tolterodine in the 1990s. This added competition has driven the research and development of newer agents and novel delivery systems to where it is today. Without the introduction of tolterodine to spur interest into the area of the sustained release medications in an effort to improve the side effect profile, it is hard to know where we would be currently. But as attention has turned to the newer agents, we turn back to our original question: what role do the IR agents have today?

Clearly there are several clinical situations where IR medications can still play a role and provide improvement for the patient. For example, IR agents are ideal for patients who either do not want or do not need continual therapy but whose main concern is the risk of embarrassment in public due to an incontinent episode. IR medications can also serve as a supplement for those patients on ER formulations who need a boost at night to improve nocturia or during social functions. When cost is a significant consideration for a patient, for example a spinal cord injury patient already on numerous medications, the availability of a less costly generic formulation may become important in the long term.

CONCLUSIONS

Most of the immediate release agents are less commonly used nowadays. Oxybutynin and tolterodine remain in our contemporary armamentarium for OAB. With their short duration of action, known side effect profile, acceptable cost, and versatility, both oxybutynin and tolterodine IR formulations remain attractive alternatives for the practitioner.

REFERENCES

1. Abrams P. Describing bladder storage function: overactive bladder syndrome and detrusor overactivity. Urology 2003; 62 (Suppl 5B): 28–37.
2. Abrams P, Cardozo L, Fall M et al. The standardisation of terminology of lower urinary tract function: report from the Standardisation Subcommittee of the International Continence Society. Neurourol Urodyn 2002; 21: 167–78.
3. Dmochowski RR, Sanders SW, Appell RA, Nitti VW, Davila GW. Bladder-health diaries: an assessment of 3-day vs 7-day entries. BJU Int 2005; 96: 1049–54.
4. van Melick HHE, Gisolf KWH, Eckhardt MD, van Venrooij GEPM, Boon TA. One 24-hour frequency-volume chart in a woman with objective urinary motor urge incontinence is sufficient. Urology 2001; 58: 188–92.
5. Ku JH, Jeong IG, Lim DJ et al. Voiding diary for the evaluation of urinary incontinence and lower urinary tract symptoms: prospective assessment of patient compliance and burden. Neurourol Urodyn 2004; 23: 331–5.
6. Fitzgerald MP, Ayuste D, Brubaker L. How do urinary diaries of women with an overactive bladder differ from those of asymptomatic controls? BJU Int 2005; 96: 365–67.
7. Cardozo L, Coyne KS, Versi E. Validation of the urgency perception scale. BJU Int 2005; 95: 591–6.
8. Coyne K, Revicki D, Hunt T et al. Psychometric validation of an overactive bladder symptom and health-related quality of life questionnaire: the OAB-q. Qual Life Res 2002; 11: 563–74.
9. Ekstrom B, Andersson K, Mattiasson A. Urodynamic effects of the intravesical instillation of atropine and phentolamine in patients with detrusor hyperactivity. J Urol 1993; 149: 155–8.
10. Glickman S, Tsokkos N, Shah PJ. Intravesical atropine and suppression of detrusor hypercontractility in the neuropathic bladder. A preliminary study. Paraplegia 1995; 33: 36–9.
11. Thuroff JW, Chartier-Kastler E, Corcos J et al. Medical treatment and medical side effects in urinary incontinence in the elderly. World J Urol 1998; 16 (Suppl 1): S48–61.
12. Nilvebrant L, Andersson KE, Gillberg PG, Stahl M, Sparf B. Tolterodine – a new bladder-selective antimuscarinic agent. Eur J Pharmacol 1997; 327: 195–207.
13. Brynne N, Dalen P, Alvan G, Bertilsson L, Gabrielsson J. Influence of CYP2D6 polymorphism on the pharmacokinetics and pharmacodynamics of tolterodine. Clin Pharmacol Ther 1998; 63: 529–39.
14. Postlind H, Danielson A, Lindgren A, Andersson SHG. Tolterodine, a new muscarinic receptor antagonist, is metabolized by cytochromes P450 2D6 and 3A in human liver microsomes. Drug Metab Dispos 1998; 26: 289–93.

15. Larsson G, Hallen B, Nilvebrant L. Tolterodine in the treatment of overactive bladder: analysis of the pooled phase II efficacy and safety data. Urology 1999; 53: 990–8.
16. Abrams P, Malone-Lee J, Jacquetin B et al. Twelve-month treatment of overactive bladder: efficacy and tolerability of tolterodine. Drugs Aging 2001; 18: 551–60.
17. Abrams P, Freeman R, Anderstrom C, Mattiasson A. Tolterodine, a new antimuscarinic agent: as effective but better tolerated than oxybutynin in patients with an overactive bladder. BJU Int 1998; 81: 801–10.
18. Drutz HP, Appell RA, Gleason D, Klimberg I, Radomski S. Clinical efficacy and safety of tolterodine compared to oxybutynin and placebo in patients with overactive bladder. Int Urogynecol J Pelvic Floor Dysfunct 1999; 10: 283–9.
19. Rentzhog L, Stanton SL, Cardozo L et al. Efficacy and safety of tolterodine in patients with detrusor instability: a dose-ranging study. BJU Int 1998; 81: 42–8.
20. Millard R, Tuttle J, Moore K et al. Clinical efficacy and safety of tolterodine compared to placebo in detrusor overactivity. J Urol 1999; 161: 1551–5.
21. Thuroff JW, Bunke B, Ebner A et al. Randomized, double-blind, multicenter trial on treatment of frequency, urgency and incontinence related to detrusor hyperactivity: oxybutynin versus propantheline versus placebo. J Urol 1991; 145: 813–17.
22. de Wachter S, Wyndaele JJ. Intravesical oxybutynin: a local anesthetic effect on bladder C afferents. J Urol 2003; 169: 1892–5.
23. Hughes KM, Lang JCT, Lazare R et al. Measurement of oxybutynin and its N-desethyl metabolite in plasma, and its application to pharmacokinetic studies in young, elderly and frail elderly volunteers. Xenobiotica 1992; 22: 859–69.
24. Waldeck K, Larsson B, Andersson KE. Comparison of oxybutynin and its active metabolite, N-desethyl-oxybutynin, in the human detrusor and parotid gland. J Urol 1997; 157: 1093–7.
25. Szollar SM, Lee SM. Intravesical oxybutynin for spinal cord injury patients. Spinal Cord 1996; 34: 284–7.
26. Lose G, Norgaard JP. Intravesical oxybutynin for treating incontinence resulting from an overactive detrusor. BJU Int 2001; 87: 767–73.
27. Dmochowski RR, Davila GW, Zinner NR et al. Efficacy and safety of transdermal oxybutynin in patients with urge and mixed urinary incontinence. J Urol 2002; 168: 580–6.
28. Davila GW, Daugherty CA, Sanders SW. A short-term, multicenter, randomized double-blind dose titration study of the efficacy and anticholinergic side effects of transdermal compared to immediate release oral oxybutynin treatment of patients with urge urinary incontinence. J Urol 2001; 166: 140–5.
29. Uckert S, Stief CG, Odenthal KP et al. Responses of isolated normal human detrusor muscle to various spasmolytic drugs commonly used in the treatment of the overactive bladder. Arzneimittelforschung 2000; 50: 456–60.
30. Guarneri L, Robinson E, Testa R. A review of flavoxate: pharmacology and mechanism of action. Drugs Today 1994; 30: 91–8.
31. Herbison P, Hay-Smith J, Ellis G, Moore K. Effectiveness of anticholinergic drugs compared with placebo in the treatment of overactive bladder: systematic review. BMJ 2003; 326: 841–7.
32. Stanton SL. A comparison of emepronium bromide and flavoxate hydrochloride in the treatment of urinary incontinence. J Urol 1973; 110: 529–32.
33. Chapple CR, Parkhouse H, Gardener C, Milroy EJG. Double-blind, placebo-controlled, crossover study of flavoxate in the treatment of idiopathic detrusor instability. BJU Int 1990; 66: 491–4.
34. Holmes DM, Montz FJ, Stanton SL. Oxybutynin versus propantheline in the management of detrusor instability. A patient-regulated variable dose trial. Br J Obstet Gynaecol 1989; 96: 607–12.
35. Coombes GM, Millard RJ. Urinary urge incontinence: randomized crossover trials of penthienate versus placebo and propantheline. Med J Aust 1996; 165: 473–6.
36. Malone DC, Okano GJ. Treatment of urge incontinence in Veterans Affairs medical centers. Clin Ther 1999; 21: 867–77.
37. Salvatore S, Khullar V, Cardozo L et al. Long-term prospective randomized study comparing two different regimens of oxybutynin as a treatment for detrusor overactivity. Eur J Obstet Gynecol Reprod Biol 2005; 119: 237–41.
38. Brown JS, Vittinghoff E, Wyman JF et al. Urinary incontinence: does it increase risk for falls and fractures? Study of Osteoporotic Fractures Research Group. J Am Geriatr Soc 2000; 48: 721–5.

39. Todorova A, Vonderheid-Guth B, Dimpfel W. Effects of tolterodine, trospium chloride, and oxybutynin on the central nervous system. J Clin Pharmacol 2001; 41: 636–44.

40. Diefenbach K, Arold G, Wollny A et al. Effects on sleep of anticholinergics used for overactive bladder treatment in healthy volunteers aged > or = 50 years. BJU Int 2005; 95: 346–9.

41. Gray SL, Lai KV, Larson EB. Drug-induced cognition disorders in the elderly: incidence, prevention and management. Drug Saf 1999; 21: 101–22.

12

Tricyclic antidepressants

Daniel Dugi and Gary E Lemack

Introduction   •   **Basic science**   •   **Clinical studies**   •   **Conclusions**

INTRODUCTION

Tricyclic antidepressants (TCAs) were among the first antidepressant medications developed, though they are now rarely used as first-line treatments. Early in their use in the 1960s and 1970s it was observed that they seemed to decrease incontinence episodes in adults and children with enuresis. Since that time, tricyclic antidepressants, particularly imipramine, have been used generally as a second-line treatment in overactive bladder (OAB) and urge incontinence. A 1999 study of Veterans Affairs medical centers found imipramine to be the third most-common drug used in urge incontinence.[1] Animal and in vitro studies support a complex mechanism of action, on the lower urinary tract as well as the central nervous system. Unfortunately, high quality clinical studies are lacking. Recently, duloxetine, a structurally unrelated compound but also an antidepressant, has shown promise for use in stress and possibly mixed incontinence.

BASIC SCIENCE

Overview

Tricyclic antidepressants have been intensely studied, but our understanding of their effects and mechanisms of action on the lower urinary tract is still incomplete. They are thought to affect human voiding by a mixture of effects on the central nervous system and on peripheral tissues. In the human central nervous system, TCAs have been found to be potent inhibitors of muscarinic, α-adrenergic, and histamine H_1 receptors.[2] Within the class of drugs, affinities for different receptors vary, e.g. the affinity of amitriptyline for muscarinic receptors is five times greater than that of imipramine.

Important in the action of TCAs is their ability to block reuptake of norepinephrine (NE) and serotonin (5-HT) at nerve terminals, increasing the concentration of these neurotransmitters. While TCAs are commonly referred to as non-selective norepinephrine/serotonin reuptake inhibitors, some are more selective than others. In rats, imipramine is selective for NE over 5-HT by a factor of 3, while its metabolite des-imipramine is selective for NE by a factor of 300. In contrast, so-called selective serotonin reuptake inhibitors (SSRIs) such as fluoxetine (Prozac®) are selective for 5-HT over NE by a factor of 10, and sertraline (Zoloft®) by a factor of 64.[3] Duloxetine, called a dual NE/5-HT reuptake inhibitor, is selective for NE over 5-HT by a factor of 9.4 in humans.[4] This reuptake blockade leads to immediate increase in the respective neurotransmitter at the synapse; it also increases stimulation of the inhibitory α_2 autoreceptor, which in time leads to *decreased* neurotransmitter release.[5]

Central nervous system effects

Increased understanding of the neurological pathways involved in voiding function illustrates how TCAs may affect overactive bladder through the central nervous system. Serotonin receptors are abundant in the central nervous system, and their activation in cat and rat models has been found to reduce reflex bladder contractions and increase the volume necessary to induce reflex voiding.[6] Antagonists of α_1[7] and α_2[8] adrenergic receptors administered intrathecally improve urine storage characteristics and decrease unstable bladder contractions.

These findings point to TCAs' actions as NE/5-HT inhibitors in their possible effects on detrusor overactivity. This reuptake alone appears to be a simplistic explanation, however. Interestingly, dual NE/5-HT reuptake inhibitors duloxetine and venlafaxine increased bladder capacity in a cat model of irritated bladder, but a combination of a selective NE reuptake inhibitor with a selective 5-HT reuptake inhibitor had no such effect.[9]

Animal experiments with TCAs demonstrate the role of the central nervous system in these drugs' effects. In a rat model, Maggi et al.[10] showed imipramine and desipramine to increase the threshold volume of the spinal voiding reflex but not to affect the supraspinal voiding reflex. When administered chronically, however, these drugs selectively raised the threshold for the supraspinal voiding reflex. This study implicates the reuptake inhibition of serotonin, as the effects were blocked when the central nervous system was depleted of 5-HT. Sohn and Kim[11] confirmed that peripherally administered imipramine diminished reflex micturition, but intrathecally administered imipramine completely abolished this reflex. Unlike the earlier study, Sohn found the effect of imipramine to be blocked by a muscarinic agonist, concluding that imipramine acts via a central anticholinergic mechanism.

In vitro studies

More is known about tricyclic antidepressants' direct effects on the lower urinary tract using in vitro models. Many studies have examined the acute effects of TCAs, mostly imipramine, on isolated strips of animal bladder in vitro. These studies, performed with concentrations of imipramine ranging from 1 to 100 times therapeutic serum levels,[12] consistently showed that imipramine reduced detrusor contractility. Labay and Boyarsky[13] found that imipramine had a direct effect on detrusor muscle, decreasing baseline muscle tone and blocking acetylcholine-induced

contractions in strips of rabbit, dog, and human detrusor.[14] Fredericks et al.[15] found that imipramine had non-competitive anticholinergic action but that oxybutynin was 100 times more potent. Olubadewo[16] confirmed non-competitive anticholinergic action at high concentrations of imipramine but found competitive inhibition at closer to therapeutic levels.

Benson et al.[17] found that imipramine decreased detrusor strip contractions by a combination of anticholinergic and antispasmodic mechanisms. The term "antispasmodic" was used to refer to direct relaxation of the muscle and inhibition of barium-induced contractions, thought to be mediated through a calcium pathway. Olubadewo found that imipramine caused direct relaxation of detrusor strips not replicated by cholinergic blockade, and it prevented calcium-induced detrusor contractions.[16] Malkowicz et al.[18] also noted inhibition of calcium-induced contractions by imipramine, and Akah[19] found that high calcium levels reversed TCA-induced detrusor strip relaxation, further suggesting that imipramine's effect on the bladder involved calcium inhibition.

Bladder efferent signaling

Part of the effect of TCAs has been attributed to a "local anesthetic" effect on nerves of the bladder.[17] Fredericks et al.[15] reported that imipramine decreased the amplitude of nerve action potentials similar to tetracaine. The significance of these findings is not known.

Live animal lower urinary tract models

Studies of the effects of TCAs on whole bladders and live animals further illustrate their effects. Khanna et al.[20] demonstrated that imipramine increased the urethral resting pressure in live female dogs. This change was completely blocked by phenoxybenzamine, indicating that the urethral pressure changes were mediated by increased α-adrenergic stimulation. Creed and Tulloch[21] performed bladder and urethral pressure studies in anesthetized dogs in response to pelvic nerve stimulation. They found that imipramine increased urethral resting tone, decreased resting bladder tone, and decreased the response of both bladder and urethra to pelvic nerve stimulation. Imipramine also decreased the contractile response of the bladder to close administration of acetylcholine, 5-HT, and histamine, but did not block the rise in urethral pressure in response to histamine. These findings suggested that imipramine's action was likely not due to its anticholinergic effects. This is supported by earlier work[22] which showed that imipramine lowered intravesical pressure but did not significantly decrease salivary gland production in response to direct nerve stimulation, suggesting that the drug effect at the organ level was not due to anticholinergic activity.

Other potential mechanisms

One other mechanism through which TCAs may affect voiding is through interaction with the production of antidiuretic hormone (ADH). Studies have found that in both children[23] and adults,[24] imipramine induces increased ADH production. While this may play some role in overactive bladder, this mechanism is likely more important in explaining imipramine's role in controlling nocturnal enuresis.

Duloxetine studies

In contrast to the direct effects of imipramine on the bladder and urethra, duloxetine appears to exert much of its effect at the central rather than the peripheral level. Thor and Katofiasc[25] demonstrated in an acetic acid-irritated cat bladder model that while duloxetine increased bladder capacity, diminished reflex voiding, and raised coordinated urethral tone, there was no effect on bladder contractions when generated by direct pelvic nerve stimulation. The increased urethral tone induced by duloxetine, eight times that of control, was linked to $5\text{-}HT_2$ and α_1-adrenergic receptors. Interestingly, all of these effects were only found in cats with acetic acid-irritated bladders, implying that duloxetine's effect requires afferent (sensory) input in a central nervous system-mediated mechanism.

CLINICAL STUDIES

The depth and quality of clinical studies of TCAs in overactive bladder is poor. The author of one of the few double-blind studies performed noted

in 1968, "The history of this treatment is typical of that of many psychotropic drugs, namely initial enthusiastic case reports, then even more enthusiastic uncontrolled studies, followed by an equivocal series of double-blind experiments."[26] Regrettably, double-blind, controlled studies of the size and quality necessary to answer the question of the role of TCAs in overactive bladder have not been performed.

The first reported utility of TCAs in incontinence was in 1960[27] when it was noted that imipramine decreased adult and pediatric enuresis in a patient taking the antidepressant. Since that time, there have been several uncontrolled trials that reflect on the use of TCAs in overactive bladder. In 1972 Cole and Fried[28] reported less incontinence and improved voiding in eight patients with neurogenic bladder. Clinical improvement generally occurred 7–10 days after treatment started, and symptoms resumed on discontinuation of imipramine. Later, Rabey et al.[29] treated 16 patients with multiple sclerosis who had detrusor overactivity, utilizing imipramine and propantheline. Urodynamic studies were performed before treatment and then 15–30 days later. Fifteen of the 16 patients had an increase in the reflex bladder contraction volume, and 14 of the 16 had increased urethral pressure profiles.

A few uncontrolled studies have been done in patients with non-neurogenic detrusor overactivity. Castleden et al.[30] treated 10 incontinent elderly patients who had urodynamically confirmed overactivity with escalating doses of imipramine. Six patients regained continence; seven patients had repeat urodynamics. Of those repeating urodynamics who had a clinical response to imipramine, there was a statistically significant increase in urethral pressure, volume to first contraction, and bladder capacity, and a decrease in pressure at bladder capacity. Barker and Glenning[31] later evaluated 74 patients with urge, stress, or mixed incontinence by urodynamics, treated with imipramine and propantheline. Cure or major or minor improvements were observed in 31%, 32%, and 7%, respectively. They noted that the greatest improvements were in patients with either normal findings or detrusor overactivity on urodynamics. Another prospective uncontrolled trial[32] gave quality of life questionnaires to 25 patients with urodynamically proven urge-predominant incontinence, before and after treatment with imipramine. At an average 6 weeks' follow-up, they found clinical improvement or cure in 73% and a 79% reduction in incontinence episodes.

Imipramine has also been studied in uncontrolled trials in women with stress incontinence. Gilja et al.[33] evaluated 30 women with pure stress incontinence treated with imipramine for 4 weeks. Seventy-one percent of patients regained continence, while 29% noted no improvement. They found statistically significant increases in urethral closure pressure after treatment, as well as increases in functional urethral length. Patients with successful treatment had increased functional urethral lengths that did not change with stress, while those who failed treatment had shortening of the urethra with stress. These findings were confirmed more recently by Lin et al.,[34] who treated 40 women with pure stress incontinence with imipramine for 3 months. Urodynamics was performed before and after treatment. They found that 35% of patients were cured according to pad weight test, and an additional 25% had more than 50% improvement. This study also found statistically significant improvements in urethral closing pressure and functional urethral length among patients with treatment success versus patients who failed treatment. The only pretreatment parameter that correlated with successful treatment was a higher urethral closing pressure.

Few randomized, controlled trials exist examining the use of TCAs in overactive bladder or incontinence. More of historical than practical interest, in 1968 Milner and Hills[26] reported a randomized placebo-controlled study of imipramine, desipramine, or nortriptyline in 212 enuretic patients confined to a psychiatric hospital, some of whom had epilepsy. Patients were given one of the study drugs or placebo. The number of times a patient passed the night with or without enuresis was compared during times of active treatment or no active treatment. They found statistically significant improvements in the number of dry nights for the study drugs, particularly for imipramine and nortriptyline, in the subset of patients who were "mentally subnormal" females or schizophrenic females. Of more modern relevance was a study by Jarvis[35] which studied 50 women with incontinence due to detrusor overactivity, receiving either instruction in bladder retraining or imipramine and flavoxate for 4 weeks. Both groups showed improvements in frequency, nocturia, urgency, and urge and stress incontinence, but interestingly, the bladder retraining group had statistically significant improvement over the drug treatment group.

Few trials have evaluated TCAs in a placebo-controlled fashion. Castleden et al.[36] performed a double-blind placebo-controlled study of imipramine versus placebo in 33 patients with urodynamically confirmed detrusor overactivity incontinence. Using resolution of incontinence and time to resolution as their primary endpoints, they found no significant differences between the two groups in those endpoints. Lose et al.[37] studied doxepin, a less-commonly used TCA, in a randomized placebo-controlled crossover study of 19 women with detrusor overactivity who had failed previous pharmacologic therapy. There were statistically significant improvements in the doxepin group for night-time voiding frequency and incontinence episodes, as well as volume at first sensation and bladder capacity. There was no difference in daytime frequency. Also, significantly more women preferred doxepin to placebo.

More recently, duloxetine has shown promise as a treatment for incontinence. Several well-designed multicenter placebo-controlled studies have shown the efficacy of duloxetine in stress urinary incontinence.[38–42] A secondary analysis[43] of an early duloxetine study[38] evaluated a subset of 171 women who had mixed urinary incontinence out of a total study population of 553 women with predominantly symptoms of stress incontinence. Patients were randomized to receive duloxetine in one of three doses or placebo over a 12-week treatment period. Both groups, stress incontinence and mixed incontinence, showed statistically significant improvements in weekly incontinent episode frequency compared to placebo.

CONCLUSIONS

Tricyclic antidepressants, particularly imipramine, have been used since the 1960s to treat incontinence. Basic science studies of the effects of TCAs in humans and animals suggest prevention of urinary incontinence in overactive bladder via effects on the central nervous system as well as the lower urinary tract directly. No well-designed clinical trials of TCAs have been performed, although several small uncontrolled trials suggest that clinical efficacy is reasonable in patients with overactive bladder. Duloxetine, currently not approved for use in incontinence in the United States, has been demonstrated in large, well-designed studies to decrease stress urinary incontinence, and it may hold promise for use in patients with mixed incontinence.

REFERENCES

1. Malone DC, Okano GJ. Treatment of urge incontinence in Veterans Affairs medical centers. Clin Ther 1999; 21: 867–77.

2. Richelson E, Nelson A. Antagonism by antidepressants of neurotransmitter receptors of normal human brain in vitro. J Pharmacol Exp Ther 1984; 230: 94–102.

3. Bolden-Watson C, Richelson E. Blockage by newly-developed antidepressants of biogenic amine uptake into rat brain synaptosomes. Life Sci 1993; 52: 1023–9.

4. Bymaster FP, Dreshfield-Ahmad LJ, Threlkeld PG et al. Comparative affinity of duloxetine and venlafaxine for serotonin and norepinephrine transporters in vitro and in vivo, human serotonin receptor subtypes, and other neuronal receptors. Neuropsychopharmacology 2001; 25: 871–80.

5. Garcia AS, Barrera G, Burke TF et al. Autoreceptor-mediated inhibition of norepinephrine release in rat medial prefrontal cortex is maintained after chronic desipramine treatment. Journal of Neurochemistry 2004; 91: 683–93.

6. De Groat W. Influence of central serotonergic mechanisms on lower urinary tract function. Urology 2002; 59 (5 Suppl): 30–6.

7. Persson K, Pandita RK, Spitsbergen JM et al. Spinal and peripheral mechanism contributing to hyperactive voiding in spontaneously hypertensive rats. Am J Physiol 1998; 275: R1366–73.

8. Ishizuka O, Mattiasson A, Andersson KE. Role of spinal and peripheral alpha 2 adrenoceptors in micturition in normal conscious rats. J Urol 1996; 156: 1853–7.

9. Katofiasc MA, Nissen J, Audia J, Thor KB. Comparison of the effects of serotonin selective, norepinephrine selective, and dual serotonin and norepinephrine reuptake inhibitors on lower urinary tract function in cats. Life Sci 2002; 71: 1227–36.

10. Maggi CA, Borsini F, Lecci A et al. Effect of acute or chronic imipramine on spinal and supraspinal micturition reflexes in rats. J Pharmacol Exp Ther 1989; 248: 278–85.

11. Sohn UD, Kim CY. Suppression of the rat micturition reflex by imipramine. J Auton Pharmacol 1997; 17: 35–41.

12. Orsulak PJ. Therapeutic monitoring of antidepressant drugs: guidelines updated. Ther Drug Monit 1989; 11: 497–507.

13. Labay P, Boyarsky S. Urinary bladder contractility: action of imipramine. Arch Phys Med Rehabil 1974; 55: 166–70.

14. Labay P, Boyarsky S. The action of imipramine on the bladder musculature. J Urol 1973; 109: 385–7.

15. Fredericks CM, Green RL, Anderson GF. Comparative in vitro effects of imipramine, oxybutynin, and flavoxate on rabbit detrusor. Urology 1978; 12: 487–91.

16. Olubadewo JO. The effect of imipramine on rat detrusor muscle contractility. Arch Int Pharmacodyn Ther 1980; 245: 84–94.

17. Benson GS, Sarshik SA, Raezer DM, Wein AJ. Bladder muscle contractility: comparative effects and mechanisms of action of atropine, propantheline, flavoxate, and imipramine. Urology 1977; 9: 31–5.

18. Malkowicz SB, Wein AJ, Ruggieri MR, Levin RM. Comparison of calcium antagonist properties of antispasmodic agents. J Urol 1987; 138: 667–70.

19. Akah PA. Tricyclic antidepressant inhibition of the electrical evoked response of the rat urinary bladder strip—effect of variation in extracellular Ca^{2+} concentration. Arch Int Pharmacodyn Ther 1986; 284: 231–8.

20. Khanna OP, Elkouss G, Heber D, Gonick P. Imipramine hydrochloride, pharmacodynamic effects on lower urinary tract of female dog. Urology 1975; 6: 48–51.

21. Creed KE, Tulloch AGS. The action of imipramine on the lower urinary tract of the dog. Br J Urol 1982; 54: 5–10.

22. Tulloch GS, Creed KE. A comparison between propanetheline and imipramine on bladder and salivary gland function. Br J Urol 1979; 51: 359–62.

23. Tomasi PA, Siracusano S, Monni AM, Mela G, Delitala G. Decreased nocturnal urinary antidiuretic hormone excretion in enuresis is increased by imipramine. BJU Int 2001; 88: 932–7.

24. Puri VN. Increased urinary antidiuretic hormone excretion by imipramine. Exp Clin Endocrinol 1986; 88: 112–14.

25. Thor KB, Katofiasc MA. Effects of duloxetine, a combined serotonin and norepinephrine reuptake inhibitor, on central neural control of lower urinary tract function in the chloralose-anesthetized female cat. J Pharmacol Exp Ther 1995; 274: 1014–24.

26. Milner G, Hills NF. A double-blind assessment of antidepressants in the treatment of 212 enuretic patients. Med J Aust 1968; 1: 943–7.

27. MacLean REG. Imipramine hydrochloride (Tofranil) and enuresis. Am J Psychiatry 1960; 117: 551.

28. Cole AT, Fried FA. Favorable experiences with imipramine in the treatment of neurogenic bladder. J Urol 1972; 107: 44–5.

29. Rabey JM, Moriel EZ, Farkas A et al. Detrusor hyperreflexia in multiple sclerosis. Alleviation by a combination of imipramine and propantheline, a clinico-laboratory study. Eur Neurol 1979; 18: 33–7.

30. Castleden CM, George CF, Renwick AG, Asher MJ. Imipramine—a possible alternative to current therapy for urinary incontinence in the elderly. J Urol 1981; 125: 318–20.

31. Barker G, Glenning PP. Treatment of the unstable bladder with propantheline and imipramine. Aust NZ J Obstet Gynaecol 1987; 27: 152–4.

32. Woodman PJ, Misko CA, Fischer JR. The use of short-form quality of life questionnaires to measure the impact of imipramine on women with urge incontinence. Int Urogynecol J Pelvic Floor Dysfunct 2001; 12: 312–15.

33. Gilja I, Radej M, Kovacic M, Parazajder J. Conservative treatment of female stress incontinence with imipramine. J Urol 1984; 132: 909–11.

34. Lin HH, Sheu BC, Lo MC, Huang SC. Comparison of treatment outcomes for imipramine for female genuine stress incontinence. Br J Obstet Gynaecol 1999; 106: 1089–92.

35. Jarvis GJ. A controlled trial of bladder drill and drug therapy in the management of detrusor instability. Br J Urol 1981; 53: 565–6.

36. Castleden CM, Duffin HM, Gulati RS. Double-blind study of imipramine and placebo for incontinence due to bladder instability. Age Ageing 1986; 15: 299–303.

37. Lose G, Jorgensen L, Thunedborg P. Doxepin in the treatment of female detrusor overactivity: a randomized double-blind crossover study. J Urol 1989; 142: 1024–6.

38. Norton PA, Zinner NR, Yalcin I, Bump RC. Duloxetine versus placebo in the treatment of stress urinary incontinence. Am J Obstet Gynecol 2002; 187: 40–8.

39. van Kerrebroeck P, Abrams P, Lange R et al. Duloxetine versus placebo in the treatment of European and Canadian women with stress urinary incontinence. BJOG 2004; 111: 249–57.

40. Millard RJ, Moore K, Rencken R, Yalcin I, Bump RC. Duloxetine vs placebo in the treatment of stress urinary incontinence: a four-continent randomized clinical trial. BJU Int 2004; 93: 311–8.

41. Dmochowski RR, Miklos JR, Norton PA et al. Duloxetine versus placebo for the treatment of North American women with stress urinary incontinence. J Urol 2003; 170: 1259–63.

42. Ghoniem GM, Van Leeuwen JS, Elser DM et al. A randomized controlled trial of duloxetine alone, pelvic floor muscle training alone, combined treatment and no active treatment in women with stress urinary incontinence. J Urol 2005; 173: 1647–53.

43. Bump RC, Norton PA, Zinner NR, Yalcin I. Mixed urinary incontinence symptoms: urodynamic findings, incontinence severity, and treatment response. Obstet Gynecol 2003; 102: 76–83.

13

Propiverine hydrochloride in the treatment of idiopathic and neurogenic detrusor overactivity: efficacy, tolerability, and safety profile

Manfred Stöhrer, Gerd Mürtz, Guus Kramer, and Herbert Rübben

Introduction • **Pharmacology** • **Efficacy** • **Tolerability and safety** • **Post-marketing drug surveillance** • **Recent advances** • **Summary** • **Acknowledgments**

INTRODUCTION

Only six antimuscarinics have been recommended with level of evidence 1 and grade A of recommendation for the treatment of detrusor overactivity by the Committee on Pharmacological Treatment chaired by Andersson during the 3rd International Consultation on Incontinence.[1] Propiverine hydrochloride (in the following abbreviated as propiverine) is one of these recommended antimuscarinics.

Propiverine has been launched in a number of countries in Europe, Asia, Africa, and South America with special focus on Germany and Japan, being the most frequently prescribed antimuscarinic drug there.

PHARMACOLOGY

Propiverine, a benzylic acid derivative, is a compound with multiple effects on the urinary bladder smooth muscle and its innervation. In recent studies, the parent drug and its main human metabolites were shown to reduce human detrusor muscle contractility, evoked by several stimuli, to about 15% of predrug administration control and affect L-type Ca^{2+} currents.[2] An age-dependency of sensitivity to the pharmacological action was not observed.[3,4]

Further pharmacodynamic and pharmacokinetic properties were reviewed in a previous paper.[5] After oral administration propiverine is rapidly and almost completely absorbed. The absolute bioavailability of 15 mg propiverine, when administered orally, amounts to 40%. A mean terminal elimination half-life of about 14 hours was reported. The plasma protein binding of propiverine amounts to approximately 90%, whereas the main metabolite is bound at a level of about 60% to plasma proteins.

The drug undergoes an extensive first pass effect. Three major metabolites have been detected, with the N-oxide being the predominant one. These metabolites occur in humans in the plasma and/or urine in concentrations high enough to exert a defined pharmacodynamic effect.

Repeated oral dosing within the therapeutic range (e.g. 20 mg twice daily) leads to a steady state mean trough level of about 60 ng/ml in healthy volunteers after 4–5 days. Despite the low renal clearance, below 1 ml/min for propiverine and its main metabolite propiverine *N*-oxide, drug accumulation does not occur after long-term treatment.

Preclinical studies elucidating the pharmacodynamic effects of propiverine were performed with various model systems in vitro and in vivo. Several radioligand binding studies demonstrated the affinity of propiverine to muscarinic receptors. However, it has significantly lower affinity for the cardiac M_2 receptors in comparison to routine reference drugs.

Studies with urinary bladder strips of various species showed an inhibiting effect of propiverine on acetylcholine and KCl-induced contractions. Additionally, propiverine was also observed to interact directly with calmodulin causing an inhibition of the activity of actomyosin adenosine triphosphatase (ATPase), also resulting in relaxation of the smooth muscle of the urinary bladder.

The in vivo effect of propiverine on the urinary bladder was investigated in various animal species. In the dog, the maximum bladder volume increased and inhibiting effects on electrically induced periodic contractions of the detrusor were shown. In the rat, maximum bladder volume was also increased significantly. In the minipig, propiverine was effective as tolterodine to reduce the maximum bladder pressure with comparable tolerability profile with respect to salivation, blood pressure, and heart rate.[6]

In summary, pharmacodynamic investigations showed antimuscarinic and additional effects on calcium influx and calcium homeostasis in urinary bladder preparations, thus proving a dual mode of action of propiverine in relaxing detrusor smooth muscle.

EFFICACY

In the past, the acknowledged terminology of the International Continence Society was based on urodynamic evaluation. Thus, detrusor instability, with no evident neurological cause, and detrusor hyperreflexia, with proven neurological cause, were differentiated.[7] Recently, the terminology has shifted from a urodynamic to a clinical perspective: overactive bladder (OAB) syndrome is considered the key clinical entity encompassing urgency, with or without urge incontinence, usually with frequency and nocturia. However, if detrusor function is assessed, and involuntary detrusor contractions during filling cystometry are verified, the term detrusor overactivity is also applicable. It is further qualified as neurogenic, when there is a relevant neurological condition, and as idiopathic detrusor overactivity, when there is no defined cause.[8]

In order to avoid misinterpretation of terminology, in this review recent terms are used, in case older terms could be replaced unambiguously. Otherwise, symptoms, signs, urodynamic observations, and conditions associated with lower urinary tract dysfunction are cited according to the terminology applicable at the time of study conduct. Key studies of the noted different clinical entities and patient populations are highlighted in the following discussion.

Neurogenic detrusor overactivity

Unequivocally, patients suffering from neurogenic detrusor overactivity, in most cases because of spinal cord injury, are not susceptible to placebo effects. Undoubtedly, propiverine is among the most thoroughly investigated antimuscarinics with respect to neurogenic detrusor overactivity, both in adults and in children.

A dose-optimizing study in patients with neurogenic detrusor overactivity[9] showed a decreased micturition frequency in 54% of the patients following 15 mg/day, and in about 80% following 30–60 mg/day.

A proof-of-concept-study by Stöhrer et al.[10] evaluated the efficacy of propiverine (15 mg three times daily) compared to placebo in 113 patients suffering from neurogenic detrusor overactivity caused by spinal cord injury. This double-blind, randomized, prospective, multi-center trial comprised visits at baseline and after 14 days of treatment. The majority of patients emptied their bladder via intermittent catheterization. The maximum cystometric bladder capacity increased significantly in the propiverine group, on average by 104 ml (pre: 262 ± 132 ml; post: 336 ± 143 ml, $p < 0.001$). This effect was paralleled by a significant decrease in maximum detrusor pressure (Figure 13.1). The results demonstrated the expected therapeutic benefit

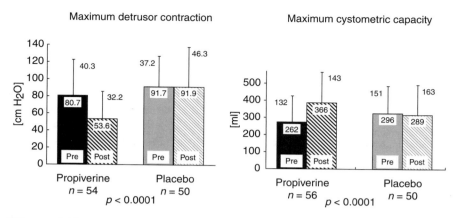

Figure 13.1 Efficacy of 15 mg three times daily (tid) propiverine compared to placebo in neurogenic detrusor overactivity. (From reference 10, with permisson)

of detrusor relaxation in neurogenic detrusor overactivity achieved by propiverine. Expectedly, no beneficial effects manifested following placebo.

Also, Japanese authors have presented efficacy evidence of propiverine in neurogenic detrusor overactivity: Takayasu et al.[11] conducted a double-blind, placebo-controlled multicentric study in 70 neurogenic patients, comparing 20 mg propiverine once daily and placebo for 2 weeks of treatment. In accordance with the European study results, maximum detrusor pressure decreased, and maximum bladder capacity increased as compared to placebo.

Propiverine was also compared to oxybutynin for neurogenic detrusor overactivity in a randomized, double-blind, multicenter study.[12] Patients were eligible if suffering from neurogenic detrusor overactivity, as defined by the International Continence Society (ICS) as a patient with known neurological disorder who also presents with detrusor overactivity. Eligibility also required a maximum cystometric capacity of less than 300 ml. After a 1-week run-in period, propiverine 15 mg three times daily (tid) or oxybutynin 5 mg tid was allocated. Urodynamic parameters were assessed as primary efficacy outcomes before and after at least 21 days of treatment. In total, 131 patients were recruited at 20 study centers. The maximum cystometric capacity was increased significantly in the propiverine group from 198 ± 110 to 309 ± 166 ml, and in the oxybutynin group from 164 ± 64 to

298 ± 125 ml. Similarly, maximum detrusor pressure during the filling phase was lowered significantly in both groups: in the propiverine group from 56.8 ± 36.2 to 37.8 ± 31.6 cmH$_2$O, and in the oxybutynin group from 68.6 ± 34.5 to 43.1 ± 29.2 cmH$_2$O. There was no significant difference in these urodynamic changes between treatment groups. For clinical parameters, the 24-hour micturition frequency decreased in the propiverine group from 10.9 to 7.9 and in the oxybutynin group from 12.0 to 9.5 episodes. Twenty-four-hour incontinence episodes were reduced in the propiverine group from 3.9 to 2.3 and in the oxybutynin group from 3.3 to 2.0. In conclusion, propiverine and oxybutynin were equally effective in increasing bladder capacity and lowering bladder pressure in patients with neurogenic detrusor overactivity. The same held true for clinical parameters.

All studies consistently demonstrated that propiverine is effective in neurogenic detrusor overactivity by increasing functional bladder capacity and decreasing detrusor pressure. Thus, a low-pressure situation in the bladder is created and continence, a treatment aim secondary to pressure reduction, is achieved, mostly in combination with intermittent catheterization.[7,10,12] Treatment periods of 2–3 weeks have been criticized as being too short. However, at least in this condition (neurogenic detrusor overactivity), these treatment periods are sufficient to demonstrate rapid onset of action. Extended treatment periods cannot be justified due to the risk of secondary complications following placebo treatment.[7]

Idiopathic detrusor overactivity

The efficacy of different propiverine dosages was evaluated in 185 patients suffering from urgency and/or urge incontinence in an open-label, randomized, multicenter parallel group study for 21 days.[13] Some 80% of patients suffered from detrusor instability verified by urodynamics. Bladder capacity and bladder compliance increased, and detrusor pressure decreased dose-dependently. Daily doses of 15–30 mg showed the most favorable efficacy/tolerability ratio.

The efficacy of propiverine (15 mg tid) in patients suffering from frequency, urgency, and urge incontinence was compared to those of oxybutynin (5 mg twice daily (bid)) and placebo in a randomized, double-blind, multicenter study conducted by Madersbacher et al.[14] A total of 366 patients (propiverine 149, oxybutynin 145, placebo 72) were recruited. Efficacy was assessed by micturition charts and urodynamics prior to and after 4 weeks of treatment. Both frequency of micturition and episodes of urgency decreased significantly following propiverine or oxybutynin, compared to placebo treatment. Urodynamic parameters showed a significant increase of the maximum cystometric bladder capacity for propiverine (pre: 222 ± 77; post: 311 ± 125 ml) and oxybutynin (pre: 226 ± 75; post: 322 ± 123 ml)

in comparison to placebo (pre: 211 ± 77; post: 263 ± 93 ml).

Propiverine was compared to tolterodine with respect to efficacy and impact on quality of life (QoL) in patients with idiopathic detrusor overactivity.[15] In this randomized, double-blind, multicenter clinical trial 202 patients with idiopathic detrusor overactivity were treated either with twice-daily regimens of 15 mg propiverine or 2 mg tolterodine over a 28-day treatment period. The primary efficacy outcome, maximum cystometric capacity, increased significantly in both groups. Secondary efficacy outcomes, i.e. voided volume per micturition, volume at first urge, and frequency–volume chart parameter also showed relevant improvements (Table 13.1). QoL improved comparably in both treatment groups (Figure 13.2). In conclusion, this study demonstrated equal improvement of efficacy and QoL with 15 mg propiverine twice-daily and 2 mg tolterodine twice-daily treatment regimens for the symptoms of detrusor overactivity.

Another double-blind, randomized, crossover study[16] in 41 women with urodynamically proven detrusor instability compared propiverine (15 mg bid) and tolterodine (2 mg bid) over a 6-week period. Based on QoL scores, micturition frequencies, and incontinence episodes, a trend towards more improved efficacy in the propiverine-treated compared to the tolterodine-treated patients was documented. Significantly superior efficacy compared to tolterodine could not be achieved due to the small patient number.

Table 13.1 Differences of post-treatment vs baseline in outcome parameters of frequency–volume charts for propiverine and tolterodine treatment. (From reference 15)

	Propiverine 15 mg bid	Tolterodine 2 mg bid	p Value (t test)
Voided volume per micturition (ml)	+31.35 ± 60.83	+27.65 ± 56.27	0.71
Urgency episodes (n)	−3.34 ± 3.07	−2.80 ± 3.73	0.37
Voiding episodes (n)	−3.07 ± 2.29	−2.95 ± 2.88	0.80
Leakage episodes (n)	−1.07 ± 1.79	−1.00 ± 1.53	0.82
Change of pads (n)	−0.40 ± 1.95	−0.39 ± 1.22	0.98

bid, twice daily

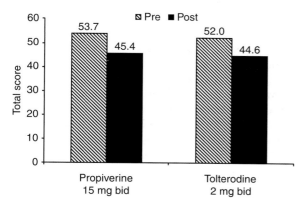

Figure 13.2 Quality of life (King's Health Score) following 15 mg twice daily (bid) propiverine ($n = 100$) compared to 2 mg bid tolterodine ($n = 102$). (From reference 15, with permission)

OAB symptoms secondary to operative procedures (e.g. transurethral resection of the prostate (TURP)) on the lower urinary tract have been shown to resolve following propiverine treatment. In a randomized prospective trial, propiverine, given for the first 10 days postoperatively, demonstrated an increased bladder capacity in 80% of the patients with 60 mg and in 60% with 30 mg, compared to 33% with placebo.[17] This was confirmed by Park et al.[18] in an open-label study. Despite only limited evidence in controlled studies, clinical experience verifies beneficial effects of propiverine in patients with OAB symptoms after TURP.

In conclusion, several placebo- and reference-controlled prospective, randomized studies have shown propiverine, oxybutynin, and tolterodine to be equieffective in patients suffering from idiopathic detrusor overactivity or overactive bladder syndrome. With respect to QoL, propiverine and tolterodine exert comparably beneficial effects.

Elderly

Several studies, although some of them were performed without placebo control, have demonstrated the efficacy of propiverine in the elderly: Dorschner et al.[19] investigated propiverine in 98 elderly (67.7 ± 6.3 years of age) patients suffering from urgency and/or urge incontinence in a double-blind, multicenter, placebo-controlled, randomized study. After 4 weeks of treatment, propiverine caused significant reductions in micturition frequency, paralleled by significant increases in average voided volume, and significant reductions in incontinence episodes, compared to placebo.

Mori et al.[20] focused on 46 demented elderly (80.8 years of age on average) suffering from urinary incontinence. Propiverine, administered for 2 weeks, improved both the cystometric bladder capacity in 46.3% and incontinence episodes in 40% of the patients. Otomo et al.[21] confirmed these results in 31 demented elderly patients. Welz-Barth[22] reported beneficial effects of propiverine over a 4-week treatment period in 39 patients with frequency, urgency, and urge incontinence, who had suffered a stroke.

Children

To the best of our knowledge, propiverine represents the antimuscarinic which is by far the best documented with respect to its pediatric use, both in neurogenic and in idiopathic detrusor overactivity.

Children with neurogenic detrusor over-activity are treated with antimuscarinics and intermittent catheterization as the gold standard regimen. Grigoleit et al.[23] confirmed the efficacy of propiverine in 74 children and adolescents suffering in most cases from myelomeningocele, all treated for 2 years and 4 months on average. The primary efficacy outcomes improved significantly: maximum cystometric capacity increased from 161.2 ± 97.3 to 252.2 ± 117.2 ml, maximum detrusor pressure decreased from 43.8 ± 39.2 to 27.1 ± 26.4 cmH$_2$O, and bladder compliance improved from 7.6 ± 6.4 to 17.0 ± 16.2 ml/cmH$_2$O. Phasic detrusor overactivity was abolished in 63%, and incontinence resolved in 54%. Propiverine was effective even in those cases unresponsive to other antimuscarinics. Especially with respect to the extensive total surveillance period of almost 172 patient-years, these results are impressive.

Schulte-Baukloh and co-workers[24] confirmed the efficacy of propiverine in 20 children suffering from neurogenic detrusor overactivity in a prospective study. All urodynamic parameters – reflex volume, maximum detrusor pressure, maximum cystometric bladder capacity, and bladder compliance – measured before and after 3–6 months of a twice-daily propiverine regimen, improved significantly.

In a comparative multicenter study, 255 children with neurogenic detrusor overactivity (199 myelomeningocele, 46 spinal cord injury, 10 different diagnoses) were evaluated retrospectively. All children had been treated with antimuscarinics (127 propiverine, 128 oxybutynin). This study by Madersbacher et al.[25] is the largest pediatric study comparing antimuscarinics in this condition, and showed that the clinically most relevant efficacy outcome parameter, maximum detrusor pressure, was on average significantly reduced in both treatment groups. However, detrusor pressure was lowered to values below 40 cmH$_2$O in 74% in the propiverine group as compared to only 50% of the oxybutynin group. This difference demonstrated effective pressure reductions manifesting more frequently following propiverine than following oxybutynin, especially in myelomeningocele-children. It is hypothesized that these more beneficial effects of propiverine may be due to its dual mode of action with antimuscarinic and calcium-modulating effects.

With respect to incontinence suggestive of idiopathic detrusor overactivity, Marschall-Kehrel et al.[26] proposed an empirically derived treatment algorithm in children unresponsive to urotherapy (Figure 13.3). In a first treatment period, propiverine monotherapy (0.4 mg/kg/day bid; Mictonetten®) was applied for 4 weeks. After reevaluation in cases of only partial response, adjuvant measures over another 12 weeks were added in a second treatment period: selective α-adrenoceptor antagonists for functional bladder outflow obstruction, desmopressin for excessive nocturnal urine production, and biofeedback for increased pelvic floor activity during micturition. This treatment algorithm, incorporating symptom-oriented additional measures in partial responders following propiverine monotherapy, improved outcomes to give an approximately 90% success rate.

A pharmacoepidemiological study by Alloussi et al.[27] evaluated 621 children suffering from urinary incontinence suggestive of idiopathic detrusor overactivity (437 propiverine, 184 oxybutynin). Continence, the primary outcome, demonstrated statistically equivalent efficacy of both antimuscarinics. However, a trend towards superior efficacy was manifested in those

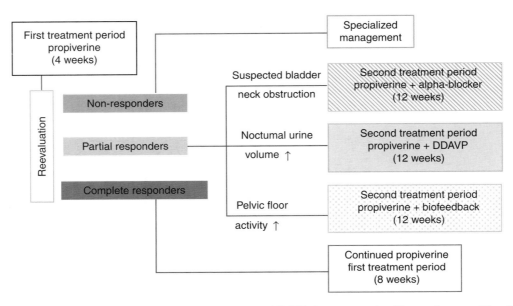

Figure 13.3 Treatment algorithm for incontinent children. DDAVP, desmopressin. (From reference 26, with permission)

individuals receiving higher doses of propiverine. Adequate diagnosis, body weight-adapted and titrated dosages, and treatment periods of at least 4 months were considered key factors for treatment success.

Another pediatric treatment algorithm, focusing on nocturnal enuresis, elucidated that in children non-responsive to first-line desmopressin treatment an adjuvant application of propiverine in cases in which nocturnal diuretic volume exceeded functional bladder capacity, improved treatment outcomes significantly (reference 28 ICS award for best clinical presentation).

Men with overactive bladder and concomitant symptoms of benign prostatic syndrome

The combined application of α-adrenoceptor antagonists and propiverine presents an innovative and promising option for alleviating lower urinary tract symptoms. However, prior to treatment, a significant degree of bladder outflow obstruction, possibly anticipating urinary retention, must be excluded.

Propiverine was the first antimuscarinic administered concomitantly with tamsulosin, comparing this add-on therapy to tamsulosin monotherapy.[29] In this prospective, randomized, 4-week multicenter trial, 134 benign prostatic hyperplasia (BPH) patients with obstructive and OAB symptoms were included. Unfortunately, the assumed infravesical obstruction was not verified by pressure–flow studies. Improvement rates of daytime frequency, urinary incontinence, and urgency were more significant with combination therapy (Figure 13.4). Interestingly, post-void residual and maximal uroflow were not affected significantly. The authors concluded that the combination of propiverine and tamsulosin improved irritative without deteriorating obstructive symptoms.

In a prospective, randomized comparative study, Lee et al.[30] evaluated propiverine combined with doxazosin in 228 men with OAB and urodynamically proven bladder outlet obstruction. Improvement rates with respect to urinary frequency, average micturition volume, and storage and urgency International Prostate Symptom Score (IPSS) symptoms were more significant with combination treatment compared to doxazosin monotherapy (Figure. 13.4). Post-void residual was increased following propiverine and doxazosin, but no case of acute urinary retention developed.

Reflecting these recent therapeutic advances we advocate the development of treatment algorithms in men suffering concomitantly from OAB and benign prostatic syndrome (BPS): for daily practice, α-adrenoceptor antagonists present the first approach. In unresponsive cases, propiverine, because of its proven efficacy also in this condition, could be added. Nevertheless, safety precautions require close monitoring, encompassing post-void residual, maximal uroflow, and preferably also sonographic evaluation of

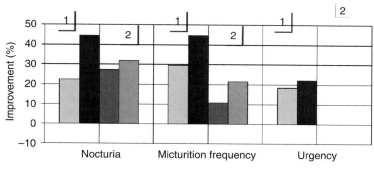

Figure 13.4 Improvement (%) of clinical symptoms following treatment with 0.2 mg/day tamsulosin monotherapy and in combination with 20 mg/day propiverine (1, from reference 29) and treatment with 4 mg/day doxazosin monotherapy and in combination with 20 mg/day propiverine. (2, from reference 30) (See also color plate section).

detrusor thickness to exclude significant bladder outflow obstruction.

Long-term efficacy

Numerous long-term studies conducted in Japan and Europe (Table 13.2) in adult patients gave evidence that efficacy is maintained for periods of 1 year, with a tendency to increase with time. Consistent clinical and urodynamic improvements were reported in these studies, covering more than 500 patient-years of propiverine treatment. Excellent long-term efficacy can be claimed also for children and adolescents.[23]

TOLERABILITY AND SAFETY

Adverse events: overall evaluation

The tolerability and safety evaluation of propiverine is based on clinical, pharmacokinetic, and pharmacodynamic studies conducted in Europe and 36 clinical studies conducted in Japan. A total of 7100 patients were exposed to propiverine in all clinical trials conducted in Europe; in controlled clinical trials 1177 patients and volunteers were exposed to propiverine, 708 were treated with placebo, and 806 with other comparator drugs.

Different dose schedules in Europe (Mictonorm®, Detrunorm® 15 mg bid recommended in OAB, 15 mg tid recommended in neurogenic detrusor overactivity) and Japan (20 mg once daily) must be taken into account when evaluating tolerability. The proposed lower doses in Japan compared to Europe are attributable to a much lower mean body weight in the Japanese compared to the European population. The majority of European patients were treated with either 45 mg/day (41.1%) or 30 mg/day (42.9%).

Very common (≥ 10%) and common (≥ 1% to < 10%) typical antimuscarinic adverse events (AEs) following propiverine treatment include especially dry mouth, accommodation disorders, affected vision, and constipation. The incidence of AEs was expectedly higher in the propiverine group compared to the placebo group. In most studies substantial incidence rates of AEs are also associated with placebo treatment. Therefore, if placebo-adjusted AE rates are calculated, side effects such as dryness of mouth manifested in only 6.9% of patients (when subtracting placebo occurrence rates). This finding reflects that AEs are extremely placebo-ingestion related, especially in OAB patients: Madersbacher et al.[14] reported that 30% of placebo-treated patients complained about dry mouth, and Takayasu et al.[11] even reported identical incidence rates for propiverine and placebo.

Furthermore, incidence rates of dry mouth, the most frequent antimuscarinic AE, depended considerably on its method of evaluation: spontaneous reporting of AE resulted in moderate incidence rates of only 2%,[19] whereas active questioning resulted in much higher incidence rates.

Adverse events with respect to etiology, gender, and age

In OAB patients, AEs were reported more frequently than in patients suffering from neurogenic conditions. Incidence rates were higher in females than in males. Assessment of tolerability revealed fewer AEs in responsive compared to unresponsive patients. Interestingly, no clinically relevant differences in incidence rates of AEs existed in elderly compared to younger patients (Table 13.3). However, children compared to adults complained even markedly less about AEs: Hoashi[43] reported an extremely low incidence rate of 1% for propiverine in Japanese children.

Adverse events: propiverine versus oxybutynin

A comparative tolerability assessment of propiverine, oxybutynin, and placebo was conducted by Madersbacher et al.[14] in patients suffering from OAB. Incidence rates of AEs were significantly lower for propiverine 15 mg tid than for oxybutynin 5 mg bid. Furthermore, taking into account severity gradings (Figure 13.5), severe dryness of the mouth manifested statistically less often with propiverine (12%) compared to oxybutynin (25%), but more often than with placebo (4%). Interestingly, severe dryness of the mouth increased with time following oxybutynin (18% after 1, 25% after 4 weeks), whereas it remained unchanged following propiverine (13% after 1, 12% after 4 weeks).

Japanese studies are consistent with these findings: Kondo et al.[44] reported AE rates of

Table 13.2 Long-term tolerability of propiverine in clinical studies conducted in Japan and Germany. (Adapted from reference 5)

Reference	Recruited patients (n) (safety/efficacy evaluation)	Patients (n) > 6 months' treatment	Patients (n) > 12 months' treatment	Surveillance period (days) Average	Surveillance period (days) Maximum
Kagawa[31]	87 (75/69)	26	15	168	807
Yoshida[32]	116 (89/82)	33	21	Intended 1 year	
Ohmori[33]	53 (52/52)	20 (71–234 days)	Not evaluable	78.4	234
Noguchi[34]	147 (141/122)	81	57	241	604
Oeda[35]	34 (32/32)	11	7	Intended initially 1 year	
Tanabe[36]	49 (42/38) (elderly)	24	14	245	Intended 1 year
Takaki[37]	120 (107/101)	12	28	Intended 1 year	
Takaki[38]	32	14 (24 weeks)	1	159	
Watanabe[39]	23	8	Not reported	125	349
Voigt[40]	29	29	29	Maximum 10 years	
Madersbacher[41]	464 (464/454)	464	330	266	NA
Overall	1154	722	502	NA	807

NA, not applicable

Table 13.3 Incidence of adverse events in elderly (*n* = 1282) compared to younger patients (*n* = 3108) after 12 weeks of propiverine treatment. (Adapted from reference 42)

Adverse event	Elderly patients > 65 years (n = 1282)	Younger patients ≤ 65 years (n = 3108)
Dry mouth (%)	26.4	25.9
Accommodation disorders (%)	6.7	6.2
Constipation (%)	9.0	7.0
Tiredness (%)	5.7	6.0
Dizziness (%)	3.1	2.6

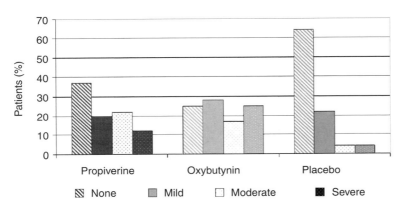

Figure 13.5 Severity of dryness of the mouth in 366 patients with urgency/urge incontinence following a 4-week treatment with propiverine 15 mg three times daily (tid), oxybutynin 5 mg twice daily (bid) or placebo. (From reference 14, with permission). (See also color plate section).

6.2–16.7% in their own and patient series of other investigators following propiverine, compared to 24.5% following oxybutynin treatment. These results in adults agree with results achieved in children: 3.9 and 9.4% following propiverine compared to 16.3 and 17.5% following oxybutynin are indicative of the distinctly superior tolerability profile of propiverine, AE rates being consistently two- to four-fold higher with oxybutynin.[27,41] Also, in the study of Batinic et al.,[45] propiverine was superior to oxybutynin and even as tolerable as placebo.

Adverse events: propiverine versus tolterodine

Propiverine and tolterodine are equally tolerable. In vivo studies in the mini-pig[6] showed no difference regarding dryness of mouth: propiverine decreased electrically stimulated salivation by 61%, tolterodine by 56%. Also, in patients

with idiopathic detrusor overactivity, Jünemann et al.[15] detected no differences: 42/100 patients exposed to propiverine and 43/102 patients exposed to tolterodine experienced adverse events (Figure 13.6). Dry mouth presented as the most common AE, which occurred in 20 patients of the propiverine group and in 19 patients of the tolterodine group (Figure 13.6). The most frequent AEs, as classified by organ systems according to the World Health Organization (Table 13.4), showed that propiverine and tolterodine are comparable with respect to tolerability.

Long-term tolerability

Acceable tolerability of propiverine was also shown under conditions of long-term administration in 11 open-label, multicenter clinical studies (Table 13.2). A 10-year follow-up of propiverine treatment was presented by Voigt et al.:[40] improved tolerability under long-term treatment may be a special feature of propiverine, a phenomenon so far not documented in other antimuscarinics.

Post-void residual

Antimuscarinics have been thought to increase the post-void residual due to possibly diminishing detrusor contractility. In some cases this might result even in urinary retention if additional factors coexist, e.g. detrusor–sphincter dyssynergia

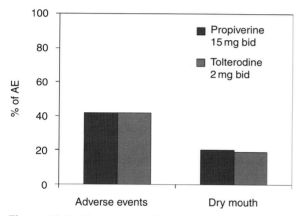

Figure 13.6 Percentage of patients with adverse events (AEs) and percentage of patients with dry mouth following propiverine (*n* = 100) and tolterodine (*n* = 102) treatment. (From reference 15, with permission)

in patients with neurogenic detrusor overactivity, or bladder outflow obstruction in patients with BPS. Accordingly, studies enrolling patients with neurogenic detrusor overactivity[10,12] as well as studies enrolling men with bladder outflow obstruction[30] showed an increased post-void residual following propiverine treatment. However, in patients with OAB symptoms, propiverine did not increase the post-void residual, as was shown consistently in several randomized, prospective, double-blind, pivotal studies.[14,19] Post-marketing drug surveillance showed a clinically relevant increase of post-void residual only in a minor percentage of 0.3%.[42,46] Also, in in vivo studies, propiverine, in contrast to oxybutynin, did not negatively affect the post-void residual.[11]

In conclusion, in patients with OAB and concomitant BPS, precautions are advisable. In patients with neurogenic detrusor overactivity, an increment or induction of post-void residual is no topic of concern if intermittent catheterization is practiced. In patients suffering from OAB, propiverine usually does not affect the post-void residual.

Cognition and psychomotor performance

Propiverine treatment did not significantly impair any of 16 psychometric tests as compared to placebo.[47] These results provide evidence that propiverine in therapeutic doses does not interfere with central nervous functions. Recently, Japanese

Table 13.4 Number of adverse events classified by organ systems following treatment with 15 mg bid propiverine (*n* = 100) and 2 mg bid tolterodine (*n* = 102). (From reference 15)

	Propiverine	Tolterodine
Gastrointestinal disorders	37	34
Accommodation disorders	9	7
General disorders and administration site conditions	6	4
Nervous system disorders	5	4
Cardiac disorders	1	6
Renal and urinary disorders	4	1
Psychiatric disorders	2	2

bid, twice daily

authors[48] investigated 32 elderly patients with neurological diseases (multiple cerebral infarction, dementia, Parkinson's disease, Alzheimer's disease) exposed to a 2-month period of propiverine treatment. No cognitive impairment was induced, and mental and motor functions were not affected by propiverine, even in these aged patients with dementia and motor dysfunction such as parkinsonism.

Cardiac safety

The cardiac safety of propiverine was assessed in a series of three placebo-controlled studies in accordance to recent guidance: (1) in 24 healthy women,[49] (2) in 98 elderly patients, among whom 24% presented with higher grades of Lown classification,[19] and (3) in 24 patients suffering from ischemic heart disease.[49] Patients included in all studies were considered to be at enhanced cardiac risk due to an age-related disposition (1, 2 above) or concomitant disease (2, 3 above). Long-term 24-hour electrocardiograms (ECGs) 12-lead resting ECGs, and other measures were conducted. No relevant differences between propiverine and placebo were shown with respect to heart rate, PQ interval, QRS interval, QT interval, or frequency-corrected QT interval. These results are in accordance with those derived from animal studies and long-term clinical exposure. Propiverine, in repetitive therapeutic dosages of 15 mg tid, has no effect on cardiac repolarization and does not raise any concerns with regard to cardiac safety, even in patients at increased risk of developing cardiac arrhythmia.

Ophthalmological safety

With respect to ophthalmological safety, in particular glaucoma, propiverine is the only antimuscarinic extensively investigated. The results of placebo-controlled, double-blind studies in primary open-angle as well as in angle-closure glaucoma patients showed no elevation of intraocular pressure.[50] Therefore, propiverine is safe in open-angle and controlled angle-closure glaucoma. However, due to the general expectation that antimuscarinics possibly increase intraocular pressure, an existing or developing glaucoma should be diagnosed before or monitored during the treatment.

Renal and hepatic impairment

Severe renal impairment does not significantly alter the disposition of propiverine and its main metabolite, propiverine-N-oxide, as deduced from a single-dose study in 12 patients with creatinine clearance < 30 ml/min.[51] No dose adjustment is to be recommended as long as the total daily dose does not exceed 30 mg/day.

With respect to hepatic impairment, steady state pharmacokinetics was evaluated in 12 patients with mild to moderate impairment of liver function due to fatty liver disease as compared to 12 healthy controls.[52] It can be concluded that in patients with mild impaired hepatic function there is no need for dose adjustments. However, no data are available in severe hepatic impairment.

Drug–drug Interaction

Only slight pharmacokinetic interactions are possible with other drugs metabolized by cytochrome P450 3A4 (CYP3A4). However, a very pronounced increase of concentrations for such drugs is not expected, as propiverine may be considered a weak inhibitor. Therefore, these effects are not of clinical relevance in comparison to classical enzyme inhibitors. Increased effects of propiverine due to concomitant medication with tricyclic antidepressants (e.g. imipramine), tranquilizers (e.g. benzodiazepines), anticholinergics, amantadine, neuroleptics (e.g. phenothiazines), and β-adrenoceptor agonists (β-sympathomimetics) have to be taken into consideration. Conversely, decreased effects of propiverine due to concomitant medication with cholinergic drugs might occur.

POST-MARKETING DRUG SURVEILLANCE

Two major post-marketing drug surveillance studies have been conducted in Europe, comprising 4390 and 2932 patients over 12-week treatment periods, respectively.[42,53] Daytime incontinence episodes (pre: 3.5; post: 1.0), daytime frequency (pre: 9.1; post: 5.8), and nocturia (pre: 2.6; post: 1.0) decreased according to Alloussi et al.[42] Comparable efficacy results were reported in the second study, e.g. daytime incontinence episodes improved from 3.6 to 1.2 episodes. Consistently, in both studies, patients with solitary OAB and patients with concomitant stress urinary incontinence showed almost comparable efficacy outcomes.

Treatment periods of 12 weeks for these almost 7300 patients add up to approximately 1700 patient-years. Previously unobserved adverse events were not detected.

Socioeconomic targets were also met by propiverine treatment: 40% of patients could substantially diminish, and 20% of patients could completely suspend pad use. The percentage of patients suspending pad use was two-fold higher following propiverine treatment (35.8 vs. 78.4) according to Alloussi et al.[42]

RECENT ADVANCES

In succession to propiverine immediate release (IR), an extended release (ER) formulation will follow in the very near future. This 30-mg ER formulation was evaluated by Jünemann et al.[54] in a double-blind, double-dummy, randomized, placebo-controlled study. Three parallel groups exposed 988 patients with OAB to propiverine IR 15 mg twice daily, propiverine ER 30 mg once daily, or placebo. A run-in period of 7 days preceded the 32-day treatment, a period being considered as sufficient to demonstrate onset of efficacy.

The primary efficacy outcome, incontinence episodes/24 hours, demonstrated both preparations to be efficacious compared to placebo. The efficacy of propiverine ER seemed to be slightly superior to that of propiverine IR. This finding is concordant to findings in ER formulations of other antimuscarinics. Results for the secondary outcomes support the primary outcome (Table 13.5). Improvements in the key clinical parameters were also reflected in quality of life, which was assessed by the King's Health Questionnaire.

With regard to tolerability, 38.5% of the patients experienced AEs in the IR, 34.3% in the ER, and 20.3% in the placebo group. Twenty-six (2.6%) patients terminated the study prematurely due to an AE: 14 (3.5%) in the IR, 11 (2.8%) in the ER, and one (0.5%) in the placebo group. Gastrointestinal disorders and nervous system disorders were the most frequent AEs leading to premature withdrawal. Overall, dry mouth

Table 13.5 Outcome parameters of frequency–volume charts comparing immediate release (IR = 15 mg bid) and extended release (ER = 30 mg once daily) propiverine vs. placebo in 988 patients with overactive bladder before (V0) and after (V1) a 32-day treatment. (From reference 54)

	Propiverine IR 2 × 15 mg	Propiverine ER 1 × 30 mg	Placebo
Incontinence episodes/24 h (n)	V0: 3.3 ± 2.7 V1: 1.1 ± 2.1 $p = 0.0007$	V0: 3.4 ± 2.8 V1: 0.9 ± 1.7 $p < 0.0001$	V0: 3.5 ± 3.6 V1: 1.7 ± 2.8
Micturitions/24 h (n)	V0: 12.8 ± 3.1 V1: 9.1 ± 3.3 $p = 0.0002$	V0: 12.7 ± 3.4 V1: 9.1 ± 3.1 $p = 0.0002$	V0: 13.4 ± 4.4 V1: 10.3 ± 3.9
Urge episodes/24 h (n)	V0: 6.1 ± 3.4 V1: 4.1 ± 3.7 $p = 0.1106$ (NS)	V0: 6.4 ± 4.1 V1: 3.8 ± 3.3 $p = 0.0028$	V0: 6.1 ± 4.1 V1: 4.4 ± 4.1
Volume voided/micturition (ml)	V0: 142.4 ± 52.0 V1: 188.9 ± 79.2 $p = 0.0039$	V0: 143.6 ± 54.8 V1: 183.7 ± 68.2 $p = 0.0667$ (NS)	V0: 144.2 ± 59.4 V1: 173.5 ± 90.0
Quality of life King's Health Score (total score)	V0: 60.5 ± 18.9 V1: 40.4 ± 21.7 $p = 0.0022$	V0: 60.1 ± 18.1 V1: 40.6 ± 21.9 $p = 0.0499$	V0: 57.4 ± 18.0 V1: 44.2 ± 21.3

bid, twice daily; NS, not significant

presented as the most frequent AE (22.8% IR, 21.7% ER, 6.4% placebo). Ophthalmological complaints such as abnormal accommodation or vision were experienced by 6.6% in the IR, 7.2% in the ER, and 2.5% in the placebo group. Each of the other organ system classes accounted for fewer than 5% of the patients. No additional kind of AE compared to the IR formulation occurred.

In conclusion, propiverine IR 15 mg bid and propiverine ER 30 mg once a day are effective, well tolerated, and safe in OAB patients. Tolerability assessment demonstrated advantages of the propiverine ER compared to the propiverine IR formulation.

SUMMARY

Propiverine is an antimuscarinic with the unique feature of a dual mode of action, comprising both antimuscarinic and musculotropic properties. Placebo- and reference-controlled clinical studies have evidenced equieffectiveness of propiverine compared to oxybutynin and tolterodine in adult and pediatric patients with neurogenic and idiopathic detrusor overactivity. Its tolerability profile is distinctly superior to that of oxybutynin and comparable to that of tolterodine. Adverse events observed were those known for this class of drugs, self-limited and reversible.

At the same time, according to the International Consultation on Incontinence, propiverine is internationally acknowledged for the treatment of detrusor overactivity, fulfilling the criteria of evidence-based medicine.

ACKNOWLEDGMENTS

We acknowledge the support of K Billy, M Bräter, D Koch, and B Tegelkamp.

REFERENCES

1. Andersson KE, Appell R, Cardozo L et al. Pharmacological treatment of urinary incontinence. In: Abrams P, Cardozo L, Khoury S, Wein A, eds. Incontinence. Plymouth, UK: Health Publication Ltd, 2005: 809–54.
2. Wuest M, Hecht J, Christ T et al. Pharmacodynamics of propiverine and three of its main metabolites on detrusor contraction. Br J Pharmacol 2005; 145: 608–19.
3. Wuest M, Braeter M, Schoeberl C, Ravens U. Juvenile pig detrusor: effects of propiverine and three of its metabolites. Eur J Pharmacol 2005; 524: 145–8.
4. Wuest M, Morgenstern K, Graf EM et al. Cholinergic and purinergic responses in isolated human detrusor in relation to age. J Urol 2005; 173: 2182–9.
5. Madersbacher H, Mürtz G. Efficacy, tolerability and safety profile of propiverine in the treatment of the overactive bladder (non-neurogenic and neurogenic). World J Urol 2001; 19: 324–35.
6. Scheepe JR, Braun PM, Bross S et al. Ein standarisiertes in-vivo-Modell zur Evaluierung anticholinerger Effekte auf die Blasenkontraktion, den Speichelfluss und das Elektromyogramm der Harnblase [A standardised model for in-vivo investigations of anticholinergic effects on bladder function, salivation and electromyographic characteristics of the detrusor]. Aktuel Urol 2000; 31: 311–16.
7. Stöhrer M, Castro-Diaz D, Chartier-Kastler E et al. Guidelines on Neurogenic Lower Urinary Tract Dysfunction. http://www.uroweb.org/files/uploaded_files/guidelines/neurogenic.pdf. Arnhem, The Netherlands: European Association of Urology, 2003.
8. Abrams P, Cardozo L, Fall M et al. The standardisation of terminology of lower urinary tract function: report from the Standardisation Subcommittee of the International Continence Society. Neurourol Urodyn 2002; 21: 167–78.
9. Mazur D, Göcking K, Wehnert J et al. Klinische und urodynamische Effekte einer oralen Propiverintherapie bei neurogener Harninkontinenz, [Clinical and urodynamic effects of oral propiverine therapy in neurogenic urinary incontinence. A multicentre study for optimising dosage]. Urologe A 1994; 33: 447–52.
10. Stöhrer M, Madersbacher H, Richter R et al. Efficacy and safety of propiverine in SCI-patients suffering from detrusor hyperreflexia – a double-blind, placebo-controlled clinical trial. Spinal Cord 1999; 37: 196–200.
11. Takayasu H, Ueno A, Tsuchida S et al. Clinical evaluation of propiverine hydrochloride (P4) against pollakisuria and urinary incontinence – a multicenter, placebo-controlled double-blind study. Prog Med 1990; 153: 459–71.

12. Stöhrer M, Mürtz G, Kramer G et al. Propiverine compared to oxybutynin in neurogenic detrusor overactivity – results of a randomized, double-blind, multicenter clinical study. Eur Urol 2007; 51: 235–42.

13. Mazur D, Wehnert J, Dorschner W et al. Clinical and urodynamic effects of propiverine in patients suffering from urgency and urge incontinence. A multicentre dose-optimising study. Scand J Urol Nephrol 1995; 29: 289–94.

14. Madersbacher H, Halaška M, Voigt R et al. A placebo-controlled, multicentre study comparing the tolerability and efficacy of propiverine and oxybutynin in patients with urgency and urge incontinence. BJU Int 1999; 84: 646–51.

15. Jünemann K-P, Halaška M, Rittstein T et al. Propiverine versus tolterodine: efficacy and tolerability in patients with overactive bladder. Eur Urol 2005; 48: 478–82.

16. Constantine G. A double blind randomised trial of tolterodine v propiverine in the treatment of bladder instability. Presented at 9th Annual Meeting of the UK ICS, 4–5 April, 2002, Sheffield, UK.

17. Dorschner W, Höfner K, Dieterich F, Jacob J. Die Wirkung des Anticholinergikums Mictonorm® auf den unteren Harntrakt. 1. Mitteilung: Der Einfluß auf die Blasenkapazität [The effects of the anticholinergic drug Mictonorm® on the lower urinary tract]. Dtsch Gesundheitswesen 1982; 37: 889–93.

18. Park YC, Sugiyama T, Kurita T et al. Efficacy and safety of propiverine hydrochloride (BUP-4® tablets) in patients with pollakiuria and urinary incontinence which do not respond to prostatectomy. Voiding Disord Digest 1998; 6: 217–26.

19. Dorschner W, Stolzenburg JU, Griebenow R et al. Efficacy and cardiac safety of propiverine in elderly patients – a double-blind, placebo-controlled clinical study. Eur Urol 2000; 37: 702–8.

20. Mori S, Kojima M, Sakai Y, Nakajima K. Bladder dysfunction in dementia patients with urinary incontinence: evaluation by cystometry and treatment with propiverine hydrochloride. Jpn J Geriatr 1999; 36: 489–94.

21. Otomo E, Maruyama S, Kobayashi I et al. Clinical evaluation of propiverine hydrochloride (P-4) on urinary disturbances due to neurological diseases. Yakuri to Chiryo 1990; 18: 1731–40.

22. Welz-Barth A, Rettig K, Mürtz G et al. Urinary incontinence – a partial deficiency after stroke requiring therapy. Eur J Geriatr 2002; 4: 68–74.

23. Grigoleit U, Mürtz G, Laschke S et al. Efficacy, tolerability and safety of propiverine hydrochloride in children and adolescents with congenital or traumatic neurogenic detrusor overactivity – a retrospective study. Eur Urol 2006; 49: 1114–20.

24. Schulte-Baukloh H, Mürtz G, Henne T et al. Urodynamic effects of propiverine hydrochloride in children with neurogenic detrusor overactivity: a prospective analysis. BJU Int 2006; 97: 355–8.

25. Madersbacher H, Mürtz G, Alloussi S et al. Efficacy and safety of propiverine in comparison to oxybutynin in children with neurogenic detrusor overactivity – an observational cohort study. Abstract presented at 44th Annual Scientific Meeting of the International Spinal Cord Society (ISCoS), 4–8 October, 2005, Munich, Germany, 28–9.

26. Marschall-Kehrel A-D, Mürtz G, Kramer G et al. An empirical treatment algorithm for incontinent children. J Urol 2004; 171: 2667–71.

27. Alloussi S, Mürtz G, Braun R et al. Efficacy, tolerability and safety of propiverine hydrochloride in comparison to oxybutynin in children with idiopathic detrusor overactivity – a multicenter observational cohort study. Presented at 35th Annual Meeting of the ICS, 28 August–2 September, 2005, Montreal, Canada.

28. Marschall-Kehrel A-D, Mürtz G, Kramer G, Juenemann K-P. A suggested treatment algorithm in nocturnal enuresis with emphasis on partial responders. 33rd Annual Meeting of the ICS, 5–9 October 2003 Florence, Italy. Neurourol Urodyn 2003; 22: 441–2.

29. Saito H, Yamada T, Oshima H et al. A comparative study of the efficacy and safety of tamsulosin hydrochloride alone and combination of propiverine hydrochloride and tamsulosin hydrochloride in the benign prostatic hypertrophy with pollakisuria and/or urinary incontinence. Jpn J Urol Surg 1999; 12: 525–36.

30. Lee K-S, Choo M-S, Kim D-Y et al. Combination treatment with propiverine hydrochloride plus doxazosin controlled release gastrointestinal therapeutic system formulation for overactive bladder and coexisting benign prostatic obstruction: a prospective, randomized, controlled multicenter study. J Urol 2005; 174: 1334–8.

31. Kagawa S, Naruo S, Kojima K et al. Study of long-term administration of propiverine hydrochloride (BUP-4® tablets) in patients with pollakiuria and urinary incontinence. Nishinihon J Urol 1998; 60: 57–64.

32. Yoshida M, Takahashi W, Ueda S et al. Long-term administration of propiverine hydrochloride (BUP-4® tablets) for the treatment of patients with urinary frequency and incontinence. Nishinihon J Urol 1997; 59: 885–92.

33. Ohmori H, Ohashi T, Oheda T et al. Study on therapeutic and adverse effect of propiverine hydrochloride for patients with urinary frequency and incontinence. Nishinihon J Urol 1990; 52: 241–7.

34. Noguchi K, Masuda M, Noguchi S et al. Long-term administration study of propiverine hydrochloride (BUP-4® tablets) in pollakiuria and urinary incontinence. Hinyokika Kiyo 1998; 44: 687–93.

35. Oeda T, Kumon T, Ohmori H et al. Long-term administration study on propiverine hydrochloride (BUP-4® tablets) in patients with pollakiuria and urinary incontinence. Nishinihon J Urol 1998; 60: 163–9.

36. Tanabe N, Ueno A, Nomura T et al. Study on therapeutic and adverse events of propiverine hydrochloride for patients with urinary frequency and incontinence in the long-term treatment. Jpn J Urol Surg 1997; 10: 809–17.

37. Takaki R, Hanyu S, Nishiyama T et al. Safety and efficacy of long-term treatment with propiverine hydrochloride in patients with frequency and urinary incontinence. Jpn J Urol Surg 1995; 8: 1109–20.

38. Takaki R, Sato A, Takahashi H et al. Long-term administration of propiverine hydrochloride (P-4) for the treatment in patients with urinary frequency and incontinence. Jpn J Urol Surg 1990; 3: 321–7.

39. Watanabe H, Kojima M, Azuma Y, Saito M. Clinical evaluation of propiverine hydrochloride in patients with pollakisuria and urinary incontinence. J New Remedies Clin 1990; 39: 699–706.

40. Voigt R, Halaška M, Martan A et al. Erfolgreiche Langzeittherapie der Harninkontinenz und Drangsymptomatik [Long-time application of anticholinergic drugs for treating urgency]. ÄP UrologieNephrologie 2000; 1: 18–20.

41. Madersbacher H, Hessdoerfer E, Martan A et al. Safety, tolerability and efficacy of propiverine long-term treatment. Presented at 35th Annual Meeting of the ICS, 28 August–2 September, 2005, Montreal, Canada.

42. Alloussi S, Schönberger B, Mürtz G et al. Behandlung des Urge-Sydroms mit Propiverin in der therapeutischen Praxis: Wirksamkeit und Verträglichkeit bei 4390 Patienten [Treatment of the urge-syndrome with propiverine in therapeutical practice: tolerability and efficacy in 4390 patients]. Urologe B 2000; 40: 367–73.

43. Hoashi E, Yokoi S, Akashi S et al. Safety and usefulness of propiverine hydrochloride (BUP-4® tablets) in children with special reference to enuresis. Shonika Rinsho 1998; 51: 173–9.

44. Kondo A, Kobayashi M, Kato T et al. Clinical effects of BUP-4® tablets on urge or mixed incontinence and analysis of the incontinence symptom score. Jpn J Urol Surg 1997; 10: 895–901.

45. Batinic D, Mürtz G, Martin F et al. Efficacy and tolerability of propiverine in children suffering from overactive bladder – a double-blind, randomised, clinical trial versus oxybutynin and placebo. Presented at Joint Meeting of the ICCS and APAPU, 10–13 December, 2002, Hong Kong, China.

46. Alloussi S, Madersbacher H, Siegert J et al. Residual urine and urinary retention due to anticholinergic therapy? Results with propiverine. 30th Annual Meeting of the International Continence Society, 28–31 August 2000. Neurourol Urodyn 2000; 19: 494–6.

47. Kluge A, Vohs K, Siegert J et al. Effect of propiverine on psychomotor performance. Presented at 26th Annual Meeting of the ICS, 27–30 August, 1996, Athens, Greece.

48. Uchiyama T, Sakakibara R, Liu Z et al. The effects of anticholinergic drugs on cognitive impairment, mental dysfunction and motor dysfunction in patients with neurological disease. Presented at 35th Annual Meeting of the ICS, 28 August–2 September, 2005, Montreal, Canada.

49. Eckl K, Tsvitbaum N, Biletsky S et al. The effect of propiverine on cardiac safety in healthy female subjects (A) and in patients suffering from ischaemic heart disease (B). Presented at 35th Annual Meeting of the ICS, 28 August–2 September, 2005, Montreal, Canada.

50. de Mey C, Petkova N, Rankova C et al. Safety of propiverine hydrochloride in glaucoma. Presented at XVIIIth EAU Congress, 12–15 March, 2003, Madrid, Spain.

51. Schug B, Wonnemann M, Donath F, Blume H. Safety and tolerability of propiverine hydrochloride (Mictonorm®) in patients with severe renal impairment. 55th Congress of the DGU, 21–24 September 2005 Düsseldorf, Germany. Der Urologe 2005; 44 (Suppl 1), S77.

52. Siepmann M, Nokhodian A, Thümmler D, Kirch W. Pharmacokinetics and safety of propiverine in patients with fatty liver disease. Eur J Clin Pharmacol 1998; 54: 767–77.

53. Alloussi S, Goepel M, Richter AE et al. Therapie der Detrusorhyperaktivität mit Propiverin. [Therapy for overactive detrusor using propiverine]. Urologe A 2005; 44: 382–6.

54. Jünemann K-P, Hessdoerfer E, Unamba-Oparah I et al. Propiverine hydrochloride immediate (IR) and extended release (ER): comparison of efficacy and tolerability in patients with overactive bladder. Neurourol Urodyn 2004; 23: 599–600 (abstr 143).

14

Extended release oral oxybutynin

Rodney A Appell

Introduction   •   **Antimuscarinic (anticholinergic) drugs**   •   **Oxybutynin**   •   **Extended release oxybutynin**

INTRODUCTION

The functions of the lower urinary tract, to store and periodically release urine, are dependent on the activity of smooth and striated muscles in the urinary bladder, urethra, external urethral sphincter, and the pelvic floor. The bladder and the urethra constitute a functional unit, which is controlled by a complex interplay between the central and peripheral nervous systems and local regulatory factors.[1–3] Bladder emptying and urine storage involve a complex pattern of efferent and afferent signaling in parasympathetic, sympathetic, and somatic nerves. These nerves are parts of reflex pathways which either maintain the bladder in a relaxed state, enabling urine storage at low intravesical pressure, or initiate micturition by relaxing the outflow region and contracting the bladder smooth muscle. The postganglionic neurons in the pelvic nerve mediate the excitatory input to the human detrusor smooth muscle by releasing acetylcholine (ACh), which acts upon muscarinic receptors. Most of the *sensory* innervation of the bladder and urethra reaches the spinal cord via the pelvic nerve and dorsal root ganglia. The most important afferents for the micturition process are myelinated Aδ fibers and unmyelinated C fibers traveling in the pelvic nerve to the sacral spinal cord, conveying information from receptors in the bladder wall to the spinal cord. The Aδ fibers respond to passive distention and active contraction, thus conveying information about bladder filling.[4] C fibers have a high mechanical threshold and respond primarily to chemical irritation of the bladder mucosa[5] or cold.[6]

A disturbed filling/storage function can, at least theoretically, be improved by agents, which decrease detrusor activity, increase bladder capacity, and/or increase outlet resistance.[7]

As pointed out previously, bladder control disorders can be divided into two general categories: disorders of filling/storage and disorders of voiding.[7] Storage problems can occur as a result of weakness or anatomic defects in the urethral outlet, causing stress urinary incontinence, which may account for one-third of cases. Failure to store also occurs if the bladder is unstable or overactive, and this may affect > 50% of incontinent men and 10–15% of incontinent young women. Overactive bladder (OAB) can occur as a result of sensitization of afferent nerve terminals in the bladder or outlet region, or changes of the bladder smooth muscle secondary to denervation or to damage to central nervous system (CNS) inhibitory pathways as can be seen in various neurological disorders, such as multiple sclerosis, cerebrovascular disease, Parkinson's disease, brain tumors, and spinal cord injury. OAB and/or detrusor overactivity (DO)[8] may also occur in elderly patients due to changes in the brain and/or bladder during aging.

Normal bladder contraction in humans is mediated mainly through stimulation of muscarinic receptors in the detrusor muscle via the neurotransmitter acetylcholine, and hence the attempts to treat overactivity via pharmacologic agents which block the effects of acetylcholine at the detrusor muscarinic receptor level. In the human bladder, where the mRNAs for all five pharmacologically defined muscarinic receptors, M_1–M_5, have been demonstrated,[9] there is a predominance of mRNAs encoding M_2 and M_3 receptors.[9,10] Both M_2 and M_3 receptors can be found on detrusor muscle cells, where M_2 receptors predominate at least 3 : 1 over M_3 receptors, but also in other bladder structures, which may be of importance for detrusor activation. Thus, muscarinic receptors can be found on urothelial cells, on suburothelial nerves, and on other suburothelial structures, possibly interstitial cells.[11,12] However, in human as well as animal detrusor, the M_3 receptors are believed to be the most important for contraction.[11,13] No differences between genders can be demonstrated in rat and human bladders.[14] The functional role for the M_2 receptors has not been clarified. Thus, one can comprehend the emphasis on attempting to use pharmacologic agents which preferentially block the M_3 muscarinic receptor. While the muscarinic receptor functions may be changed in different urological disorders, such as outflow obstruction, neurogenic bladders, bladder overactivity without overt neurogenic cause, and diabetes,[15] it is not always clear what the changes mean in terms of changes in detrusor function. It appears that OAB may be the result of several different mechanisms, both myogenic[16] and neurological,[17] but most probably, both factors contribute to the genesis of the disease.

ANTIMUSCARINIC (ANTICHOLINERGIC) DRUGS

Many drugs have been tried, but the results are often disappointing, partly due to poor treatment efficacy and/or side effects. The development of pharmacologic treatment of the different forms of urinary incontinence has been slow, and the use of some of the currently prescribed agents is based more on tradition than on evidence from results of controlled clinical trials.[3] Pharmacologic and/or physiologic efficacy evidence means that a drug has been shown to have its desired effects in relevant preclinical experiments or in healthy volunteers or in experimental situations in patients.

Antimuscarinics block, more or less selectively, muscarinic receptors. The common view is that in OAB/DO, the drugs act by blocking the muscarinic receptors on the detrusor muscle, which are stimulated by acetylcholine, released from activated cholinergic (parasympathetic) nerves.

This then results in a decrease in the ability of the bladder to contract. However, antimuscarinic drugs act mainly during the storage phase, decreasing urge and increasing bladder capacity, and during this phase, there is normally no parasympathetic input to the lower urinary tract.[18] Furthermore, antimuscarinics are usually competitive antagonists. This implies that when there is a massive release of acetylcholine, as during micturition, the effects of the drugs should be decreased, otherwise the reduced ability of the detrusor to contract would eventually lead to urinary retention. Undeniably, high doses of antimuscarinics can produce urinary retention in humans, but in the dose range needed for beneficial effects in OAB/DO, there is little evidence for a significant reduction of the voiding contraction. The question is whether there are other effects of antimuscarinics that can contribute to their beneficial effects in the treatment of OAB/DO.[19] Muscarinic receptor functions may change in bladder disorders associated with OAB/DO, implying that mechanisms, which normally have little clinical importance, may be upregulated and contribute to the pathophysiology of OAB/DO.[20]

Muscarinic receptors are found on bladder urothelial cells where their density can be even higher than in detrusor muscle. The role of the urothelium in bladder activation has attracted much interest,[21] but whether the muscarinic receptors on urothelial cells can influence micturition has not yet been established. Acetylcholine may be released from both neuronal and non-neuronal sources (e.g. the urothelium) and directly or indirectly (by increasing detrusor smooth muscle tone) excite afferent nerves in the suburothelium and within the detrusor. This mechanism may be important in the pathophysiology of OAB and a possible target for antimuscarinic drugs.

Several studies have supported that antimuscarinics can depress involuntary bladder contractions.[22–25] On the other hand, there are several reports of insufficient efficacy of antimuscarinics given orally to patients with DO.[26–29] It is unclear to what extent this can be attributed to low bioavailability of the drugs used, to side effects limiting the dose that can be given, or to a resistance phenomenon.

Generally, antimuscarinics can be divided into tertiary and quaternary amines.[30] They differ with regard to lipophilicity, molecular charge, and even molecular size (tertiary compounds generally having higher lipophilicity and molecular charge than quaternary agents). Atropine, tolterodine, oxybutynin, propiverine, darifenacin, and solifenacin are tertiary amines. They are generally well absorbed from the gastrointestinal tract and should theoretically be able to pass into the CNS, dependent on their individual physicochemical properties. High lipophilicity, small molecular size, and low charge will increase the possibilities to pass the blood–brain barrier. Quaternary ammonium compounds, such as propantheline and trospium, are not well absorbed, pass into the CNS to a limited extent, and have a low incidence of CNS side effects.[31] They still produce well-known peripheral antimuscarinic side effects, such as blurred vision, constipation, tachycardia, and dryness of mouth. Many antimuscarinics (all currently used tertiary amines) are metabolized by the cytochrome P450 enzyme system to active and/or inactive metabolites.[30] The most commonly involved P450 enzymes are CYP2D6 and CYP3A4. The metabolic conversion creates a risk for drug–drug interactions, resulting in either reduced (enzyme induction) or increased (enzyme inhibition, substrate competition) plasma concentration/effect of either the antimuscarinic and/or interacting drug.

Antimuscarinics are still the most widely used treatment for urge and urge incontinence.[20] However, currently used drugs lack selectivity for the bladder,[32] and effects on other organ systems may result in side effects, which limit their usefulness. For example, all antimuscarinic drugs are contraindicated in untreated narrow angle glaucoma.

Theoretically, drugs with selectivity for the bladder could be obtained, if the subtype(s) mediating bladder contraction, and those producing the main side effects of antimuscarinic drugs, were different. Unfortunately, this does not seem to be the case. One way of avoiding many of the antimuscarinic side effects is to administer the drugs intravesically. However, this is practical only in a limited number of patients.

OXYBUTYNIN

Clinical practice and the literature support the efficacy of antimuscarinic medications for the treatment of OAB, beginning with oxybutynin. In fact, the immediate release form of oxybutynin (OXY-IR) is recognized for its efficacy, and the newer antimuscarinic agents are all compared to it once efficacy over placebo has been determined. Although most patients respond favorably to antimuscarinic medication, smaller percentages achieve total dryness. In general, the new formulations of oxybutynin and other antimuscarinic agents offer patients efficacy roughly equivalent to that of OXY-IR, and the advantages of the newer formulations lie in improved dosing schedules and side-effect profile.[33–35]

With respect to oxybutynin, an extended release (OXY-ER) once-daily oral formulation gained approval by the US Food and Drug Administration (FDA) in 1999. Again, the data support this newer formulation of oxybutynin as effective in the treatment of OAB, with significant reductions in urge incontinence, but only a small number of patients reach total dryness. For this reason, in addition to side effects and cost, very few continue to remain on the medications for a full year, once they have been prescribed.

The chemical oxybutynin is a tertiary amine antimuscarinic agent with combined local anesthetic and muscle relaxant properties.[36] As a muscarinic receptor antagonist, it has a higher affinity for M_1 and M_3 receptors than for other muscarinic subtypes, and its effects may be primarily attributed to the (R)-enantiomer.[37] It is well absorbed, but undergoes extensive upper gastrointestinal and first pass hepatic metabolism via the cytochrome P450 system (CYP3A4) into multiple metabolites. However, the primary metabolite, N-desethyl-oxybutynin (DEO) has pharmacologic properties similar to those of the parent compound, and has been implicated as the major cause of the troublesome side effect of dry mouth associated with the administration of oxybutynin. OXY-IR results in a reduction of urinary frequency by 50% and urge incontinence episodes by up to 70% , but the prevalence of dry mouth varies between 12 and 70% depending on dosage.[38] Oxybutynin and DEO are highly lipophilic which aids in absorption, but will also have a higher penetration into the CNS by allowing enhanced crossing of the blood–brain barrier more readily than other tertiary amines. Electroencephalography (EEG) studies have demonstrated an enhanced ability for oxybutynin to gain access to the CNS via the blood–brain barrier,[31,39,40] where oxybutynin is associated with changed power density in the alpha ranges and quantitative EEG (qEEG) bands.

EXTENDED RELEASE OXYBUTYNIN

In an effort to improve the dosing schedule and the side effect profile, an extended release once-daily oral formulation of oxybutynin (OXY-ER) was developed. OXY-ER uses an osmotic delivery system (OROS®; Alza) to release the medication at a fixed rate over 24 hours. This eliminates the serum concentration fluctuations that contribute to the intolerable side effects associated with OXY-IR.[3] Physically, OXY-ER resembles a conventional tablet, but it consists of two core compartments: a drug layer containing the active ingredient (oxybutynin) and a push layer containing osmotically active compounds. Both are wholly surrounded by a semipermeable membrane with a laser-drilled hole on the drug side. Water in the gastrointestinal tract enters the tablet and mixes with the oxybutynin to form a suspension. Water also enters the push layer through the semipermeable membrane via osmosis. The push layer expands and pushes the suspended drug out of the laser-drilled hole into the gastrointestinal tract for absorption. Aside from the convenience of once-daily administration, OXY-ER eliminates the three times daily peak-to-trough serum concentration fluctuation associated with OXY-IR. Such marked variation in oxybutynin level is thought to contribute to the intolerable dose-dependent side effects of the drug. Studies with adult volunteers have shown a smoother peak-to-trough fluctuation of plasma concentration with each dosing of OXY-ER. The plasma level rises slowly over 4–6 hours and remains fairly constant over the 24-hour dosing interval.[41,42] Steady-state concentration is reached by day 3 of administration. In addition, the peak serum concentration of oxybutynin in this extended release formulation is 2.5 times lower than that of the conventional formulation.[41] A lower peak value and more stable serum concentration are the pharmacokinetic hallmarks of OXY-ER.

In addition, OXY-ER is mostly metabolized in the large intestine where it is not influenced by the cytochrome P450 enzyme system, thus bypassing the gut-mediated drug metabolism. This results in reduced levels of the primary metabolite, DEO, and, therefore, fewer adverse effects. OXY-IR undergoes extensive first pass metabolism in the upper gastrointestinal tract, producing high serum levels of the primary metabolite DEO, the primary cause of intolerable side effects. In contrast, OXY-ER is protected inside its non-disintegrating capsule and is released at a steady rate for 24 hours, spending only 3–5 hours in the upper gastrointestinal tract. Most of the active compound oxybutynin is released in the colon, where first pass metabolism is much less extensive than in the small bowel.[43,44] As a result, first pass metabolism is proportionally reduced and, thus, the serum ratio of DEO/oxybutynin is reduced and less severe dry mouth may be expected.[42] This hypothesis is supported by a study that showed the mean bioavailability was higher for oxybutynin (153%) and lower for DEO (69%) with OXY-ER than with OXY-IR.[41]

A more stable serum concentration together with less first pass metabolism may explain the improved tolerability of OXY-ER over OXY-IR. OXY-ER caused less suppression of saliva output and less severe dry mouth than OXY-IR in healthy volunteers.[41,42] Whereas patients taking OXY-ER and OXY-IR had similar reductions in urge incontinence (83% and 76–87%, respectively) and total incontinence episodes (80–81% and 75–86%, respectively), indicating equivalent clinical efficacy,[45,46] the incidence and severity of dry mouth were lower in the OXY-ER group. Dry mouth of any severity was reported by 68% and 87% in the OXY-ER and OXY-IR groups, respectively ($p = 0.04$).[45] Moderate or severe dry mouth occurred in 25% and 46%, respectively ($p = 0.03$). Dry mouth was still the most common side effect of OXY-ER (68%) followed by somnolence (38%), constipation (30%), and blurred vision (28%). With the exception of dry mouth, OXY-ER and OXY-IR were comparable in terms of the rates of systemic side effects.

Clinical trials demonstrate equivalent efficacy between OXY-IR and OXY-ER in reducing the number of incontinence episodes and number of voidings per day, with improved tolerability of the OXY-ER.[25–28] In studies of up to 12 weeks in duration, discontinuation rates due to adverse effects were only 7% for OXY-ER compared to

27% for OXY-IR.[24] The once-daily dosing has also been demonstrated to improve patient compliance with taking the medication.[41,42] OXY-ER is usually begun at 10 mg/day (5 mg in the elderly) and the dose may be titrated up to 30 mg/day. Unfortunately, the side effects increase as the dose increases. For patients whose bladder symptoms have been stabilized on OXY-IR, switching to OXY-ER reduces the side effects without compromising clinical efficacy.[47]

Maximum clinical benefit is achieved by the fourth week, and is sustained through 12 weeks of maintenance therapy. The optimal dosage appears to be between 5 and 15 mg daily. In one trial, 70.8% of participants chose a maintenance dose of 5–15 mg, while 17% used a dose of 25–30 mg daily.[48] Although the latter doses are significantly higher, only 5.4% of these patients discontinued treatment due to antimuscarinic side effects.[48] OXY-ER may provide important therapeutic options for motivated patients who require a higher dose to achieve optimal relief of OAB symptoms without experiencing excessive side effects (e.g. neurogenic bladder patients).

Furthermore, OXY-ER appears to be safe in the elderly. In a long-term, open-label, community-use study, there was a very low incidence of CNS side effects, including changes in mental acuity and memory.[49] Over 50% of patients in that community-based study were over 65 years of age. The drug demonstrated comparable efficacy across all age groups. In a different open-label study evaluating urge incontinence, nearly equal numbers of patients older and younger than 65 years old achieved complete urinary continence (46) and, in addition, the rates of dry mouth were similar. These results are important, since urge urinary incontinence is not only prevalent among the elderly (affecting 12–38% over the age of 60),[50] but is also the second leading cause of patient admissions to nursing homes.[51]

Historically, only 18–22% of patients remain on long-term (> 6 months) treatment with OXY-IR,[9,10] whereas 60% of those on OXY-ER remain on the drug at 12 months.[49]

Newer extended release formulations of oxybutynin are in clinical development. These systems use alternative delivery methods to obtain once-daily dosing with a reduction in tolerability-related issues as compared to the immediate release form of oxybutynin chloride. These new systems are often termed controlled release or CR. Instead of an osmotic delivery system, a cellulose matrix system which combines sodium alginate, cellulose, and aliphatic alcohol in an enteric coated tablet forms the basis of oxybutynin CR. The bioavailability of drug delivered by this system is similar to that of the immediate release formulations, with a 75% reduction in peak plasma levels as compared to the immediate release cogener. Once-daily dosing with 15 mg CR oxybutynin resulted in less frequent and less bothersome dry mouth than with immediate release (IR) oxybutynin ingested in a regimen of 5 mg three times daily.[52] Also, stimulated salivary secretion was greater with the CR form as opposed to the IR form.

In randomized, controlled trials as comparison with IR oxybutynin, no significant differences in degree of efficacy were noted, but significant reductions were found as compared to baseline in urinary urgency and incontinence, and a significant improvement in volume voided, with the CR formulation.[53,54] Initial dosing at 15 mg/day was evaluated in these trials as compared to 5 mg three times daily of the IR formulation. Although total dry mouth rates were not dissimilar between CR and IR formulations, tolerability and persistence with therapy were superior with the CR formulation.[53]

In an effort to evaluate the dose response for the CR formulation, another trial assessed efficacy/tolerability-driven dose changes in a controlled population. After an initial starting dose of 5 mg CR/day, dose increases or decreases were allowed around a dosing range of 5–15 mg/day.[55] After a 2-week lead-in period, subjects were randomized in a 1 : 1 : 1 schema to starting doses of 5, 10, or 15 mg CR oxybutynin. Three-day diary analysis of changes in frequency, incontinence episodes (primary outcomes), volume voided, and urinary urgency (secondary outcomes) was used to assess efficacy. Subjects also completed a four-point satisfaction questionnaire. Adverse events were collected using a general non-leading question and then graded as to severity if reported positively by the initial question. Dry mouth severity was rated using the Data Mining Surveillance System (DMSS) scale, which had previously been validated.[55] Tolerability was also assessed using a one-item subjective patient appraisal question.

Of the initial 237 patients, 190 completed the trial. All efficacy outcomes were more significantly benefited by the 15-mg dose as compared to either the 5- or 10-mg dose. These efficacy benefits were reflected in patient satisfaction scores. There was a dose-dependent effect on dry mouth as reported by DMSS evaluations, with increasing dry mouth being noted with ascending dose. Of those studied, 92% found the 5-mg dose tolerable as compared to 82% with the 15-mg dose. Dry mouth ranged from 56% to 70% with dosing, yet when balanced against efficacy 52% of those receiving the 15-mg dose reported the best efficacy/tolerability balance (as compared to 35 and 36% respectively for the 5- and 10-mg doses). The authors concluded that a dose–response relationship was noted with this delivery system, and that 15 mg/day CR oxybutynin provided the best balance of effect and side effects.

The advent of other types of delivery systems allowing once-daily dosing will further advance our knowledge about extended release oxybutynin. The ease of once-daily dosing accompanied by the improvement in tolerability provided by these systems has improved the pharmacologic activity of oxybutynin and allowed easier use of the pharmacologic entity for bothersome symptoms of OAB.

REFERENCES

1. Andersson K-E. Pharmacology of lower urinary tract smooth muscles and penile erectile tissues. Pharmacol Rev 1993; 45: 253–308.
2. de Groat WC, Yoshimura N. Pharmacology of the lower urinary tract. Ann Rev Pharmacol Toxicol 2001; 41: 691–721.
3. Andersson K-E, Wein AJ. Pharmacology of the lower urinary tract: basis for current and future treatments of urinary incontinence. Pharmacol Rev 2004; 56: 581–631.
4. Janig W, Morrison JF. Functional properties of spinal visceral afferents supplying abdominal and pelvic organs, with special emphasis on visceral nociception. Prog Brain Res 1986; 67: 87–114.
5. Habler H, Janig W, Koltaenburg M. Activation of unmyelinated afferent fibres by mechanical stimuli and inflammation of the urinary bladder in the cat. J Physiol 1990; 425: 545–62.
6. Fall M, Lindstrom S, Mazieres L. A bladder-to-bladder cooling reflex in the cat. J Physiol 1990; 427: 281–300.
7. Wein AJ. Neuromuscular dysfunction of the lower urinary tract and its treatment. In: Walsh PC, Retik AB, Vaughan ED Jr, Wein AJ, eds. Campbell's Urology, 7th edn. Philadelphia: WB Saunders, 1998; 953–1006.
8. Abrams P, Cardozo L, Fall M et al. The standardization of terminology of lower urinary tract function. Neurourol Urodyn 2002; 21: 167–78.
9. Sigala S, Mirabella G, Peroni A et al. Differential gene expression of cholinergic muscarinic receptor subtypes in male and female normal human urinary bladder. Urology 2002; 60: 719–25.
10. Yamaguchi O, Shisda K, Tamura K et al. Evaluation of mRNAs encoding muscarinic receptor subtypes in human detrusor muscle. J Urol 1996; 156: 1208–13.
11. Chess-Williams R, Chapple CR, Yamanishi T et al. The minor population of M3-receptors mediate contraction of human detrusor muscle in vitro. J Auton Pharmacol 2001; 21: 243–8.
12. Gillespie JI, Harvey IJ, Drake MJ. Agonist and nerve induced phasic activity in the isolated whole bladder of the guinea-pig: evidence for two types of bladder activity. Exp Physiol 2003; 88: 343–57.
13. Andersson K-E, Arner A. Urinary bladder contraction and relaxation: physiology and pathophysiology. Physiol Rev 2004; 84: 935–86.
14. Kories C, Czborra C, Fletcher C et al. Gender comparison of muscarinic receptor expression and function in rat and human urinary bladder: differential regulation of M2 and M3 receptors? Naunyn Schmiedebergs Arch Pharmacol 2003; 367: 524–31.
15. Andersson K-E. New roles for muscarinic receptors in the pathophysiology of lower urinary tract symptoms. BJU Int 2000; 86 (Suppl 2): 36–42.
16. Brading AF. A myogenic basis for the overactive bladder. Urology 1997; 50 (Suppl 6A): 57–67.
17. de Groat WC. A neurologic basis for the overactive bladder. Urology 1997; 50 (Suppl 6A): 36–52.
18. Morrison J, Steers WD, Brading A et al. Neurophysiology and neuropharmacology. In: Abrams P, Khoury S, Wein A, eds. Incontinence, 2nd edn. Plymouth, UK: 2002: 83–163.
19. Andersson K-E, Yoshida M. Antimuscarinics and the overactive detrusor – which is the main mechanism of action? Eur Urol 2003; 43: 1–5.

20. Andersson K-E. Antimuscarinics for treatment of overactive bladder. Lancet Neurol 2004; 3: 46–53.

21. Andersson K-E. Bladder activation: afferent mechanisms. Urology 2002; 59(5 Suppl 1): 43–50.

22. Low JA. Urethral behavior during the involuntary detrusor contraction. Am J Obstet Gynecol 1977; 128: 32–42.

23. Cardozo LD, Stanton SL. An objective comparison of the effects of parenterally administered drug in patients suffering from detrusor instability. J Urol 1979; 122: 58–9.

24. Blaivas JG, Labib KB, Michalik J et al. Cystometric response to propantheline in detrusor hyperreflexia: therapeutic implications. J Urol 1980; 124: 259–62.

25. Naglo AS, Nergardh A, Boreus LO. Influence of atropine and isoprenaline on detrusor hyperactivity in children with neurogenic bladder. Scand J Urol Nephrol 1981; 15: 97–102.

26. Ritch AES, Castleden CM, George CF et al. A second look at emepronium bromide in urinary incontinence. Lancet 1977; 1: 504–6.

27. Walter S, Hansen J, Hansen L et al. Urinary incontinence in old age. A controlled trial of emepronium bromide. Br J Urol 1982; 54: 249–51.

28. Bonnesen T, Tikjob G, Kamper AL et al. Effect of emepronium bromide on symptoms and urinary bladder function after transurethral resection of the prostate. A double-blind randomized trial. Urol Int 1984; 39: 318–20.

29. Zorzitto ML, Jewett MAS, Fernie GR et al. Effectiveness of propantheline bromide in the treatment of geriatric patients with detrusor instability. Neurourol Urodyn 1986; 5: 133–40.

30. Guay DR. Clinical pharmacokinetics of drugs used to treat urge incontinence. Clin Pharmacokinet 2003; 42: 1243–85.

31. Pietzko A, Dimpfel W, Schwantes U et al. Influence of trospium chloride and oxybutynin on quantitative EEG in healthy volunteers. Eur J Clin Pharmacol 1994; 47: 337–43.

32. Eglen RM, Hegde SS, Watson N. Muscarinic receptor subtypes and smooth muscle function. Pharmacol Rev 1996; 48: 531–65.

33. Appell RA, Sand P, Dmochowski R et al. Prospective randomized, controlled trial of extended-release oxybutynin chloride and tolterodine tartrate in the treatment of overactive bladder: results of the OBJECT study. Mayo Clin Proc 2001; 76: 358–63.

34. Diokno AC, Appell RA, Sand PK et al. Prospective, randomized, double-blind study of the efficacy and tolerability of the extended-release formulations of oxybutynin and tolterodine for overactive bladder; result of the OPERA trial. Mayo Clin Proc 2003; 78: 687–95.

35. Dmochowski RR, Davila GW, Zinner NR et al. Efficacy and safety of transdermal oxybutynin in patients with urge and mixed urinary incontinence. J Urol 2002; 168: 580–6.

36. Yarker YE, Goa KL, Fitton A. Oxybutynin. A review of its pharmacodynamic and pharmacokinetic properties, and its therapeutic use in detrusor instability. Drugs Aging 1995; 6: 243–62.

37. Norona-Blob L, Kachur JF. Enantiomers of oxybutynin: in vitro pharmacological characterization at M1, M2 and M3 muscarinic receptors and in vivo effects on urinary bladder contraction, mydriasis and salivary secretion in guinea pigs. J Pharmacol Exp Ther 1991; 256: 562–7.

38. Douchamps J, Derenne F, Stockis A, et al. The pharmacokinetics of oxybutynin in man. Eur J Clin Pharmacol 1988; 35: 515–20.

39. Pak RW, Petrou SP, Staskin DR. Trospium chloride: aquaternary amine with unique phamacologic properties. Curr Urol Rep 2003; 4(6): 436–40.

40. Todorova A, Vonderheid-Guth B, Dimpfel W. Effects of tolterodine, trospium chloride, and oxybutynin on the central nervous system. J Clin Pharmacol 2001; 41: 636–44.

41. Gupta SK, Sathyan G. Pharmacokinetics of an oral once-a-day controlled release oxybutynin formulation compared with immediate-release oxybutynin. J Clin Pharmacol 1999; etc. 39: 289–96.

42. Sathyan G, Chancellor MB, Gupta SK. Effect of OROS controlled release delivery on the pharmacokinetics and pharmacodynamics of oxybutynin chloride. Br J Clin Pharmacol 2001; 52: 409–17.

43. Anderson RU, Mobley D, Blank B et al. Once daily controlled versus immediate release oxybutynin chloride for urge urinary incontinence. J Urol 1999; 161: 1809–12.

44. Ilett KF, Tee LBG, Reeves PT et al. Metabolism of drugs and other xenobiotics in the gut lumen and wall. Pharmacol Ther 1990; 46: 67–93.

45. Paine MF, Khaighi M, Fisher JM et al. Characterization of interintestinal variations in human CYP3A-dependent metabolism. J Pharmacol Exp Ther 1997; 283: 1552–62.

46. Versi E, Appell RA, Mobley D et al. Dry mouth with conventional and controlled-release oxybutynin in urinary incontinence. Obstet Gynecol 2000; 95: 718–21.

47. Birns J, Lukkari E, Malone-Lee JG. A randomized controlled trial comparing the efficacy of controlled release oxybutynin tablets (10 mg once daily) with conventional oxybutynin tablets (5 mg twice daily) in patients whose symptoms were stabilized on 5 mg twice daily of oxybutynin. BJU Int 2000; 85: 793–8.

48. Gleason DM, Susset J, White C et al. Evaluation of a new one-daily formulation of oxybutynin in the treatment of urinary urge incontinence. Urology 1999; 54: 420–3.

49. Appell RA, Diokno A, Antoci J et al. One-year, prospective, open-label trial of controlled-release oxybutynin for overactive bladder in a community-based population [Abstract]. Neurourol Urodyn 2000; 19: 526, (abstr 117).

50. Thomas TM, Plymat KR, Blannun J et al. prevalence of urinary incontinence. Br Med J 1980; 281: 1243–5.

51. Chamberlain TM, Stephenson DW, Appell RA et al. Urinary incontinence in the long-term care patient. Consultant Pharmacist 1990; 5: 173–8.

52. Reiz JL, Darke AC. Steady state pharmacokinetics and pharmacodynamics of once daily controlled release oxybutynin and immediate release oxybutynin. Can J Clin Pharmacol 2003; 10: 131.

53. Barkin J, Corcos J, Radomski SB et al. A randomized, double blind, paralled group comparison of controlled and immediate release oxybutynin chloride in urge urinary incontinence. Clin Ther 2004; 26: 1026–36.

54. Radomski SB, Caley B, Reiz JL et al. Pilot evaluation of a new formulation of once daily controlled release oxybutynin in the treatment of urinary incontinence. Curr Med Res Opin 2004; 20: 249–53.

55. Corcos J, Casey R, Patrick A et al. A double-blind randomized dose-response study comparing daily doses of 5, 10 and 15 mg controlled-release oxybutynin: balancing efficacy with severity of dry mouth. BJU Int 2006; 97: 520–7.

15

Tolterodine in the management of overactive bladder

Jonathan S Starkman, Karl J Kreder, and Roger R Dmochowski

Introduction • **Dosage** • **Mechanism of action** • **Metabolism** • **Drug interactions**
• **Efficacy data for tolterodine in management of overactive bladder** • **Tolterodine in special populations**
• **Conclusion**

INTRODUCTION

Overactive bladder (OAB) is a common symptom complex of the lower urinary tract characterized by urinary frequency, urgency, urge incontinence, and nocturia.[1] While it is generally accepted that OAB symptomatology is widely underreported for a variety of reasons, it is estimated that OAB affects up to 33 million adults in the United States, with a third experiencing urinary urge incontinence.[2,3] Symptoms of OAB are known to have a negative impact on health-related quality of life, leading to limitations in daily activities, withdrawal from social situations, embarrassment, anxiety, and depression.[4-6] There are documented health risks associated with OAB, as it has been shown that postmenopausal women with urinary incontinence have a significantly higher risk of falling and sustaining a fracture.[7] Furthermore, there is a huge financial burden associated with OAB, with total costs related to urinary incontinence exceeding $25 billion per year.[8]

Although OAB is a syndrome for which no identifiable cause has been determined, the pathophysiological abnormalities underlying detrusor overactivity are reasonably well understood and effective treatments for OAB are currently available. While there are a variety of available treatment options for OAB, it is extremely important to individualize therapy, with consideration given to each patient's lifestyle, cognitive ability, and expectations. Realistic goals should be outlined and discussed with patients prior to the initiation of any form of therapy. The management of OAB has become standardized to some degree, and because it is the least invasive approach, behavioral therapies are often recommended as first line treatment. Behavioral therapies include a combination of pelvic floor muscle exercises (with or without biofeedback), pelvic floor electrical stimulation, fluid restriction, dietary modification, and timed/prompted voiding. Oftentimes, patient compliance with these conservative, non-invasive treatments declines with time as they require more effort on the part of the patient to be effective.[9] Pharmacotherapy for OAB is also extremely effective, with muscarinic receptor antagonists demonstrating efficacy in the reduction of OAB symptoms in numerous randomized clinical trials. In addition, several studies have shown that combination therapy with medications and behavioral techniques provide superior outcomes to those with either treatment alone.[10,11]

Despite the existence of effective treatments for OAB, at any given time only a fraction of patients are receiving therapy. A recent European survey found that only 27% of patients seeking treatment for OAB were currently receiving medication at the time of the survey.[12] Reasons for this disparity are likely multifactorial, including issues related to cost of therapy, patient and physician attitudes, a heterogeneous patient population with respect to symptom severity and response to therapy, and side effects related to medication. Furthermore, both neurogenic and myogenic mechanisms may play important roles in the bladder's responsiveness to particular agents and interventions.[13]

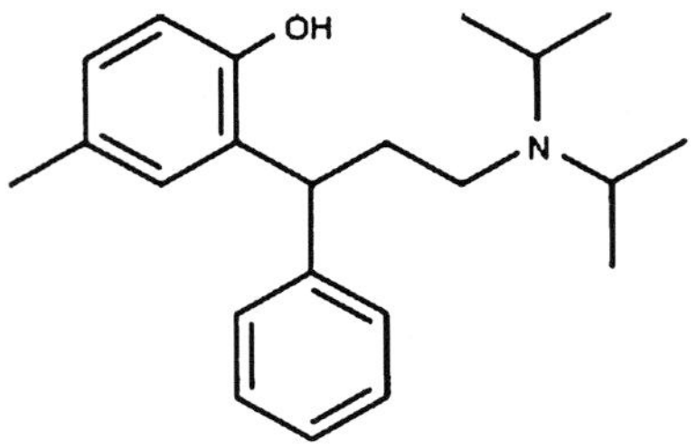

DOSAGE

The optimal dose of tolterodine immediate release formulation (IR) in clinical practice has been shown to be 2 mg administered twice daily.[14,15] Dose-ranging studies have shown that >4 mg per day results in an unacceptably high incidence of residual urine (secondary to depressed detrusor contractility) and dry mouth, while the incidence of adverse events at a dose ≤2 mg twice daily (4 mg/day) was comparable to that with placebo.[15] Tolterodine extended release formulation (ER) is administered as a sustained release capsule delivering a 4-mg total daily dose of tolterodine. This dosing regimen was largely extrapolated to an equivalent 24-hour dosage of tolterodine IR.

MECHANISM OF ACTION

When assessing treatment options for OAB, muscarinic receptor antagonists are currently considered the standard of care. Five different receptor types (M_1–M_5) have currently been identified, which vary in distribution throughout the body depending on the particular organ system. In the bladder the predominant receptors are the M_2 and M_3 subtypes. Studies using animal experiments have demonstrated that detrusor contractility occurs by M_3 receptor-mediated smooth muscle contraction via hydrolysis of phosphatidylinositol and release of intracellular calcium.[16–18] Furthermore, there is also evidence that M_2 receptor-mediated contractions occur via the inhibition of cyclic adenosine monophosphate (cAMP)-mediated relaxation of detrusor smooth muscle.[19] As a result, by binding to the M_2 and M_3 muscarinic receptors of urothelial and detrusor smooth muscle cells, tolterodine exerts its therapeutic effect by interrupting

Figure 15.1   Chemical structure of tolterodine tartrate.

signal transduction pathways that culminate with a detrusor contraction.

Tolterodine, a synthetic tertiary amine with a molecular weight of 475.6 daltons and a pK_a value of 9.9, is administered as a tartrate salt (Figure 15.1). Tolterodine and its major 5-hydroxymethyl metabolite (5-HM) are competitive, pure muscarinic receptor antagonists. Tolterodine effectively inhibits carbachol-induced contractions of human and guinea-pig bladder strips in a concentration-dependent, competitive manner.[20] Unlike oxybutynin, which preferentially binds to the M_3 receptor ($M_3 > M_2$), tolterodine does not exhibit muscarinic receptor subtype specificity. The non-selective binding properties of tolterodine have been demonstrated in in vitro studies using Chinese hamster ovarian cells expressing human muscarinic receptors (M_1– M_5).[20,21] Furthermore, radioligand binding studies have shown that tolterodine has an eight-fold lower affinity for muscarinic receptors (M_3) in the guinea-pig parotid gland when compared to oxybutynin. Thus, tolterodine exhibits a relative functional selectivity for the bladder over the salivary glands in vivo that is not attributable to specific muscarinic receptor subtype selectivity.[22,23] This has important clinical implications, as tolterodine has the potential for comparable efficacy and improved tolerability in comparison to oxybutynin.

METABOLISM

Following oral administration, tolterodine is rapidly absorbed from the gastrointestinal tract and undergoes first pass metabolism in the liver. Tolterodine may be administered with food or under fasting conditions with similar efficacy, as bioequivalence has been observed for the active moiety (unbound tolterodine plus 5-HM) under both circumstances.[24] Tolterodine metabolism follows two pathways once taken up by the liver (Figure 15.2). The principal metabolic pathway results in extensive hydroxylation of tolterodine's 5-methyl group by the CYP2D6 microsome, forming the active 5-hydroxymethyl metabolite (5-HM).[25]

As a result of a genetic polymorphism, approximately 7% of the Caucasian population is deficient with respect to this isoenzyme (CYP2D6) and termed poor metabolizers. Thus, tolterodine metabolism proceeds via the CYP3A4-mediated pathway in this population, forming N-dealkylated tolterodine.[26] Pharmacokinetic studies have shown that tolterodine is metabolized at a slower rate in poor metabolizers than in extensive metabolizers; this results in significantly higher plasma levels of tolterodine and virtually undetectable levels of 5-HM.[9] The pharmacological properties of 5-HM are identical to those of the parent compound, while other metabolites are not considered to contribute to the pharmacological effects of tolterodine; therefore, the pharmacokinetic differences between extensive and poor metabolizers are unlikely to result in any relevant differences in clinical response. As a result, tolterodine dosage is the same regardless of the patient's metabolic phenotype.[27]

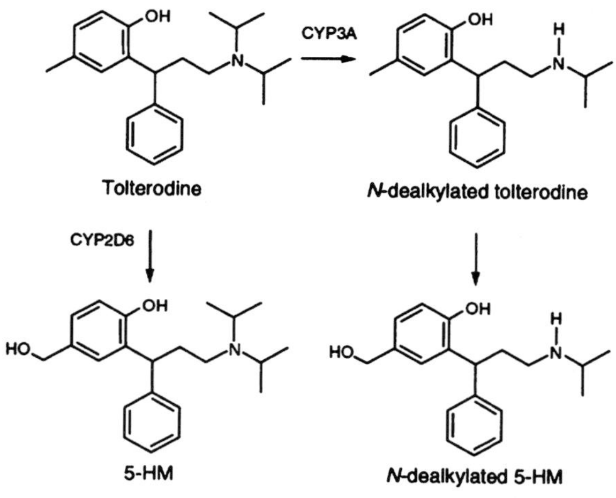

The excretion of tolterodine and its metabolites is primarily renal (77%), with a small percentage excreted in the feces (17%).[28] The elimination half-life of tolterodine and 5-HM is 2–3 hours in normal metabolizers and increases to 9–10 hours in poor metabolizers. Studies have shown that only 5–15% of renally excreted drug is actually tolterodine and 5-HM, with the majority comprising of 5-carboxylic acid metabolites.[28] Although this is the case, the effects of renal dysfunction on tolterodine pharmacokinetics have not been well documented, and it is recommended that caution be exercised when administering tolterodine to patients with significant renal insufficiency. With respect to liver dysfunction, studies in patients with hepatic cirrhosis have shown that tolterodine serum concentrations and elimination half-life are increased, compared to healthy volunteers.[29] There were no serious adverse events; however, patients with hepatic impairment had twice the exposure to pharmacologically active drug. Dosage reduction (maximum 1 mg twice daily) is therefore recommended in patients with evidence of significant liver disease.

DRUG INTERACTIONS

Currently there are limited data available concerning drug–drug interactions with tolterodine and other prescribed medications. Drugs that inhibit CYP2D6 can potentially alter the pharmacokinetics of tolterodine and 5-HM; serum levels thus parallel those seen in poor metabolizers. This was specifically investigated using fluoxetine, a potent CYP2D6 inhibitor.[30] Despite changing the pharmacokinetic profile, patients' exposure to the active moiety (unbound tolterodine plus 5-HM) remained constant; therefore, dosage adjustments are not currently recommended. Another study investigated the effects of tolterodine on the metabolism of other cytochrome P450 metabolized drugs, specifically debrisoquine (index of CYP2D6), omeprazole (index of CYP2C19 and CYP3A4), and caffeine (index of CYP1A2).[31] Tolterodine administered twice daily had no observed effect on the activities of these cytochrome isoenzymes, and the authors concluded that tolterodine is unlikely to significantly alter the metabolism of substrates of these isoenzymes. Furthermore, there

Figure 15.2   Metabolic pathways of tolterodine.

is literature documenting safe coadministration of tolterodine with warfarin,[32] oral contraceptives,[33] thiazide and loop diuretics,[34] tricyclic antidepressants,[34] and duloxetine.[35] Although formal pharmacological studies administering tolterodine simultaneously with CYP3A4 inhibitors have not been performed, it is recommended that patients taking a known CYP3A4 inhibitor receive a maximum dose of 1 mg twice daily. This is due to the fact that metabolism proceeds through CYP3A4-mediated dealkylation of tolterodine in poor metabolizers, which could potentially lead to significantly higher serum levels of tolterodine.[36]

Tolterodine ER

Despite the fact that tolterodine IR has shown comparable efficacy and improved tolerability in comparison to oxybutynin, the analysis of pharmacy claims data reveals that less than one-third of patients continue either agent beyond 6 months.[37] Data such as this were a major factor leading to the development of an extended release formulation of tolterodine.

The extended release (ER) formulation of tolterodine was developed to facilitate patient compliance with a once-daily dosing regimen and improve tolerability. A state-of-the-art drug delivery system utilizing an encapsulated microsphere formulation of tolterodine allows stable and sustained release of drug over the entire physiologic pH range (Figure 15.3). Tolterodine ER is a capsule containing identical tolterodine ER beads. Each bead contains an insoluble core, a sealcoat polymer layer, a drug layer, a prolonged release polymer layer comprising 85% ethyl cellulose, and an overcoat layer (Figure 15.4).[38] Tolterodine is slowly released across the semipermeable polymer layer providing prolonged release of drug throughout the 24-hour dosing interval. The insoluble bead core is excreted unchanged in the stool. As with the IR formulation, tolterodine ER is extensively metabolized in the liver via the CYP2D6 pathway, forming the active metabolite 5-HM.

Pharmacokinetics of tolterodine IR and tolterodine ER

The multiple-dose pharmacokinetics of tolterodine IR and ER were analyzed in a study by Olsson and Szamosi[39] using 19 healthy volunteers. CYP2D6 genotyping using polymerase chain reaction (PCR) determined that 14 patients were extensive metabolizers and five patients were poor metabolizers. A comparison of predose and steady state serum concentrations revealed that steady state was reached by day 6 for both tolterodine IR and tolterodine ER. Tolterodine IR is rapidly absorbed, reaching maximum serum concentrations within 0.5–2 hours after oral administration. Conversely, tolterodine ER has a more gradual serum concentration–time profile, achieving maximum concentrations over a 2–6 hour window. Compared with 2 mg twice-daily IR dosing, once-daily 4 mg ER dosing yields a lower peak concentration (C_{max}) (75% of IR C_{max}) and a higher C_{min} (1.5 times greater than that with tolterodine IR). As a result, the fluctuation index values were lower for tolterodine ER, which reflects its therapeutic stability over the

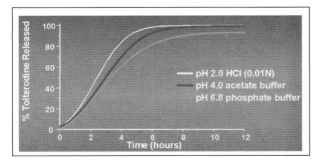

Figure 15.3   Tolterodine ER release as a function of pH. (See also color plate section).

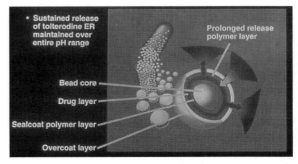

Figure 15.4   Tolterodine ER drug delivery system.

24-hour dosing interval. The 5-HM serum concentration-time profile parallels both tolterodine formulations in extensive metabolizers (Figure 15.5). As expected tolterodine serum concentrations are higher in poor metabolizers with respect to both IR and ER administration (Figure 15.6). The median steady state pharmacokinetic parameters of tolterodine and its 5-HM metabolite are summarized in Table 15.1. Although there were specific pharmacokinetic differences observed between the two tolterodine formulations, area under the curve (AUC) values were consistent with pharmacokinetic equivalence, thus allowing a smooth transition from one agent to the other in clinical practice (Table 15.2).

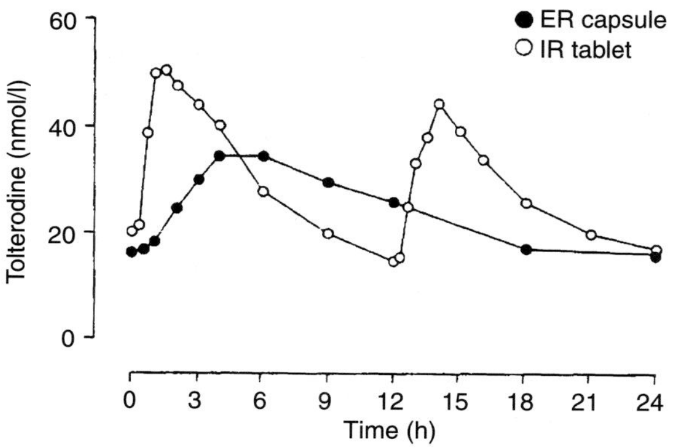

Figure 15.6 Tolterodine serum concentration vs time profile in poor metabolizers.

EFFICACY DATA FOR TOLTERODINE IN MANAGEMENT OF OVERACTIVE BLADDER

Tolterodine was the first muscarinic receptor antagonist specifically developed for the treatment

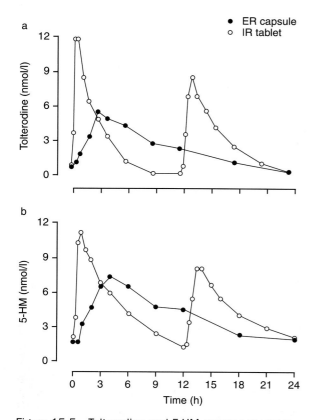

Figure 15.5 Tolterodine and 5-HM serum concentrations vs time profile in extensive metabolizers.

of OAB. Observed functional selectivity of tolterodine for the bladder translates into clinical efficacy and improved tolerability for patients. Numerous comparative, randomized studies have demonstrated that tolterodine IR (2 mg twice daily (bid)) is equally as effective compared with oxybutynin IR (5 mg three times daily (tid)) in ameliorating the bothersome symptoms of OAB.[40,41] Studies have also shown that tolterodine is well tolerated during long-term treatment.[42] Furthermore, tolterodine ER (4 mg once daily) offers convenient once-daily dosing, which improves the tolerability of drug therapy even further.[43] In the following sections we review important clinical trial data for both tolterodine IR and ER formulations.

Tolterodine IR

Early studies of the IR formulation of tolterodine have demonstrated that it is effective in ameliorating overactive bladder symptoms. A large, double-blind, placebo controlled trial has established the efficacy and tolerability of tolterodine IR compared to placebo.[44] One-thousand and twenty-two patients with ≥5 urge incontinence episodes/week and ≥8 voids/day were randomized to tolterodine IR 2 mg twice daily ($n = 514$) or placebo ($n = 508$). Patients were well matched with respect to demographic and clinical characteristics, as well as prior history of responsiveness to antimuscarinic therapy. With respect to micturition variables, tolterodine IR resulted in

Table 15.1 Tolterodine Median Steady State Pharmacokinetic Parameters

Parameter	Extensive metabolizers (n = 13) ER capsule 4 mg once daily	IR tablet 2 mg twice daily	Poor metabolizers (n = 4) ER capsule 4mg once daily	IR tablet 2mg twice daily
Tolterodine				
AUC24 (nmol/L·h)	52 (17–793)	80 (12–716)	570 (479–2203)	685 (538–2123)
C_{max} (nmol/L)	6.1 (1.1–59)	Morning: 12 (1.2–57)	35 (28–130)	Morning: 51 (40–143)
		Evening: 9.2 (1.5–50)		Evening: 45 (34–99)
C_{min} (nmol/L)	0.34 (0.03–19)	0.22 (0.006–14)	15 (12–71)	15 (12–65)
FI	2.0 (0.91–4.1)	3.5 (1.4–5.9)	0.76 (0.62–0.96)	1.2 (0.88–1.5)
t_{max} (h)	4 (2–6)	Morning: 1 (0.33–1.5)	4 (3–6)	Morning: 1 (0.67–1.5)
		Evening: 1.5 (0.67–3)		Evening: 1.8 (1.5–3)
$t\frac{1}{2}z$ (h)	6.2 (3.2–14)	2.8 (1.6–9.1)	11 (8.9–41)	8.7 (7.6–17)
5–HM				
AUC24 (nmol/L·h)	94 (38–187)	105 (41–199)	ND	ND
C_{max} (nmol/L)	7.3 (2.9–13)	Morning: 11 (5.3–19)	ND	ND
		Evening: 8.2 (4.1–15)		
C_{min} (nmol/L)	1.6 (0.09–4.4)	1.1 (0.18–4.1)	ND	ND
FI	1.5 (0.72–2.9)	2.6 (0.74–4.0)	ND	ND
t_{max} (h)	4 (2–6)	Morning: 1 (0.33–2)	ND	ND
		Evening: 1.5 (1-4)		
$t\frac{1}{2}z$ (h)	10 (3.1–18)	5.0 (3.2–13)	ND	ND

AUC_{24} = area under the serum concentration-time curve from time zero to 24 hours; C_{max} = maximum observed serum concentration; C_{min} = minimum observed serum concentration; ER = extended release; FI = fluctuation index [(Cmax – C_{min})/(AUC24/24)]; IR = immediate release; ND = not determined (serum concentrations lower than limit of quantification); $t\frac{1}{2}z$ = terminal half-life; t_{max} = time to C_{max}

Adapted from Olsson B and Szamosi J. Multiple dose pharmacokinetics of a new once daily extended release formulation versus immediate release tolterodine. Clin Pharmacokinet 2001; 40: 227–35.

a significant improvement in urge incontinence episodes/week (-10.6 vs. -6.9; $p = 0.0005$), micturition frequency (-1.7 vs. -1.2; $p = 0.0079$), and average voided volume ($+29$ ml vs. $+14$ ml; $p = 0.0001$) compared with placebo treatment. Following 12 weeks of treatment, 61% of tolterodine treated patients reported an improvement in their overall bladder condition as compared to 43% of placebo treated patients ($p = 0.001$). In general, tolterodine IR was well tolerated throughout the study period. Dry mouth was the most frequently observed adverse event and was reported more frequently among patients treated with tolterodine (30% vs. 8%). The majority of cases of dry mouth were mild to moderate in intensity, with only 2% of tolterodine treated patients experiencing severe dry mouth. Other adverse events were reported with less frequency and less variability between groups (constipation, 7% vs. 4%; headache, 4% vs. 5%; central nervous system (CNS), 3.9% vs. 3.4%). The study concluded that tolterodine IR 2 mg twice daily provides effective control of OAB symptoms with acceptable tolerability.

Drutz et al.[45] conducted a randomized, multicenter, placebo controlled trial comparing the

Table 15.2 Median Steady State Pharmacokinetic Parameters of active moiety (unbound tolterodine + 5-HM) following tolterodine administration

Parameter	ER capsule 4mg once daily	IR tablet 2mg twice daily	Geometric mean ratio (90% CI)
AUC_24 (nmol/L·h)	26 (13–52)	28 (14–60)	0.97 (0.90–1.04)
C_{max} (nmol/L)	2.7 (0.77–3.7)	3.2 (1.0–5.5)	0.74 (0.65–0.84)
C_{min} (nmol/L)	0.53 (0.03–1.7)	0.32 (0.01–23.2)	1.43 (0.55–3.76)

Active moiety = sum of unbound concentrations of tolterodine + 5-hydroxymethyl metabolite in extensive metabolizers (n = 13) and unbound tolterodine alone in poor metabolizers (n = 4); **Geometric mean ration** = values represent the ratios for the ER capsule relative to the IR tablet; C_{max} values for tolterodine IR represent the highest concentration found after morning and evening dosing; AUC_{24} = area under the serum concentration-time curve from time zero to 24 hours; **CI** = confidence interval; C_{max} = maximum observed concentration; C_{min} = minimum observed concentration
Adapted from Olsson B and Szamosi J. Multiple dose pharmacokinetics of a new once daily extended release formulation versus immediate release tolterodine. Clin Pharmacokinet 2001; 40: 227–35.

efficacy and safety of tolterodine IR, oxybutynin IR, and placebo in 277 patients with OAB. Significant decreases in daily micturition frequency were observed for all treatment groups relative to baseline ($p = 0.026$ for placebo and $p < 0.001$ for tolterodine and oxybutynin), with tolterodine 2 mg bid demonstrating superiority relative to placebo ($p = 0.036$). With respect to daily incontinence episodes, all three treatment groups demonstrated significant improvement from baseline ($p = 0.013$ for placebo and $p < 0.001$ for tolterodine and oxybutynin), although there were no differences between groups. Both tolterodine and oxybutynin demonstrated significant improvements in voided volume compared to placebo (+34 ml and +50 ml vs. +12 ml; $p = 0.0075$ and $p = 0.0001$). Furthermore, 65% of oxybutynin and 63% of tolterodine treated patients noted a ≥50% reduction in incontinence episodes, with 22% and 21% experiencing complete continence. As in other OAB clinical trials, dry mouth was the most frequently reported adverse event in all treatment groups, with the incidence being significantly higher in the oxybutynin treated patients (69% (O-IR), 30% (T-IR), and 15% (placebo); $p < 0.001$). While most cases of dry mouth were mild, the percentage of patients experiencing moderate to severe dry mouth was much higher with oxybutynin (44% (O-IR) vs. 9% (T-IR) and 7% (placebo)). Fifty-seven patients withdrew from the study, with most withdrawals related to adverse events ($n = 34$). Significantly more patients withdrew in the

oxybutynin group in comparison to tolterodine ($p = 0.002$) and placebo ($p = 0.026$). The study concluded that while the efficacies of oxybutynin and tolterodine appear equivalent, the significantly improved tolerability of tolterodine may allow for safe and long-term effective treatment.

The OBJECT (Overactive Bladder: Judging Effective Control and Treatment) trial was a prospective, randomized, controlled trial comparing the relative safety and efficacy of oxybutynin ER and tolterodine IR.[46] Three-hundred and seventy-eight patients with at least seven up to 50 urge incontinence episodes per week and ≥10 voids per day were randomized, and 332 completed the study. The study found that both oxybutynin ER and tolterodine IR significantly improved urge incontinence episodes, total incontinence episodes, and micturition frequency at 12 weeks compared to baseline ($p < 0.001$). At study completion, oxybutynin ER was significantly more effective than tolterodine IR for all outcome measures: urge incontinence episodes ($p = 0.03$), total incontinence ($p = 0.02$), and daily micturition frequency ($p = 0.02$). Dry mouth was the most frequent complication observed (28.1% (O-ER) vs. 33.2% (T-IR); $p = 0.32$), and the incidence of moderate to severe dry mouth was also similar (10.2% vs. 10.9%; $p = 0.87$). Overall, all other complications occurred at low rates and with similar frequency. Furthermore, study discontinuation related to adverse events was also similar between active treatment groups (7.6% vs. 7.8%; $p = 0.99$). The study concluded that oxybutynin ER was more efficacious and demonstrated comparable tolerability to tolterodine IR in the treatment of OAB.

Harvey et al.[47] conducted a meta-analysis of randomized clinical trials comparing tolterodine IR and oxybutynin IR. Four studies ultimately met study inclusion criteria and were included in the pooled analysis.[45, 48–50] The study found that both drugs demonstrated significant improvement in micturition diary parameters relative to baseline. The reduction in voids/day was similar for both oxybutynin IR and tolterodine IR (weighted mean difference (WMD), 0.00; 95% confidence interval (CI), −0.38 to 0.38), while there was noted to be a statistically significant reduction in incontinence episodes per day (WMD, 0.41; CI, 0.04 to 0.77) and an increase in voided volume (8.24 ml; 95% CI, −14.11 to −2.38) in favor of oxybutynin IR. With respect to adverse events, the relative risk of dry mouth was 50% less for patients taking tolterodine (relative risk (RR), 0.54; 95% CI, 0.48 to 0.61), and tolterodine IR treated patients were 67% less likely to complain of moderate to severe dry mouth. Furthermore, the risk of study withdrawal was 37% less for patients treated with tolterodine IR (RR, 0.63; 95% CI, 0.46 to 0.88). The authors concluded from the analysis that both drug treatments improve micturition diary parameters, with efficacy marginally in favor of oxybutynin. This may not be clinically significant, however, given the fact that tolerability was superior with tolterodine IR.

Tolterodine ER

A large double-blind, multicenter, randomized, placebo-controlled trial evaluated the comparative efficacy and tolerability of tolterodine ER 4 mg once daily ($n = 507$), tolterodine IR 2 mg twice daily ($n = 514$), or placebo ($n = 508$).[51] Approximately 81% of patients were women, and 50% of patients in each treatment group had a history of prior pharmacotherapy. All treatment arms were well matched with respect to demographics and baseline micturition parameters. Both tolterodine ER and tolterodine IR demonstrated significant improvements in all measured micturition diary variables, including urge incontinence episodes per week (−11.8 (ER), $p = 0.0001$ and −10.6 (IR), $p = 0.0005$ vs. placebo), voluntary

micturitions per day (−1.7 (ER), $p \leq 0.0005$ and −1.6 (IR), $p \leq 0.0002$ vs. placebo), total micturitions per day (−3.5 (ER) and −3.3 (IR), both $p \leq 0.0005$ vs. placebo), and average voided volume (+34 ml (ER) and +29 ml (IR), both $p < 0.0001$ vs. placebo). The median reduction in incontinence episodes as a percentage of baseline values was 71% for tolterodine ER, 60% for tolterodine IR, and 33% for placebo, with the ER formulation being 18% more efficacious than the IR formulation ($p < 0.05$).

During the study, common adverse events related to treatment included dry mouth, constipation, and headache. With the exception of dry mouth, all other side effects occurred with equal frequency in the active treatment and placebo groups (Table 15.3). Dry mouth occurred in 23%, 30%, and 8% for tolterodine ER, tolterodine IR, and placebo, respectively. Overall, patients taking tolterodine ER had a 23% reduction in dry mouth compared to tolterodine IR ($p < 0.02$). The vast majority of cases of dry mouth were rated by patients as mild to moderate, with only 1.8% complaining of severe dry mouth. The study concluded that tolterodine ER was superior to tolterodine IR with respect to overall efficacy and tolerability, offering patients a safe and effective once-daily treatment option.

The OPERA (Overactive Bladder: Performance of Extended Release Agents) trial specifically evaluated the comparative safety and efficacy of oxybutynin ER and tolterodine ER.[52] This was a double-blind, active-control study that randomized 790 women with 21–60 urge incontinence episodes per week to oxybutynin ER 10 mg/day ($n = 391$) or tolterodine ER 4 mg/day ($n = 399$) given for 12 weeks. Oxybutynin ER resulted in numerically superior voiding diary outcomes in comparison to tolterodine ER, although not all measured endpoints resulted in statistical significance. Both treatment groups produced similar reductions in urge incontinence episodes per week (37.1 to 10.8 (O-ER) vs. 36.7 to 11.2 (T-ER); $p = NS$) and total incontinence episodes per week (43.4 to 12.3 vs. 42.4 to 13.8; $p = NS$). Treatment with oxybutynin ER demonstrated more efficacy in reducing micturition frequency (71.1 to 25.2 vs. 66.4 to 28.4; $p = 0.003$) and more patients reported complete continence (23% vs. 16.8%; $p = 0.03$). Dry mouth was the most common adverse event observed in both groups, with a

Table 15.3   Treatment related adverse events

Adverse Event	Tolterodine ER 4 mg qd (n = 505)	Treatment Group Tolterodine IR 2 mg bid (n = 512)	Placebo (n = 507)
Parasympathetic			
Dry mouth	118 (23)	156 (30)	39 (8)
Xerophthalmia	17 (3)	12 (2)	10 (2)
Abnormal vision	6 (1)	4 (1)	2 (0.5)
Dry skin	2 (0.5)	6 (1)	1 (0.5)
Gastrointestinal			
Constipation	30 (6)	35 (7)	22 (4)
Dyspepsia	15 (3)	16 (3)	7 (1)
Abdominal pain	19 (4)	13 (3)	8 (2)
Diarrhea	10 (2)	16 (3)	11 (2)
Flatulence	10 (2)	14 (3)	9 (2)
Nausea	7 (1)	10 (2)	10 (2)
Nervous System			
Headache	32 (6)	19 (4)	23 (5)
Somnolence	14 (3)	13 (3)	9 (2)
Dizziness	11 (2)	9 (2)	5 (1)
Fatigue	11 (2)	6 (1)	4 (1)
Insomnia	7 (1)	2 (0.5)	9 (2)
Urinary			
Urinary tract infection	16 (3)	13 (3)	20 (4)
Dysuria	5 (1)	8 (2)	1 (0.5)
General			
Peripheral edema	7 (1)	7 (1)	4 (1)

Adapted from Van Kerrebroeck P, Kreder K, Jonas U, Zinner N, Wein A. Tolterodine once-daily: superior efficacy and tolerability in the treatment of overactive bladder. Urology 2001; 57: 414–21.

greater number of patients reporting dry mouth in the oxybutynin ER group (29.7% vs. 22.3%; $p = 0.02$). The majority of cases were classified as mild (no influence on daily activities or requiring intervention); therefore, 93% of oxybutynin and 95% of tolterodine treated patients would be classified as having clinically insignificant dry mouth when analyzed concomitantly with patients who did not experience this complication. Other anticholinergic side effects did not differ between groups, and included constipation, diarrhea, and headache. CNS adverse effects such as dizziness, somnolence, insomnia, and depression were noted in 1–4% of patients for both drug formulations.

Different results were obtained from the Antimuscarinic Clinical Effectiveness Trial (ACET), which evaluated the comparative efficacy and safety of extended release tolterodine and oxybutynin.[53] Twelve-hundred and eighty-nine patients were enrolled in a non-randomized fashion to tolterodine ER (2 mg, $n = 333$; 4 mg, $n = 336$) or oxybutynin ER (5 mg, $n = 313$; 10 mg, $n = 307$). A greater percentage of patients perceived an improved bladder condition with tolterodine ER 4 mg compared with the other drug regimens (70% vs. 60% (T-ER, 2 mg); 59% (O-ER, 5 mg); 60% (O-ER, 10 mg); all $p < 0.01$ vs. T-ER, 4 mg). Dry mouth was the most common adverse event and patients reported significantly less severe dry mouth with tolterodine ER compared to oxybutynin ER; furthermore, more patients in the oxybutynin ER (10 mg) group withdrew from the study due to tolerability issues, compared to the tolterodine ER (4 mg) group (13% vs. 6%; $p = 0.001$).

Following a 12-week multicenter randomized placebo controlled trial, patients were offered the opportunity to enroll in a 1-year open label extension trial using 4 mg tolterodine ER once daily.[54] Of the 1377 patients who completed the 12-week study, 1077 (78%) chose to continue in the 1-year open label extension trial. The objective of this study was to examine the long-term safety, tolerability, and efficacy of extended release tolterodine. Efficacy was evaluated from micturition diaries and the patient's perception of bladder condition after 3 and 12 months of treatment, whereas safety was assessed after 3, 6, 9, and 12 months of treatment. Seventy-five percent of patients who entered the 1-year study completed 1 year of therapy with tolterodine. Dry mouth was the most common adverse event, which occurred in 12.9% of patients as compared to 23% in the 12-week trial. When dry mouth did occur it tended to be mild in severity. Other adverse events occurred in fewer than 5% of patients. The authors concluded that tolterodine ER in a dose of 4 mg per day displayed a favorable long-term safety, tolerability, and efficacy profile.

The STAR study was a prospective, double-blind, randomized clinical trial comparing two new-generation antimuscarinics at their recommended daily dosage, namely solifenacin 5 mg or 10 mg once daily and tolterodine ER 4 mg once daily. [55] This study randomized 1177 patients with OAB (≥ 8 voids per 24 hours, ≥ 1 incontinence episode per 24 hours, or ≥ 1 urgency episode per 24 hours) to solifenacin ($n = 578$) and tolterodine ER ($n = 599$). At 4 weeks patients were given the option to increase medication dosage but were dummied, as upward dose titration is approved only for solifenacin. Comparable reductions in micturitions per 24 hours were observed with both agents (-2.45 (solifenacin) vs. -2.24 (tolterodine ER); $p = 0.004$ for non-inferiority). In terms of secondary voiding diary parameters, solifenacin resulted in statistically significant improvements in urgency ($p = 0.035$), urge incontinence ($p = 0.001$), and overall incontinence ($p = 0.006$) compared to tolterodine ER. Seventy-four percent of solifenacin treated patients experienced a $\geq 50\%$ reduction in incontinence episodes, versus 67% for tolterodine ER ($p = 0.021$), and a greater percentage of patients achieved continence with solifenacin (59% vs. 49%; $p = 0.006$). Furthermore, solifenacin resulted in larger improvements in voided volume, number of incontinence pads used, and patient's perception of their bladder condition. The majority of adverse events were mild to moderate, with dry mouth being the most commonly reported side effect related to treatment in both treatment groups. The incidence of severe dry mouth was similar regardless of agent (1.7% vs. 1.5%), as was the rate of study withdrawal (3.5% vs. 3.0%). The authors attributed the favorable results to the flexible dosing available with solifenacin, allowing clinicians to achieve a balance in optimizing efficacy with improved tolerability.

The comparative efficacy and safety of transdermal oxybutynin (OXY-TDS), oral tolterodine, and placebo was assessed in another double-blind, multicenter study.[56] Three-hundred and sixty-one patients with OAB symptoms responsive to standard antimuscarinic medications underwent a washout phase with subsequent randomization to transdermal oxybutynin (3.9 mg/day, twice weekly), extended release (ER) tolterodine (4 mg daily), or placebo. Study outcomes were based on voiding diaries, incontinence-specific quality of life, and tolerability/safety. The two active treatment groups were similar in terms of efficacy, demonstrating statistically significant changes in daily incontinence episodes, average voided volume, and disease-specific quality of life, compared to placebo. One-hundred and twenty patients were continent upon completion of the study, including 47 (39%), 47 (39%), and 26 (22%) patients receiving OXY-TDS, tolterodine ER, and placebo (both $p = 0.014$ vs. placebo).

While all measured efficacy outcomes showed comparable improvement, systemic adverse events occurred more frequently with tolterodine ER (23.6%) compared to OXY-TDS (19%) and placebo (12%). The majority of these were classified as mild and moderate. Dry mouth occurred in 4.1% of patients receiving OXY-TDS and 7.3% of patients receiving tolterodine ER, compared to 1.7% with placebo (OXY-TDS, $p = 0.2678$; tolterodine ER, $p = 0.0379$). Constipation occurred in 3.3% and 5.7% of OXY-TDS and tolterodine ER treated patients, respectively. The study demonstrated that OXY-TDS is similar to tolterodine ER in treating patients with OAB symptoms, while maintaining a low anticholinergic side effect profile that is comparable to that with placebo.

The 037 Study Group evaluated the effect of tolterodine ER on night-time micturitions in patients with overactive bladder.[57] This study evaluated the efficacy and tolerability of a night-time dosing regimen on urgency-related micturitions. The 850 patients enrolled into this 12-week, randomized, controlled study were instructed to take their medication within 4 hours of going to bed. Patients were asked to rate the degree of urgency for each micturition in their voiding diary using a five-point rating scale. Micturitions were than classified as non-overactive bladder voids (1 or 2 on the scale) or OAB voids (3, 4, or 5 on the scale). The trial demonstrated that tolterodine reduced the total number of nocturnal micturitions, but compared to placebo this difference was not statistically significant. However, tolterodine ER significantly reduced overactive bladder-related (3, 4, 5 on the scale) and severe overactive bladder-related micturitions (4, 5 on the scale) compared with placebo. The adverse events associated with night-time dosing were few, with dry mouth reported by 9% of patients, versus 2% for placebo, and constipation in 3% versus 2% in the placebo group. Serious adverse events occurred in 1.2% of patients in each treatment arm. The authors concluded that tolterodine ER significantly reduced nocturnal micturitions due to overactive bladder. Additionally, night-time dosing was associated with fewer adverse events and therefore should be considered as a dosing alternative to reduce the potential occurrence of antimuscarinic side effects such as dry mouth.

Tolterodine IR and ER: quality of life

While clinical efficacy and safety measures will continue to play an important role in OAB clinical trials, they fail to address the patient's perspective of disease burden and outcomes. These patient-derived measures are increasingly becoming more important when critically assessing the effectiveness of specific treatment and the healthcare delivery system as a whole.[58] There have been several studies specifically evaluating the effects of tolterodine as it relates to health related quality of life (HRQoL). Using the King's Health Questionnaire (KHQ) and the Medical Outcomes Study Short Form 36 (SF-36), Pleil et al.[59] demonstrated statistically significant improvements in numerous HRQoL domains (incontinence impact, role limitations, and symptom severity endpoints), which were consistent with the clinical

efficacy of tolterodine IR relative to placebo. Kelleher et al.[60] randomized patients to treatment with tolterodine ER ($n = 507$) or placebo ($n = 508$) and observed statistically significant improvements in bladder control and decreased symptom severity as measured with the KHQ. These authors found that the improvements in HRQoL were sustained during a 12-month open-label extension involving 1077 patients.[61] Thus, treatment of OAB with tolterodine IR and ER can result in measurable improvements in a wide variety of quality of life domains which reflect the patient's perception of the effect of treatment.

TOLTERODINE IN SPECIAL POPULATIONS

Pediatric patients

Urinary incontinence in the pediatric population may be due to both neurogenic and non-neurogenic mechanisms. Idiopathic urinary incontinence or dysfunctional voiding (detrusor overactivity during the filling phase) is the most common type of incontinence in children, with the precise etiology remaining unknown. Pharmacotherapy and behavioral therapy with/without biofeedback have traditionally been the most widely accepted forms of treatment. As tolterodine is postulated to have a superior side-effect profile to that of oxybutynin, there has been much interest in treating both neurogenic and non-neurogenic detrusor overactivity in pediatric patients with tolterodine.

Munding et al.[62] demonstrated that adult doses of tolterodine IR (1 mg, 2 mg, 4 mg bid) in combination with behavioral therapy were safe and efficacious in reducing incontinence episodes in children with a primary diagnosis of dysfunctional voiding. In their study, 22/30 children (73%) were cure/improved and only four (13.3%) experienced adverse events, with one discontinuing treatment due to diarrhea. Hjalmas et al.[63] performed a dose-escalation study in children with OAB symptoms and found that voiding diary parameters were improved in all treatment groups, with the greatest efficacy observed at the 1-mg and 2-mg dosages. Although most adverse events were not considered drug related, they occurred more often in the 2-mg group, and therefore the authors determined the optimal dose in children to be 1 mg twice daily.

Tolterodine has also shown efficacy in treating myelomeningocele patients with neurogenic detrusor overactivity. Goessl et al.[64] evaluated 22 children with neurogenic detrusor overactivity and found significant improvements in cystometric capacity, bladder compliance, and maximum detrusor pressure ($p < 0.001$). In those patients that crossed over from oxybutynin to tolterodine, tolterodine demonstrated equal efficacy in comparison to oxybutynin with respect to measured urodynamic parameters.

Nijman et al.[65] evaluated the results from two large, randomized controlled trials in children aged 5–10 years with urinary urge incontinence suggestive of detrusor overactivity. A total of 224 and 487 were randomized to placebo and tolterodine (2 mg daily). Tolterodine was well tolerated during the 12-week study period, with dry mouth and constipation occurring infrequently. While there was no statistically significant difference in the primary outcome measure (incontinence episodes per week) due to a significant placebo response, children weighing less than 35 kg had the most benefit from treatment with tolterodine. As a result, the authors suggested that a weight-adjusted dosing regimen may optimize the benefit of therapy in older and heavier children.

Several investigators have specifically evaluated the performance of tolterodine therapy in children failing oxybutynin. Bolduc et al.[66] evaluated 34 children with a mean age of 8.9 years who were crossed over from oxybutynin to tolterodine due to anticholinergic side effects. The authors found that efficacy was similar with respect to questionnaire and voiding diary parameters. Twenty (59%) patients reported no adverse effects, six described similar but tolerable side effects, and eight patients discontinued therapy due to bothersome side effects. The study concluded that tolterodine was well tolerated, allowing 77% of patients who could not tolerate oxybutynin to continue pharmacotherapy without significant adverse effects.

Elderly patients

It has been well established that both the incidence and the prevalence of OAB symptoms increase with age. The diagnosis and management of OAB in older geriatric patients is often complicated by medical comorbidities and related medications, mobility disorders, cognitive impairment, bowel habits, and fluid intake. Furthermore, muscarinic receptor antagonists can exacerbate chronic medical conditions (e.g. constipation, glaucoma, dementia . . .) leading to bothersome adverse effects related to therapy.[67] There have been several clinical studies specifically addressing the safety and efficacy of tolterodine in elderly patients with OAB.

Malone-Lee et al.[68] evaluated 177 patients (age $\geq$ 65 years) with OAB symptoms in a randomized, double-blind, placebo controlled trial investigating the clinical safety and efficacy of two dosages of tolterodine IR. There were no serious drug-related adverse events during the study with either dosage of tolterodine IR. Overall, 2%, 3%, and 1% of placebo, tolterodine 1 mg, and tolterodine 2 mg treated patients experienced a serious adverse event unrelated to treatment. There were no cases of urinary retention, as well as no differences in laboratory parameters, electrocardiogram (ECG) variables, and ECG morphology. Dry mouth was the most commonly reported adverse event and was statistically more likely in tolterodine treated patients (30% (1 mg) and 48% (2 mg) vs. 9%; $p = 0.013$ vs. placebo). Other adverse events (gastrointestinal, dizziness, headache, and abnormal visual accommodation) were less likely and were not significantly different when compared to placebo. Most adverse events were classified as mild to moderate, with only 3% and 2% of tolterodine and placebo treated patients withdrawing from the study. Statistically significant effects on micturition parameters were observed, particularly for tolterodine IR (2 mg twice daily). Overall, it appears that tolterodine IR is both safe and effective in older patients with OAB symptomatology.

A subanalysis of data from a large randomized clinical trial of tolterodine ER[51] evaluated the comparative efficacy and safety of tolterodine ER 4 mg once daily in older (age $\geq$ 65) and younger patients (age $<$ 65).[69] There were no differences in efficacy as determined via micturition diary and incidence of adverse events with respect to age. As would be expected, dry mouth was the most common side effect and there were no central nervous system, visual, cardiac (ECG), or laboratory safety concerns noted. Withdrawal rates were similar, irrespective of age. Furthermore, data from a large open-label, observational study of 2250 patients found no significant age-associated differences with respect to tolerability.[70] The study did, however, find that efficacy was slightly diminished in older patients, with baseline symptom severity being the best predictor of response.

Mixed urinary incontinence

Urinary urge incontinence (UUI) and stress urinary incontinence (SUI) are both common disorders of the lower urinary tract that are distinctly different with respect to pathophysiology, as well as treatment. Most OAB randomized clinical trials have excluded patients with a significant stress incontinence component. However, there are a few published studies evaluating the effectiveness of tolterodine in patients with mixed urinary incontinence (MUI).

A double-blind, randomized, placebo-controlled trial in 854 women with urge-predominant mixed urinary incontinence demonstrated that the presence of stress incontinence had no demonstrable effect on tolterodine ER ability to reduce urge incontinence episodes or improve other micturition variables.[71] Kreder et al.[72] investigated the comparative efficacy of tolterodine in 239 patients with urge-predominant MUI and 755 patients with urge incontinence alone. Following 16 weeks of therapy, baseline to endpoint improvements in all voiding diary parameters were statistically significant for both the MUI and UI groups ($p < 0.001$), with no intergroup differences ($p = 0.39$). Lastly, Michel et al.[73] observed that patients with MUI achieve equal benefit from pharmacotherapy with tolterodine IR as patients with pure OAB if SUI is mild to moderate (type I and II SUI). Patients with type III SUI had slightly diminished efficacy as measured by micturition diary parameters, but still responded favorably in comparison to baseline. Taken together, these studies appear to indicate that patients with mixed symptomatology can achieve salutary benefits from both tolterodine IR and ER formulations.

Male patients with lower urinary tract symptoms

There has been much interest in the utilization of muscarinic receptor antagonists in the management of male patients with irritative lower urinary tract symptoms (LUTS) and concomitant benign prostatic hyperplasia (BPH). BPH is a common cause of bothersome LUTS in men, and the prevalence has been shown to increase with age. While voiding symptoms are more prevalent, OAB symptoms including frequency, urgency, and urge incontinence have a tendency to cause more bother, and reportedly affect 40–70% of patients with bladder outlet obstruction (BOO).[74,75] Thus, effective management of OAB symptoms represents an important endpoint in men with BPH and BOO. Although transurethral resection of the prostate (TURP) has generally been considered the most effective therapy to manage BPH-related LUTS, uroselective α_1-adrenoceptor antagonists are often given as first line treatment due to their efficacy in improving symptom scores and quality of life outcomes. Alpha-blockers have demonstrated excellent efficacy in improving voiding symptoms via decreasing bladder outlet resistance via smooth muscle relaxation. Due to the limited density of α receptors in the detrusor smooth muscle, there is limited benefit in managing OAB symptoms with alpha-blockers.

While antimuscarinic receptor blockers have clearly demonstrated adequate safety and efficacy in women with OAB, there has been some concern with effects on detrusor contractility and subsequent urinary retention in male patients with LUTS secondary to BOO. Although some investigators have suggested that muscarinic receptor antagonists may precipitate urinary retention,[76] a recent study of 2 mg tolterodine twice daily in men with BPH showed significant efficacy in treating detrusor overactivity without effecting urinary flow rate or increasing the incidence of urinary retention.[77] A study by Kaplan et al.[78] evaluated a 6-month treatment regimen of tolterodine ER in 43 men with LUTS/BPH who had previously failed alpha-blocker therapy. Thirty-nine men (91%) completed the study and demonstrated significant improvements in both primary and secondary efficacy endpoints. Twenty-four-hour micturition frequency decreased from 9.8 to 6.3 voids ($p < 0.03$) and nocturia episodes decreased from 4.1 to 2.9 nightly ($p < 0.01$). Furthermore, there were significant improvements in the American Urological Association (AUA) symptom index (-6.1, $p < 0.001$), peak flow (Q_{max}) (+1.9 ml/s, $p < 0.001$), and post-void residual urine volume (-22 ml, $p < 0.03$). When AUA symptom scores were stratified into storage symptoms (items 2, 4, and 7) and voiding symptoms (items 1, 3, 5, and 6), tolterodine ER resulted in significant improvements in all individual symptoms following 6 months of treatment. Tolterodine ER had no effect on erectile function in participating men, and mean scores on the International Index of Erectile Function (IIEF) erectile function domain actually increased with treatment (12.7 to 19.6; +6.9). During the period of study, four men (9%) discontinued tolterodine ER therapy because of intolerable dry mouth.

Another more recent study evaluated the efficacy and tolerability of tolterodine ER in men with overactive bladder and urinary urge incontinence.[79] A post hoc analysis of data from the 12-week tolterodine ER registration trial included 163 men randomized to placebo versus tolterodine ER. Reductions in weekly UI episodes were significantly greater in the tolterodine ER group compared to the placebo group (-11.9 vs. -5.9, $p = 0.02$; -71% vs. -40%, $p < 0.05$). A greater reduction in daily micturition frequency was observed for tolterodine ER (-1.7 vs. -1.4; -12% vs. -4%) although the difference was not statistically significant. Overall, a larger percentage of men experienced treatment benefit with tolterodine compared to placebo (63% vs. 46%, $p = 0.04$). Dry mouth was the only adverse event with increased incidence compared to placebo (16% vs. 7%). Although one patient withdrew due to symptoms suggestive of urinary retention, none of the patients completing the study developed acute urinary retention necessitating catheterization. The study concluded that muscarinic receptor antagonists can effectively treat OAB symptoms in men without perpetuating voiding difficulties via inhibition of detrusor contractility.

A unique study by Lee et al.[80] examined the effects of doxazosin with or without tolterodine in men with BOO and OAB. They found that about half of the men with symptomatic BOO had OAB symptoms, and that those with detrusor overactivity tended to be older and have higher International Prostate Symptom Scores (IPSS). While 79% of men with symptomatic BOO and no OAB improved with doxazosin alone, only 35% with BOO and OAB were improved with monotherapy. The addition of tolterodine 2 mg twice daily was effective in improving symptoms in 73% of patients with BOO and OAB. Thus, the addition of tolterodine was successful in salvaging patients with BOO and OAB who would have otherwise failed monotherapy with an α_1 receptor blocker.

A prospective, randomized study compared tamsulosin alone to combination treatment with tamsulosin and tolterodine IR in patients with BOO and concomitant detrusor overactivity.[81] While both treatment groups demonstrated improvements in maximum flow rate and volume at first contraction, only the patients receiving combination treatment with tolterodine IR demonstrated statistically significant improvements in quality of life scores (Urolife™ BPH questionnaire; $p = 0.0003$) following therapy. Furthermore, there were improvements in maximum detrusor pressure and maximum unstable contraction pressure with combination therapy. As there were no instances of acute urinary retention or changes in flow rate or post-void residual, combination therapy with an alpha-blocker and tolterodine IR seems to be a safe and viable treatment modality for patients with BOO and concomitant detrusor overactivity.

CONCLUSION

In clinical trials, both tolterodine IR and ER have shown superior efficacy to placebo and comparable efficacy to other muscarinic receptor antagonists. Systemic anticholinergic adverse effects are infrequent, with dry mouth being most commonly reported. Tolterodine has predictable pharmacokinetic absorption and elimination parameters as shown in both in vitro and in vivo studies. Consistent plasma concentrations of tolterodine ER avoid labile peak and trough concentrations seen with the IR formulation, improving patient compliance with therapy. Both tolterodine IR and ER remain excellent treatment options for patients experiencing bothersome OAB symptoms.

REFERENCES

1. Wein AJ, Rovner ES. Definition and epidemiology of overactive bladder. Urology 2002; 60 (5 Suppl 1): 7–12; discussion 12.

2. Burgio KL, Ives DG, Locher JL, Arena VC, Kuller LH. Treatment seeking for urinary incontinence in older adults. J Am Geriatr Soc 1994; 42: 208–12.

3. Dugan E, Roberts CP, Cohen SJ et al. Why older community-dwelling adults do not discuss urinary incontinence with their primary care physicians. J Am Geriatr Soc 2001; 49: 462–5.

4. Bogner HR, Gallo JJ, Sammel MD et al. Urinary incontinence and psychological distress in community-dwelling older adults. J Am Geriatr Soc 2002; 50: 489–95.

5. Ouslander JG. Management of overactive bladder. N Engl J Med 2004; 350: 786–99.

6. Steers WD, Lee KS. Depression and incontinence. World J Urol 2001; 19: 351–7.

7. Brown JS, Vittinghoff E, Wyman JF et al. Urinary incontinence: does it increase risk for falls and fractures? Study of Osteoporotic Fractures Research Group. J Am Geriatr Soc 2000; 48: 721–5.

8. Wagner TH, Hu TW. Economic costs of urinary incontinence. Int Urogynecol J Pelvic Floor Dysfunct 1998; 9: 127–8.

9. Dmochowski R. Improving the tolerability of anticholinergic agents in the treatment of overactive bladder. Drug Saf 2005; 28: 583–600.

10. Burgio KL, Goode PS, Locher JL et al. Predictors of outcome in the behavioral treatment of urinary incontinence in women. Obstet Gynecol 2003; 102: 940–7.

11. Mattiasson A, Blaakaer J, Hoye K, Wein AJ. Simplified bladder training augments the effectiveness of tolterodine in patients with an overactive bladder. BJU Int 2003; 91: 54–60.

12. Milsom I, Abrams P, Cardozo L et al. How widespread are the symptoms of an overactive bladder and how are they managed? A population-based prevalence study. BJU Int 2001; 87: 760–6.

13. Dmochowski RR. The puzzle of overactive bladder: controversies, inconsistencies, and insights. Int Urogynecol J Pelvic Floor Dysfunct 2006; 17: 650–8.

14. Jonas U, Hofner K, Madersbacher H, Holmdahl TH. Efficacy and safety of two doses of tolterodine versus placebo in patients with detrusor overactivity and symptoms of frequency, urge incontinence, and urgency: urodynamic evaluation. The International Study Group. World J Urol 1997; 15: 144–51.

15. Rentzhog L, Stanton SL, Cardozo L et al. Efficacy and safety of tolterodine in patients with detrusor instability: a dose-ranging study. Br J Urol 1998; 81: 42–8.

16. Andersson KE, Yoshida M. Antimuscarinics and the overactive detrusor—which is the main mechanism of action? Eur Urol 2003; 43: 1–5.

17. Chess-Williams R, Chapple CR, Yamanishi T, Yasuda K, Sellers DJ. The minor population of M3-receptors mediate contraction of human detrusor muscle in vitro. J Auton Pharmacol 2001; 21: 243–8.

18. Fetscher C, Fleichman M, Schmidt M, Krege S, Michel MC. M(3) muscarinic receptors mediate contraction of human urinary bladder. Br J Pharmacol 2002; 136: 641–3.

19. Chapple CR, Yamanishi T, Chess-Williams R. Muscarinic receptor subtypes and management of the overactive bladder. Urology 2002; 60 (5 Suppl 1): 82–8; discussion 88–9.

20. Nilvebrant L, Andersson KE, Gillberg PG, Stahl M, Sparf B. Tolterodine—a new bladder-selective antimuscarinic agent. Eur J Pharmacol 1997; 327: 195–207.

21. Nilvebrant L, Hallen B, Larsson G. Tolterodine—a new bladder selective muscarinic receptor antagonist: preclinical pharmacological and clinical data. Life Sci 1997; 60: 1129–36.

22. Hills CJ, Winter SA, Balfour JA. Tolterodine. Drugs 1998; 55: 813–20; discussion 821–2.

23. Nilvebrant L. Tolterodine and its active 5-hydroxymethyl metabolite: pure muscarinic receptor antagonists. Pharmacol Toxicol 2002; 90: 260–7.

24. Olsson B, Brynne N, Johansson C, Arnberg H. Food increases the bioavailability of tolterodine but not effective exposure. J Clin Pharmacol 2001; 41: 298–304.

25. Postlind H, Danielson A, Lindgren A, Andersson SH. Tolterodine, a new muscarinic receptor antagonist, is metabolized by cytochromes P450 2D6 and 3A in human liver microsomes. Drug Metab Dispos 1998; 26: 289–93.

26. Brynne N, Dalen P, Alvan G, Bertilsson L, Gabrielsson J. Influence of CYP2D6 polymorphism on the pharmacokinetics and pharmacodynamics of tolterodine. Clin Pharmacol Ther 1998; 63: 529–39.

27. Nilvebrant L. The mechanism of action of tolterodine. Rev Contemp Pharmacother 2000; 11: 13–27.

28. Brynne N, Stahl MM, Hallen B et al. Pharmacokinetics and pharmacodynamics of tolterodine in man: a new drug for the treatment of urinary bladder overactivity. Int J Clin Pharmacol Ther 1997; 35: 287–95.

29. Rahimy MH, Narang PK, Scheinman S. A phase I, open label, safety and pharmacokinetic study of tolterodine in patients with hepatic cirrhosis. Document 9600328. New York: Pharmacia and Upjohn, 1996.

30. Brynne N, Svanstrom C, Aberg-Wistedt A, Hallen B, Bertilsson L. Fluoxetine inhibits the metabolism of tolterodine-pharmacokinetic implications and proposed clinical relevance. Br J Clin Pharmacol 1999; 48: 553–63.

31. Brynne N, Bottiger Y, Hallen B, Bertilsson L. Tolterodine does not affect the human in vivo metabolism of the probe drugs caffeine, debrisoquine and omeprazole. Br J Clin Pharmacol 1999; 47: 145–50.

32. Gillberg PG, Sundquist S, Nilvebrant L. Comparison of the in vitro and in vivo profiles of tolterodine with those of subtype-selective muscarinic receptor antagonists. Eur J Pharmacol 1998; 349: 285–92.

33. Olsson B, Landgren BM. The effect of tolterodine on the pharmacokinetics and pharmacodynamics of a combination oral contraceptive containing ethinyl estradiol and levonorgestrel. Clin Ther 2001; 23: 1876–88.

34. Ruscin JM, Morgenstern NE. Tolterodine use for symptoms of overactive bladder. Ann Pharmacother 1999; 33: 1073–82.

35. Hua TC, Pan A, Chan C et al. Effect of duloxetine on tolterodine pharmacokinetics in healthy volunteers. Br J Clin Pharmacol 2004; 57: 652–6.

36. Brynne N, Forslund C, Hallen B, Gustafsson LL, Bertilsson L. Ketoconazole inhibits the metabolism of tolterodine in subjects with deficient CYP2D6 activity. Br J Clin Pharmacol 1999; 48: 564–72.

37. Lawrence M, Guay DR, Benson SR, Anderson MJ. Immediate-release oxybutynin versus tolterodine in detrusor overactivity: a population analysis. Pharmacotherapy 2000; 20: 470–5.

38. Detrol® LA package insert. New London, CT: Pharmacia, 2005.

39. Olsson B, Szamosi J. Multiple dose pharmacokinetics of a new once daily extended release tolterodine formulation versus immediate release tolterodine. Clin Pharmacokinet 2001; 40: 227–35.

40. Clemett D, Jarvis B. Tolterodine: a review of its use in the treatment of overactive bladder. Drugs Aging 2001; 18: 277–304.

41. Abrams P. Evidence for the efficacy and safety of tolterodine in the treatment of overactive bladder. Expert Opin Pharmacother 2001; 2: 1685–701.

42. Abrams P, Malone-Lee J, Jacquetin B et al. Twelve-month treatment of overactive bladder: efficacy and tolerability of tolterodine. Drugs Aging 2001; 18: 551–60.

43. Swift S, Garely A, Dimpfl T, Payne C. A new once-daily formulation of tolterodine provides superior efficacy and is well tolerated in women with overactive bladder. Int Urogynecol J Pelvic Floor Dysfunct 2003; 14: 50–4; discussion 54–5.

44. Chancellor M, Freedman S, Mitcheson HD, Primus G, Wein A. Tolterodine, an effective and well tolerated treatment for urge incontinence and other overactive bladder symptoms. Clin Drug Invest 2000; 19: 83–91.

45. Drutz HP, Appell RA, Gleason D, Klimberg I, Radomski S. Clinical efficacy and safety of tolterodine compared to oxybutynin and placebo in patients with overactive bladder. Int Urogynecol J Pelvic Floor Dysfunct 1999; 10: 283–9.

46. Appell RA, Sand P, Dmochowski R et al. Prospective randomized controlled trial of extended-release oxybutynin chloride and tolterodine tartrate in the treatment of overactive bladder: results of the OBJECT Study. Mayo Clin Proc 2001; 76: 358–63.

47. Harvey MA, Baker K, Wells GA. Tolterodine versus oxybutynin in the treatment of urge urinary incontinence: a meta-analysis. Am J Obstet Gynecol 2001; 185: 56–61.

48. Abrams P, Freeman R, Anderstrom C, Mattiasson A. Tolterodine, a new antimuscarinic agent: as effective but better tolerated than oxybutynin in patients with an overactive bladder. Br J Urol 1998; 81: 801–10.

49. Malone-Lee J, Shaffu B, Anand C, Powell C. Tolterodine: superior tolerability than and comparable efficacy to oxybutynin in individuals 50 years old or older with overactive bladder: a randomized controlled trial. J Urol 2001; 165: 1452–6.

50. Van Kerrebroeck P, Serment G, Dreher E. Clinical efficacy and safety of tolterodine compared to oxybutynin in patients with overactive bladder. Neurourol Urodyn 1997; 16: 478–9.

51. Van Kerrebroeck P, Kreder K, Jonas U, Zinner N, Wein A. Tolterodine once-daily: superior efficacy

and tolerability in the treatment of the overactive bladder. Urology 2001; 57: 414–21.

52. Diokno AC, Appell RA, Sand PK et al. Prospective, randomized, double-blind study of the efficacy and tolerability of the extended-release formulations of oxybutynin and tolterodine for overactive bladder: results of the OPERA trial. Mayo Clin Proc 2003; 78: 687–95.

53. Sussman D, Garely A. Treatment of overactive bladder with once-daily extended-release tolterodine or oxybutynin: the antimuscarinic clinical effectiveness trial (ACET). Curr Med Res Opin 2002; 18: 177–84.

54. Kreder KJ, Mayne C, Jonas U. Long-term safety, tolerability and efficacy of extended-release tolterodine in the treatment of overactive bladder. Eur Urol 2002; 41: 588–95.

55. Chapple CR, Martinez-Garcia R, Selvaggi L et al. A comparison of the efficacy and tolerability of solifenacin succinate and extended release tolterodine at treating overactive bladder syndrome: results of the STAR trial. Eur Urol 2005; 48: 464–70.

56. Dmochowski RR, Sand PK, Zinner NR et al. Comparative efficacy and safety of transdermal oxybutynin and oral tolterodine versus placebo in previously treated patients with urge and mixed urinary incontinence. Urology 2003; 62: 237–42.

57. Rackley R, Weiss JP, Rovner ES, Wang JT, Guan Z, on behalf of the 037 Study Group. Nighttime dosing with tolterodine reduces overactive bladder-related nocturnal micturitions in patients with overactive bladder and nocturia. Urology 2006; 67: 731–6.

58. Kobelt G, Kirchberger I, Malone-Lee J. Review. Quality-of-life aspects of the overactive bladder and the effect of treatment with tolterodine. BJU Int 1999; 83: 583–90.

59. Pleil AM, Reese PR, Kelleher CJ, Okano GJ. Health related quality of life of patients with overactive bladder receiving immediate-release tolterodine. Eur J Health Econ 2001; 2: 69–74.

60. Kelleher CJ, Reese PR, Pleil AM, Okano GJ. Health-related quality of life of patients receiving extended-release tolterodine for overactive bladder. Am J Manag Care 2002; 8 (19 Suppl): S608–15.

61. Kelleher CJ, Kreder KJ, Pleil AM, Burgess SM, Reese PR. Long-term health-related quality of life of patients receiving extended-release tolterodine for overactive bladder. Am J Manag Care 2002; 8 (19 Suppl): S616–30.

62. Munding M, Wessells H, Thornberry B, Riden D. Use of tolterodine in children with dysfunctional voiding: an initial report. J Urol 2001; 165: 926–8.

63. Hjalmas K, Hellstrom AL, Mogren K, Lackgren G, Stenberg A. The overactive bladder in children: a potential future indication for tolterodine. BJU Int 2001; 87: 569–74.

64. Goessl C, Sauter T, Michael T et al. Efficacy and tolerability of tolterodine in children with detrusor hyperreflexia. Urology 2000; 55: 414–18.

65. Nijman RJ, Borgstein NG, Ellsworth P, Djurhuus JC. Tolterodine treatment for children with symptoms of urinary urge incontinence suggestive of detrusor overactivity: results from 2 randomized, placebo controlled trials. J Urol 2005; 173: 1334–9.

66. Bolduc S, Upadhyay J, Payton J et al. The use of tolterodine in children after oxybutynin failure. BJU Int 2003; 91: 398–401.

67. Ouslander JG. Geriatric considerations in the diagnosis and management of overactive bladder. Urology 2002; 60 (5 Suppl 1): 50–5; discussion 55.

68. Malone-Lee JG, Walsh JB, Maugourd MF. Tolterodine: a safe and effective treatment for older patients with overactive bladder. J Am Geriatr Soc 2001; 49: 700–5.

69. Zinner NR, Mattiasson A, Stanton SL. Efficacy, safety, and tolerability of extended-release once-daily tolterodine treatment for overactive bladder in older versus younger patients. J Am Geriatr Soc 2002; 50: 799–807.

70. Michel MC, Schneider T, Krege S, Goepel M. Does gender or age affect the efficacy and safety of tolterodine? J Urol 2002; 168: 1027–31.

71. Khullar V, Hill S, Laval KU et al. Treatment of urge-predominant mixed urinary incontinence with tolterodine extended release: a randomized, placebo-controlled trial. Urology 2004; 64: 269–74; discussion 74–5.

72. Kreder KJ Jr, Brubaker L, Mainprize T. Tolterodine is equally effective in patients with mixed incontinence and those with urge incontinence alone. BJU Int 2003; 92: 418–21.

73. Michel MC, de la Rosette JJ, Piro M, Goepel M. Does concomitant stress incontinence alter the efficacy of tolterodine in patients with overactive bladder? J Urol 2004; 172: 601–4.

74. Hyman MJ, Groutz A, Blaivas JG. Detrusor instability in men: correlation of lower urinary tract

symptoms with urodynamic findings. J Urol 2001; 166: 550–2; discussion 53.

75. Knutson T, Schafer W, Fall M, Pettersson S, Dahlstrand C. Can urodynamic assessment of outflow obstruction predict outcome from watchful waiting?—A four-year follow-up study. Scand J Urol Nephrol 2001; 35: 463–9.

76. Chapple CR. Pharmacological therapy of benign prostatic hyperplasia/lower urinary tract symptoms: an overview for the practising clinician. BJU Int 2004; 94: 738–44.

77. Abrams P. Tolterodine therapy in men with bladder outlet obstruction and symptomatic detru-sor overactivity is not associated with urinary safety concerns. J Urol 2002; 167 (Suppl): 266 (abstr 1048).

78. Kaplan SA, Walmsley K, Te AE. Tolterodine extended release attenuates lower urinary tract symptoms in men with benign prostatic hyperplasia. J Urol 2005; 174: 2273–5; discussion 2275-6.

79. Roehrborn CG, Abrams P, Rovner ES et al. Efficacy and tolerability of tolterodine extended-release in men with overactive bladder and urgency urinary incontinence. BJU Int 2006; 97: 1003–6.

80. Lee JY, Kim HW, Lee SJ et al. Comparison of doxazosin with or without tolterodine in men with symptomatic bladder outlet obstruction and an overactive bladder. BJU Int 2004; 94: 817–20.

81. Athanasopoulos A, Gyftopoulos K, Giannitsas K et al. Combination treatment with an alpha-blocker plus an anticholinergic for bladder outlet obstruction: a prospective, randomized, controlled study. J Urol 2003; 169: 2253–6.

16

Trospium chloride

David R Staskin

Introduction • Chemistry • Pharmacology • Clinical studies
• Post-marketing surveillance • Conclusions

INTRODUCTION

Overactive bladder (OAB) – defined by the International Continence Society (ICS) as urinary urgency, with or without urgency incontinence, usually with urinary frequency and nocturia[1] – is thought to affect around 33 million adults in the USA.[2] The ICS definition reflects the varying symptomatology experienced by patients with OAB – for example, some patients (~37%) experience urgency incontinence (termed OAB-wet), whereas others do not (termed OAB-dry).[2]

OAB has a significant, detrimental impact on quality of life (QoL), and can also impose financial and physical and mental health burdens on individual patients, their families, and caregivers.[3–7] The defining symptom of OAB – urgency – is associated with the most significant burden in terms of symptom bother.[8] In addition, patients with urgency incontinence experience significant decreases in overall QoL, as well as poor physical and mental health and a significant financial burden.[9]

The pathophysiology of OAB is complex and not fully understood. Three main theories have been proposed. The myogenic theory purports that involuntary detrusor contractions are the result of smooth muscle changes.[10] The neurogenic theory suggests that the symptoms of OAB result from alterations to central inhibitory pathways in the brain or spinal cord, or sensitization of afferent nerve terminals in the urothelium.[11]

The autonomous theory proposes that OAB results from an increase in autonomous activity involving non-micturition contractions and phasic sensory discharge.[12] In practice, the pathophysiology may differ between individual patients and may involve one or more of the proposed mechanisms.[13] In support of the idea that OAB is a heterogeneous condition with differing pathophysiologies is the observation that among patients with cystometrically detectable detrusor contractions, only half of the patients are actually able to feel urgency along with abnormal bladder contractions.[14]

The current standard of care for OAB with or without urgency incontinence is pharmacotherapy with an antimuscarinic agent. In the USA, antimuscarinic agents approved for the treatment of OAB in adults include oxybutynin[15] and tolterodine,[16] and most recently darifenacin,[17] solifenacin,[18] and trospium chloride.[19,20]

Trospium is an orally administered, quaternary amine antimuscarinic agent that has been available in Europe for over 20 years. In May 2004, trospium was granted a license in the USA for the treatment of OAB with symptoms of urgency incontinence, urgency, and urinary frequency. Trospium is the only quaternary amine among the antimuscarinic agents approved for the treatment of OAB, and it is this unique chemical structure and the differences in its pharmacokinetic profile that set trospium apart from the other agents in this class.

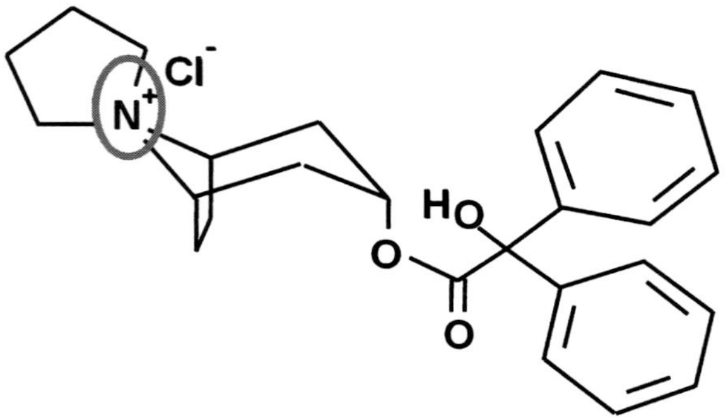

Figure 16.1 The chemical structure of trospium highlighting the quaternary amine ring.

CHEMISTRY

Trospium is a hydrophilic, quaternary ammonium derivative of atropine with a molecular weight of 427.97 and an empiric formula of $C_{25}H_{30}ClNO_3$ (Figure 16.1). The solubility of trospium in water is approximately 0.5 g/ml, and, in its natural form, trospium is a fine, colorless to slightly yellow crystalline solid. Trospium is supplied as 20-mg tablets for oral administration.

PHARMACOLOGY

Pharmacokinetic profile

Trospium is mainly absorbed via the gut by a poorly understood process that may involve P-glycoprotein systems and saturable binding to the intestinal mucosa.[21] Less than 10% of an oral dose of trospium is absorbed via the gastrointestinal tract, and the mean bioavailability is estimated at ~10%. Absorption is not affected by age or gender;[21] however, food reduces the bioavailability and it is recommended that trospium be taken on an empty stomach or at least 1 hour before meals.[21,22] The peak plasma concentration of trospium (~4 ng/ml) is reached in approximately 4–5 hours following oral administration of a 20-mg immediate release formulation, with a mean elimination half-life of between 10 and 20 hours.[21]

Trospium has a plasma half-life of around 20 hours and is excreted largely unchanged via the kidneys (~60% of the absorbed dose), with the remainder as inactive metabolites.[21,22] Although the mean renal clearance of trospium is four-fold higher than the average glomerular filtration rate – suggesting an active tubular secretion process – trospium does not appear to compete with other drugs excreted primarily via the kidneys, such as digoxin.[21,23]

There is little evidence of tissue or organ accumulation during repeated oral dosing of trospium, and the majority of the absorbed dose is distributed systemically bound to plasma proteins.[21,22] Of note is the observation that trospium does not appear to penetrate the central nervous system, most likely as a consequence of its low lipophilicity and ionization at low pH.[21,24,25]

Lack of metabolism via the hepatic cytochrome P450 enzyme pathway

In vivo studies indicate that the majority of trospium is not metabolized and appears in the urine in unchanged form. A small portion (15%) is metabolized via partial ester hydrolysis to form the inactive metabolites azonia-spiro-nortropanol and benzylic acid,[21] a process that does not involve the hepatic cytochrome P (CYP)-450 isozyme system.

As trospium is not metabolized via the hepatic CYP450 system, at therapeutic dose levels it exerts only negligible inhibitory effects against the key hepatic isozymes most frequently involved in drug metabolism, including CYP3A4, CYP2D6, CYP1A2, CYP2E1, CYP2C19, CYP2C9, and CYP2A6.[26,27] A consequence of this is that no clinically relevant drug–drug interactions have been identified when coprescribing trospium with other medications metabolized via the hepatic CYP450 system, and to date none have been reported.[21,22,27]

The role of the M_2/M_3 muscarinic receptor subtypes in micturition

Regulation of normal micturition is controlled by both afferent (sensory) and efferent (motor) neural pathways in combination with a variety of central and peripheral neurotransmitters, including acetylcholine, which interacts with muscarinic receptors in the detrusor muscle, thereby facilitating bladder contraction.[28] Of the five known human muscarinic receptors (M_1–M_5), the postsynaptic M_2 and M_3 receptors are found with greatest abundance within the bladder smooth muscle at a ratio of approximately 3 : 1 ($M_2 : M_3$). A role for the M_3 receptors in mediating direct contractile responses of the bladder smooth muscle has been demonstrated both in pharmacologic and animal-modeled gene-knockout studies. A functional role of the M_2 receptors appears to be mediation of an indirect contractile response by reversing cyclic adenosine monophosphate (cAMP)-dependent β-adrenoceptor-mediated relaxation.[28] In addition, evidence from gene-knockout studies, using combinations of molecules with differing affinities for one or more receptor subtypes, suggests that the M_2 receptors may also operate by enhancing the M_3-mediated contractions, although the mechanisms underlying this are at present unclear.[28] Recent data suggest that the role of the M_2 receptors in mediating bladder contractions may increase in patients with neurogenic bladder dysfunction, and also with age.[29,30]

Balanced selectivity for the M_2/M_3 muscarinic receptor subtypes

Among the available antimuscarinic agents currently approved for the treatment of OAB, trospium is unusual in that it binds to all five muscarinic receptors with similar affinity (Table 16.1).[31,32] In comparison with other antimuscarinic agents, trospium has the greatest affinity for the M_1, M_2, and M_3 receptors.[31,32] Given that smooth muscle contraction involves both the M_3 receptors (directly) and the M_2 receptors (indirectly via reversal of relaxation and through crosstalk with the M_3 receptors), it follows that blockade of both receptor subtypes may

provide both enhancement of the accommodation response and inhibition of the contractile response. This effect may be distinct from that seen with selective or predominant inhibition of M_3 receptors, as provided by other antimuscarinic agents for the treatment of OAB.

The ability of trospium to reverse cholinergically induced bladder smooth muscle contraction has been demonstrated in in vitro studies.[33–36] Trospium causes relaxation of cultured detrusor myocytes[35] and effects a dose-related reversal of cholinergically induced porcine and human bladder smooth muscle contraction.[33,34]

It has been suggested that inhibition of the M_2 receptor subtype may result in cardiac adverse effects, as M_2 is the predominant isoform present in the human heart. In a single-blind randomized placebo-controlled trial, however, trospium at doses up to 100 mg twice daily was not associated with an increased QT interval.[37] Furthermore, in two large-scale clinical trials involving over 1000 patients, the mean increase in heart rate compared with placebo was 3–4 beats per minute, which was not considered to be clinically significant. In these trials, no cardiac side effects were observed in $\geq 1\%$ of the study population.[37] The absence of cardiac effects may in part be due to the low systemic availability of trospium as a result of its low permeability across biological membranes, most likely because the molecule is ionized at neutral pH.

While inhibition of the M_1 receptor subtype in the central nervous system (CNS) has been implicated in the cognitive side effects of other antimuscarinic agents, the reported inability of trospium to cross the blood–brain barrier means that the

Table 16.1 Muscarinic receptor (M) binding affinities of trospium and selected antimuscarinic agents used for the treatment of overactive bladder[31,32]

| Agent | Muscarinic receptor subtype binding affinity (pK$_i$) | | | | |
	M_1	M_2	M_3	M_4	M_5
Trospium	9.1	9.2	9.3	9.0	8.6
Darifenacin	8.2	7.4	9.1	7.3	8.0
Oxybutynin	8.7	7.8	8.9	8.0	7.4
Tolterodine	8.8	8.0	8.5	7.7	7.7
Solifenacin	7.6	6.9	8.0	—	—

affinity of trospium for the M_1 receptor subtype is not regarded as a significant safety concern.[38–40] This has been confirmed in clinical studies, which have shown a lack of cognitive side effects with trospium therapy.[41–44] Furthermore, in the 20 years that trospium has been available in Europe, no case reports detailing adverse cognitive effects have been documented.

Local activity via afferent pathways

As described previously, the majority of the absorbed dose of trospium is excreted unchanged via the kidneys and, as such, a relatively high proportion of the active parent drug is found in the urine. The significance of active compound in the urine has only recently come to light, following developments in our understanding of the functions of the bladder urothelium. Where once the urothelium was believed to be a passive barrier, preventing transfer of substances from urine into the underlying tissues, emerging evidence indicates that urothelial and suburothelial cells exhibit specialized sensory and signaling properties.[45,46] These properties may allow cells of the urothelium to engage in reciprocal communication with neighboring cells, as well as afferent nerves of the bladder wall.[38,47,48]

The presence of muscarinic receptors on the urothelial cells – interestingly at a density even higher than in the detrusor muscle[49] – opens the possibility that direct topical action of trospium on urothelial cells may contribute to the physiologic effects seen with this agent. Experiments involving instillation of antimuscarinic agents directly into the bladder provide us with compelling evidence to support this notion. Fröhlich and colleagues[50] observed that intravesical instillation of either oxybutynin or trospium into the bladders of patients with urgency or urgency incontinence resulted in a significant increase in maximal bladder capacity and a decrease in bladder pressure.[50] More recently, Kim and colleagues[51] observed that continuous infusion into the bladders of rats of the antimuscarinic agents oxybutynin, trospium, tolterodine, and dimethindene at clinically meaningful concentrations suppressed carbachol-induced bladder overactivity.[51]

As the majority of antimuscarinic agents currently approved for the treatment of OAB are extensively metabolized, and thus little active compound is excreted in the urine, the ability to provide local inhibitory effects via the urothelium may be limited to trospium. The importance of the excreted urine concentration of trospium is demonstrated in a further study by Kim and colleagues,[52] in which human urine collected following ingestion of therapeutic doses of trospium, tolterodine, or oxybutynin was instilled into rat bladders. In contrast to the previous study, in which all of the antimuscarinic agents provided similar afferent effects,[51] in this study, only the urine containing trospium suppressed the carbachol-induced overactivity.[52] This is the first study to report that the excreted concentration of trospium after oral ingestion of 20 mg in humans had a significant effect in a rat model of detrusor overactivity. The results provide support for the proposal that trospium may have activity via urothelium-mediated afferent pathways.

CLINICAL STUDIES

Efficacy

The ability of trospium to ameliorate bladder symptoms of urgency, frequency, and urgency incontinence has been confirmed in a variety of patient populations in comparison with placebo and other antimuscarinic agents in a series of European studies.[53–57] In addition, two randomized, placebo-controlled, multicenter studies have been conducted in the USA in adults diagnosed with OAB.[19,20] It is these trials that formed the basis of the approval of this agent for the treatment of OAB in the USA.

In the two US studies, 1181 adult patients (aged > 18 years) with symptoms of OAB (including urgency incontinence) for at least 6 months' duration were randomly assigned to receive either placebo or trospium 20 mg twice daily for up to 3 months.[19,20] In addition to the standard parameters investigated in trials on OAB therapy – frequency, volume voided, urgency incontinence episodes – the US trials investigated the severity of the urgency episodes using the validated Indevus Urgency Severity Scale.[58] Given that urgency is the central and defining symptom of OAB, it may seem obvious that the effects of therapy on this symptom should be closely investigated; however, the majority of studies to date evaluating the effects of OAB therapy have

Table 16.2 US studies among patients with overactive bladder treated with trospium 20 mg twice daily[19,20,22]

Efficacy endpoint	Rudy et al.[19]			Zinner et al.[20]		
	Placebo (n = 325)	Trospium (n = 323)	p Value	Placebo (n = 256)	Trospium (n = 253)	p Value
Urgency severity score						
Baseline	1.75	1.79		1.8	1.8	
Change from baseline	−0.02	−0.21	< 0.0001	−0.04	−0.22	≤ 0.001
Urinary frequency/24 h						
Baseline	13.2	12.9		12.9	12.7	
Change from baseline	−1.76	−2.67	< 0.001	−1.29	−2.37	≤ 0.001
Urgency incontinence episodes/week*						
Baseline	27.3	26.9		30.1	27.3	
Change from baseline	−12.1	−16.1	< 0.001	−13.9	−15.1	≤ 0.05

*Difference assessed by rank analysis of variance while all others were assessed by analysis of variance

been limited to the measurement of the presence or absence of the symptom rather than the severity of the urgency experience.

Trospium significantly reduced urgency severity, episodes of urgency incontinence, and urinary frequency, and improved bladder capacity compared with placebo from the first week of treatment onwards (Table 16.2).[19,20,22] These improvements were paralleled by improvements in QoL among women, as measured using the Incontinence Impact Questionnaire (IIQ), which evaluates impact on travel, physical activity, social relationships, and emotional health.[20] Similar improvements in total IIQ score were not seen in men, however, as the scale has not been validated for use in males, and hence further work is needed to clarify this result.

Additional analyses were conducted on the data from these two studies in order to examine more closely the onset of action of trospium compared with placebo in terms of reducing the symptoms of OAB.[59–61] Significant reductions in daily void volume and the number of daily urgency incontinence episodes emerged within the first 7 days of treatment for patients treated with trospium, with separation from placebo emerging as early as day 3 of treatment for micturition frequency in one study[61] and from day

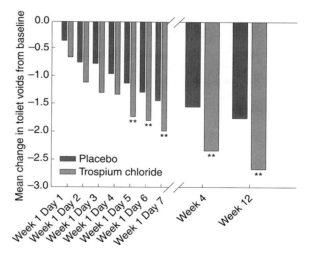

Figure 16.2 Onset of action of trospium as measured by the reduction in the number of daily micturitions among adult patients with overactive bladder treated with trospium 20 mg twice daily or placebo for up to 12 weeks. **p value for treatment comparability statistically significant. Weekly data (weeks 4 and 12) are average findings across 7 days of diary data. (From reference 60, with permission).

5 onwards in the second (Figure 16.2).[60] In addition, patients treated with trospium experienced a significant reduction in the severity of urgency symptoms from day 3 onwards.[60]

The data from these two studies have been reanalyzed using the recently validated OAB-Symptom Composite Score (OAB-SCS).[62] The OAB-SCS combines scores for changes in urgency severity per toilet void, daily voids, and urgency incontinence frequency to yield a single composite score reflecting changes in all the core symptoms of OAB. As such, the OAB-SCS reflects patients' experience of OAB as a whole rather than as a collection of individual symptoms. In the study by Zinner and colleagues,[62] patients treated with trospium reported a mean 10-point improvement in their OAB-SCS compared with a 5-point improvement among patients who received placebo, suggesting that patients treated with trospium experienced noticeable improvements in all their symptoms, including urgency severity (Figure 16.3).[62]

In two key European placebo-controlled studies that included 517 adult patients with cystometrically confirmed OAB, trospium produced significant improvements in the maximum cystometric bladder capacity and urinary volume at the first unstable contraction (Table 16.3).[53,54] Patients were also asked to assess the efficacy of their treatment, and in a meta-analysis of the results from the two studies, patients treated with trospium reported significantly greater clinical improvement than did those who received placebo ($p < 0.0001$).[63]

Trospium has also been compared with other currently available antimuscarinic agents, including tolterodine and oxybutynin (Table 16.4).[55-57] Adult patients with urge syndrome who were treated with trospium 20 mg twice daily experienced greater improvements in their daily micturition frequency than did patients treated with tolterodine (2 mg twice daily) or those who received placebo.[56] Two studies that compared trospium with oxybutynin revealed comparable efficacy according to urodynamic measures between the two agents during both short-term (2 weeks)[57] and longer-term (52 weeks)[55] therapy, although patients were more likely to experience adverse events when treated with oxybutynin than with trospium and, as such, a risk–benefit assessment favors trospium.

Safety and tolerability

Trospium is well tolerated in the clinical setting (Table 16.5).[22] In the placebo-controlled US-based studies, dry mouth and constipation were the most commonly reported adverse events overall. Combined data from the trials of Rudy and colleagues[19] and Zinner and colleagues[20] indicated that 20.1% of patients treated with trospium 20 mg twice daily experienced dry mouth compared with 5.8% of patients who received placebo.[22] Constipation was also reported more frequently by patients treated with trospium (9.6% of patients compared with 4.6% of patients in the placebo group).[22] In one of these two studies, patients were given the option of continuing with, or switching to, trospium for a further 9 months.[64] Dry mouth (11.3% of patients) and constipation (8.8% of patients) remained the most commonly reported adverse events during the extension phase.[64] Comparable tolerability has been reported in the European placebo-controlled studies.[53,54] In the study conducted by Alloussi and colleagues, gastrointestinal disorders were the most commonly reported adverse events overall (trospium 6.2% of patients, placebo 1.0% of patients), with dry mouth accounting for the majority of these adverse events.[53] The incidence of dry mouth and constipation seen with trospium compares favorably with that seen for other antimuscarinic agents approved for the treatment of OAB.

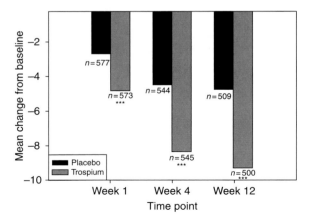

Figure 16.3 Mean change in overactive bladder (OAB) Symptom Composite Scores from baseline among adult patients with OAB treated with trospium 20 mg twice daily or placebo for up to 12 weeks. ***p value < 0.001 for treatment comparability from analysis of variance (ANOVA). (From reference 62, with permission).

Table 16.3 European placebo-controlled clinical studies among adult patients with overactive bladder treated with trospium 20 mg twice daily (bid)[53,54]

Study	Study population	Design	Treatments	Endpoints	Key findings
Alloussi et al.[53]	n = 309 Adults > 18 years with urodynamically confirmed detrusor instability	3-week, multicenter, placebo-controlled trial	Trospium 20 mg bid (n = 210) Placebo (n = 99)	Maximum cystometric bladder capacity Volume at first unstable contraction	Significant increase in maximum bladder capacity ($p = 0.0001$ vs. placebo; per-protocol analysis) More pronounced increase in volume at first unstable contraction ($p = 0.0027$ vs. placebo)
Cardozo et al.[54]	n = 208 Adults 18–70 years with urodynamically confirmed detrusor instability	3-week, multicenter, placebo-controlled trial	Trospium 20 mg bid (n = 104) Placebo (n = 104)	Maximum cystometric bladder capacity Volume at first unstable contraction	Significant increase in maximum cystometric bladder capacity ($p \leq 0.05$ vs. placebo) Significant increase in volume at first unstable contraction ($p \leq 0.05$ vs. placebo)

Table 16.4 European active comparator-controlled clinical studies among adult patients with overactive bladder (OAB)-type symptoms treated with trospium 20 mg twice daily (bid)[55-57]

Study	Study population	Design	Treatments	Endpoints	Key findings
Junemann and Al-Shukri[56]	n = 234 Subjects with a medical history of pollakisuria > 10/day, nocturia, and imperative desire to void	3-week, multicenter, placebo- and active comparator-controlled trial	Trospium 20 mg bid Tolterodine 2 mg bid Placebo	Change from baseline in daily micturition frequency	Trospium reduced micturition frequency compared with placebo ($p \leq 0.01$)
Halaska et al[55]	n = 358 Subjects with urge syndrome (undue frequency of micturition, nocturia, overwhelming urge, wetting) or urge urinary incontinence	52-week, multicenter, active comparator-controlled trial	Trospium 20 mg bid Oxybutynin 5 mg bid	Maximum cystometric bladder capacity Volume at first uninhibited detrusor contraction Volume at first sensation to void	No significant difference between trospium and oxybutynin at 52 weeks in: • maximum cystometric bladder capacity • volume at first unstable contraction • volume at first sensation to void • decrease from baseline in micturition frequency and urgency episodes
Madersbacher et al[57]	n = 95 Adults with spinal cord injuries and detrusor hyperreflexia	2-week active comparator-controlled trial	Trospium 20 mg bid Oxybutynin (5 mg three times daily)	Maximum cystometric bladder capacity	Significant increase in maximum cystometric bladder capacity ($p \leq 0.001$ from baseline) No significant difference between trospium and oxybutynin

Table 16.5 Adverse events (% of patients) reported more frequently among patients treated with trospium 20 mg twice daily than among those who received placebo (occurring in ≥ 1% of patients in any treatment group)[22]		
Adverse event	Trospium 20 mg bid (n = 591)	Placebo (n = 590)
Gastrointestinal disorders		
Dry mouth	20.1	5.8
Constipation	9.6	4.6
Upper abdominal pain	1.5	1.2
Constipation aggravated	1.4	0.8
Dyspepsia	1.2	0.3
Flatulence	1.2	0.8
Nervous system disorders		
Headache	4.2	2.0
General disorders		
Fatigue	1.9	1.4
Renal and urinary disorders		
Urinary retention	1.2	0.3
Eye disorders		
Dry eyes	1.2	0.3

Lack of central nervous system effects

In a subanalysis of the US-based phase III study described previously,[19] patients treated with trospium did not report any relevant increase in daytime sleepiness during the study period (assessed using the Stanford Sleepiness Scale).[43] Moreover, there was no appreciable age-related effect on daytime sleepiness during treatment with trospium in this study.[43] In a separate study among healthy volunteers aged ≥ 50 years, duration and latency of rapid eye movement (REM) sleep following a single oral dose of trospium were comparable with those of individuals who received placebo.[65] In comparison, treatment with oxybutynin or tolterodine resulted in a significant reduction in REM sleep of ~15% and

a slightly (but not significantly) greater REM latency compared with placebo.[65]

The potential effect of trospium on other measures of CNS function has also been explored. Among 12 healthy volunteers, multichannel electroencephalography did not reveal any significant decreases in alpha and $beta_1$ wave activity following intravenous or oral administration of trospium, while significant decreases were noted following oxybutynin administration.[42] These results were subsequently confirmed in a placebo-controlled, single-blind comparison of oxybutynin, tolterodine, and trospium.[44]

POST-MARKETING SURVEILLANCE

The availability of trospium in Europe for over 20 years has yielded data from > 10 000 patients involved in more than 20 clinical trials. Patients with a variety of OAB-like and other irritable bladder symptoms, including irritable bladder, urge incontinence, pollakisuria, nocturia, and urge syndrome, have received trospium and continue to report significant improvements across the core symptoms of OAB during therapy.[66] In addition, patients have also reported a reduced requirement for incontinence aids and improvements in QoL.[67,68] Consistent with observations in the clinical trial setting, dry mouth is the most commonly reported adverse event in post-marketing studies, being reported by 4.1% of patients.[66]

ONCE DAILY PREPARATION

At the time of this publication (Feb 2007), a once-daily preparation of trospium chloride is pending approval at the Food and Drug Administration. The extended release formulation is based on a combination of timed and pH dependent disintegration of bead coating which provides a controlled release of trospium over a 24-hour period. One of the pivotal Phase III studies has been accepted for publication[69]. Patients (n = 601) were randomized to trospium once-daily (TXR, n = 298) or placebo (P, n = 303). TXR treatment resulted in significant improvements over placebo in all primary and secondary efficacy outcomes at Week 1 and throughout the 12 week study (Table 16.6). The most common AE's were dry mouth (TXR = 8.7% vs. P = 3.0%) and constipation (TXR = 9.4% vs. P = 1.3%), while CNS AE's

Table 16.6 Key primary and secondary efficacy endpoints for trospium chloride once-daily (rank analysis of variance intent-to-treat:last observation carried forward) (study 018 data on file Indevus Pharmaceuticals, Lexington, MA)

Endpoint	Placebo (n = 300)	Trospium XR (n = 292)	p-value
Urinary frequency/day			
Baseline	12.74 (0.15)	12.78 (0.15)	NS
Change from baseline[a]			
Week 1	−1.24 (0.13)	−1.66 (0.14)	< 0.0092
Week 12	−1.99 (0.16)	−2.81 (0.15)	< 0.0001
No. of UUI episodes/week			
Baseline	28.98 (1.25)	28.77 (1.27)	NS
Change from baseline[a]			
Week 1	−8.66 (0.95)	−13.03 (0.91)	0.0003
Week 12	−13.49 (1.09)	−17.34 (1.18)	0.0024
Average volume voided (mL/void/day)			
Baseline	155.93 (3.01)	151.03 (2.91)	NS
Change from baseline			
Week 1	12.07 (2.11)	21.61 (2.76)	0.0036
Week 12	18.89 (2.79)	29.77 (3.16)	0.0039
No. of urgency voids/day			
Baseline	11.80 (0.17)	11.86 (0.17)	NS
Change from baseline[a]			
Week 1	−1.34 (0.16)	−1.90 (0.16)	0.0033
Week 12	−2.12 (0.19)	−3.11 (0.17)	< 0.0001
Urgency severity score/void			
Baseline	1.87 (0.03)	1.88 (0.03)	NS
Change from baseline[a]			
Week 1	−0.10 (0.02)	−0.21 (0.02)	0.0002
Week 12	−0.18 (0.03)	−0.32 (0.03)	0.0004

(TXR = 2.0% vs. P = 3.3%) were less than placebo (Table 16.7). No clinically meaningful changes in laboratory, physical examination, or ECG parameters were noted. The once daily trospium chloride formulation provided statistically and clinically significant improvement in the key symptoms of OAB (urgency, frequency, and UUI). The previously reported efficacy of the BID preparation was maintained, while "class effect" anticholinergic AE's occurred at comparatively low levels, especially dry mouth, elicited at the lowest reported rate in the oral drug class.

CONCLUSIONS

Trospium has proved effective in reducing the symptoms of OAB and improving QoL,

with an onset of clinical effect for the majority of parameters observed within the first week of treatment. The unique pharmacologic properties of this compound may confer a number of potential clinical benefits. First, as a quaternary amine, trospium has low lipophilicity and is ionized at neutral pH. These properties limit the transfer of trospium across biological membranes, including those of the blood–brain barrier. Lack of penetration into the CNS results in a low likelihood of cognitive adverse events being associated with trospium treatment. Second, the presence of significant amounts of unchanged trospium in the urine may allow it to provide local effects via afferent pathways. Topical activity, mediated via afferent receptors of the urothelium, may contribute to the improved clinical profile of

Table 16.7 Incidence of all treatment emergent adverse events judged at least possibly related and reported in ≥ 1.0% of patients treated with trospium chloride once-daily (study 018 data on file Indevus Pharmaceuticals, Lexington, MA)

Adverse event	Number of patients (%)	
	Placebo (n = 303)	Trospium XR (n = 298)
Total patients with at least 1 TEAE at least possibly related	53 (17.5)	80 (26.8)
Gastrointestinal disorders		
Dry mouth	9 (3.0)	26 (8.7)
Constipation	4 (1.3)	28 (9.4)
Abdominal pain	2 (0.7)	3 (1.0)
Abdominal pain lower	3 (1.0)	3 (1.0)
Abdominal distension	1 (0.3)	3 (1.0)
Constipation aggravated	3 (1.0)	3 (1.0)
Nausea	2 (0.7)	3 (1.0)
Dyspepsia	3 (1.0)	6 (2.0)
Nervous system disorders		
Headache	8 (2.6)	3 (1.0)
Vision blurred	2 (0.7)	3 (1.0)
General disorders		
Dry skin	0	3 (1.0)
Eye disorders		
Dry eye	1 (0.3)	4 (1.3)
Renal and urinary disorders		
Urinary tract infection	3 (1.0)	6 (2.0)
Urinary retention	1 (0.3)	4 (1.3)

TEAE = treatment-emergent adverse event.

this agent compared with other antimuscarinic agents that are more extensively metabolized, particularly in terms of abnormal urgency sensations, an earlier onset of clinical effect, and prolonged efficacy. Finally, the lack of metabolism via the hepatic CYP450 enzyme system allows trospium to be confidently prescribed alongside the majority of commonly used medications without concern for adverse metabolic drug–drug interactions.

REFERENCES

1. Abrams P, Cardozo L, Fall M et al. The standardisation of terminology in lower urinary tract function: report from the Standardisation Sub-Committee of the International Continence Society. Urology 2003; 61: 37–49.

2. Stewart WF, Van Rooyen JB, Cundiff GW et al. Prevalence and burden of overactive bladder in the United States. World J Urol 2003; 20: 327–36.

3. Abrams P, Kelleher CJ, Kerr LA, Rogers RG. Overactive bladder significantly affects quality of life. Am J Manag Care 2000; 6 (11 Suppl): S580–90.

4. Hu TW, Wagner TH. Health-related consequences of overactive bladder: an economic perspective. BJU Int 2005; 96 (Suppl 1): 43–5.

5. Liberman JN, Hunt TL, Stewart WF et al. Health-related quality of life among adults with symptoms of overactive bladder: results from a US community-based survey. Urology 2001; 57: 1044–50.

6. Voytas J. The role of geriatricians and family practitioners in the treatment of overactive bladder and incontinence. Rev Urol 2002; 4 (Suppl 4): S44–9.

7. Wu EQ, Birnbaum H, Marynchenko M et al. Employees with overactive bladder: work loss burden. J Occup Environ Med 2005; 47: 439–46.

8. Coyne K, Payne C, Bhattacharyya SK et al. The impact of urinary urgency and frequency on health-related quality of life in overactive bladder: results from a national community survey. Value Health 2004; 7: 455–63.

9. Coyne K, Revicki D, Hunt T et al. Psychometric validation of an overactive bladder symptoms and health-related quality of life questionnaire: the OAB-q. Qual Life Res 2002; 11: 563–74.

10. Brading AF. A myogenic basis for the overactive bladder. Urology 1997; 50 (Suppl 6A): 57–67.

11. De Groat WC. A neurologic basis for the overactive bladder. Urology 1997; 50 (Suppl 6A): 36–52.

12. Gillespie JI. The autonomous bladder: a view of the origin of bladder overactivity and sensory urge. BJU Int 2004; 93: 478–83.

13. Goldberg RP, Sand PK. Pathophysiology of the overactive bladder. Clin Obstet Gynecol 2002; 45: 182–92.

14. Wyndaele JJ, Van Meel TD, De Wachter S. Detrusor overactivity. Does it represent a difference if patients feel the involuntary contractions? J Urol 2004; 172: 1915–18.

15. Gleason DM, Susset J, White C, Munoz DR, Sand PK. Evaluation of a new once-daily formulation of oxbutynin for the treatment of urinary urge incontinence. Ditropan XL Study Group. Urology 1999; 54: 420–3.

16. Clemett D, Jarvis B. Tolterodine: a review of its use in the treatment of overactive bladder. Drugs Aging 2001; 18: 277–304.

17. Chapple CR. Darifenacin: a novel M3 muscarinic selective receptor antagonist for the treatment of overactive bladder. Expert Opin Investig Drugs 2004; 13: 1493–500.

18. Chapple CR, Rechberger T, Al-Shukri S et al. Randomized, double-blind placebo- and tolterodine-controlled trial of the once-daily antimuscarinic agent solifenacin in patients with symptomatic overactive bladder. BJU Int 2004; 93: 303–10.

19. Rudy D, Cline K, Harris R, Goldberg K, Dmochowski R. Multicenter Phase III trial studying trospium chloride in patients with overactive bladder. Urology 2006; 67: 275–80.

20. Zinner N, Gittelman M, Harris R et al. Trospium chloride improves overactive bladder symptoms: a multicenter Phase III trial. J Urol 2004; 171: 2311–15.

21. Doroshyenko O, Jetter A, Odenthal KP, Fuhr U. Clinical pharmacokinetics of trospium chloride. Clin Pharmacokinet 2005; 44: 701–20.

22. Sanctura™ prescribing information. Esprit Pharma and Indevus Pharma Inc. July 2004. Available at www.sanctura.com.

23. Sandage B, Sabounjian L, Shipley J et al. Predictive power of an in vitro system to assess drug interactions of an antimuscarinic medication: a comparison of in vitro and in vivo drug–drug interaction studies of trospium chloride with digoxin. J Clin Pharmacol 2006; 46: 776–84.

24. Langguth P, Mutschler E. Lipophilisation of hydrophilic compounds: consequences of transepidermal and intestinal transport of trospium chloride. Arzneimittelforschung 1987; 37: 1362–6.

25. Langguth P, Kubos A, Krumbiegel G et al. Intestinal absorption of the quaternary trospium chloride: permeability-lowering factors and bioavailabilities for oral dosage forms. Eur J Pharm Biopharm 1997; 43: 265–72.

26. Breuel HP, Murtz G, Bondy S, Horkulak J, Gianetti BM. Safety and tolerance of trospium chloride in the high dose range. Arzneimittelforschung 1993; 43: 461–4.

27. Beckmann-Knopp S, Rietbrock S, Weyhenmeyer R et al. Inhibitory effects of trospium chloride on cytochrome P450 enzymes in human liver microsomes. Pharmacol Toxicol 1999; 85: 299–304.

28. Hegde SS. Muscarinic receptors in the bladder: from basic research to therapeutics. Br J Pharmacol 2006; 147: S80–7.

29. Pontari MA, Braverman AS, Ruggieri MR Sr. The M2 muscarinic receptor mediates in vitro bladder contractions from patients with neurogenic bladder dysfunction. Am J Physiol Regul Integr Comp Physiol 2004; 286: R874–80.

30. Ruggieri MR, Tibb A, Braverman AS. Age-induced changes in muscarinic receptor subtypes mediating urinary bladder contraction. Presented at International Continence Society Annual Scientific Meeting, 23–27 August, 2004, Paris, France.

31. Napier C, Gupta P. Darifenacin is selective for the human recombinant M_3 receptor subtype. Neurourol Urodyn 2002; 21: A445.

32. Ikeda K, Kobayashi S, Suzuki M et al. M3 receptor antagonism by the novel antimuscarinic agent solifenacin in the urinary bladder and salivary gland. Naunyn Schmeidebergs Arch Pharmacol 2002; 366: 97–103.

33. Uckert S, Stief CG, Odenthal KP et al. Comparison of the effects of various spasmolytic drugs on isolated human and porcine detrusor smooth muscle. Arzneimittelforschung 1998; 48: 836–9.

34. Uckert S, Stief CG, Odenthal KP et al. Responses of isolated normal human detrusor muscle to various spasmolytic drugs commonly used in the treatment of the overactive bladder. Arzneimittelforschung 2000; 50: 456–60.

35. Eckert RE, Wilhelm A, Schwantes U et al. Modulation der zytoplasmatischen Ca-konzentration isolierter Myozyten des detrusor vesicae durch anticholinergika. Akt Urol 1995; 26: 4–6.

36. Erbsloh J. [Clinical-pharmacological examination of a new compound from the nortropine series by means of cystometry]. Arzneimittelforschung 1967; 17: 1532–3. [in German]

37. Dmochowski R, Staskin DR. The Q-T interval and antimuscarinic drugs. Curr Urol Rep 2005; 6: 405–9.

38. Andersson KE. Potential benefits of muscarinic M_3 receptor selectivity. Eur Urol Suppl 2002; 1: 23–8.

39. Pak RW, Petrou SP, Staskin DR. Trospium chloride: a quaternary amine with unique pharmacologic properties. Curr Urol Rep 2003; 4: 436–40.

40. Scheife R, Takeda M. Central nervous system safety of anticholinergic drugs for the treatment of overactive bladder in the elderly. Clin Ther 2005; 27: 144–53.

41. Herberg KW. General and traffic safety and the effects of incontinence medication: new studies on the safety potential of urological anticholinergics. Med Welt 1999; 50: 217–22.

42. Pietzko A, Dimpfel W, Schwantes U et al. Influences of trospium chloride and oxybutynin on quantitative EEG in healthy volunteers. Eur J Clin Pharmacol 1994; 47: 337–43.

43. Staskin DR, Harnett MD. Effect of trospium chloride on somnolence and sleepiness in patients with overactive bladder. Curr Sci 2004; 5: 423–6.

44. Todorova A, Vonderheid-Guth B, Dimpfel W. Effects of tolterodine, trospium chloride and oxybutynin on the central nervous system. J Clin Pharmacol 2001; 41: 636–44.

45. Birder L. Role of the urothelium in bladder function. Scand J Urol Nephrol Suppl 2004; (215): 48–53.

46. Birder LA. More than just a barrier: urothelium as a drug target for urinary bladder pain. Am J Physiol Renal Physiol 2005; 289: F489–95.

47. Andersson KE. Antimuscarinics for treatment of overactive bladder. Lancet Neurol 2004; 3: 46–53.

48. Andersson KE, Yoshida M. Antimuscarinics and the overactive detrusor – which is the main mechanism of action? Eur Urol 2003; 43: 1–5.

49. Hawthorn MH, Chapple CR, Cock M, Chess-Williams R. Urothelium-derived inhibitory factor(s) influences on detrusor muscle contractility in vitro. Br J Pharmacol 2000; 129: 416–19.

50. Fröhlich G, Burmeister S, Wiedemann A et al. Intravesical instillation of trospium chloride, oxybutynin and verapamil for relaxation of the bladder detrusor muscle. A placebo controlled, randomized clinical test. Arzneimittelforschung 1998; 48: 486–91. [in German]

51. Kim YT, Yoshimura N, Masuda H et al. Antimuscarinic agents exhibit local inhibitory effects on antimuscarinic receptors in bladder-afferent pathways. Urology 2005; 65: 238–42.

52. Kim YT, Yoshimura N, Masuda H et al. Intravesical instillation of human urine after oral administration of trospium, tolterodine and oxybutynin in a rat model of detrusor overactivity. BJU Int 2006; 97: 400–3.

53. Alloussi S, Laval K-U, Eckert R et al. Trospium chloride in patients with motor urge syndrome (detrusor instability): a double-blind, randomised, multicentre, placebo-controlled study. J Clin Res 1998; 1: 439–41.

54. Cardozo L, Chapple CR, Toozs-Hobson P et al. Efficacy of trospium chloride in patients with detrusor instability: a placebo-controlled, randomized, double-blind, multicentre clinical trial. BJU Int 2000; 85: 659–64.

55. Halaska M, Ralph G, Wiedemann A et al. Controlled, double-blind, multicentre clinical trial to investigate long-term tolerability and efficacy of trospium chloride in patients with detrusor instability. World J Urol 2003; 20: 392–9.

56. Junemann KP, Al-Shukri S. Efficacy and tolerability of trospium chloride and tolterodine in 234 patients with urge syndrome: a double-blind, placebo-controlled, multicentre clinical trial. Abstract Neurourol Urodyn 2000; 19: 488–90.

57. Madersbacher H, Stohrer M, Richter R et al. Trospium chloride versus oxybutynin: a randomized, double-blind, multicenter trial in the treatment of detrusor hyper-reflexia. Br J Urol 1995; 75: 425–56.

58. Nixon A, Colman S, Sabounjian L et al. A validated patient reported measure of urinary urgency severity in overactive bladder for use in clinical trials. J Urol 2005; 174: 604–7.

59. Garely A, for the Trospium Study Group. Trospium chloride demonstrated rapid onset of effect for multiple overactive bladder symptoms in female patients. J Pelvic Med Surg 2005; 11 (Suppl 1): S41.

60. Rudy D, Cline K, Harris R et al. Time to onset of improvement in symptoms of overactive bladder using antimuscarinic treatment. BJU Int 2006; 97: 540–6.

61. Sand P, Dmochowski R. Trospium chloride improves symptoms of overactive bladder within one week. Abstract presented at International Continence Society Annual Meeting, 5–9 October, 2003, Florence, Italy (abstr no. 370).

62. Zinner N, Harnett M, Sabounjian L et al. The overactive bladder-symptom composite score: a composite symptom score of toilet voids, urgency severity and urge urinary incontinence in patients with overactive bladder. J Urol 2005; 173: 1639–43.

63. Fröhlich G, Bulitta M, Strosser W. Trospium chloride in patients with detrusor overactivity: meta-analysis of placebo-controlled, randomized, double-blind, multi-center clinical trials on the efficacy and safety of trospium chloride twice daily. Int J Clin Pharmacol Ther 2002; 40: 295–303.

64. Zinner N. Long-term efficacy with continued trospium chloride use. Presented at the American Urogynecological Society Annual Scientific Meeting, 29–31 July, 2004, San Diego, USA.

65. Diefenbach K, Arnold G, Wollny A et al. Effects on sleep of anticholinergics used for overactive bladder treatment in healthy volunteers aged ≥ 50 years. BJU Int 2005; 95: 346–9.

66. Hoefner K, Oelke M, Machtens S, Grunewald V. Trospium chloride – an effective drug in the treatment of overactive bladder and detrusor hyperreflexia. World J Urol 2001; 19: 336–43.

67. Raz S, Erikson DR. SEAPI QMM incontinence classification system. Neurourol Urodyn 1992; 11: 187–99.

68. Wiedemann A, Monser C, Braun W, Zumbe J. [Socio-economic aspects of urinary incontinence – saving potential through anticholinergics]. Urologe B 1998; 38: 154–9.

69. Staskin D, Sand P, Zinner N, Dmochowski RO. Once-daily trospium chloride is effective and well tolerated for the treatment of overactive bladder: results from a multicenter Phase III trial. J Urol (in press Sep 2007).

17

Darifenacin

Christopher R Chapple

Introduction • Pharmacological profile • Clinical efficacy of darifenacin • Tolerability and safety of darifenacin • Quality of life improvement with darifenacin • Summary • Acknowledgments

INTRODUCTION

The majority of symptoms of overactive bladder syndrome (OAB) are thought to result from over-activity of the detrusor muscle, which is known to be mediated by acetylcholine-mediated stimulation of muscarinic M_3 receptors in the bladder.[1] Most of the currently available antimuscarinic agents are not selective for the M_3 receptor subtype, resulting in unwanted adverse events. In the cardiovascular system, for example, the M_2 receptor subtype can mediate parasympathetically driven bradycardia and a decrease in cardiac output; in the brain the role of cortical M_1 receptors in cognition is well documented (M_1 receptor blockade would therefore be expected to impair central nervous system (CNS) function); in the salivary glands both M_1 and M_3 receptors control secretion; in the eye, M_3 and M_5 receptors mediate ciliary muscle contraction. Hence, theoretically, a drug with selectivity for the M_3 receptor subtype should demonstrate strong efficacy in OAB with few adverse events related to blockade of other muscarinic receptor subtypes, in particular fewer cognitive adverse events, reduced or no effect on heart rate, less severe dry mouth, and fewer visual disturbances.[2,3]

Darifenacin is a muscarinic M_3 selective receptor antagonist used for the treatment of OAB. Darifenacin prolonged release (Enablex®/Emselex®) 7.5 and 15 mg once daily (od) is approved for OAB treatment in the USA, EU, and various rest-of-world markets.

PHARMACOLOGICAL PROFILE

Chemistry and pharmacodynamics

Darifenacin is a positively charged tertiary amine with one stereochemical center (Figure 17.1). It has a molecular weight of 507.5 Da, is supplied as a hydrobromide salt, and has solubility across the physiological pH range that exceeds 0.6 ng/ml.[4] The formulations used commercially are once-daily prolonged release tablets containing 7.5 or 15 mg of active drug.

In vitro studies with ^{3}H-darifenacin have shown that it binds to the M_3 receptor subtype in a competitive and reversible manner with a binding affinity greater than that of the other muscarinic receptor subtypes.[5–8] In a study in Chinese hamster ovary (CHO)-K1 cells expressing M_1–M_5 receptors, darifenacin showed 9–59-fold greater affinity for the M_3 receptor subtype relative to the other muscarinic receptor subtypes (Figure 17.2).[6] The question is therefore posed as to what degree of relative muscarinic receptor subtype selectivity is necessary to result in a reduction in antimuscarinic side-effects. Whilst the selectivity of darifenacin over M_2 receptors is 59-fold, the selectivity over M_1 receptors is nine-fold.

In vitro data have suggested that the M_3 receptor selectivity of darifenacin may be translated into functional selectivity in human tissue.[9–11] For example, darifenacin has displayed potent activity (greater than that seen with tolterodine and oxybutynin) in contractile studies involving

(S)-2-{1-[2-(2,3-dihydrobenzofuran-5-yl)ethyl]-3-pyrrolidinyl}-2,
2-diphenylacetamide hydrobromide

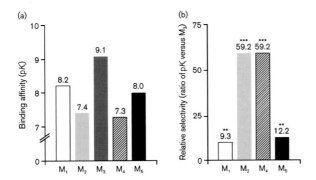

$C_{28} H_{30} N_2 O_2.HBr$

This arm confers
the M_3 selectivity

Figure 17.1 Chemical structure of darifenacin.

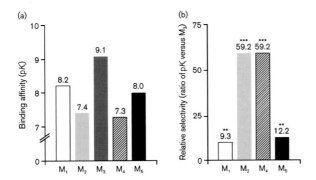

Figure 17.2 (a) In vitro muscarinic receptor binding affinities (pK_i) of darifenacin at human recombinant receptor subtypes M_1–M_5 in Chinese hamster ovary (CHO)-K1 cells and (b) relative selectivity (ratio of K_i values) for each subtype compared to that of M_3 receptors. ***$p < 0.001$ vs. M_3.

human isolated urinary bladder, and has demonstrated a pA_2 (antagonistic activity) value of 9.34 in human isolated detrusor smooth muscle.[10,11] Such data do, however, need to be confirmed by appropriate clinical studies.

Since both the M_1 and M_3 receptor subtypes are thought to play a role in the control of mucous (lubricant) secretions of the salivary glands,[3,12,13] a sparing effect on the M_1 subtype could limit the effect of treatment on salivary flow. Indeed, darifenacin has been shown to cause a smaller reduction in salivary flow and was associated with a lower incidence of dry mouth compared

with oxybutynin immediate release (IR) (a muscarinic antagonist non-selective for M_3 over M_1 receptors) in two separate comparative studies.[14,15] Since the M_1 receptors are also thought to be involved in memory and cognitive function,[16,17] this M_1 sparing effect could limit effects on memory and cognitive function, compared with a less sensitive agent.[3] Evidence suggesting that this is true with darifenacin is discussed below (see "Cognitive safety").

M_2 receptors are the predominant subtype found in the heart, and antagonism of these receptors can lead to tachycardia. This does not appear to be of concern with darifenacin, as may be expected from an M_2 receptor-sparing profile. Please refer to the "Cardiac safety" section for further information on the cardiovascular effects of darifenacin.

Functional selectivity will also be influenced by local concentrations of the active drug. An autoradiographic study in rats by Devineni et al.[18] reported low levels of ^{14}C-darifenacin in the brain following a single intravenous injection (Figure 17.3), suggesting minimal CNS penetration. In addition, a study reported by the same group showed that darifenacin is a substrate for the P-glycoprotein-mediated efflux transporter (a property not reported for other currently available antimuscarinic agents);[19] thus, any darifenacin crossing the blood–brain barrier and entering the CNS can be actively transported back out, thereby reducing the potential for CNS adverse events. These findings, combined with darifenacin's lipophilicity, molecular size, and positive molecular charge, indicate that CNS concentrations are likely to be low, reducing the potential for CNS adverse effects.

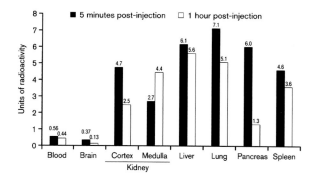

Figure 17.3 Concentrations of ^{14}C-darifenacin in selected organs of the rat measured using autoradiography following a single intravenous injection of 4 mg/kg.

Pharmacokinetics

Darifenacin is rapidly and completely absorbed from the gastrointestinal tract following oral administration with the prolonged release formulation, achieving maximum plasma concentrations after approximately 7 hours.[4,20,21] Food has no effect on absorption.[4] Steady-state plasma levels are achieved within 6 days of once-daily administration of darifenacin; it is highly bound to plasma proteins (98% in humans) and is extensively distributed into tissues, with a volume of distribution of 163 l.[4,20] An overview of the pharmacokinetics of darifenacin is presented in Table 17.1.

Darifenacin undergoes extensive first pass metabolism, with 15% and 19% bioavailability following oral administration of the 7.5- and 15-mg doses, respectively.[21] Darifenacin is primarily metabolized by the cytochrome P450 enzymes CYP3A4 and CYP2D6. The drug has three main routes of metabolism (Figure 17.4): monohydroxylation

Table 17.1 Summary of key pharmacokinetic parameters of darifenacin[4]	
Parameter	Value
Time to maximum concentration (T_{max})	~7 hours
Half-life ($t_{1/2}$)	11.9 hours
Oral bioavailability	
7.5 mg	15%
15 mg	19%
Affected by food	No
Plasma-protein bound	98%
Volume of distribution	163 l
Drug–drug interactions	*Recommendation*
Potent CYP3A4 inhibitors (e.g. ketoconazole, itraconazole, ritonavir, nelfinavir, clarithromycin, nefazodone)	Combination contraindicated or daily dose should not exceed 7.5 mg[4,22]
Moderate CYP3A4 inhibitors (e.g. erythromycin, diltiazem, fluconazole, verapamil)	No dosing adjustment recommended[4]
Potent CYP2D6 inhibitors (e.g. parotexine, terbinafine, cimetidine, quinidine)	No dosing adjustment recommended[4]
Special populations	*Recommendation*
Older patients	No dosing adjustment recommended[4]
Patients with renal impairment	No dosing adjustment recommended[4]
Patients with mild hepatic impairment	No dosing adjustment recommended[4,23]
Patients with moderate hepatic impairment	Dose should not exceed 7.5 mg od[4]
Patients with severe hepatic impairment	Not recommended[4,23]

od, once daily

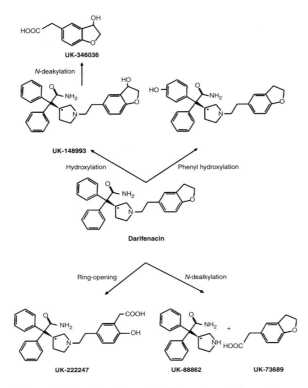

Figure 17.4 Structure of darifenacin and its major metabolites, together with its metabolic pathways in humans.

in either the dihydrobenzfuran or the diphenyl-acetamide moiety; opening of the dihydrobenz-furan ring; or *N*-dealkylation at the pyrrolidine nitrogen.[20] Metabolism via multiple routes compared with metabolism via a single route has the potential advantage that if concomitant comedi-cations affect one route, metabolism can still occur via the ongoing activity of other pathways. The main metabolite, UK-148993, is 50-fold less potent than darifenacin and hence does not con-tribute significantly to the overall clinical effect of the drug.[21]

Excretion of darifenacin is rapid (within 48 hours following a single dose) and balanced between urine (~60%) and feces (~40%) in humans; only a small amount (3%) is excreted unchanged.[4,20]

Coadministration of certain metabolic enzyme inhibitors or inducers of these enzymes may affect darifenacin exposure. It is recommended that darifenacin should be used with caution when coadministered with potent CYP3A4 inhi-bitors (e.g. ketoconazole, itraconazole, ritonavir,

nelfinavir, clarithromycin, and nefazodone).[4,21] Darifenacin has been shown to have no clini-cally relevant effects on the pharmacokinetics of the CYP3A4 substrate midazolam or a commonly used combination oral contraceptive (0.15 mg levonorgestrel, 0.03 mg ethinylestradiol).[4,23]

The potential for drug–drug interactions mediated by other routes is low: darifenacin coadministration may lead to a small increase in exposure to digoxin (possibly by competition for the P-glycoprotein transporter) but dose adjust-ment is not necessary; darifenacin did not alter the effects of warfarin on prothrombin time.[4]

Pharmacokinetics in special populations

Studies have demonstrated that there is no need for darifenacin dose adjustment according to age or gender.[4] Similarly, the low renal clearance of darifenacin means that renal impairment does not affect the pharmacokinetics of the drug.[23] Dose adjustment is not necessary for those patients with mild hepatic impairment, but for patients with moderately impaired hepatic func-tion the dose of darifenacin should not exceed 7.5 mg od.[23] Furthermore, no studies have been conducted in patients with severe hepatic impair-ment, and as such darifenacin is not recom-mended for these patients (Table 17.1).[4,23]

CLINICAL EFFICACY OF DARIFENACIN

On the basis of clinical findings from preliminary studies, the clinical efficacy of darifenacin has been evaluated in a number of well-conducted and extensive clinical studies in adults with OAB (Table 17.2: studies I–XI).

Urodynamic efficacy studies

In a study involving patients with OAB and detrusor overactivity, no differences were obser-ved between patients taking darifenacin 15 mg od or oxybutynin 2.5 mg tid on ambulatory uro-dynamics following 7 days' treatment (study I).[14] In an additional study involving patients with urodynamically verified OAB, 2 weeks' treat-ment with the same doses of either drug showed similar significant reductions in the number of incontinence episodes per week compared with placebo ($p < 0.05$) (study II).[15]

Table 17.2 Key clinical studies with darifenacin

Study	Design	Patients	Dose and duration	Publication
I	Phase II Multicenter Double-blind Randomized Two-way crossover	$n = 65$ randomized Male/female: 44/21 Age: 20–75 years	Darifenacin IR 2.5 mg tid/oxybutynin 2.5 mg tid ($n = 16$) Darifenacin PR 15 mg od/oxybutynin 5 mg tid ($n = 24$) Darifenacin PR 30 mg od/oxybutynin 5 mg tid ($n = 25$) 7 days for each treatment	Chapple and Abrams, 2005[14]
II	Phase II Multicenter Double-blind Randomized Placebo-controlled Four-way crossover	$n = 76$ randomized Male/female: 5/71 Age: 33–84 years	Darifenacin PR 15 mg od Oxybutynin 5 mg tid Placebo ($n = 58$) 2 weeks' treatment, according to a randomized sequence	Zinner et al., 2005[15]
III	Phase IIIb Multicenter Double-blind Randomized Placebo-controlled Parallel-group	$n = 561$ randomized Male/female: 85/476 Age: 19–88 years Recruited from studies A1371041 and A1371047	Darifenacin PR 3.75 mg od ($n = 53$) Darifenacin PR 7.5 mg od ($n = 229$) Darifenacin PR 15 mg od ($n = 115$) Placebo ($n = 164$) 12 weeks	Haab et al., 2004[24]
IV	Phase III Multicenter Double-blind Randomized Placebo-controlled Parallel-group	$n = 439$ randomized Male/female: 64/375 Age: 21–88 years	Darifenacin PR 7.5 mg od ($n = 108$) Darifenacin PR 15 mg od ($n = 107$) Darifenacin PR 30 mg od ($n = 115$) Placebo ($n = 109$) 12 weeks	Hill et al., 2006[25]
V	Phase III Multicenter Double-blind Randomized Placebo-controlled Parallel-group	$n = 680$ randomized Male/female: 112/568 Age: 21–93 years	Darifenacin PR 15 mg od ($n = 112$) Darifenacin PR 30 mg od ($n = 230$) Tolterodine IR 2 mg bid ($n = 223$) Placebo ($n = 115$) 12 weeks	Romanzi et al., 2005[26]
VI	Phase IIIb Multicenter Double-blind Randomized	$n = 395$ randomized Male/female: 62/333	Darifenacin PR 7.5 mg od with option to titrate up to 15 mg od after week 2 ($n = 268$)	Steers et al., 2005[27]

Table 17.2 *Continued*				
Study	Design	Patients	Dose and duration	Publication
	Placebo-controlled Parallel-group Flexible dose	Age: 22–89 years	Placebo ($n = 127$)	
VII	Phase IIIb Multicenter Open-label Long term	$n = 716$ randomized Male/female: 107/609 Age: 19–89 years	Patients completing studies III or VI received darifenacin PR 7.5/15 mg od (individualized) ($n = 716$) 24 months	Haab et al., 2006[28]
VIII	Phase II Randomized Double-blind Double-dummy Placebo-controlled Four-way crossover	$n = 27$ randomized Male/female: 27/0 Age:19–44 years	Darifenacin PR 7.5 mg od ($n = 27$) Darifenacin PR 15 mg od ($n = 25$) Dicyclomine 20 mg od ($n = 24$) Placebo ($n = 24$) 7 days	Kay and Wesnes, 2005[29]
IX	Phase II Randomized Double-blind Placebo-controlled Three-period crossover	$n = 129$ randomized Male/female: 54/75 Age: 65–84 years	Darifenacin PR 3.75 mg od ($n = 72$) Darifenacin PR 7.5 mg od ($n = 74$) Darifenacin PR 15 mg od ($n = 65$) Darifenacin IR 5 mg od ($n = 71$) Placebo ($n = 69$) 14 days' treatment each for 3 out of 5 treatments	Lipton et al., 2005[30]
X	Phase IV Multicenter Randomized Double-blind Double-dummy Placebo-controlled Parallel-group	$n = 150$ randomized Male/female: 57/93 Age: 60–83 years	Darifenacin PR 7.5/15 mg od ($n = 49$) Oxybutynin ER 10/15/20 mg od ($n = 50$) Placebo ($n = 51$) 3 weeks	Kay et al., 2006[31]
XI	Phase IV Randomized Double-blind Parallel-group Placebo and active-controlled Multiple-dose	$n = 188$ Male/female: 83/105 Age: 46–65 years	Darifenacin 15 mg od ($n = 47$) Darifenacin 75 mg od ($n = 46$) Moxifloxacin 400 mg od ($n = 48$) Placebo ($n = 47$) 7 days	Serra et al., 2005[32]

IR, immediate release; PR, prolonged release; tid, three times daily; od, once daily; bid, twice daily

Fixed-dose studies

A pooled analysis has been conducted on data from three pivotal darifenacin studies (studies III–V), which included a total of 1059 patients with OAB.[33] All three studies had a similar study design, where patients were randomized to receive either darifenacin 7.5 mg or matching placebo (n = 337 and 273, respectively), or darifenacin 15 mg or matching placebo (n = 334 and 388, respectively). After 12 weeks of treatment, darifenacin 7.5 and 15 mg significantly reduced (both $p < 0.01$) the median number of incontinence episodes per week (the primary efficacy endpoint) compared with placebo (Table 17.3).[33] Improvements in OAB symptoms were observed within 2 weeks' treatment, as exemplified in the individual studies (studies III and IV) (Figure 17.5).[4,24,25] There was a significant dose–response trend in studies in which the darifenacin 7.5- and 15-mg doses were evaluated ($p < 0.001$ and $p = 0.002$ using one-sided analysis based on Jonckheere's test, and $p < 0.001$ for both studies at every visit using the Poisson generalized linear mixed-effects model).[26] Secondary efficacy endpoints were also significantly improved with both darifenacin doses compared with placebo, including the number/severity of urgency episodes, micturition frequency, increased bladder capacity and the number of incontinence episodes requiring a change of clothes/pads (Table 17.3).

One of the three double-blind 12-week studies included in the pooled analysis included a tolterodine treatment arm, compared with darifenacin 15 mg and placebo (study V). Using a Poisson generalized linear mixed effects model, darifenacin was shown to significantly reduce incontinence episodes per week compared to placebo ($p < 0.05$) at all timepoints, with increasing effect over time, whereas tolterodine only caused significant reductions compared to placebo ($p < 0.05$) at early timepoints (Table 17.4).[26]

Evaluation of the pooled clinical data in the format of responder rates, i.e. the proportion of patients achieving a predefined reduction in incontinence episodes per week, produced equally positive findings. The proportion of patients achieving a $\geq 70\%$ reduction from baseline in incontinence episodes per week at week 12 was 48% and 57% for darifenacin 7.5 and 15 mg, respectively, compared with matching placebo values of 33% and 39% ($p < 0.001$).[33] A more stringent responder rate cut-off point of $\geq 90\%$ yielded 27% and 28% responders to darifenacin 7.5 and 15 mg but only 17% in each of the placebo groups ($p < 0.005$).[33]

Flexible-dosing studies

Allowing patients to tailor the dose of darifenacin to their particular requirements may confer considerable benefit, as highlighted in a flexible-dose study (study VI).[27] In this double-blind, placebo-controlled study, 395 patients were randomized to receive darifenacin 7.5 mg od ($n = 268$) or matching placebo ($n = 127$) for 2 weeks, and were then permitted to up-titrate to 15 mg (or matching placebo) if additional efficacy was required and the 7.5-mg dose was well tolerated; the standard OAB efficacy and safety parameters were recorded for the 12-week duration of the study. Significantly more patients responded to darifenacin than to placebo in terms of reduction in incontinence episodes per week and normalization of micturition at week 2, with further benefit being observed at week 12 (Figure 17.6). Dose titration allowed those patients with a good response on darifenacin 7.5 mg at week 2 to maintain and increase their response at week 12 to the same degree as has been reported in the pooled analysis of the fixed dose studies,[33] while patients with a less than optimal response at week 2 achieved a much improved reduction in incontinence episodes per week at week 12 following escalation to the 15-mg dose (Figure 17.6).[27]

The benefits of dose individualization can also be seen in a long-term non-comparative, 24-month, open-label extension study (study VII)[28] which enrolled patients from two 12-week placebo-controlled (feeder) studies. Patients entering the extension study received darifenacin 7.5 mg od for 2 weeks (irrespective of treatment in the feeder studies), after which voluntary up-titration to darifenacin 15 mg was permitted, as was subsequent down-titration to 7.5 mg if necessary. Persistence with darifenacin was high, and two-thirds of patients (475/716) who entered the extension phase completed the 24-month period (equivalent to a persistence rate of 66.3% and 1089.9

Table 17.3 Effect of once-daily treatment with darifenacin either 7.5 or 15 mg once daily (od) or matching placebo for 12 weeks on efficacy variables in patients with overactive bladder (OAB) and older (≥ 65 years) patients with OAB[33,34]

Variable/treatment group	No. of evaluable patients	Median change from baseline (%)	Median difference from placebo (95% CI)	p Value*
Incontinence episodes/week				
Overall group				
darifenacin 7.5 mg	335	−8.8 (−68.4)	−2.0 (−3.6, −0.7)	0.004
placebo	271	−7.0 (−53.8)		
darifenacin 15 mg	330	−10.6 (−76.8)	−3.2 (−4.5, −2.0)	< 0.001
placebo	384	−7.5 (−58.3)		
≥ 65 years				
darifenacin 7.5 mg	97	−11.2 (−66.7)	−5.9 (−9.1, −2.2)	< 0.001
placebo	72	−4.8 (−34.8)		
darifenacin 15 mg	109	−10.8 (−75.9)	−4.1 (−6.4, −1.6)	< 0.001
placebo	108	−6.8 (−44.8)		
No. of micturitions/day				
Overall group				
darifenacin 7.5 mg	335	−1.6 (−16.6)	−0.8 (−1.1, −0.4)	< 0.001
placebo	271	−0.9 (−9.1)		
darifenacin 15 mg	330	−1.9 (−17.4)	−0.8 (−1.1, −0.4)	< 0.001
placebo	385	−1.0 (−9.9)		
≥ 65 years				
darifenacin 7.5 mg	97	−1.8 (−18.0)	−1.3 (−2.0, −0.8)	< 0.001
placebo	72	−0.6 (−7.0)		
darifenacin 15 mg	109	−1.8 (−17.0)	−1.1 (−1.6, −0.5)	< 0.001
placebo	109	−1.0 (−9.0)		
No. of urgency episodes/day				
Overall group				
darifenacin 7.5 mg	335	−2.0 (−29.0)	−0.8 (−1.3, −0.4)	< 0.001
placebo	271	−1.0 (−14.3)		
darifenacin 15 mg	330	−2.3 (−29.0)	−0.9 (−1.3, −0.5)	< 0.001
placebo	384	−1.2 (−16.7)		
≥ 65 years				
darifenacin 7.5 mg	97	−2.1 (−26.0)	−1.7 (−2.6, −0.9)	< 0.001
placebo	72	−0.6 (−7.0)		
darifenacin 15 mg	109	−2.4 (−26)	−1.5 (−2.3, −0.8)	< 0.001
placebo	108	−0.8 (−10)		
Mean severity of urgency episodes/day[†]				
Overall group				
darifenacin 7.5 mg	335	−7.8 (−14.2)	−4.0 (−6.6, −1.6)	0.001
placebo	270	−4.2 (−7.8)		
darifenacin 15 mg	329	−9.3 (−16.1)	−4.9 (−7.1, −2.7)	< 0.001
placebo	383	−4.5 (−8.0)		

Table 17.3 *Continued*

Variable/treatment group	No. of evaluable patients	Median change from baseline (%)	Median difference from placebo (95% CI)	p value*
Bladder capacity (average volume voided/micturition, ml)				
Overall group				
darifenacin 7.5 mg	322	15.0 (9.6)	10 (3, 17)	0.007
placebo	255	8.0 (4.9)		
darifenacin 15 mg	320	27.0 (17.5)	20 (14, 27)[††]	< 0.001
placebo	366	6.0 (3.9)		
≥ 65 years				
darifenacin 7.5 mg	93	14.0 (10.0)	15 (2, 26)	0.018
placebo	68	2.0 (1.0)		
darifenacin 15 mg	107	27.0 (18.0)	26 (15, 36)	< 0.001
placebo	104	2.0 (1.0)		
Mean no. of incontinence episodes/week resulting in change of clothing/pads[†]				
Overall group				
darifenacin 7.5 mg	333	−4.0 (−77.1)	−1.8 (−2.8, −0.9)	< 0.001
placebo	270	−2.0 (−47.7)		
darifenacin 15 mg	324	−4.8 (−78.6)	−2.0 (−3.0, −1.1)	< 0.001
placebo	378	−2.7 (−55.1)		
Mean no. of nocturnal awakenings/week for overactive bladder[†]				
Overall group				
darifenacin 7.5 mg	334	−1.7 (−14.9)	−0.7 (−1.4, 0.2)	0.13
placebo	269	−0.8 (−9.5)		
darifenacin 15 mg	329	−1.9 (−20.5)	−0.7 (−1.4, 0.0)	0.06
placebo	382	−1.1 (−13.4)		

*P value calculated using Wilcoxon test, stratified by study; [†]no data for older population reported; [††]significantly different between doses ($P = 0.0093$)

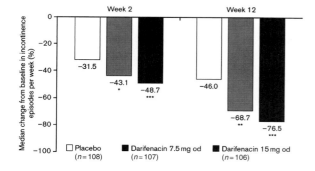

Figure 17.5 Median change from baseline in incontinence episodes per week in patients with overactive bladder (OAB) after 2 and 12 weeks' treatment with darifenacin 7.5 and 15 mg or placebo. *$p < 0.05$; **$p < 0.01$; ***$p < 0.001$ vs. placebo (stratified Wilcoxon test); od, once daily.

patient-years of exposure). Efficacy of darifenacin was maintained over the 24-month period, including significant improvements in the median number of incontinence episodes per week (median reduction 84.4% at 24 months; $p < 0.001$ vs. feeder-study baseline) (Figure 17.7), and after 24 months more than 40% of patients achieved a ≥ 90% reduction in incontinence episodes per week (study VII).[28]

Efficacy in subpopulations

The efficacy of darifenacin has also been demonstrated across various subpopulations. In a female population analysis of the pooled 12-week double-blind, placebo-controlled studies, the number of incontinence episodes was reduced by 69.3%

			Reduction in incontinence episodes, treatment 1 vs.
Week	Treatment 1	Treatment 2	treatment 2 (%)
2	Darifenacin	Placebo	27.3*
	Tolterodine	Placebo	16.9*
	Darifenacin	Tolterodine	12.5
6	Darifenacin	Placebo	30.5*
	Tolterodine	Placebo	18.9*
	Darifenacin	Tolterodine	14.2
12	Darifenacin	Placebo	32.7*
	Tolterodine	Placebo	17.1
	Darifenacin	Tolterodine	18.8*

Table 17.4 Reduction in incontinence episodes per week in patients with overactive bladder (OAB) receiving either darifenacin 15 mg once daily (od), tolterodine 2 mg twice daily (bid), or placebo[26]

*$p < 0.05$

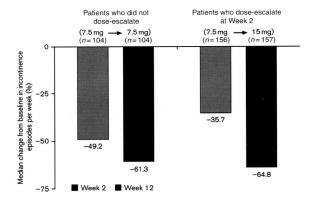

Figure 17.6 Median percentage change from baseline in the number of incontinence episodes per week during treatment with darifenacin at weeks 2 and 12, according to dose-escalation status. (From reference 27, with permission)

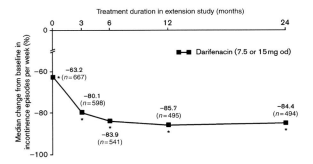

Figure 17.7 Median change from baseline in incontinence episodes per week in patients with overactive bladder (OAB) after 24 months' open-label treatment with darifenacin 7.5/15 mg. *$p < 0.001$ vs. feeder-study baseline.

with darifenacin 7.5 mg od ($p < 0.001$ vs. placebo) and by 75.3% ($p < 0.001$ vs. placebo) with darifenacin 15 mg od in 900 female patients with OAB (≥ 18 years).[35]

Another subpopulation analysis was performed on 107 men (aged 22–86 years) with OAB who took part in the 2-year extension study described above. The results showed that darifenacin significantly improved OAB symptoms after 24 months of treatment, which included a significant median reduction in the number of incontinence

episodes per week (–90.9%; $p < 0.001$ vs. feeder-study baseline).[36]

Focusing on older patients with OAB, an analysis was performed on patients ≥ 65 years included within the pooled analysis of three phase III double-blind trials. Following 12 weeks of treatment with darifenacin 7.5 or 15 mg od, there was a significant improvement in all OAB symptoms in these patients. Specifically, the median reduction in incontinence episodes per week in older patients was 66.7% with darifenacin 7.5 mg od ($p < 0.001$ vs. placebo) and 75.9% with darifenacin 15 mg od ($p < 0.001$ vs.

placebo).[34] This result was comparable to that achieved in the overall OAB patient population (study VII).[28] Furthermore, in the 2-year extension study described above, an analysis was carried out to determine the efficacy of darifenacin 7.5 or 15 mg od in patients aged ≥ 65 years. The 214 patients included in this analysis received darifenacin 7.5 mg od for 2 weeks, which was followed by dose individualization (either 7.5 or 15 mg od). Improvements in OAB symptoms were seen with both doses of darifenacin, with reductions in the number of incontinence episodes/week of 59.1% at the end of the feeder studies and of 83.7% at the end of the extension study, compared with feeder-study baseline ($p < 0.001$).[37] As before, these results were comparable with the overall patient population data (study VII).[28]

TOLERABILITY AND SAFETY OF DARIFENACIN

Tolerability

The commercially available doses of 7.5 and 15 mg have been well tolerated in all studies where safety and tolerability were examined. Adverse events (AEs) have generally appeared to be dose-related and mild to moderate in severity. In the pooled analysis of 1049 patients in three phase III studies, the most common AEs were dry mouth (7.5 mg, 20%; 15 mg, 35%; placebo, 8%) and constipation (7.5 mg, 15%; 15 mg, 21%; placebo, 6%), which resulted in low rates of discontinuation overall (7.5 mg, 0.6%; 15 mg, 2.1%; placebo, 0.3%). In addition, only 22%, 30%, and 25% of patients receiving treatment with 7.5 mg or 15 mg darifenacin or placebo, respectively, needed to use laxatives, which included stool-softeners, bulk-forming agents (fiber supplements), and osmotic and stimulant laxatives in this pooled analysis.[33]

As discussed previously, a flexible-dosing regimen allows patients to choose the most appropriate dose of darifenacin, and treatment is tailored to each patient based on their sensitivity to drug treatment. Thus, more 'sensitive' patients can be treated with the lowest dose that gives the desired effect, which would reduce the risk of unwanted effects. Thus, in a study using this type of dosing regimen, the all-causality incidence of dry mouth at week 2 was highest in the group of patients who were most sensitive to darifenacin, choosing to remain on a dose of darifenacin 7.5 mg od (17.6%), while it was lower in both the up-titration and the placebo groups (7.5% and 7.1%, respectively). However, by week 12, when both sensitive and less sensitive patients had received their optimal doses, the incidence of dry mouth was similar in the two darifenacin groups (20.4% vs. 17.5%, respectively) (study VI).[27]

After completion of this study, some of these patients were entered into an open-label, non-comparative, 2-year extension study with the same flexible-dosing protocol. Darifenacin 7.5 and 15 mg od was well tolerated, and the most commonly reported AEs were again dry mouth and constipation (all-causality rates: 23.3% and 20.9%, respectively), leading to discontinuation in 1.3% and 2.4% of patients, respectively (study VII).[28] These results were similar to those at week 12 of the double-blind phase.[24,27] Constipation infrequently required intervention, and the use of fiber supplements, stool softeners, or laxatives was initiated by only 5.6% of patients during the extension (comprising 32 patients who reported constipation as an AE and eight who did not) (study VII).[28] An analysis of bowel habits completed at the start and end of the open-label extension study revealed that there was little difference between feeder-study end and extension study in bowel habits in the overall population. However, in the group of patients who reported constipation as an AE, minor changes in bowel habits were seen. This suggests that constipation reporting was related to minor changes in bowel habits rather than true constipation (study VII).[28]

In studies comparing darifenacin with other antimuscarinic agents, darifenacin was found to be at least as well tolerated as the comparator agent. In a crossover study in adults with OAB, oxybutynin IR 5 mg tid was associated with a significantly higher rate of dry mouth compared with darifenacin 15 mg od (36% vs. 13%; $p < 0.05$) or placebo (5%; $p < 0.05$).[15] Indeed, four patients receiving oxybutynin IR discontinued as a result. The incidence of constipation was similar for both darifenacin (10%) and oxybutynin IR (8%), but blurred vision (3%) and dizziness (2%) were reported only with oxybutynin IR (study II).[15]

In a separate crossover study of darifenacin 15 mg od and oxybutynin IR 5 mg tid, a significantly (p = 0.0002) greater salivary flow rate was seen with darifenacin than with oxybutynin – this was paralleled by a higher incidence of dry mouth in the oxybutynin group compared with the darifenacin group (study I).[14]

Darifenacin 7.5 and 15 mg od has also been compared with tolterodine 2 mg twice daily (bid) in a pooled analysis of three phase III fixed-dose studies, and the tolerability profiles of the two drugs were comparable. In this analysis dry mouth was the most common AE in all groups (7.5 mg, 20%; 15 mg, 35%; tolterodine, 27%; placebo, 8%) followed by constipation (7.5 mg, 15%; 15 mg, 21%; tolterodine, 10%; placebo, 5%).[38] The overall use of constipation remedies (laxatives, stool softeners or fiber supplements) was similar in the darifenacin 7.5 mg od and placebo groups (5.9% and 6.2%, respectively) and darifenacin 15 mg od and tolterodine 2 mg bid groups (9.6% and 10.3%, respectively).[38] Discontinuation associated with constipation in this pooled analysis was also comparable for darifenacin 7.5 mg od (0.6%) and placebo (0.3%) and for darifenacin 15 mg od (1.2%) and tolterodine 2 mg bid (1.8%).[38]

Cognitive safety

Some antimuscarinic therapies have the potential to affect cognitive function due to the non-selective inhibition of M_1 muscarinic receptors,[3] which is particularly problematic in OAB because of the large proportion of older patients who are predisposed towards age-related cognitive decline.[39] In the randomized, placebo-controlled clinical trials, CNS adverse events with darifenacin were comparable to those with placebo.[23] This result was similar to that seen in a 2-year extension study where long-term darifenacin treatment resulted in a low incidence of CNS adverse events, which was again comparable to placebo (study VII).[28]

In a study of healthy male subjects completing a battery of cognitive function tests, darifenacin (7.5 and 15 mg od) for 6 days had similar effects to placebo, whereas the M_1 agonist agent dicyclomine (20 mg four times daily), used as a positive control, significantly impaired performance in five out of 12 assessments (study VIII) (Figure 17.8a).[29]

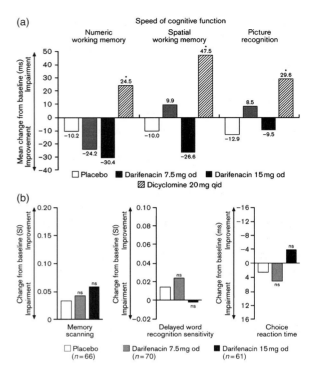

Figure 17.8 Effect of darifenacin on cognitive functioning in: (a) healthy volunteers; and (b) healthy volunteers $\geq$ 65 years of age. *$p < 0.05$ vs. placebo; od, once daily; qid, four times daily; SI, Système International standard units; ns, not significant.

Similarly, in 129 older ($\geq$ 65 years) subjects with no or mild cognitive impairment there were no significant differences between either dose of darifenacin (7.5 and 15 mg od) and placebo in the primary (memory scanning sensitivity, speed of choice time, and word recognition sensitivity) and secondary endpoints (study IX) (Figure 17.8b).[30] In addition, in this study darifenacin did not cause clinically relevant changes in alertness, contentment, or calmness, and was well tolerated.

The effects of darifenacin and oxybutynin extended release (ER) on cognitive function (particularly memory) were compared in 150 subjects $\geq$ 60 years of age in a multicenter, double-blind, double-dummy, parallel-group, 3-week study (study X).[31] Doses of oxybutynin ER were 10 mg od during week 1, increasing to 15 mg then 20 mg od by week 3; darifenacin was administered at 7.5 mg od in weeks 1 and 2, and then 15 mg od in week 3. There was no significant difference between darifenacin and placebo in terms of the primary endpoint – delayed recall on Name–Face Association Test – at week 3 (mean difference –0.06, $p = 0.908$). In contrast, oxybutynin ER resulted in memory impairment, with significantly lower scores than with placebo and darifenacin (mean differences –1.30, $p = 0.011$; and –1.24, $p = 0.022$, respectively) for delayed recall on the Name–Face Association Test at week 3 (study X) (Figure 17.9).[31] Additional tests of delayed recall indicated significant memory impairment with oxybutynin ER versus placebo at certain timepoints, while darifenacin was similar to placebo throughout. Interestingly, no between-treatment differences were detected in self-rated memory, demonstrating that subjects were unaware of any memory deterioration.

Cardiac safety

The phase III clinical trial program did not report any cardiovascular AEs with darifenacin that were more frequent than with placebo.[33] In the elderly subpopulation from the pooled phase III fixed-dose studies, the incidence of cardiovascular AEs during darifenacin therapy was similar to that with placebo, and did not increase with increasing dose.[34] Furthermore, the incidence of any cardiovascular AEs during long-term

darifenacin therapy for OAB was no different from that reported during the 12-week phase III studies (study VII).[28]

Kay and Wesnes (study VIII)[29] found that in a double-blind, four-way crossover study involving 27 healthy male volunteers, darifenacin (7.5 mg and 15 mg od) had similar effects to placebo on heart rate for 6 days (4 hours post-dose: 7.5 mg, 59.7 beats per minute (bpm); 15 mg, 58.6 bpm; placebo, 60.6 bpm) and heart rate variability (4 hours post-dose: 7.5 mg, 35.3%; 15 mg, 32.4%; placebo, 32.8%). In contrast, at 4 hours after the dose, dicyclomine (20 mg four times daily) significantly decreased heart rate (55.8 bpm; $p < 0.01$) and increased heart rate variability (44.7%; $p < 0.01$).

The potential for darifenacin to cause QT/QTc prolongation, a predictor of ventricular tachyarrhythmia (torsades de pointes), which can be fatal, has been evaluated in a 7-day study in 188 healthy volunteers randomized to receive either the maximum dose (15 mg) or a supramaximal dose (75 mg), using moxifloxacin 400 mg od as the positive control (study XI).[32] Neither dose of darifenacin prolonged the QTc (corrected QT) interval compared with baseline (15 mg, –2.6 ms; 75 mg, –6.3 ms; placebo, –2.6 ms), unlike moxifloxacin, which increased it by 10.3 ms ($p < 0.001$). Darifenacin is therefore not expected to increase the risk of torsades de pointes.

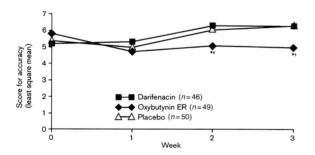

Figure 17.9 Effects of darifenacin, oxybutynin extended release (ER), and placebo on accuracy of delayed recall on the Name–Face Association Test at each timepoint. Scores on Name–Face Association Test can range from 0 to 14, with average values declining from 11.5 (20–29 years old) to 6.1 (70+ years old) across various age groups. The average score for subjects aged 60–69 years is 6.6. *$p < 0.05$ vs. placebo; †$p < 0.05$ vs. darifenacin (analysis of covariance (ANCOVA), adjusted for baseline score, age, and sex). Patient numbers reflect baseline values.

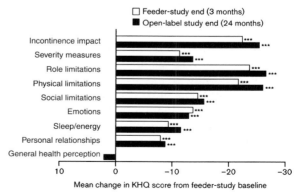

Figure 17.10 Improvements in quality of life (assessed using the King's Health Questionnaire, KHQ) in overactive bladder (OAB) patients receiving darifenacin 7.5/15 mg for 12 weeks or 24 months ***$p < 0.001$ vs. feeder-study baseline.

QUALITY OF LIFE IMPROVEMENT WITH DARIFENACIN

The combination of efficacy and tolerability seen with darifenacin has been paralleled by improvements in patient-reported outcome measures, indicating that the reductions in OAB symptoms are recognized and meaningful to the patients themselves. In the pooled analysis of phase III fixed-dose studies, quality of life was assessed using the King's Health Questionnaire (KHQ) and significant improvements were observed versus placebo.[40] In a 24-month open-label extension study, involving patients from two 12-week feeder studies who received darifenacin either 7.5 or 15 mg od, significant improvements were observed in eight out of nine of the KHQ domains at 3 months, and were maintained or improved further at 24 months (Figure 17.10).[41] These findings help to ensure patient compliance and treatment persistence, both of which help in maintaining long-term efficacy with darifenacin therapy for OAB.

SUMMARY

Extensive evidence from robust clinical trials has demonstrated that darifenacin 7.5 and 15 mg od provides significant clinical benefit across the range of symptoms of OAB in the overall patient population, as well as specifically in the older OAB patient population. Furthermore, darifenacin 7.5 and 15 mg od provides a tolerability profile that is similar to that of other antimuscarinic agents, with events that are typically mild in severity and easily managed; there is no meaningful impact on bowel habits and, again, the AE profile in the older population resembles that of the overall population. The long-term tolerability profile with darifenacin is comparable to that seen in the 12-week clinical studies, and there is a low propensity for CNS or cardiac adverse effects. Overall, darifenacin provides strong efficacy combined with good tolerability, particularly with regards to cognitive and cardiac safety, making the drug an interesting and potentially valuable alternative approach to the treatment of OAB, especially in older patients.

ACKNOWLEDGMENTS

Preparation of the manuscript was supported by Novartis Pharma AG. Editorial and project management services were provided by ACUMED®.

REFERENCES

1. Fetscher C, Fleichman M, Schmidt M, Krege S, Michel MC. M_3 muscarinic receptors mediate contraction of human urinary bladder. Br J Pharmacol 2002; 136: 641–3.
2. Andersson KE. Antimuscarinics for treatment of overactive bladder. Lancet Neurol 2004; 3: 46–53.
3. Andersson KE. Potential benefits of muscarinic M_3 receptor selectivity. Eur Urol Suppl 2002; 1 (Suppl): 23–8.
4. Enablex® prescribing information. East Hanover, NJ: Novartis Pharmaceuticals Corp, 2005.
5. Moriya H, Takagi Y, Nakanishi T et al. Affinity profiles of various muscarinic antagonists for cloned human muscarinic acetylcholine receptor (mAChR) subtypes and mAChRs in rat heart and submandibular gland. Life Sci 1999; 64: 2351–8.
6. Napier C, Gupta P. Darifenacin is selective for the human recombinant M_3 receptor subtype. Neurourol Urodyn 2002; 21: A445 (abstr).
7. Napier C, Laskey P, Gupta P, Clarke NP. Competitive and reversible interaction of darifenacin with human recombinant M_3 receptors. Eur Urol Suppl 2003; 2: A780 (abstr).
8. Smith CM, Wallis RM. Characterisation of [^{3}H]-darifenacin as a novel radioligand for the study of muscarinic M_3 receptors. J Recept Signal Transduct Res 1997; 17: 177–84.
9. Chua CB, Harriss DR, Marsh KA, Hill SJ, Bates CP. Effect of darifenacin on muscarinic responses in normal and unstable human detrusor smooth muscle cells. Neurourol Urodyn 1997; 16: 355–6.
10. Miyamae K, Yoshida M, Murakami S et al. Pharmacological effects of darifenacin on human isolated urinary bladder. Pharmacology 2003; 69: 205–11.
11. Yoshida M. Comparison of pharmacological effects on various antimuscarinic drugs on human isolated urinary bladder. Neurourol Urodyn 2001; 20: 462–3 (abstr 57).
12. Gautam D, Heard TS, Cui Y, et al. Cholinergic stimulation of salivary secretion studied with M_1

and M_3 muscarinic receptor single- and double-knockout mice. Mol Pharmacol 2004; 66: 260–7.

13. Mei L, Roeske WR, Izutsu KT, Yamamura HI. Characterization of muscarinic acetylcholine receptors in human labial salivary glands. Eur J Pharmacol 1990; 176: 367–70.

14. Chapple CR, Abrams P. Comparison of darifenacin and oxybutynin in patients with overactive bladder: assessment of ambulatory urodynamics and impact on salivary flow. Eur Urol 2005; 48: 102–9.

15. Zinner N, Tuttle J, Marks L. Efficacy and tolerability of darifenacin, a muscarinic M_3 selective receptor antagonist (M_3 SRA), compared with oxybutynin in the treatment of patients with overactive bladder. World J Urol 2005; 23: 248–52.

16. Anagnostaras SG, Murphy GG, Hamilton SE et al. Selective cognitive dysfunction in acetylcholine M_1 muscarinic receptor mutant mice. Nat Neurosci 2003; 6: 51–8.

17. Messer WS Jr, Bohnett M, Stibbe J. Evidence for a preferential involvement of M_1 muscarinic receptors in representational memory. Neurosci Lett 1990; 116: 184–9.

18. Devineni D, Skerjanec A, Woodworth TG. Low central nervous system (CNS) penetration by darifenacin, a muscarinic M_3 selective receptor antagonist, in rats. Proc Br Pharmacol Soc Summer 2005 (abstr 092P) http://www.pa2online.org/abstracts/Vol3Issue2abst092P.pdf

19. Skerjanec A, Devineni D. Affinity of darifenacin for the p-glycoprotein efflux pump: a mechanism contributing to the CNS sparing profile? Abstract presented at British Pharmacological Society Winter Meeting, 14–16 December, 2004, Newcastle, UK.

20. Beaumont KC, Cussans NJ, Nichols DJ, Smith DA. Pharmacokinetics and metabolism of darifenacin in the mouse, dog, rat and man. Xenobiotica 1998; 29: 63–75.

21. Kerbusch T, Wählby U, Milligan PA, Karlsson MO. Population pharmacokinetic modelling of darifenacin and its hydroxylated metabolite using pooled data, incorporating saturable first-pass metabolism, CYP2D6 genotype and formulation-dependent bioavailability. Br J Clin Pharmacol 2003; 56: 639–52.

22. Emselex European Public Assessment Report (EPAR). Scientific Discussion. European Medicines Agency (EMEA), http://www.emea.eu.int/humandocs/Humans/EPAR/emselex/emselex.htm, 2005.

23. Skerjanec A. The clinical pharmacokinetics of darifenacin. Clin Pharmacokinet 2006; 45(4): 325–350.

24. Haab F, Stewart L, Dwyer P. Darifenacin, and M_3 selective receptor antagonist, is an effective and well-tolerated once-daily treatment for overactive bladder. Eur Urol 2004; 45: 420–9.

25. Hill S, Khullar V, Wyndaele J-J, Lheritier K; Darifenacin Study Group. Dose response with darifenacin: a novel once-daily M3 selective receptor antagonist for the treatment of overactive bladder: results of a fixed-dose study. Int Urogynecol J Pelvic Floor Dysfunct 2006; 17: 239–47.

26. Romanzi LJ, DelConte A III, Kralidis G. Impact of darifenacin compared with tolterodine on incontinence episodes in patients with overactive bladder. Obstet Gynecol 2005; 105: 88S (abstr 3522).

27. Steers W, Corcos J, Foote J, Kralidis G. An investigation of dose titration with darifenacin, an M3 selective receptor antagonist. BJU Int 2005; 95: 580–6. [Erratum in BJU Int 2005; 95: 1385–6.]

28. Haab F, Corcos J, Siami P et al. Long-term darifenacin treatment for overactive bladder: results of a 2-year, open-label extension study. BJU Int 2006; 98: 1025–32.

29. Kay GG, Wesnes KA. Pharmacodynamic effects of darifenacin, a muscarinic M_3 selective receptor antagonist for the treatment of overactive bladder, in healthy volunteers. BJU Int 2005; 96: 1055–62.

30. Lipton RB, Kolodner K, Wesnes K. Assessment of cognitive function in the elderly population: effects of darifenacin (an M_3 selective antimuscarinic agent under investigation for the treatment of overactive bladder). J Urol 2005; 173: 493–8.

31. Kay GG, Crook T, Rekeda L et al. Differential effects of the antimuscarinic agents darifenacin and oxybutynin ER on memory in older subjects. Eur Urol 2006; 50: 317–26.

32. Serra DB, Affrime MB, Bedigian MP et al. QT and QTc interval with standard and supratherapeutic doses of darifenacin, a muscarinic M_3 selective receptor antagonist for the treatment of overactive bladder. J Clin Pharmacol 2005; 45: 1038–47.

33. Chapple C, Steers W, Norton P et al. A pooled analysis of three phase III studies to investigate the efficacy, tolerability and safety of darifenacin, a muscarinic M_3 selective receptor antagonist, in the treatment of overactive bladder. BJU Int 2005; 95: 993–1001.

34. Foote J, Glavind K, Kralidis G, Wyndaele JJ. Treatment of overactive bladder in the older patient: pooled analysis of three phase III studies of darifenacin, an M_3 selective receptor antagonist. Eur Urol 2005; 48: 471–7.

35. Kerr L, DelConte A. The effects of darifenacin on the improvement of symptoms of overactive bladder among female patients. J Endourol 2004; 18(Suppl 1): MP18–19 (abstr).

36. Zellner M, Lheritier K, Kawakami FT, Freedman S. Efficacy, tolerability and safety of long-term darifenacin treatment in men with overactive bladder: a 2-year, open-label, extension study. Abstract presented at World Congress of Men's Health and Gender, 30 September–1 October, 2005, Vienna, Austria.

37. Haab F, Hill S, Lheritier K, Kawakami FT, Gittelman M. Long-term treatment of overactive bladder with darifenacin in older patients: analysis of responder rates in a 2-year, open-label extension study. Poster presented at 21st Annual Meeting of the European Association of Urologists, 5–8 April, 2006, Paris, France.

38. Thomas S, Romanzi L, Lheritier K. Constipation and associated intervention in patients with overactive bladder treated with darifenacin or tolterodine. Int Urogynecol J 2005; 16(Suppl 2):S101 (abstr 306)

39. Crook TH, Lebowitz D, Pirozzolo FJ et al. Recalling names after introduction: changes across the adult life span in two cultures. Dev Neuropsychol 1993; 9: 103–13.

40. Chapple C, Kelleher C, Perrault L. Darifenacin, an M_3 selective receptor antagonist, improves quality of life in patients with overactive bladder. Prog Urol 2004; 14(Suppl 3): 22 (abstr 67).

41. Young J, Lheritier K, Steel M, Dwyer P. QoL outcomes during long-term treatment with darifenacin for overactive bladder (OAB): a 2-year open-label extension study. Qual Life Res 2005; 14: 2036, P-36/1678 (abstr).

18

Solifenacin succinate

Karl J Kreder and Roger R Dmochowski

Introduction • Chemistry and pharmacokinetics • Mechanism of action • Drug–drug interactions
• Clinical trials • Summary

INTRODUCTION

The International Continence Society (ICS) defines overactive bladder syndrome (OAB) as comprising the symptoms of urinary urgency, with or without urge incontinence and usually accompanied by diurnal frequency and nocturia.[1] This condition (syndrome) is estimated to affect up to 22% of American adults, with higher rates encountered in elderly demographic estimates.[2,3] Multiple treatment options for OAB exist, including isolated behavioral therapy, isolated pharmacologic therapy, combined behavioral and pharmacologic therapy (presumably most common), and surgical therapy for pharmacologic failures or due to pharmacologic intolerance. Pharmacologic therapy has been the main form of treatment for the overactive bladder for approximately three decades. This treatment has depended heavily on the use of antimuscarinic agents, first introduced with the advent of oxybutynin in the 1970s. Newer agents provide the convenience of once-a-day dosing due to longer-acting pharmacodynamic profiles directly attributed to delivery systems. Well-designed meta-analyses have revealed that sustained-release agents have improved side-effect profiles as compared to shorter-acting agents. Solifenacin succinate is a new antimuscarinic agent which has two existing doses, 5 mg and 10 mg, and is administered as a once-daily dosing regimen.

CHEMISTRY AND PHARMACOKINETICS

Solifenacin succinate is an antimuscarinic compound and a member of the tertiary amine group of antimuscarinic agents. The chemical formula and structure are shown in Figure 18.1. The molecular weight of the compound is 480.55.

Multiple studies have been performed in otherwise healthy, younger patients to evaluate the pharmacokinetics of this compound. In multiple dosing studies (5 mg, 10 mg, 20 mg, and 30 mg) performed in healthy young men, the time to maximum concentration (t_{max}) for solifenacin varied from 2.9 hours for the 20-mg dose to 5.8 hours for the 5-mg dose. The half life ($t_{1/2}$) was 45 hours and 64 hours respectively for the two dosing intervals.[4] Steady state serum levels of solifenacin were reached after 10 days of continuous therapy.

Metabolism and elimination

Solifenacin undergoes extensive hepatic metabolism predominantly by the CYP3A4 enzyme pathway. In healthy volunteers, only 15% of carbon-14 radiolabeled solifenacin (parent compound) is recovered in its intact state in the urine. Some 69.2% of the radioactive solifenacin is recovered as metabolites of the parent compound, and an additional 22.5% is recovered in feces.[5]

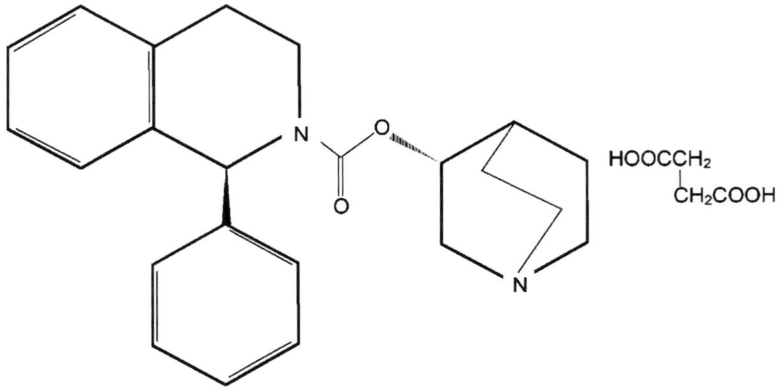

Figure 18.1 Structural formula of solifenacin succinate.

Relatively older patients (aged 65–80) have been found in at least one study to have average urinary concentration (AUC) and maximum concentration (C_{max}) 16% and 20% higher than younger study volunteers aged 18–55.[6] Clinical trials, however, have shown similar efficacy and safety between patients arbitrarily segregated by 65 years of age or greater.[7] There does not appear to be a gender requirement for dose adjustment; however, pharmacokinetics are lacking for different racial groups. In the presence of severe renal impairment, there is approximately a 2.1-fold increase in the AUC and 1.6 increase in the $t_{1/2}$ encountered with acute dosing of solifenacin.[8] In those patients with moderate hepatic impairment (Child's class B), there is approximately a 2-fold increase in the $t_{1/2}$ and a 35% increase in the average urinary concentration when it is administered acutely in those individuals.

MECHANISM OF ACTION

Although five types of muscarinic receptors exist in the human body, it has been shown that the M_2 and M_3 receptors play the most significant role in bladder function.[9–11] Approximately three-quarters to 80% of the muscarinic receptors in the bladder are M_2 and approximately 20–25% are of the M_3 type. It is generally presumed that the M_3 receptor, although present in lesser numbers in the human bladder, is that which is most responsible for normal bladder contraction in the healthy human bladder. The M_2 receptor as of yet has an undefined function, but may be involved in bladder relaxation. Direct M_3 receptor activation results in detrusor muscle contraction via phosphoinositide hydrolysis. Activation of the M_2 receptor may actually counteract sympathetically mediated smooth muscle relaxation, thereby creating an environment for bladder contraction.[12] In neurogenic voiding dysfunction, the M_2 receptor has been found to play a more significant role in detrusor overactivity related to this condition.[5] Muscarinic receptors exist throughout the human body; the M_3 receptor is present in substantial concentrations in the salivary gland (parotid) as well as in the intestine, and therefore the antimuscarinic effect at the level of these receptors may have an adverse influence on both intestinal and salivary gland function, leading to xerostomia and constipation.

Ikeda et al. compared differences in binding characteristics between two similar antimuscarinic agents, being solifenacin and oxybutynin, in rodent models using guinea pigs and mice.[5] In binding assays, the pK_i values of solifenacin for M_1, M_2, and M_3 were 7.6, 6.9, and 8.0 for each specific receptor. For oxybutynin in these animal models, the similar values were 8.6, 7.7, and 8.9, respectively. This group also studied the tissue selectivity between the lower urinary tract (specifically the bladder) and salivary gland in the detrusor of the guinea pig and also in the submandibular gland of the mouse. The test was stimulated with carbachol, and release of intracellular calcium was determined. The study authors determined that calcium released from detrusor cells was potentially inhibited by solifenacin (pK_i = 8.4) and oxybutynin (pK_i = 8.6); however, salivary glands were antagonized to a greater extent by oxybutynin (pK_b = 8.8) as opposed to solifenacin (pK_b = 7.4). As this activity was responsive to M_3 stimulation, the authors concluded that solifenacin may have relative salivary gland-sparing activity during acute administration.

Ohtake et al. also evaluated bladder selectivity of the compound solifenacin in the male Wistar rat, to compare salivary versus bladder selectivity.[13] The authors compared the results for solifenacin to those of other commonly available antimuscarinic compounds, including tolterodine, oxybutynin, darifenacin, and atropine. In this study, both solifenacin and tolterodine demonstrated selectivity for bladder smooth muscle cells over salivary gland cells; however, oxybutynin, darifenacin, and atropine did not demonstrate this selectivity. All of the studied agents inhibited carbachol-induced intracellular calcium increase in both bladder smooth muscle cells and also salivary gland cells, and this effect was noted to occur in a dose-dependent fashion. The authors also noted that solifenacin and tolterodine, in a dose-dependent fashion, inhibited carbachol-induced intravesical bladder pressure elevation and salivary gland secretion with functional selectivity for the bladder over the salivary gland. The other studied compounds did not demonstrate this selectivity. The authors then, on the basis of this rodent model, concluded that the selectivity for urinary bladder activity of solifenacin was greater than that of tolterodine, which in turn was greater than that of oxybutynin. Oxybutynin was found to be equal to darifenacin and atropine in overall selectivity for the urinary bladder.

Kobayashi et al. examined the same compounds in a primate model (monkey) using smooth muscle bladder cells and also submandibular gland cells.[14] They noted that the pK_i ratios of submandibular gland/bladder cells of the various agents were 2.1 for solifenacin, 0.65 for tolterodine, 0.51 for oxybutynin, and 0.46 for darifenacin. These authors also concluded that solifenacin demonstrated the greatest bladder selectivity of the studied agents. These authors did not study atropine.[14]

DRUG–DRUG INTERACTIONS

The primary metabolic pathway for solifenacin is the hepatic CYP3A4 pathway; therefore, inhibitors or inducers of this pathway may affect solifenacin pharmacokinetics. Uchida et al. examined the effects of food ingestion on the pharmacokinetic profile of solifenacin in a randomized crossover study of 24 healthy men (all under the age of 45) with body weights not exceeding 100 kg and body mass index (BMI) ≤ 30.[15] These study subjects received a 10-mg acute dose in both a fasting and a fed state in sequential periods. Subsequently, the same dose was administered to the second group of patients in a fed state during the first period and fasting state during the second period. Measured parameters included C_{max}, AUC, $t_{\frac{1}{2}max}$, and t_{max}. The authors found that in all patients there was no effect of fed state upon study drug absorption.[15] Michel et al. studied the interaction of solifenacin and warfarin in 12 young healthy males and also in 12 male and female study subjects.[16] The administration of 10 mg once daily with a single oral dose of 25 mg of warfarin or 0.25 mg loading dose of digoxin followed by 1.25 mg was well tolerated, and did not appear to affect the pharmacokinetics.[16]

CLINICAL TRIALS

Multiple studies have been performed studying the effect of solifenacin in men. Chapple et al. reported a large multicenter randomized trial involving 1281 patients with typical overactive bladder symptoms.[7] Of the initial study group, 1077 were actually reported from the standpoint of outcomes. After placebo run-in, patients were randomized to receive tolterodine 2 mg twice a day (bid), placebo, or solifenacin 5 or 10 mg on a once-a-day basis for 12 weeks in a double-blind fashion. Voiding diaries were used to evaluate study outcomes at baseline, week 4, and week 12. The main efficacy variables analyzed were change from baseline and mean number of urgency episodes, incontinence episodes, and urgency incontinence episodes. In this large trial, patients treated with solifenacin demonstrated a significant decrease from baseline and number of urgency episodes on a daily basis compared to placebo (placebo 33%, solifenacin 5 mg 52%, solifenacin 10 mg 55%, $p < 0.001$).[7]

Solifenacin ingestion resulted in significant reductions in incontinence episodes versus placebo, with 5 mg dosing resulting in a decrease of 1.42 episodes per day ($p = 0.008$) and 10 mg resulting in a reduction of 1.45 episodes per day ($p = 0.0038$). Table 18.1 summarizes the effects

Table 18.1 Number of patients discontinuing treatment before study completion and the treatment-related major anticholinergic side-effects (1077 patients). From reference 7, with permission

Characteristic	Placebo	Solifenacin (once daily)		Tolterodine 2 mg (twice daily)	Total
		5 mg	10 mg		
n	267	279	268	263	1077
Discontinuing (n (%))					
Adverse event	10 (3.7)	9 (3.2)	7 (2.6)	5 (1.9)	31 (2.9)
Consent withdrawal	10 (3.7)	11 (3.9)	7 (2.6)	8 (3.0)	36 (3.3)
Lost to follow-up	2 (0.7)	1 (0.4)	2 (0.7)	6 (2.3)	11 (1.0)
Protocol violation	5 (1.9)	4 (1.4)	0	3 (1.1)	12 (1.1)
Insufficient response	2 (0.7)	2 (0.7)	1 (0.4)	3 (1.1)	8 (0.7)
Patient died	0	0	1 (0.4)	1 (0.4)	2 (0.2)
Other	3 (1.1)	1 (0.4)	1 (0.4)	0	5 (0.5)
Total	32 (12.0)	28 (10.0)	19 (7.1)	26 (9.9)	105 (9.7)
Major side-effects (n (%))					
Dry mouth	13 (4.9)	39 (14.0)	57 (21.3)	49 (18.6)	
Constipation	5 (1.9)	20 (7.2)	21 (7.8)	7 (2.6)	
Blurred vision	7 (2.6)	10 (3.6)	15 (5.6)	4 (1.5)	

From Chapple CR, Rechberger T, Al-Shukri S, Meffan P, Everaert K, Huang M, Ridder A, on behalf of the YM-905 Study Group. Randomized, double-blind placebo - and tolterodine - controlled trial of the once-daily antimuscarinic agent solifenacin in patients with symptomatic overactive bladder. BJU Int 2004; 93(3): 303–10, with permission.

reported in this trial. Another head-to-head trial of solifenacin and tolterodine (STAR) was reported by Chapple et al.[17] The primary endpoint of this study was powered for non-inferiority, and solifenacin was studied in 5 mg and 10 mg dosing versus tolterodine in its standard 4-mg dose, with or without a placebo addition. After 1 month on the initial starting dose, patients were allowed to escalate their dose of solifenacin after medical approval from 5 mg to 10 mg. Similarly, patients in the tolterodine arm were allowed to escalate to an additional 4-mg placebo pill if they felt that their symptoms warranted this. The study trial design is included in Figure 18.2. Solifenacin was found to be as equally effective as tolterodine ($p = 0.004$, non-inferiority) from the standpoint of the primary endpoint of reduction of micturition frequency (Figure 18.3). When compared to the 4-mg extended-release tolterodine (Table 18.2), solifenacin demonstrated significant improvements in secondary outcome measures including urge incontinence ($p = 0.001$), overall incontinence ($p = 0.006$), and urgency ($p = 0.035$).

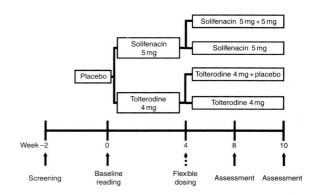

Figure 18.2 STAR Trial study design. From Chapple CR, Martinez-Garcia R, Selvaggi L, Toozs-Hobson, Warnack W, Drogendijk T et al. A comparison of the efficacy and tolerability of solifenacin succinate and extended release tolterodine at treating overactive bladder syndrome: results of the STAR trial. Eur Urol 2005; 48(3): 464–70, with permission.

Table 18.2 Secondary endpoints from the STAR (solifenacin and tolterodine) trial

Endpoint	Solifenacin mean change from baseline	Tolterodine mean change from baseline	p Value solifenacin vs. tolterodine
Incontinence episodes/24 h	−1.60	−1.11	0.006
Urge incontinence episodes/24 h	−1.42	−0.83	0.001
Pads used/24 h	−1.72	−1.19	0.002
Urgency episodes/24 h	−2.85	−2.42	0.035
Volume voided/micturition (ml)	+37.95	+31.00	0.010

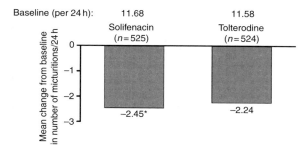

Figure 18.3 Baseline to endpoint change in overactive bladder symptoms from the STAR trial. $*p = 0.004$ for non-inferiority vs. tolterodine.

Forty-nine percent of those patients receiving tolterodine were clinically continent (no incontinence episodes on 3-day diary) at the end of the trial, as compared to 59% of the solifenacin patients ($p = 0.006$). It should be noted that these numbers were pooled numbers and did not specifically report differences between 5 mg and 10 mg of solifenacin versus tolterodine. Overall discontinuation rates were 5.9% for solifenacin and 7.3% for tolterodine.

In another trial, Cardozo et al. reported 1091 enrolled and 907 actually treated patients in a multinational randomized placebo-controlled trial of 5 mg and 10 mg of solifenacin compared to placebo.[18] This was a 12-week trial with the primary efficacy variable being change from baseline in the mean number of micturitions per 24 hours. Secondary efficacy variables evaluated included change from baseline to end of study in the number of urgency episodes per 24 hours, urge incontinence, all incontinence, voided volume per micturition, and nocturia. Study evaluation was performed via 3-day diary record-keeping. Solifenacin 5-mg and 10-mg doses were statistically significantly different from placebo in the mean number of micturitions per 24 hours (placebo 1.59 micturitions per day reduction; solifenacin 5 mg 2.37 reduction in micturitions per day; and solifenacin 10 mg 2.81 reductions per day). The other primary and secondary outcome events are summarized in Table 18.3.

The authors reported overall xerostomia rates of 2.3% in the placebo group and 7.7% of patients receiving 5 mg of solifenacin, and 23.1% of those patients receiving 10 mg of solifenacin. Overall constipation rates were 2% with placebo, 3.7% with 5 mg of solifenacin, and 9.1% with 10 mg of solifenacin. Interestingly, visual disturbance (blurring of vision) was not noted to any greater degree in patients on active agents as compared to those on placebo.

In another large trial, Haab et al. reported patients with an extended exposure to the active agent solifenacin.[19] These patients were patients followed upon completion of a previous 12-week study trial. Of the 1802 patients who completed the 12-week trial, 1637 (91%) elected to enter the extension trial. All patients were initially started on solifenacin 5 mg and then were allowed to dose adjust either up or subsequently down at weeks 16, 20, and 40 (Figure 18.4). Three-day voiding diaries were used to establish efficacy, and were completed at baseline as well as each follow-up visit and the end of the study. Efficacy values evaluated included change from baseline in mean number of urgency episodes per day, micturitions per day, all incontinence episodes, urgency incontinence episodes, volume voided per micturition, and nocturia episodes. Eighty-one percent

Table 18.3 Change from baseline to 12-week endpoint in voiding frequency, urgency episodes, and urge incontinence for patients in the mixed urinary incontinence cohort, and the actual and percentage changes in overactive bladder symptoms at open-label endpoint by double-blind treatment

		Solifenacin	
Variable	Placebo	5 mg	10 mg
Voiding frequency			
n	430	159	452
Mean (SEM):			
baseline voids/24 h	11.5 (0.14)	12.2 (0.28)	11.7 (0.15)
actual change from baseline, voids/24 h	−1.4 (0.13)	−2.5 (0.25)†	−2.6 (0.13)†
Mean % change from baseline	−10	−19	−21
Median % change from baseline	−12	−21	−22
Urgency			
n	423	155	445
Mean (SEM):			
baseline no. of urgency episodes	6.2 (0.18)	6.1 (0.38)	6.3 (0.20)
actual change from baseline	−2.1 (0.17)	−3.4 (0.36)†	−3.4 (0.18)†
Mean % change from baseline	−32	−52	−52
Median % change from baseline	−42	−73	−69
Urge incontinence			
n	365	113	373
Mean (SEM):			
baseline no. of urge incontinence episodes	3.0 (0.15)	3.1 (0.27)	3.2 (0.16)
actual change from baseline	−1.3 (0.13)	−1.6 (0.23)*	−1.9 (0.14)†
Mean % change from baseline	−34	−46	−59
Median % change from baseline	−64	−82	−94
All groups + open-label solifenacin			
Mean (SEM) [%] change from original baseline to 52-week endpoint			
n	107	129	120
Voids/24 h	−1.74 (0.31) [−13]	−3.06 (0.27) [−23]	−3.30 (0.28) [−25]
n	81	91	88
Episodes of urge incontinence	−1.63 (0.42) [−32]	−1.67 (0.29) [−54]	−2.08 (0.28) [−69]
n	104	125	118
Episodes of urgency	−2.33 (0.30) [−44]	−3.45 (0.33) [−59]	−4.17 (0.38) [−69]

*$p < 0.05$ vs. placebo; †$p < 0.001$ vs. placebo

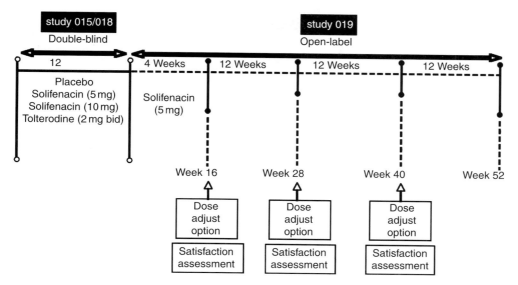

Figure 18.4 Open label extension study design. From Haab F, Cardozo L, Chapple C, Ridder AM, for the Solifenacin Study Group. Long-term open-label solifenacin treatment associated with persistance with therapy in patients with overactive bladder syndrome. Eur Urol 2005; 47: 376–84, with permission.

Table 18.4 **Number of patients with expected solifenacin treatment-emergent anticholinergic side-effects by severity for all patients.*** From reference 19, with permission

	Patients on solifenacin 5 mg at AE report (n = 1633)	Patients on solifenacin 10 mg at AE report (n = 1114)	All patients on solifenacin (n = 1633)
Dry mouth (n (%))			
mild	132 (8.1)	122 (11.0)	235 (14.4)
moderate	28 (1.7)	56 (5.0)	82 (5.0)
severe	6 (0.4)	16 (1.4)	22 (1.3)
Constipation (n (%))			
mild	56 (3.4)	49 (4.4)	96 (5.9)
moderate	19 (1.2)	27 (2.4)	44 (2.7)
severe	5 (0.3)	12 (1.1)	17 (1.0)
Blurred vision (n (%))			
mild	49 (3.0)	39 (3.5)	85 (5.2)
moderate	16 (1.0)	9 (0.8)	25 (1.5)
severe	2 (0.1)	1 (0.1)	3 (0.2)

AE, adverse event
*Adverse events during solifenacin treatment were recorded during 52 weeks of treatment for all patients in the extension study

of those patients initially enrolled completed the 40-week drug exposure experience. Mean incontinence episodes increased by 66% during study performance. The overall mean number of micturitions per 24 hours decreased by 23%, with nocturic episodes decreasing by 32% and urgency episodes on a 24-hour basis decreasing by 63%. The volume voided per micturition increased by

31% and overall nocturia (nocturnal frequency) decreased by 50%. There was a median decrease of 100% in urge incontinent episodes during this trial. Of the patients who had urge incontinence at baseline after 52 weeks, 60% of those patients were dry on therapy and 74% of patients rated their overall efficacy as satisfactory at the study end. Overall side-effects are summarized in Table 18.4

In another study specifically evaluating quality of life effect, Kelleher et al. analyzed data on quality of life from a pooled analysis of two 12-week multinational double-blind controlled trials included with a 40-week open-label extension of these 12-week trials. Patients were randomized to placebo and active drug at the 5-mg and 10-mg doses.[20] The King's Health Questionnaire was used to evaluate individual bladder problems; it was administered at the start of the blinded portion of each trial and also at weeks 4 and 12 during therapy. A total of 1890 patients were analyzed during the 12-week study. Significant differences in quality of life were noted in those patients exposed to solifenacin versus placebo in all domains, except for personal relationships, after the 12-week trial. When evaluating data from the extension trial (40-week), patients on both 5-mg and 10-mg doses of solifenacin had significant improvements in their quality of life from the start of the open-label period to the end of the trial period. This overall improvement was 17% for general health perception and 35–48% for improvement of other domains.

A recent post hoc analysis of 3298 subjects taking part in 12-week registration trials of solifenacin was undertaken to assess the effect of active drug on mixed incontinence. A total of 1041 subjects with mixed symptoms were identified. In double-blind controlled trials, 43% (5 mg) and 49% (10 mg) of subjects became continent at the study end. In open-label trials, 52% became continent and 34% reported resolution of symptomatic urgency at the study end. The authors suggested that these findings supported the use of solifenacin in the mixed incontinence population, given a magnitude of response not too dissimilar from that of the urge incontinence-only population.[21]

In another pooled analysis of patients aged over 65, solifenacin efficacy and tolerability were analyzed specific to an older study population. In four studies, 1041 subjects were identified, with a mean age of 71.2 years. Incontinence, urgency, and frequency were all statistically improved as compared to placebo, and these benefits were maintained long term in open-label analysis. Adverse events most commonly included dry mouth and constipation, and were of mild to moderate intensity. The authors concluded that solifenacin was well tolerated and efficacious in this specific sub-population.[22]

Recently, the effect of solifenacin on the symptom of urgency has been rigorously assessed in a trial entitled VENUS (VESIcare® Efficacy and Safety in PatienTs with Urgency Study).[23] The VENUS trial design was randomized, double-blind, and placebo-controlled, and assessed patients with or without incontinence with at least one urgency episode per day during 3-day diary record keeping. The primary efficacy variable was change from baseline in the mean number of urgency episodes per 24 hours. Warning time was also assessed on the day immediately preceding the baseline and 12-week diary records.

Seven hundred and thirty-nine patients were entered into the trial, with 372 receiving solifenacin. At weeks 4 and 8, subject dosing could be maintained, increased, or decreased depending upon subject perception of therapy. At the study end, solifenacin subjects experienced a mean decrease of 3.91 urgency episodes as compared to 2.73 for placebo ($p < 0.001$). Warning time median length also increased from baseline significantly in the solifenacin group (31.5 seconds) as compared to the placebo-ingesting subjects (12.0 seconds, $p = 0.032$). Overall, warning time increased by almost 2 minutes (186.4 seconds) in the solifenacin group, as compared to 54.7 seconds in the placebo arm. The authors concluded that solifenacin is effective for subjective urgency, and also produces a measurable response (increase) in warning time.

SUMMARY

Solifenacin has been shown in clinical trials to be an effective and well-tolerated treatment option for those patients with the overactive bladder syndrome. Data support an increase in overall functional bladder capacity with a decrease in the bothersome symptoms of urinary incontinence, frequency, and urgency. In non-human animal studies, data support the selectivity of solifenacin for the bladder over the salivary gland, thus possibly supporting clinical data which demonstrate a decrease in dry mouth and constipation with this compound in clinical trials.

REFERENCES

1. Abrams P, Cardozo L, Fall M et al. The standardisation of terminology in lower urinary tract function: report from the Standardisation Subcommittee of the International Continence Society. Urology 2003; 61: 37–49.
2. Stewart W, Herzog R, Wein A. Prevalence and impact of overactive bladder in the U.S.: results from the NOBLE program. Neurourol Urodyn 2001; 20: 406–8.
3. Versi E. Screening initiative confirms widespread prevalence of overactive bladder in American adults. Int Urogynecol J 2001; 12: S13.
4. Smulders RA, Krauwinkel WJ, Swart PJ, Huang M. Pharmakokinetics and safety of solifenacin succinate in healthy young men. J Clin Pharmacol 2004; 44: 1023–33.
5. Ikeda K, Kobayashi S, Suzuki M et al. M₃ receptor antagonism by the novel antimuscarinic agent solifenacin in the urinary bladder and salivary gland. Arch Pharmacol 2002; 366: 97–103.
6. Krauwinkel WJ, Smulders RA, Mulder H, Swart PJ, Taekema-Roelvink ME. Effect of age on the pharmacokinetics of solifenacin in men and women. Int J Pharmacol Ther 2005; 43: 227–38.
7. Chapple CR, Rechberger T, Al-Shukri S et al., on behalf of the YM-905 Study Group. Randomized, double-blind placebo- and tolterodine-controlled trial of the once-daily antimuscarinic agent solifenacin in patients with symptomatic overactive bladder. BJU Int 2004; 93: 303–10.
8. Prescribing information: VESIcare®. Philadelphia, PA and Research Triangle Park, NC: Astellas Pharma, US, Inc and the GlaxoSmithKline Group of Companies, 2004.
9. Andersson K-E, Wein AJ. Pharmacology of the lower urinary tract: basis for current and future treatments of urinary incontinence. Pharmacol Rev 2004; 56: 581–631.
10. Yamaguchi O, Shishido K, Tamura K et al. Evaluation of mRNAs encoding muscarinic receptor subtypes in human detrusor muscle. J Urol 1996; 156: 1208–13.
11. Sigala S, Mirabella G, Peroni A et al. Differential gene expresion of cholinergic muscarinic receptor subtypes in male and female normal human urinary bladder. Urology 2002; 60: 719–25.
12. Nakamura T, Kimura J, Yamaguchi O. Muscarinic M2 receptors inhibit Ca2+ -activated K+ channels in rat bladder smooth muscle. Int J Urol 2002; 9: 689–96.
13. Ohtake A, Ukai M, Hatanaka T et al. In vitro and in vivo tissue selectivity profile of solifenacin succinate (YM905) for urinary bladder over salivary gland in rats. Eur J Pharmacol 2004; 492: 243–50.
14. Kobayashi S, Ikeda K, Miyata K. Comparison of in vitro selectivity profiles of solifenacin succinate (YM905) and current antimuscarinic drugs in bladder and salivary glands: a Ca²⁺ mobilization study in monkey cells. Life Sci 2004; 74: 843–53.
15. Uchida T, Krauwinkel WJ, Mulder H, Smulders RA. Food does not affect the pharmacokinetics of solifenacin, a new muscarinic receptor antagonist: results of a randomized crossover trial. Br J Clin Pharmacol 2004; 58: 4–7.
16. Michel MC, Minematsu T, Hashimoto T, den Hoven WV, Swart PJ. In vitro studies on the potential of solifenacin for drug–drug interactions: plasma protein binding and MDR1 transport. Br J Clin Pharmacol 2005; 59: 647 (abstr).
17. Chapple CR, Martinez-Garcia R, Selvaggi L et al. A comparison of the efficacy and tolerability of solifenacin succinate and extended release tolterodine at treating overactive bladder syndrome: results of the STAR trial. Eur Urol 2005; 48: 464–70.
18. Cardozo L, Lisec M, Millard R et al. Randomized, double-blind placebo controlled trial of the once daily antimuscarinic agent solifenacin succinate in patients with overactive bladder. J Urol 2004; 172: 1919–24.
19. Haab F, Cardozo L, Chapple C, Ridder AM, for the Solifenacin Study Group. Long-term open-label solifenacin treatment associated with persistence with therapy in patients with overactive bladder syndrome. Eur Urol 2005; 47: 376–84.
20. Kelleher CJ, Cardozo L, Chapple CR, Haab F, Ridder AM. Improved quality of life in patients with overactive bladder symptoms treated with solifenacin. BJU Int 2005; 95: 81–5.

21. Satskin D, Te A. Short and long term efficacy of solifenacin treatment in patients with symptoms of mixed urinary incontinence. BJU Int 2006; 92: 1256–61.

22. Wagg A, Wyndaele JJ, Sieber P. Efficacy and tolerability of solifenacin in elderly subjects with overactive bladder syndrome: a pooled analysis. Am J Geriatr Phamacother 2006; 4: 14–24.

23. Toglia M, Andoh M, Hussain I. Solifenacin improved warning time significantly compared to placebo in patients with overactive bladder. Proc Int Continence Soc 2006; 25: 123A.

19

Transdermal oxybutynin (Oxytrol™)

G Willy Davila

Introduction • Transdermal oxybutynin • Pharmacokinetics • Clinical efficacy
• Safety and tolerability • Conclusions

INTRODUCTION

Oral anticholinergic medications are the mainstay of pharmacotherapy for overactive bladder (OAB). Antimuscarinic properties of these drugs block acetylcholine-induced stimulation of the postganglionic parasympathetic muscarinic receptor sites in animal[1,2] and human tissues.[3] Various agents are currently used for OAB therapy, all with demonstrated efficacy in the treatment of OAB. However, their effectiveness is limited by their systemic anticholinergic side effects. An improved understanding of muscarinic receptor subtypes and their anatomic location can help to explain this phenomenon.[4] Both M_2 and M_3 receptors are present in the bladder. M_2 receptors (80% of the receptor concentration in the bladder) are responsible for detrusor relaxation, while M_3 receptors control detrusor contraction. About 90% of the muscarinic receptors in the salivary glands are of the M_3 variety.[5] The concomitant stimulation of these muscarinic receptors in salivary glands and the bowel by anticholinergic agents leads to the well-recognized adverse side effects of dry mouth and constipation.

Oxybutynin pharmacologic effects on the bladder

Oxybutynin (OXY) has been used for decades to control symptoms of urinary incontinence (UI) and is likely the most commonly used drug for this purpose worldwide. With spasmolytic and antimuscarinic properties, OXY has a direct relaxant effect on the bladder.[6]

OXY has been characterized as a selective muscarinic antagonist[7] with a 10-fold higher affinity for M_3 receptors than for M_2 receptors.[4] Therefore, this agent acts directly on the primary receptor responsible for detrusor contraction, explaining the drug's effectiveness in reducing urge incontinence episodes. It also acts on the primary receptors located in the salivary gland, explaining the associated incidence of dry mouth (87%) experienced by patients who take oral OXY.[8]

Upon oral intake, OXY formulations undergo extensive hepatic and gastrointestinal metabolism to form the primary recognized active metabolite, N-desethyl-oxybutynin (DEO). Following oral administration of the OXY, DEO can be measured in the circulation at levels 4–10 times higher than that of the parent compound.

Oral OXY is very effective in reducing the number of weekly UI episodes, as demonstrated in multiple controlled trials. Although effectiveness is high, so is the incidence of dry mouth – up to 87% for extended release OXY and 68% for immediate release OXY.[8] Investigations into other OXY drug delivery systems, such as intravesical, intravaginal, or transdermal, are aimed at reducing the incidence of anticholinergic side effects while maintaining beneficial effects on OAB.

Rationale for transdermal drug delivery systems

Patches or transdermal drug delivery systems to deliver drugs continuously through the skin into the circulation have been available for over 25 years. These systems maintain constant drug-plasma levels and may simplify drug administration. The first patch was Transderm Scop™, marketed by CIBA, which released the anti-motion sickness drug, scopolamine. Nitroglycerin patches for angina prophylaxis soon followed. Today, a wide array of drugs including anti-hypertensives, contraceptive hormones, and hormone replacement therapy agents are effectively administered by transdermal delivery.

Transdermal drug delivery patches are available in two configurations: a reservoir type that controls the rate of drug delivery to the skin and a matrix type that uses the skin to control the absorption rate. Transdermal drug patches provide ease of administration, disposability, and control of drug delivery. An added benefit is that first pass metabolism by the liver is avoided, permitting reduced drug doses and a reduction in drug interactions. The serum level peaks and troughs that are typically observed with immediate release or extended release oral medications are far less frequent with transdermal administration. Fewer side effects may promote patient compliance and increased treatment efficacy.

TRANSDERMAL OXYBUTYNIN

Based on its molecular characteristics, metabolism, and side effect profile following oral administration, OXY is thought to be a desirable agent for transdermal delivery. Following oral administration, agents undergo gastrointestinal and hepatic first pass metabolism that can reduce bioavailability.[9,10] Transdermal delivery systems allow the drug to bypass the gastrointestinal and hepatic first pass metabolism, providing more consistent control of absorption into the circulation.[11] Importantly, following oral administration, inconsistent serum drug concentrations may lead to adverse effects during unnecessarily high peak concentrations and subtherapeutic levels at trough times.[9] During transdermal therapy, more controlled absorption results in the ability to administer lower dosages and achieve therapeutic blood levels at a steady state over extended periods of time.[12,13] These lower dosages can lead to a reduction in dose-related side effects and ultimately lead to improved patient adherence. Because of its efficacy-limiting metabolite-related adverse effects, a transdermal delivery system for

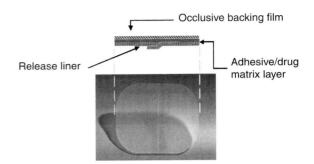

Figure 19.1 Side and top views of transdermal oxybutynin matrix system. (From reference 14, with permission)

OXY (TD-OXY) was developed in the early 1990s. The oxybutynin transdermal system (Oxytrol™; Watson Pharmaceuticals) delivers oxybutynin as the free base (not as a hydrochloride salt, as does the oral formulation).

TD-OXY is a matrix-type patch composed of three layers.[14] (Figure 19.1). The first layer consists of a thin backing film made of flexible and occlusive polyester/ethylene-vinyl acetate that ensures physical integrity and protects the middle layer, which contains the acrylic adhesive. This middle layer also contains OXY and triacetin, and United States Pharmacopeia, a skin permeability enhancer Layer three is a release liner composed of two overlapping siliconized polyester strips that can be peeled off and discarded by the patient prior to applying the adhesive/drug layer to the skin.

PHARMACOKINETICS

The average daily dose of OXY absorbed from the 39-cm^2 patch is 3.9 mg. In a study of healthy volunteers, the average plasma OXY concentration during an application of a 39-cm^2 system was 3–4 mg/ml in 24–48 hours, with steady concentrations maintained up to 96 hours (Figure 19.2). This sustained delivery makes it possible for patients to apply a single patch for 3–4 days with effective continuous maintenance of serum levels. Bioequivalency has been demonstrated for application at different body sites, including abdomen, buttock, and hip (Figure 19.2), thus resulting in a recommendation to rotate patch placement along the lower abdomen, hips, and upper buttocks.

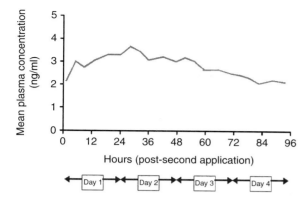

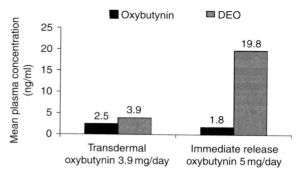

Figure 19.3 Average plasma oxybutynin and N-desethyl-oxybutynin (DEO) concentrations measured up to 96 hours after transdermal or oral (extended release) oxybutynin delivery

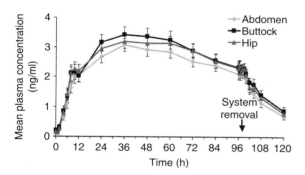

Figure 19.2 Steady-state oxybutynin concentrations following Oxytrol™ application. (From reference 14, with permission)

Once in the circulation, oxybutynin from TD-OXY is metabolized primarily by the cytochrome P450 enzymes, particularly CYP3A4, found mostly in the liver and gut wall. Its metabolites include phenylcyclohexylglycolic acid, which is pharmacologically inactive, and DEO, which is pharmacologically active. Following the oral administration of OXY, presystemic first pass metabolism results in bioavailability of approximately 6% and a relatively higher plasma concentration of the active DEO metabolite compared with that following transdermal delivery.[11,15] Transdermal administration of OXY bypasses the gastrointestinal and hepatic first pass metabolism, reducing the formation of DEO especially when compared to immediate release OXY (Figure 19.3).

A pharmacokinetic study comparing transdermal with extended release OXY demonstrated that transdermal administration resulted in considerably lower fluctuation in OXY and DEO

plasma concentrations, reduced DEO formation, and increased saliva production during the dosing period.[16] Compared with oral administration, TD-OXY is administered at lower dosages yet is absorbed at higher levels; approximately 100% of the 3.9 mg is absorbed through the skin and into the circulation.

Adhesion

Since the pharmacologic agent is located in the adhesive layer, complete patch adhesion is critical for drug dosing. Adhesion was periodically evaluated during the phase III studies.[9,17] Of the 4746 evaluations of the transdermal system, 20 (0.4%) were observed to have become completely detached and 35 (0.7%) had become partially detached. More than 98% of the systems were assessed as being at least 75% adherent and expected to deliver adequate doses of medication.

CLINICAL EFFICACY

One phase II study and two phase III studies have been undertaken and have demonstrated that TD-OXY is effective in controlling OAB symptoms, with a resultant low incidence of anticholinergic side effects.

Phase II study

The goal of the phase II study was to evaluate a maximized OXY dosage based on tolerability of dry mouth, rather than the efficacy in reducing

OAB symptoms. It was a double-blind, placebo-controlled trial of 249 urge incontinent patients who were present responders to immediate-release OXY.[9] Symptom requirements recorded in a 3-day urinary diary after prestudy treatment washout included 10 or more UI episodes, 56 or more voids, and 350 ml or less urinary void volume. The efficacy endpoints included change from baseline in the number of incontinence episodes, comparisons of daily urinary frequency, and urinary voided volume. Safety endpoints were confirmation of continued efficacy and adherence. Double-blind therapy included twice weekly application of TD-OXY, daily ingestion of oral OXY capsules, or matching placebo for 2 weeks. The dosage was sequentially increased over 6 weeks if the subject reported tolerable dry mouth symptomatology. The aim was to achieve an intolerable dry mouth. Maximum dosage reached was 20 mg/day orally and 5.2 mg/day in the transdermal group. It is possible that higher dosages may have been reached if the term of the trial was longer than 6 weeks.

Efficacy results of the study showed that daily incontinence episodes decreased similarly in both transdermal and oral treatment groups (7.2 to 2.4 (66%) and 7.2 to 2.6 (72%), respectively, $p = 0.39$).[9] A visual analog scale reduction in urinary leakage improved from washout in both groups ($p < 0.0001$) with no difference between them ($p = 0.9$). Most importantly, dry mouth occurred in significantly fewer patients in the transdermal group (38%) compared with the oral group (94%, $p < 0.001$) at the maximal achieved dosage (Figure 19.4). An anticholinergic symptoms questionnaire was used in order to capture the symptom of dry mouth in a specifically prompted fashion. Among patients in the transdermal group, 67% experienced a reduction in severity of dry mouth compared with previous oral treatment; 90% had no or mild skin erythema. Plasma concentrations of OXY increased according to dose, and reflected differences in metabolism of transdermal vs. oral administration, with DEO levels relatively low in the transdermal group. Overall, TD-OXY efficacy was comparable to that of oral OXY-IR, with a markedly lower incidence of dry mouth, giving credence to the concept of administration of OXY via transdermal routes.

Phase III studies

The first phase III study was a double-blind, placebo-controlled trial with 520 urge and mixed UI patients with the goal of identifying the optimal dosage of TD-OXY.[17] Of the 520 patients, 125 received TD-OXY 3.9 mg/day while 132 patients received a placebo patch; 130 and 133 participants received 1.3 mg/day and 2.6 mg/day TD-OXY, respectively. After a 3–4-week screening period, patients continued treatment for 12 weeks. Symptom requirements recorded in a 7-day urinary diary after the prestudy washout period included 10 or more urge UI episodes and 56 or more voids. Efficacy endpoints of the study were the change from baseline in the number of incontinence episodes, daily urinary frequency comparisons, and urinary voided volume. Safety endpoints were the confirmation of continued efficacy and patient compliance. After the 12-week double-blind period, subjects were offered enrollment in a 12-week open-label extension, during

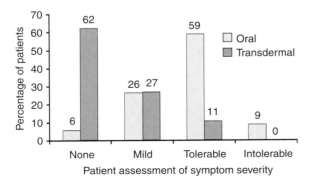

Figure 19.4 Phase II study. Dry mouth rates according to administration route.

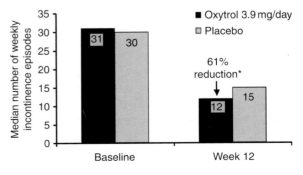

Figure 19.5 Phase III trial. Reduction in weekly incontinence episodes. $^*p = 0.0265$ vs. placebo.

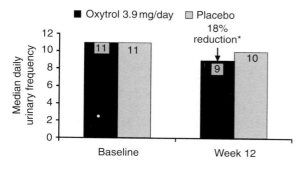

Figure 19.6 Phase III trial. Reduction in daily urinary frequency. $^*p = 0.0313$ vs. placebo.

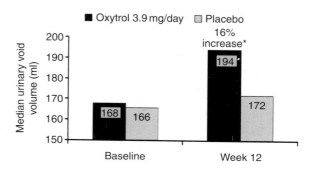

Figure 19.7 Phase III trial. Increases in urinary voided volume. $^*p = 0.0009$ vs. placebo.

Table 19.1 Incontinence episodes per day, daily micturition frequency, and average void volume at baseline, endpoint, and change from baseline, among patients taking transdermal oxybutynin, oral extended release tolterodine, or placebo[18]

	Transdermal oxybutynin* 3.9 mg/day (n = 121/119)		Tolterodine* 4 mg/day (n = 123/123)	Placebo* (n = 117/115)
Incontinence episodes (number/day)				
baseline	4		4	4
endpoint	1		1	2
change	−3		−3	−2
p vs. placebo	0.0137		0.0011	—
p vs. active comparison		0.5878		
Micturition frequency (number/day)				
baseline	12		12	12
endpoint	10		10	10
change	−2		−2	−1
p vs. placebo	0.1010		0.0025	—
p vs. active comparison		0.2761		
Average void volume (ml)				
baseline	160		150	171
endpoint	188		193	165
change	24		29	6.5
p vs. placebo	0.0023		0.0006	—
p vs. active comparison		0.7690		

*Median changes

which they could increase the TD-OXY dosage to optimally reduce OAB symptoms.

In the study, a 3.9-mg daily dose of TD-OXY significantly decreased the number of weekly incontinence episodes (median change, −19.0 vs. −15.0, $p = 0.0265$) (Figure 19.5), reduced average daily urinary frequency (median change, −2.0 vs. −1.0, $p = 0.0313$) (Figure 19.6), increased average voided volume (median change, 26 ml vs. 5.5 ml, $p = 0.0009$) (Figure 19.7), and significantly improved quality of life (Incontinence Impact Questionnaire total score, $p = 0.0327$) compared with placebo. The most common adverse event was application site pruritus (TD-OXY, 16.8%; placebo, 6.1%). The incidence of dry mouth in the transdermal group was similar to that with placebo (9.6% vs. 8.3%). In the 12-week open-label period, a sustained reduction of nearly three incontinence episodes per day was noted. Interestingly, after "self-titration" of the dosage, 59% of subjects were using a 3.9 mg/day patch size, while 39% were satisfied at a 2.6-mg/day dosage.

The second phase III study compared the efficacy and safety of TD-OXY 3.9 mg/day with oral, extended release tolterodine 4 mg/day and with placebo in 361 patients with urge or mixed incontinence.[18] In order to study a more homogeneous population, and to reduce side effect occurrence, all enrolled subjects were anticholinergic non-naive, not having been on previous pharmacotherapy for their OAB. Patients were randomized to 12 weeks of double-blind, double-dummy, placebo-controlled treatment. Endpoints included change from baseline in patient urinary incontinence symptoms, incontinence-specific quality of life (QoL), and safety.

Both TD-OXY and tolterodine significantly reduced the number of daily incontinence episodes, increased voided volume (Table 19.1), and significantly improved QoL (Incontinence Impact Questionnaire total score, $p < 0.05$; Urinary Distress Inventory–Irritative Symptoms subscale, $p < 0.05$) compared with placebo. Pairwise efficacy comparisons between active treatments demonstrated no significant differences ($p > 0.05$). The most common adverse reaction for the OXY group was application site pruritus (14% vs. 4.3% placebo), accompanied by a relatively lower incidence of dry mouth compared with toltero-dine (4.1% vs. 7.3%, respectively, vs. 1.7% for placebo; $p < 0.05$).

SAFETY AND TOLERABILITY

The most common adverse events for TD-OXY are localized application site pruritus and erythema. A low incidence of systemic anticholinergic side effects, comparable to that with placebo, was noted in all studies (Table 19.2). Notably, the incidence of dry mouth was lower than that reported in the literature for oral formulations of OXY and was similar to the incidence observed with placebo.[8] The incidence of diarrhea and constipation was not significantly different from that with placebo.

Local application site reactions

Local application site reactions with TD-OXY are generally transient and involve self-limiting, mild-to-moderate pruritus and erythema. Most patients experience either no or mild-to-moderate application site reactions. Of those who do, very few are severe, requiring patch discontinuation. Pruritus appears to be a more troublesome symptom than does erythema.

Although no trials have been conducted to compare incidence of application reactions, local tolerability reactions are generally similar with TD-OXY and those of other types of transdermal matrix products.[19,20] Studies of hormone replacement matrix and fentanyl reservoir transdermal systems have revealed higher application site reaction rates (41–53%).[21,22]

In order to reduce the chance of developing an application site reaction, patients should be

Table 19.2 Emergence of adverse events[17]		
	Transdermal oxybutynin 3.9 mg/day (n = 125)	Placebo adverse event (n = 132)
Abnormal vision	0%	1.5%
Constipation	0.8%	3.0%
Diarrhea	3.2%	2.3%
Dry mouth	9.6%	8.3%
Application site pruritus	16.8%	6.1%
Application site erythema	5.6%	2.3%

instructed to apply the system to dry, intact skin on the abdomen, hip, or buttock. A new application site should be selected with each new system to avoid reapplication at the same site within any 7-day period. Mild erythema may be seen after the patch is removed, but generally resolves within a few hours.

Skin tolerability

Topical reactions are a common concern for patients. In a study focusing on skin reactivity, skin tolerability at application sites was evaluated every 3 weeks during the double-blind period and then at 2, 4, and 12 weeks during the open-label period, independent of reported adverse events.[23] Skin tolerability was assessed by visual inspection of the most recently used application site and rated according to a four-point scale (absent to severe erythema). On study completion, patients filled in questionnaires concerning their perception of treatment benefit and their willingness to continue transdermal treatment. Results showed that 86% of patients reported either no or mild erythema. The number of days to erythema onset ranged from 29 to 39 days in the double-blind period and from 89 to 133 days during the open-label period. Additionally, in most cases, erythema was reversible and minimally perceptible 24 hours after patch removal. Overall, 93% of patients reported no significant skin erythema (Figure 19.8). During the double-blind period, 6.4% of patients withdrew from the trial while 3.4% withdrew during the open-label period because of adverse skin reactions. Pruritis at the application site may occur, and may be bothersome in up to 17.8% of patients (Figure 19.8). However, rarely is it significant enough to warrant discontinuation of therapy. The discontinuation rate did not correlate with an increase in severity of application site reactions. Most skin reactions are temporary, resolving within days of patch removal. If necessary, skin moisturizers or topical steroid ointments may be used.

A voluntary patient satisfaction questionnaire was completed in which study participants were asked to comment on their experiences with transdermal therapy during the double-blind phase of the study, as compared with previous oral therapy. The results showed that the majority of patients (67%) were satisfied with the appearance of the

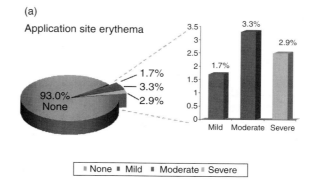

(a)

Application site erythema

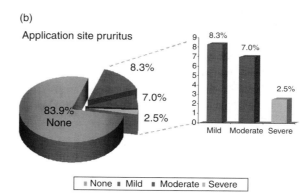

(b)

Application site pruritus

Figure 19.8 Skin erythema (a) and pruritis (b) occur in a small percentage of patients. (See also color plate section).

transdermal system (e.g. transparency, discretion) and did not find it bothersome. Sixty-eight percent described the system as easy to apply. The majority (78%) of patients found that remembering to reapply the transdermal system was the same or easier than remembering to take a pill each day. Of those patients who completed the questionnaire and who experienced application site itching, the majority (72%) reported that these symptoms disappeared within a week. Overall, 66% indicated a preference for transdermal delivery compared with oral or other treatment options.

Continuation of treatment

Treatment continuation rates have been high in TD-OXY clinical trials. The initial phase III trial involved a 12-week TD-OXY evaluation, with a 12-week open-label period and an optional 28-week safety extension period.[24] Of the original

520 patients, 86% completed the double-blind period, 92% of eligible patients continued into the open-label period, and 87% of those completed the open-label period.[25] The second phase III trial had similar findings, with 89.9% completing the double-blind phase, and 79% enrolling in and 89% completing the open-label period.

The Multicenter Assessment of Transdermal Therapy in Overactive Bladder with Oxybutynin (MATRIX) study is a 6-month, open-label, randomized, multicenter, prospective trial in a community-based population. This study is under way to assess safety, health-related quality of life, and other patient-reported outcomes in a large number of patients treated with TD-OXY. Study entry data are already being reported and providing useful data regarding the current demographics of the populations of those suffering from OAB.[26]

CONCLUSIONS

At a dose of 3.9 mg/day, TD-OXY administered in a twice-weekly regimen is an effective, safe, and well-tolerated treatment for patients with overactive bladder. Efficacy is comparable to that of other common pharmacologic treatment regimens: immediate release OXY in the phase II study, extended release OXY in the pharmacokinetic study, and tolterodine in the phase III study. OXY plasma levels are stable and correlate well with significant median reductions in the number of incontinence episodes and urinary frequency, along with an increase in voided volume. Most importantly, TD-OXY was associated with a low incidence of anticholinergic adverse events, particularly dry mouth, at a rate comparable to that with placebo. Since the high incidence of such side effects often causes patients to discontinue oral anticholinergics, the data demonstrate the unique properties of transdermal OXY delivery. Local application site reactions were generally mild, involving pruritus and erythema.

The pharmacokinetic data regarding TD-OXY further emphasize the role of the parent compound in achieving beneficial response regarding OAB symptoms, and the role of its metabolites in the development of effect-negating side effects. This may prove important in the development of future therapies for the treatment of OAB.

Patch size determines the OXY dosage delivered. As such, in its current formulation, a dosage requirement of greater than 3.9 mg/day would require a larger patch, or multiple patches, possibly increasing the rate of skin reactivity and/or making this treatment modality financially unsuitable. OXY lends itself to individualization in dosage, both on a chronic basis as well as for specific short-term usage. Since TD matrix dosing is dependent on patch surface area, many patients have increased their dosage by applying an extra patch or a portion of one.[27,28] The increased circulating OXY level can be expected to improve response rates, based on the previous phase II trial data. Other means of increasing circulating OXY include taking an additional oral dosage. This strategy has been utilized by taking half or one entire immediate release tablet, just prior to an activity when OAB symptoms would be particularly undesirable, such as airplane travel or going to a concert or opera. Rarely has extended release dosing been used for this purpose.

The use of an effective patch delivery system is well accepted by obstetricians/gynecologists and primary care physicians who are accustomed to other transdermal drug delivery applications. Urologists, on the other hand, are not as familiar with the use of matrix-type patches for drug delivery. Urologists should familiarize themselves with this novel delivery system and become aware of its potential benefits in terms of compliance with therapy due to ease of administration and reduced side effect profile.

Certain subgroups of patients will likely benefit to a greater degree from this drug delivery system. These include the elderly and those residing in nursing homes, those with a neurogenic bladder, and those with difficulty taking oral medications. No studies have yet been performed in children, and more studies are required in an adult male population. Future studies will be required to evaluate the use of TD-OXY in these subgroups.

REFERENCES

1. Levin RM, Wein AJ. Direct measurement of the anticholinergic activity of a series of pharmacological compounds on the canine and rabbit urinary bladder. J Urol 1982; 128: 396–8.

2. Kachur JF, Peterson JS, Carter JP et al. R and S enantiomers of oxybutynin: pharmacological effects in guinea pig bladder and intestine. J Pharmacol Exp Ther 1988; 247: 867–72.

3. Batra S, Biorklund A, Hedlund H, Andersson KE. Identification and characterization of muscarinic cholinergic receptors in the human urinary bladder and parotid gland. J Auton Nerv Syst 1987; 20: 129–35.

4. Nilvebrant L, Andersson KE, Gillberg PG, Stahl M, Sparf B. Tolterodine: a new bladder-selective antimuscarinic agent. Eur J Pharmacol 1997; 327: 195–207.

5. Wang P, Luthin GR, Ruggieri MR. Muscarinic acetylcholine receptor subtypes mediating urinary bladder contractility and coupling to GTP binding proteins. J Pharmacol Exp Ther 1995; 273: 959–66.

6 Nagy F, Hamvas A, Frang D. Idiopathic bladder hyperactivity treated with Ditropan (oxybutynin chloride). Int Urol Nephrol 1990; 22: 519–24.

7. Nilvebrant L, Sparf B. Different affinities of some anticholinergic drugs between the parotid gland and ileum. Scand J Gastroenterol 1982; 72 (Suppl): 69–77.

8. Anderson RU, Mobley D, Blank B et al. Once daily controlled versus immediate release oxybutynin chloride for urge urinary incontinence: OROS Oxybutynin Study Group. J Urol 1999; 161: 1809–12.

9. Davila GW, Daugherty CA, Sanders SW. A short-term, multicenter, randomized double-blind dose titration study of the efficacy and anticholinergic side effects of transdermal compared to immediate release oral oxybutynin treatment of patients with urge urinary incontinence. J Urol 2001; 166: 140–5.

10. Ranade VV. Drug delivery systems. 6. Transdermal drug delivery. J Clin Pharmacol 1991; 31: 401–18.

11. Zobrist RH, Schmid B, Feick A, Quan D, Sanders SW. Pharmacokinetics of the R- and S-enantiomers of oxybutynin and N-desethyloxybutynin following oral and transdermal administration of the racemate in healthy volunteers. Pharm Res 2001; 18: 1029–34.

12. Verma RK, Garg S. Current status of drug delivery technologies and future directions. Pharm Tech On-line 2001; 25: 1–14.

13. Bowen AJ, John VA, Ramirez ME, Good WR. Bioavailability of oestradiol from the Alora™ (0.1 mg/day) oestradiol matrix transdermal delivery system compared with Estraderm™ (0.1 mg/day). J Obstet Gynecol 1998; 18: 575–80.

14. Oxytrol™ package insert. Corona, CA: Watson Pharma, 2003.

15. Zobrist RH, Quan D, Thomas HM, Stanworth S, Sanders SW. Pharmacokinetics and metabolism of transdermal oxybutynin: in vitro and in vivo performance of a novel delivery system. Pharm Res 2003; 20: 103–9.

16. Appell RA, Chancellor M, Zobrist RH, Thomas HM, Sanders SW. Pharmacokinetics, metabolism, and saliva output during transdermal and extended-release oral oxybutynin administration in healthy subjects. Mayo Clin Proc 2003; 78: 696–702.

17. Dmochowski RR, Davila GW, Zinner NR et al. Efficacy and safety of transdermal oxybutynin in patients with urge and mixed urinary incontinence. J Urol 2002; 168: 580–6.

18. Dmochowski RR, Sand PK, Zinner NR et al. Comparative efficacy and safety of transdermal oxybutynin and oral tolterodine versus placebo in previously treated patients with urge and mixed urinary incontinence. Urology 2003; 168: 580–6.

19. Notelovitz M, Cassel D, Hille D et al. Efficacy of continuous sequential transdermal estradiol and norethindrone acetate in relieving vasomotor symptoms associated with menopause. Am J Obstet Gynecol 2000; 182: 7–12.

20. Weiss SR, Ellman Hdolker M. A randomized controlled trial of four doses of transdermal estradiol for preventing postmenopausal bone loss: Transdermal Estradiol Investigator Group. Obstet Gynecol 1999; 94: 330–6.

21. Lopes P, Rozenberg S, Graaf J, Fernandez-Villoria E, Marianowski L. Aerodiol versus the transdermal route: perspectives for patient preference. Maturitas 2001; 38 (Suppl 1): S31–9.

22. Allan L, Hays H, Jensen NH et al. Randomised crossover trial of transdermal fentanyl and sustained release oral morphine for treating chronic non-cancer pain. BMJ 2001; 322: 1154–8.

23. Newman DK. Patient perceptions of new therapeutic options for the control of overactive bladder. Abstract presented at The Society of Urologic Nurses and Associates, 2003, San Antonio, TX.

24. Dmochowski RR, Davila GW, Sanders SW. Transdermal oxybutynin and controlled-release oral tolterodine in patients with positive treatment

effect to anticholinergic therapy for overactive bladder [Abstract]. Neurourol Urodyn 2002; 21: 380.

25. Data on file. Corona, CA: Watson Pharma, 2003.

26. Sand PK, Dmochowski RR, Goldberg RP, McIlwain M, Lucente VR. Does overactive bladder impact interest in sexual activity: baseline results from the MATRIX study. Int Urogynecol J 2005; 16 (Suppl 2): S122.

27. Zinner NR, Davila G, Anderson RP. Dose modulation using oxybutynin transdermal system for overactive bladder in older adults. J Am Geriatr Soc 2004; 52 (Suppl 1): S76–7.

28. Ruscin JM, Staskin DR, Sand PK et al. Dose modulation of oxybutynin transdermal system for overactive bladder. Consult Pharm 2004; 19: 938.

20

Strategies for data comparison for drugs used in the treatment of overactive bladder

Alan J Wein and Roger R Dmochowski

Introduction   •   How do antimuscarinics work?   •   Comparing data for overactive bladder treatment
•   Conclusions and suggestions

INTRODUCTION

Overactive bladder (OAB) is defined as a symptom syndrome characterized by urgency, with or without urge incontinence, usually with frequency and nocturia. Other descriptors for this symptom complex are the urge syndrome or urgency–frequency syndrome.[1] Patients with OAB represent a substantial proportion of patients with urinary symptomatology. One-third of them suffer from incontinence.[2] As compared with women with effort-related urinary incontinence, women with urgency-related incontinence have a poor overall quality of life, perhaps related to both the volume of urine lost as well as the unpredictable nature of the leakage.[3–5]

Multiple classes of pharmacologic agents are potentially useful (meaning that they have a mechanism which is plausible on paper) to clinically decrease bladder activation and contractility or decrease sensation and thereby treat OAB. In the United States, at least, only the antimuscarinics have been "approved" for use in the treatment of OAB, implying that a proof of principle has been satisfied with respect to therapeutic response. Some[6] have argued that, although statistically significant, the differences between antimuscarinic drugs and placebo in terms of treatment results are small, and may be of questionable clinical significance, especially in view of the fact that the differences between active drugs and placebo in terms of tolerability seem to be greater. The Committee on Pharmacology at the International Consultation on Incontinence (ICI), utilizing somewhat different methodology to assess clinical effectiveness[7] has made recommendations for the treatment of overactive bladder, finding the antimuscarinic drugs to be clinically useful. The ICI committee did have the advantage, in its latest report, of more contemporary data than were available to Herbison et al.,[6] and data which assessed not only individual symptoms and urodynamic findings but also quality of life instruments and global impression scales. Antimuscarinic drugs remain the first line pharmacological treatment for overactive bladder. There is no reason to expect these agents to cure the underlying disturbance, the pathophysiology of which, though widely discussed, has not been firmly established, except in the case of certain neurologic injuries or diseases, and, even then, the sensory activators, neural paths, and efferent mechanisms are still somewhat disputed.[8]

Uroselectivity

It is an unfortunate and inconvenient fact that there are no agents in clinical use whose actions are purely selective for the lower urinary tract

(LUT). This concept is embodied by the term "uroselective", a term to our knowledge introduced by Karl-Erik Andersson.[9,10] The majority of side effects attributed to drugs facilitating bladder storage (or emptying) are the collateral effects on organ systems that share some of the same neurophysiological or neuropharmacological characteristics as the LUT. The problem is how to affect LUT function without interfering with the function of other organ systems and how to lessen or eliminate the symptoms of OAB without disturbing normal micturition. In general, drug therapy for all LUT dysfunction is hindered by a lack of uroselectivity, which explains most problems dealing with the balance with efficacy and tolerability in the pharmacotherapy of OAB. Many of the drugs utilized can be highly effective; however, the adverse effects are dose dependent and can often limit the ability to exploit a given drug's therapeutic effect. Escalating dosages may indeed increase efficacy, but, more often than not, lead to increasing unwanted effects from other organ systems, which may result in not being able to achieve a therapeutic dose sufficient to relieve symptoms satisfactorily. Improvements in uroselectivity could be approached in a number of ways, including:

- receptor selectivity
- organ selectivity
- alterations in drug delivery, metabolism, and distribution.

To employ the concept of receptor selectivity, one must first be absolutely certain of the receptors that are involved in the afferent and efferent pathways responsible for producing the symptoms under consideration. With OAB, this has not been settled, and arguments still exist regarding concepts so basic as the involvement (or noninvolvement) in man of the M_2 receptor in normal and abnormal LUT function. The concept of receptor selectivity may be of little use unless the receptor is not expressed in other organs, or unless a receptor subtype exists which is specific for the organ being treated for its afferent or efferent connections. Organ specificity may indeed be the "Holy Grail" of drug therapy for OAB. The ideal organ-selective drug would exert desirable effects only on the bladder and/or the urethra, thus eliminating side effects. Theoretically, this

is obviously a very attractive concept, but practically and clinically, it is very difficult (currently impossible) to achieve. Alternative drug delivery systems may be helpful by increasing the target concentration of an agent (e.g. intravesical or intradetrusor or suburothelial therapy) or by changing the metabolism of a drug to lower the concentration of a metabolite particularly productive of side effects. Certain drugs or their metabolites may be prevented from gaining access to a potentially troublesome site of activity (e.g. the blood–brain barrier) either by virtue of their innate characteristics or by alteration. Given our current state of imperfection of knowledge in this area, it is important to distinguish the potential laboratory or theoretical effects from real clinical effects, both beneficial and adverse. Commercial or marketing claims of the superiority of one agent over another, based either on clinical studies or on theoretical edges, should be subject to strong scrutiny. This chapter will focus on drug comparison, specifically with reference to the antimuscarinic agents, although the general principles and concepts can be applied to the comparison of any type of agents, one to another. The concepts expressed here are a mixture of fact and personal opinion, and many are shared and have been extensively discussed by us and others.

HOW DO ANTIMUSCARINICS WORK?

It is interesting that there is no universal consensus on the mechanism of antimuscarinic action in the treatment of overactive bladder, even though this drug class is the only drug class approved for therapy of OAB, at least in the United States. It is one of those interesting situations which demonstrates that long-held theories are not necessarily correct simply because of their longevity, but should be subject to periodical scrutiny. The traditional view of why antimuscarinics are effective was that normal bladder contraction was caused by the release of acetylcholine from postganglionic parasympathetic nerves, which combined with muscarinic receptors on the detrusor smooth muscle to initiate the process of excitation contraction coupling, resulting in detrusor contraction. Since OAB was assumed to be a reflection only of involuntary bladder contractions, it seemed logical that the treatment should be directed towards the antagonism of this sequence of events. There are a couple of inconvenient facts that interfere with this hypothesis:

1. In the usual doses, antimuscarinics do not seem to affect emptying in patients with OAB unless they are on the verge of urinary retention, either because of bladder decompensation or because of severe outlet obstruction. In higher doses, they certainly can produce retention, and this is in fact the goal of treatment in the case of some patients with OAB (neurogenics who wet between intermittent catheterizations, for example).
2. In a patient with OAB in whom retention is not a goal, the antimuscarinics act during the filling/storage phase of micturition and not during the emptying/voiding phase.

Antimuscarinics could therefore act by one of the following mechanisms (or a combination):

1. Directly on the smooth muscle to inhibit an emptying contraction. This mechanism is most useful in the patient with neurogenic OAB who is on intermittent catheterization but who is wet between catheterizations. More often than not, high doses of antimuscarinics are necessary to achieve this. This mechanism may also be useful in the treatment of urgency-related urinary incontinence to facilitate the inhibition that is attributed to the pelvic floor contraction component of behavioral modification.
2. Directly on the detrusor smooth muscle to inhibit "micromotion", a phenomenon hypothesized to occur because of a leak of acetylcholine from the postganglionic parasympathetic nerves during filling/ storage.[11]
3. Directly on afferent receptors in the urothelium, the interstitium, or the detrusor muscle.

It may be that a particular agent exerts its therapeutic effects differently in different patients, depending on the pathophysiology of the OAB symptom syndrome in that particular patient. However, it should be acknowledged that there is no agreement at present as to the relative importance of the M_3 and M_2 receptor component in these activities.

COMPARING DATA FOR OVERACTIVE BLADDER TREATMENT

What do we want?

Ideally we would like clinical uroselectivity, which can be defined as achieving the desired effects on bladder function (primarily reduced urgency, frequency, nocturia, and urgency incontinence, when present, relative to systemic effects). It is an inconvenient fact that muscarinic receptors exist not only in the detrusor smooth muscle, bladder interstitium, and urothelium, but also in the salivary glands, the bowel, the iris and ciliary bodies, the lacrimal glands, the heart, and the central nervous system. The ideal drug, then, would be efficacious, tolerable, and safe, meaning that, through whatever mechanism, it would be selective for the lower urinary tract. However, the ideal drug would possess more characteristics than just those (Table 20.1). Tolerability refers to side effects which are commonly more annoying than hazardous, such as dry mouth, alterations in bowel function, headache, etc. Safety in this context would refer primarily to cognitive function, cardiovascular issues, and drug–drug interactions. Compliance/persistence is a term that refers to how likely the patient is to remain on treatment. This does not mean being given the drug in the context of a study, but how apt the patient is to renew his/her prescription, especially when some payment for this must come out of pocket. The fact is that persistence at the end of 1 year in that sort of situation ranges somewhere between 10% and 20% for this class of agents.[12] If there was one agent that was equal to the

Table 20.1   The ideal drug

Includes not just
- efficacy
- tolerability
- safety

But also
- compliance/persistence
- cost
- bother
  - to patient
  - to provider

others in all other categories, and was less expensive, this would obviously be the drug of choice. Bother refers, in the case of the patient, to problems with the drug, either tolerability or safety issues, and, in the case of the provider, problems with side effects, dosing issues, etc., engendering telephone calls and excess office visits.

The ICI assessment

The International Consultation on Incontinence has a committee on pharmacology which reviews the most relevant information obtained since the previous meeting, summarizes this, and makes recommendations regarding pharmacologic management, evaluating the drugs according to a modification of the Oxford Guidelines (Table 20.2).[7] Under the category of drugs used for the treatment of overactive bladder symptoms/detrusor overactivity, the committee's assessments are seen in Table 20.3. It should be remembered that these assessments were based on data available at the time of the meeting, and that at the time this volume is published, they will be by definition incomplete, since they do not include newer

antimuscarinic agents (fesoterodine, once daily trospium, for example) or considerably updated more voluminous information on other agents (e.g. botulinum toxin). Nevertheless, it is clear, from looking at the committee's assessments and the individual discussions under each agent,

Table 20.3   International Consultation on Incontinence 2004 Assessments[7]

	Grade	Level
Antimuscarinics		
Tolterodine	1	A
Trospium	1	A
Darifenacin	1	A
Solifenacin	2	A
Propantheline	2	B
Atropine, hyoscyamine	3	C
Drugs with mixed actions		
Oxybutynin	1	A
Propiverine	1	A
Dicyclomine	3	C
Flavoxate	2	D

Table 20.2   International Consultation on Incontinence Assessments. 2004: Oxford Guidelines (modified)

Level of Evidence

Level 1: Systematic reviews, meta-analyses, good-quality randomized controlled clinical trials
Level 2: Randomized controlled clinical trials, good-quality prospective cohort studies
Level 3: Case-control studies, case series
Level 4: Expert opinion

Grades of Recommendation

Grade A: Based on level 1 evidence (highly recommended)
Grade B: Consistent Level 2 or 3 evidence (recommended)
Grade C: Level 4 studies or "majority evidence" (optional)
Grade D: Evidence inconsistent or inconclusive (no recommendation possible)

that there is no agreement as to a "best" pharmacologic agent for OAB treatment, and that the committee considered all of the "1-A" agents within a certain spectrum, possessing different characteristics, but with no clear consensus regarding a winner with respect to "clinical effectiveness" (efficacy, tolerability, safety).

What and how do we measure?

The efficacy measures which have been utilized and published are seen in Table 20.4. Some require little explanation, such as urgency associated incontinence episodes. Others, such as urgency, may be more difficult to interpret, depending upon the explanation given to the study subjects as to what they should report and record as urgency. Urodynamic parameters, such as the volume to the first involuntary bladder contraction, cystometric bladder capacity, and bladder activity index, are most useful, in our opinion, prior to large scale clinical studies to corroborate positive effects on filling/storage. Because these studies are so variable, not only from day to day, but even on the same day in a given individual, our personal feeling is that they are all but useless for comparative studies and comparisons of one drug to another. Commonly reported tolerability measures are seen in Table 20.5. Again, it makes a difference, when trying to compare one study to another, to know the actual definition(s) utilized to explain to patients what they should report as the parameter under consideration. Safety measures (which may be more theoretical than real) (see below) are listed in Table 20.6.

The edge concept

After propantheline, the first commonly utilized pharmacologic agent for overactive bladder was oxybutynin. Tolterodine followed, and, when there were basically only two drugs on the market, it was relatively easy, though the arguments were not always correct and backed up by data, to argue that one drug was "superior" to another. Now there are multiple competitors, and the only consensus that can be reached is the fact that none of these are perfect. There may be some "edges"

that one agent has over another. However, we like to think of edges as being either real or theoretical. Real edges would consist of true and unarguable differences in efficacy, tolerability, safety, compliance, and persistence. Possible theoretical edges are listed in Table 20.7. Our personal opinion is that it is entirely correct to say that when theoretical edges do not translate to real edges, there are two possibilities:

1. The proper studies simply have not been done in the proper way to demonstrate these.
2. The edge is non-existent in clinical practice.

It seems to us that theoretical edges are most valuable in instances where real edges are arguable. This is an important aspect of what we have come to know as "marketing".

Comparing parameters

One has only to pick up one of the major (or non-major) urologic journals containing articles in which drug summaries or data are discussed to see direct or indirect comparisons of one agent to another based on specific quotations of data that relate to parameters which, when written on paper, sound the same. However, there are reasonable and unreasonable ways to compare parameters, one drug to another. Our personal opinion about some of these follows.

Comparing study to study

Barring head-to-head studies, we believe comparisons are essentially worthless unless the studies cited are exactly the same except for the agents utilized. In other words, apples to apples and not apples to oranges. This applies to all studies of single agents, whether blinded, placebo controlled, or open label, but in which one drug is not directly compared to another. If one is going to compare such an article in one journal to one in another journal, the baseline criteria of the two populations must be exactly the same and the conduct of the studies (all details) exactly alike. It goes without saying that it should be easier to obtain "dryness" in a less severely affected cohort. The number of naive (never receiving

Table 20.4 Efficacy measures: overactive bladder

Parameter	Per day	Per week	Mean	Median	Explanation
Urge incontinence episodes	✓	✓	✓	✓	
Total incontinence episodes	✓	✓	✓	✓	
Frequency (total)	✓	✓	✓	✓	Both counting incontinence episodes and not; Absolute and > 8
Frequency minus nocturia	✓	✓	✓	✓	Same as above
Interval between micturitions			✓		1440 (minutes)/number per day (mean)
Interval between micturitions				✓	Minutes between each (median). Time (minutes) from urgency to void/leak
Delay (warning) time			✓	✓	(Needs sexier name)
Nocturia	✓	✓	✓	✓	Awakened from sleep plus go back. Both counting incontinence episodes and not Absolute and > "normal"
Nocturia/voids	✓	✓	✓	✓	Number from going to bed until arising Both counting incontinence episodes and not Absolute and > "normal"
Volume/void			✓	✓	Absolute and increase from placebo Voluntary void only
Urgency episodes	✓	✓	✓	✓	Both counting incontinence episodes and not
Urgency assessment					Visual analog or 3- or 5-point scale
Pad number	✓	✓	✓	✓	Different types a problem
Pad weight	✓		✓	✓	Pad test? In other words, how to weigh (before or after changing?)
Quality of life					Which tool? KHQ, I-QoL, etc.
% dry (no UUI episodes)					Need baseline: 3 days? 7 days?
% dry (no incontinence whatever)			✓	✓	As a % of those with incontinence
% dry days for those with incontinence?			✓	✓	Same as above
% no urgency					3 days? 7 days?
% urge-free days			✓	✓	
Overall impression					Visual analog or 3- or 5-point scale

Changes expressed as absolute numbers and/or percentage change: need baseline numbers – these will differ. UUI, urge urinary incontinence; KHQ, King's Health Questionnaire; I-QOL, Urinary Incontinence Quality of Life Scale.

Table 20.5   Tolerability measures: overactive bladder

Parameter	Details
Discontinuations	Number (%) – and reason why?
Dry mouth	Number (%)
	Mild/moderate/severe (total and percentage; percentage of those with dry mouth)
	Percentage discontinuing because of it
	Quantitative? (i.e. "spit test" or others)
Constipation (can also term change in bowel habits but need to assess diarrhea, gas, etc. Should do, scale or parameters needed)	Mild/moderate/severe (total and percentage; percentage of those with constipation)
	Percentage discontinuing because of it
	Percentage starting or increasing laxatives
	Decrease in number of bowel movements, increase in consistency
Dry eyes	Percentage mild/moderate/severe
	Number/percentage discontinuing because of it
Headache	Percentage mild/moderate/severe
	Number/percentage discontinuing because of it
	How to measure? Subjective/objective

Table 20.6   Safety measures: overactive bladder

Parameter	Details
Blurred vision	Percentage mild/moderate/severe
	Number/percentage discontinuing because of it
Photophobia	Same as above
Mental status	Same as above. How to measure? Subjective/objective
Somnolence, confusion	Same as above. How to measure? Subjective/objective
Depression, recall	Same as above. How to measure? Subjective/objective
Dizziness, light-headedness	Same as above. How to measure? Subjective/objective
Cardiac	Tachycardia/palpitations
	Arrhythmias
	QTc interval
Drug–drug interactions	Liver metabolism issues
	Renal excretion issues

Table 20.7 Theoretical Edges (Possible)	

• Blood-brain barrier
• Cardiac issues
• Drug-drug interactions
   – Metabolic (liver)
   – Active tubular secretion (kidney)
 	
• Urine concentrations
	• Receptor profile
	   – M3 selective
	   – "Balanced"
	   – Relatively M3 selective
	• Uroselectivity
	   – Pick a model
	• Half Life Issues
	• Titratability

antimuscarinic therapy) and non-naive patients must be approximately the same in each group. Further, of the non-naive population, the percentages of those having achieved previous "success" must be exactly the same in order to make an accurate comparison of two agents. There should be the same percentage of men and women. Many feel that it is "easier" to make men with urgency urinary incontinence dry than women. Finally, it is difficult to compare strictly European to strictly US data, especially with respect to tolerability. It has always seemed to us that, as a rule, the number of complaints regarding tolerability are fewer in European studies than in US studies. Electronic diary keeping will result, in our opinion, in a higher placebo rate than simply written diary data. We think the reason for this, though unsubstantiated, is that electronic diary keeping, in effect, results in some behavioral modification (training effect), whereas written diaries, especially if all filled out for 1 week in a spare moment, do not. As mentioned previously, parameters must be defined in exactly the same way in order to draw any reasonable conclusions regarding superiority of one agent over another, with respect to any efficacy or tolerability parameter.

Initially, there were major arguments regarding whether mean or median data should be utilized, especially when looking at urgency incontinence episode reduction. Outliers can dramatically affect the mean, whereas the median is less affected. Generally, whatever the "bigger number" is, is chosen to demonstrate efficacy. For some reason, in the United States package insert, mean numbers only are listed for oxybutynin, tolterodine, trospium, and solifenacin. Median numbers are listed for darifenacin, and,

for the oxybutynin transdermal system, both mean and median numbers.

Many feel felt that one way to level the playing field when comparing one study to another, and the studies both used a placebo comparison, is to subtract the placebo number from the drug number. In certain circumstances, this is useful, but we think an equally or more useful parameter is to look at the drug/placebo ratio. It is clear one can come up with the same numerical difference between drug and placebo, and yet have the drug/placebo ratio considerably different. We like the idea of listing both the drug minus placebo difference and the drug/placebo ratio. In most instances we consider the latter more meaningful.

Theoretical edges

There are a number of theoretical edges (see Table 20.7) that are often cited to give one agent an advantage over the other. Recognizing that the following are my personal opinions only, nevertheless, we think that there is some merit in discussing these.

Receptor profile

Arguments abound with respect to the ideal receptor antagonist profile of an antimuscarinic agent for the treatment of overactive bladder. One can essentially divide the agents up into three overlapping groups. There is one agent that is relatively M_3 specific, and it should be recognized that relative is a relative term. Some people would consider a 10 : 1 receptor affinity ratio significant, others a 100 : 1 ratio, and still others would not consider receptor selectivity as anything less than over a 100 ratio. For a "relatively"

M_3 selective drug, it would obviously be a theoretical advantage to consider all aspects of lower urinary function, with respect to cholinergic receptors, as being regulated primarily or wholly by the M_3 receptor. For the group of drugs known as "balanced" receptor antagonists (referring primarily to a balance between M_3 and M_2 blockade characteristics), it is obviously advantageous to cite series that hypothesize a large role for the M_2 receptor in the pathophysiology of the overactive bladder symptom syndrome. There is a group of drugs that, at least on paper, are primarily M_3–M_1 blockade agents, and, for these agents, because of the possible central nervous system implications (see below), one sees little relating their specific receptor blockade spectra to clinical effectiveness.

Uroselectivity

Uroselectivity is defined above. It is helpful, on a theoretical basis, to have an experimental model documenting uroselectivity (more activity related to one bladder parameter than to inhibition of a function in another organ system), and to be able to relate this to some clinical parameter. When the only two drugs commonly utilized were oxybutynin and tolterodine, there was an experimental cat model in which tolterodine had more of an action on inhibiting bladder contractility than salivation, and this was correlated in print to a slightly lower incidence of dry mouth, though not in head-to-head studies.[13] Now, each of the six agents has a model in which they are "uroselective", though the models are different, and even the organ systems to which bladder parameters are compared may be different. These include the dog, the cat, the rat, the mouse, the guinea pig, and the rabbit.

The blood–brain barrier and central nervous system considerations

If a drug did have cognitive dysfunction issues, then that would obviously be a major disadvantage for that agent. On a theoretical basis, the factors that would be considered would include:

- whether the agent or any of its active metabolites pass across the blood–brain barrier
- whether, once in the central nervous system, the agent effectively blocks the so-called

"cognition receptor", the M_1 receptor, to a significant degree
- whether the agent is actively transported out of the central nervous system, e.g. by a P-glycoprotein system.

It is relatively easy to make a chart looking at the characteristics of the oral and transdermal antimuscarinics with respect to their propensities across the blood–brain barrier, based on lipophilicity, molecular size, polarity, and transport by a P-glycoprotein system. Receptor profile has been mentioned previously, and an agent with a significant M_1 blockade propensity on paper would seem to be at a competitive disadvantage in this regard. However, all of this remains a theoretical edge unless some cognitive dysfunction can be demonstrated with respect to an individual agent. Such a trial would ideally match one drug against another, at the usually utilized and maximal recommended dosages. A positive result would transform a theoretical edge in this regard to a real edge. In this regard, it must be remembered that drug trials with antimuscarinic agents are generally not carried out in a "real life" population. In other words, these are generally reasonably healthy individuals in all other respects than the diagnosis of overactive bladder. It may be that in a "real life" population (community use), especially older individuals with concomitant diagnoses and on other medications, such problems may be more manifest. There is evidence that the blood–brain barrier may be somewhat compromised in various pathologic states and in aging.[14] There is also evidence that suggests that individuals with a high "anticholinergic load" (medications which possess anticholinergic properties) are at greater risk for cognitive dysfunction.[15] Whether this translates, however, into an increased risk for such individuals for cognitive abnormalities with certain antimuscarinic agents, taken in therapeutic dosages, is a question that has not yet been answered, or even asked in a trial situation. A positive result would clearly turn a theoretical edge into a real one in this context. No such evidence exists at present.

Urine concentration

Antimuscarinics for overactive bladder are generally metabolized by the liver or/and excreted by the kidneys. With some agents, at least, a sufficient concentration of drug/active metabolites in the urine can be achieved to cause changes in detrusor responses in a laboratory stimulation. To prove that this urinary concentration added to the effect of the serum concentration of the agent, however, one would need to show that the effect is truly additive in terms of some efficacy parameter. To be a real edge, not only would the effect have to be additive to that produced by the serum concentration of the drug, but the overall efficacy of the drug would have to be demonstrated to be greater than another drug without a significant urine concentration, in terms of efficacy or onset of action. With respect to this latter parameter, it should be noted that the only way to prove "quicker onset of action" is to actually compare one drug to another, recording data with respect to efficacy and tolerability for every day past day zero.

Note, however, that a statistically significant numerical improvement at day 2 or 3 of treatment does not necessarily translate into a clinically significant result.

Cardiac issues

There is little question that antagonism of the M_2 receptor can result in tachycardia and palpitations. There is also little question that prolongation of a corrected QT (QTc) interval can predispose to a ventricular arrhythmia, torsade de pointes. Both issues have received substantial attention with respect to the antimuscarinics, and also other agents. A cardiac "safe" drug is obviously desirable, but this raises the question as to precisely what the added risk is for a given increase in resting or exercise heart rate, and the same for a given prolongation of the QTc interval. It is certainly true, with respect to each of these parameters, that it is the outlier population that would be at greater risk, and so not just the mean increase or prolongation must be examined, but also the outliers. Could unreported cases of "sudden" death represent such instances? Perhaps, but there is no current evidence that this is the case. When discussing this topic, one must be very careful to see that the line is not crossed between reporting real data and established associations, and speculation.

Drug–drug interactions

It is possible for drug–drug interactions to occur with antimuscarinic agents, either on the basis of liver metabolism or competition for active tubular excretion in the kidneys. Drugs that are metabolized by the cytochrome system in the liver certainly have a theoretical risk of being either the perpetrator or the victim in a drug–drug interaction with another agent sharing similar enzymatic degradation, and, likewise, the same considerations apply to agents actively excreted by the renal tubules. It is certainly logical to theorize that the more such agents an individual is actively taking, the more subject an individual would be to such drug–drug interactions. However, to our knowledge, there has never been reported a significant drug–drug interaction with an antimuscarinic agent used for the treatment of overactive bladder in which the antimuscarinic agent has either been the perpetrator or the victim. This does not mean that such instances have not occurred, only that they have not been recognized and/or reported.

Half-life issues

Theoretically, a drug with a substantially longer half-life would take longer to build up a stable serum concentration, and it would take longer for the drug to "wash out" once administration was stopped. In the former case, one might expect the onset of action to be slower, and in the latter case, one might expect a significant side effect to take longer to dissipate than with a drug with a shorter half-life. Although all of this sounds logical, in order to make this claim a clinically meaningful one, one would have to prove that the onset of a significant clinical action of such a drug was in fact substantially delayed over that of other agents with a shorter half-life, and one would have to prove that a particularly bothersome side effect took significantly longer to dissipate to the point where it was not so significant. Otherwise, these issues remain, in our opinion, theoretical. On the other hand, one cannot make the claim that, with a drug possessing a longer half-life, it is fine to skip a dose or miss a dose every now and then, because the long half-life would "protect" the serum level from varying significantly under those circumstances. Again, unless one can definitely substantiate that claim with data, it remains an unproven assertion.

Titratability or flexible dosing

Our feeling is that an individual provider is either a "flexible dosing person" or not. Some people like the idea of being able to give different doses of a compound without significantly increasing the cost (one pill), while others like the concept of that one dose fits all. It seems to us, however, that if one is going to use flexible dosing correctly, the instructions or regimen must be quite clear, including: (1) the time after which the initial assessment should be made; (2) whether there is a population of individuals who should be started directly on the larger or one of larger doses of the drug. The idea behind flexible dosing seems logical. Start the patient on an initial dose, evaluate. If the patient does not have tolerability issues, and if the efficacy results have been such that greater efficacy is desired, move the patient to the higher dose. Do not move the patient to the higher dose if tolerability issues are encountered at the lower dose, or if the effect at the lower dose is sufficient for patient satisfaction.

Looking good

Although no one likes to admit it, there are ways to maximize data presentation to favor a given compound. Some of these, derived from observations as editors, and from various writings and texts follow:[16]

1. Find a theoretical edge. Try and find something that looks like a surrogate endpoint, even in a laboratory animal, that supports this.
2. Select the clinical populations for trials carefully, to show maximum efficacy and tolerability.
3. Redefine terms if necessary to either maximize or minimize effect, with respect to both efficacy parameters and tolerability parameters.
4. Carefully select data for citation and comparison. Always use your best and someone else's worst. "Cherry pick" data from different studies. Compare raw numbers or percentages if favorable. De-emphasize the placebo rates if unfavorable.
5. Completer studies always give a better result than intention to treat studies. A completer study is a study in which all individuals who drop out of the study are excluded. Since one would logically assume that a number of people drop out, not just because of protocol violations, but either because of lack of efficacy, poor tolerability, or both, this is generally favorable to the agent under consideration. An intention to treat study utilizes the data from all patients entering into the study, and utilizes a principle called last observation carried forward, which means that the last set of data available at the time the patient dropped out of the study are the data utilized. Persistence studies, usage studies, and switch studies are generally completer studies. Persistence studies perhaps constitute the most egregious misuse of the completer concept. Patients who come off a variety of studies with an agent are offered the opportunity to go on active agent (some of these will have been on placebo) and remain on this agent for long periods of time, with periodic visits. Any patients who drop out are excluded from data analysis. Claims result as to (1) the percentage of patients who actually stay on the drug; (2) how well the drug maintains its effect; (3) the long-term quality of life improvement. Clearly, with respect to each parameter, the bias inherent in doing the study this way is prejudicial to a favorable result.
6. "Usage" studies: a usage study translates into the ultimate completer study, generally without the aid of a placebo control. This is sometimes called a "seeding" study. A group of physicians, known to prescribe high numbers of a particular agent, are selected to enroll patients in a clinical study which looks at efficacy and tolerability of an agent without a placebo control. In this situation, results are generally quite good and, for the purpose of comparison with other agents, quite meaningless, in my opinion. Some feel that such studies are simply to introduce practitioners to prescribing a particular medication.

Table 20.8 Summary sheet

	30 Efficacy	10 Serum level	10 Metabolism	10 Salivary	10 Bowel	10 CNS	10 Ocular	10 Other	100 Total
Darifenacin									
Fesoterodine									
Oxybutynin									
Oxybutynin transdermal									
Propiverine									
Solifenacin									
Tolterodine									
Trospium									

Table 20.9 Summary sheet variation

	Efficacy UI episodes	Efficacy urgency	CNS		Cardiac		Dry mouth	Constipation	Drug–drug interaction		Dosing
			T	R	T	R			T	R	
Darifenacin											
Fesoterodine											
Oxybutynin patch											
Oxybutynin XL											
Solifenacin											
Tolterodine LA											
Trospium											

++, great advantage; +, advantage; ±, no real advantage or disadvantage over other drugs; −, disadvantage; −−, great disadvantage; 0, little information.
T, theoretically; R, realistically.

7. "Switch" studies: this is somewhat similar to a usage study, especially if no placebo control is utilized. High prescribing practitioners are generally recruited to enroll patients in a study, part of the entry criteria of which is that the patients have been on another particular agent, which they have discontinued, generally for a variety of reasons. Usually this translates to a completer study, and the results are generally quite good, with the claim generally being made that drug A succeeds in instances where drug B has failed. We do not recall ever seeing a negative result.

8. Devise a new parameter. This could be a single parameter or a particular scale, either related to a single efficacy parameter, such as urgency, or an overall composite score or index. All of us in the field recognize that an accepted and agreed upon "therapeutic index", which takes into consideration efficacy, tolerability, and safety, would be extremely desirable, but only if such an index were easily adaptable to the parameters in any clinical study. Such an index could truly facilitate comparison of one drug to another. If someone simply devises a new parameter or scale and no one else uses it, then, by definition, they are certainly the best with respect to that one parameter or scale.

9. Favorably compare a drug, with respect to one parameter, with another agent, where the second agent (comparator) is an "easy kill". Then, in discussion, imply that the drug is best in class with respect to that particular attribute.

10. Maximize the effect in all figures. There are obviously different ways of picturing a range that goes from 0 to 0.1, for example. If variation brackets make a comparison less favorable, leave them out.

11. If all else fails, do a data dump. One out of 20 times something significant will be found with a *p* value of less than 0.05.

12. Do not adjust for baseline differences if unfavorable.

13. If outliers help the results, leave them in; if they hurt, eliminate them.

14. If confidence intervals make a comparison less favorable, leave them out.

CONCLUSIONS AND SUGGESTIONS

In our opinion, there is presently no ideal drug for the treatment of overactive bladder. The individual informed provider will have to make up his/her mind with respect to comparisons between efficacy, tolerability, and safety parameters between the agents available. Currently, there are a number of antimuscarinic agents that exhibit proof of principle, but the individual practitioner is left to a perusal of journal articles, continuing medical education (CME) or promotional talks, and detail pieces to decide which drug or drugs will be his/her first choice. We have two suggestions. One is to construct a summary sheet of sorts, such as pictured in Table 20.8. We have simply arbitrarily assigned a maximum number of points for different parameters, a perfect score being 100. The category "Other" refers to items such as skin reactions, etc., which may be unique to a given product, at least in the mind of the provider. We have listed a variation of this system in Table 20.9. Here, one would look at the potential attributes of an agent with respect to various parameters related to efficacy, tolerability, and safety, and categorized, whether in one's mind one drug has an advantage over another, or is disadvantaged with respect to this parameter, or whether there is no particular advantage/disadvantage with respect to this one parameter. Until we have something that approximates to a "therapeutic index", that all agree upon, which can be easily utilized in every clinical study, we will have to deal with a situation in which there are multiple claims and counter-claims with respect to theoretical and real advantages, the practitioner being left to sort these out on his/her own. Hopefully, this chapter has given some insight as to how to go about this.

REFERENCES

1. Abrams P, Cardozo L, Fall M et al. The standardisation of terminology of lower urinary tract function: Report from the Standardisation Subcommittee of the International Continence Society. Neurourol Urodyn 2002; 21: 167–78.

2. Stewart W, Van Rooyen JB, Cundiff G et al. Prevalence and burden of overactive bladder in the United States. World J Urol 2003; 20: 326–36.

3. DuBeau CE, Levy B, Mangione CM et al. The impact of urge urinary incontinence on quality of life, importance of patients' perspective and explanatory style. J Am Geriatr Soc 1998; 46: 683–92.

4. Kobelt G, Kirchberger J, Malone-Lee J. Quality of life aspects of the overactive bladder and the effect of treatment with tolterodine. BJU Int 1999; 83: 583–90.

5. Simeonova Z, Milsom I, Kullendorff AM et al. The prevalence of urinary incontinence and its influence on the quality of life in women from an urban Swedish population. Acta Obstet Gynecol Scand 1999; 78: 546–51.

6. Herbison P, Hay-Smith J, Ellis G, Moore K. Effectiveness of anticholinergic drugs compared with placebo in the treatment of overactive bladder: systematic review. Br Med J 2003; 326: 841–4.

7. Andersson K-E, Appell R, Cardozo L et al. Pharmacological treatment of urinary incontinence. In: Abrams P, Cardozo L, Khoury S, Wein A, eds. Incontinence. Plymouth, UK: Health Publication Ltd, 2005: 809–54.

8. Abrams P, Drake M. Overactive bladder. In: Wein A, Kavoussi L, Novick A, Partin a, Peters C, eds. Campbell-Wash Urology. Philadelphia, PA USA: Elsevier Inc, 2007; 2079–90.

9. Andersson K-E. The overactive bladder: pharmacologic basis of drug treatment. Urology 1997; 50: 74–84.

10. Andersson K-E. The concept of uroselectivity. Eur Urol 1998; 33 (Suppl 2): 7–11.

11. Andersson KE. Antimuscarinics for the treatment of overactive bladder. Lancet Neurol 2004; 3: 46–53.

12. Levy R, Muller N. Urinary incontinence: economic burden and new choices in pharmaceutical treatment. Adv Ther 2006; 23: 556–73.

13. van Kerrebroeck P, Kreder K, Jonas U, Zinner N, Wein A. Tolterodine Study Group. Tolterodine once daily: superior efficacy and tolerability in the treatment of the overactive bladder. Urology 2001; 57: 414–18.

14. Kay G, Granville L. Antimuscarinic agents: implications and concerns in the management of overactive bladder in the elderly. Clin Ther 2005; 27: 127–38.

15. Ancelin ML, Artero S, Portet F et al. Nondejenerative mild cognitive impairment in elderly people and use of anticholinergic drugs: Longitudinal cohort study. Br Med J 2006; 332: 455–59.

16. Greenhalgy T. How to read a paper: the basics of evidence based medicine. Oxford, UK: Blackwell publishing, 2006.

21

Pharmacotherapy of overactive bladder in bladder outlet obstruction

Jonathan Sullivan and Paul Abrams

Introduction • Is it safe to use antimuscarinics in men with lower urinary tract symptoms suggestive of bladder outlet obstruction? • Do antimuscarinics alleviate symptoms in men with lower urinary tract symptoms suggestive of bladder outlet obstruction? • Should antimuscarinics be used in conjunction with treatment to reduce bladder outlet obstruction? • Other treatment options • Future research • Conclusions

INTRODUCTION

Histological benign prostatic hyperplasia (BPH) is common in aging men.[1] BPH may progress to cause benign prostatic enlargement (BPE), and cause benign prostatic obstruction (BPO), which is frequently associated with lower urinary tract symptoms (LUTS). These may include voiding symptoms such as poor flow and hesitancy, and storage symptoms characteristic of overactive bladder (OAB), such as urgency and frequency.[2] Traditionally, pharmacotherapy for LUTS in older men has centered on treatments whose primary aim is to reduce the severity of bladder outlet obstruction (BOO), with the intention of relieving all symptoms, regardless of whether storage or voiding symptoms predominate.

Many older men with LUTS have BOO on urodynamic testing, but around 40–70% of these patients also have detrusor overactivity (DO).[3–5] Although the most bothersome LUTS are the OAB symptoms such as frequency and urgency,[2] until recently the received wisdom was that "treatment with anticholinergic agents for detrusor instability related to obstruction is inappropriate and often precipitates urinary retention" (McGuire, cited by Kaplan et al.[6]).

Most clinicians therefore consider alpha-blockers and 5α-reductase inhibitors as the standard starting points for the pharmacotherapy of LUTS in older men, in those patients not responding to conservative measures such as fluid restriction, avoidance of caffeine, and so on. In selected men with more normal flow rates and little or no residual urine, particularly younger men with predominant OAB symptoms, it is reasonable to use antimuscarinics as primary treatment, but in general antimuscarinics would only be considered if the patient fails to respond to an alpha-blocker. Data are now emerging which suggest that the role of antimuscarinics should be reconsidered.

This chapter reviews the current evidence for the use of antimuscarinics as a treatment for LUTS in men with likely or proven BOO. Three key questions about the use of antimuscarinics are considered:

- are they safe?
- do they help?
- can they be used safely without additional drug treatment to reduce BOO?

Until the last few years there has been no evidence base to answer these questions, but a series of recent studies has started to provide some answers. The discussion centers on the use of antimuscarinics, but also includes some discussion of possible alternative treatments and of future research needed in this area.

IS IT SAFE TO USE ANTIMUSCARINICS IN MEN WITH LOWER URINARY TRACT SYMPTOMS SUGGESTIVE OF BLADDER OUTLET OBSTRUCTION?

For many years, the assumption has been that the answer to this question is a definite "no". Most modern randomized controlled trials of antimuscarinics include a proportion of men, usually about 20–30% of the total number of subjects, and allow an age range up to 75 or 80 years. However, in order to restrict the study population to those with idiopathic detrusor overactivity (DO) and presumably to avoid the presumed risk of provoking retention, it is standard practice to exclude patients from these trials with a suspicion of bladder outlet obstruction, defined by, for example, "clinically significant obstruction", "significant voiding difficulties", "retention", or large residual urine, typically defined as a post-void residual (PVR) of > 200 ml.[7,8] For this reason, data on the use of antimuscarinics in men with LUTS suggestive of BOO have not been available until trials have been undertaken specifically to study this group of patients. These trials are reviewed below.

Combined therapy with alpha-blockers and anticholinergics

Athanasopoulos et al. reported a study of 50 men aged 52–80 years in a 3-month study comparing tamsulosin monotherapy 0.4 mg once daily (group 1) against combination therapy with tamsulosin plus tolterodine 2 mg twice daily (group 2).[9] Patients included had mild or moderate obstruction (Schafer groups 2 and 3), and proven DO. Group allocation was randomized, but there was no blinding. Assessment of response was by the Urolife™ BPH quality of life questionnaire translated into Greek, and by repeated urodynamic studies.

There were no episodes of retention in either group. Two patients in group 2 stopped tolterodine due to dry mouth. This study suggests that the addition of tolterodine to tamsulosin is safe in the short term, but it should be noted that

patients with severe obstruction (not defined) were specifically excluded from the study.

KS Lee et al. studied 228 men aged 50–80 years with proven BOO on urodynamics, and with frequency (nine or more voids per 24 hours) and urgency episodes at least once per day.[10] Patients were excluded if the post-void residual was > 30% of the maximum cystometric capacity on baseline urodynamics. This was an 8-week, randomized, double-blind, multicenter study, with 1:2 randomization between monotherapy with doxazosin controlled release 4 mg once daily (group 1), versus combination therapy doxazosin 4 mg once daily plus propiverine 20 mg once daily (group 2). Symptoms were assessed by the International Prostate Symptom Score (IPSS).

There were no episodes of retention in either group during the study, but two patients in group 2 were withdrawn from the study due to a rise in PVR during the study to > 50% of voided volume (i.e. bladder voiding efficiency < 67%). The average PVR increased significantly in group 2 (from 29 to 50 ml, $p < 0.002$). The only significant difference in incidence of side effects was for dry mouth: 6% in group 1, 18% in group 2, $p < 0.05$, although less than a third of the affected patients in each arm discontinued the study as a result of dry mouth.

It should be noted that the majority of patients studied (50–60%) fell into the equivocal range of obstruction as defined by an Abrams–Griffiths (AG) number [now termed the bladder outlet obstruction index (BOOI)[11] of 20–40. Further-more, only 35% of the total sample had DO. Although this possibly calls into question the proportion of patients who might benefit from antimuscarinics, there is some evidence that women with symptoms of OAB but without DO on urodynamics respond to antimuscarinic therapy at the same rate as women with proven DO.[12] The typical patient in this study was only mildly obstructed and tended not to have DO. Extrapolating these results to the broader population of older men with LUTS may not be appropriate.

JY Lee et al. reported a non-blinded, non-randomized study of 144 men with BOO, comparing doxazosin monotherapy against combination therapy with doxazosin plus tolterodine.[13] The patients were divided on the basis of baseline urodynamics into those with BOO alone, and those with BOO and OAB. The design incorporated an initial 3-month period on doxazosin 2–4 mg once daily, followed by an assessment of response. For those not improved on alpha-blockers alone, tolterodine 2 mg twice daily was then added for a further 2 months, followed by reassessment.

A total of 60 patients went on to combined treatment, compared to 84 maintained on alpha-blockers alone due to satisfactory clinical response. No details of the severity of obstruction were given, other than that the AG numbers were "similar" between groups. Men with PVR > 150 or "severe obstruction" on screening were excluded (over 30% of the patients screened). Patients with OAB and BOO were older, had a higher IPSS (25 vs. 21.5) and prostate volume (35 vs. 29 ml), but no difference in prostate specific antigen (PSA) or peak flow (Q_{max}). Response was assessed simply by changes in IPSS after 3 months on alpha-blocker, and again at 5 months after further alpha-blockers or combination therapy. Reported side effects included a 27% incidence of dry mouth in those on combined therapy. Two of 16 patients with dry mouth reported it as severe and discontinued the antimuscarinics. Temporary acute retention occurred in two of 60 men (3.3%) on combined therapy. Both of these rapidly resolved after overnight catheterization and stopping antimuscarinics.

Okada et al. reported, in abstract form, the addition of propiverine to alpha-blockers in 35 patients with predominantly OAB symptoms who failed to respond to alpha-blockers alone.[14] During 12 weeks of treatment there were no cases of urinary retention requiring catheterization. PVR did not change significantly.

Antimuscarinic monotherapy

Abrams et al. compared antimuscarinic monotherapy against placebo in a recent study.[15] A total of 222 men were randomized 2 : 1 between treatment with tolterodine 2 mg twice daily or placebo for 12 weeks in a multicenter study of men aged 40 years or older with frequency (> 8 voids per 24 hours), urgency with or without incontinence, urodynamically confirmed DO, and mild to severe obstruction (BOOI $\geq$ 20). Exclusions included PVR > 40% of maximum cystometric capacity and urinary retention within the preceding 12 months.

Only one episode of acute urinary retention (AUR) was seen during the study period, in the placebo group, with none in the tolterodine group. However, two patients on tolterodine were withdrawn due to a high PVR (320 ml in one, undefined in the other). A number of other patients in each group had other changes in voiding symptoms, with no significant difference in incidence between groups.

There was no significant difference in the overall incidence of adverse events. Dry mouth was common amongst the tolterodine treated patients (24%) compared to placebo (1%), but only one of 36 patients with dry mouth considered it severe. Total urinary system adverse events were comparable between groups (13% vs. 13%). Urodynamics results showed evidence of fairly small treatment differences due to tolterodine for bladder contractility index (BCI):[11] −10 ($p < 0.005$); voiding efficiency: −7% ($p < 0.02$); and PVR: +27 ml ($p < 0.004$). Significant reductions were seen in $PdetQ_{max}$ (detrusor pressure at Q_{max}) due to tolterodine, with a difference between groups of −7 cmH$_2$O.

On central review, 7% of patients were considered unobstructed, and 33% equivocal (or mildly obstructed). In contrast to the study by KS Lee,[10] the typical patient in this study was moderately obstructed with proven detrusor overactivity.

It seems reasonable to conclude that tolterodine is relatively safe as monotherapy in patients with BOO and DO, at least over a 12-week period. As patients with severe obstruction were included, it is a little easier to generalize the finding, although the safety of tolterodine in men with moderate or large residual urine has not been established. While there were no episodes of AUR in the tolterodine group, two patients were withdrawn due to high PVR. It is not clear whether the baseline characteristics of these patients were suggestive of a higher risk of retention, e.g. higher baseline PVR, larger prostate, etc. Monitoring of PVR may be needed when using antimuscarinics as monotherapy, at least for selected patients.

Kaplan et al. have recently published a prospective open-label study using tolterodine extended release (ER) 4 mg once daily for 6 months as monotherapy in men with LUTS and "BPH" who failed on various alpha-blockers at a mean 5.7 months, due either to side effects (26%) or lack of efficacy (74%).[6] A total of 43 men aged between 50 and 83 years were recruited, with

IPSS $\geq$ 8 points, maximum flow rate 4–15 ml/s, and "BPH" on digital rectal examination (DRE). Four men discontinued tolterodine due to side effects (dry mouth). There was no significant change in erectile or ejaculatory function. There were no cases of urinary retention over 6 months, the longest follow-up reported in the literature to date.

DO ANTIMUSCARINICS ALLEVIATE SYMPTOMS IN MEN WITH LOWER URINARY TRACT SYMPTOMS SUGGESTIVE OF BLADDER OUTLET OBSTRUCTION?

Combined therapy with alpha-blockers and antimuscarinics

JY Lee et al. specifically assessed the effect of adding antimuscarinics to patients failing to respond to alpha-blockers.[13] The results suggested that the likely response to alpha-blockers was predicted by whether or not the patients had BOO alone, or whether they also had OAB, defined by Lee et al. as the presence of DO with involuntary detrusor contractions (IDCs) of > 10 cmH$_2$O on urodynamics. Of patients with BOO alone, 79% were clinically improved with alpha-blockers alone, against only 35% of those with BOO and DO. In those not responding to alpha-blockers alone, the addition of tolterodine was associated with clinical improvement in 38% in the BOO only group, and 73% of the BOO and DO group. Total IPSS was the only assessment of response reported in this study.

Athanasopoulos et al. reported only changes in quality of life as a measure of subjective outcome, without any other assessment of symptoms by questionnaire.[9] However, they also reported urodynamic data before and after treatment. In those treated with tamsulosin alone, there was a significant increase in maximum flow rate ($+1.2$ ml/s, $p = 0.0001$) and in volume at first IDC, from baseline ($+30$ ml, $p < 0.02$). Other variables did not change significantly on tamsulosin alone. For the group on tamsulosin and tolterodine, there were significant increases in Q$_{max}$ ($+1.3$ ml/s, $p = 0.002$) and in volume at first IDC ($+100$ ml, $p < 0.0001$); and there were significant decreases in maximum Pdet during micturition (-8.3 cmH$_2$O, $p < 0.01$) and maximum amplitude of IDC (-11.2 cmH$_2$O, $p < 0.0001$). Comparison between groups showed only significant differences for lower volume at first IDC, lower maximum IDC, and higher bladder capacity in favor of tolterodine. Urolife™ quality of life scores were significantly improved from baseline in the combined treatment group ($p = 0.0003$), but not after treatment with tamsulosin alone ($p = 0.836$). It is not clear why there was no improvement in quality of life in those on alpha-blockers alone.

KS Lee et al. report a different combination of alpha-blocker and antimuscarinics, comparing doxazosin monotherapy against doxazosin plus propiverine.[10] From voiding diary data significant changes in favor of combined therapy were noted for daytime frequency, total voiding frequency (but not nocturia on its own), and mean voided volume. There was no difference in total IPSS between groups, but there were significant differences between the groups in storage symptom total (IPSS questions 2, 4 and 7), and in urgency score (IPSS question 4). There was no difference in the overall bother score, but patient global satisfaction scores were significantly higher in the combined therapy group. The data provided do not include estimates of treatment effect.

Okada et al. studied patients with predominantly OAB symptoms, with non-responders to alpha-blockers treated by the addition of propiverine hydrochloride.[14] The storage symptom components of the IPSS all improved significantly, by around 40%, and there was a significant increase in Q$_{max}$ (8.7 to 9.5 ml/s) and voided volume (98 to 130 ml). The quality of life (QoL) score also improved significantly, by about 30%.

Antimuscarinic monotherapy

Abrams et al. compared tolterodine against placebo over 12 weeks.[15] Clear treatment differences were noted, with a 59-ml increase in volume at first IDC ($p < 0.003$) and a 67-ml increase in cystometric capacity ($p = 0.0001$) attributable to treatment with tolterodine. One intriguing finding in this study was a statistically significant reduction in the BOOI from 49 to 40 in the tolterodine group, compared to no change in the placebo group, 43 to 44, $p = 0.01$. The authors found no obvious explanation for this finding.

Kaplan's recent study[6] showed significant improvements in American Urological Association (AUA) symptom scores (-6.1 points, $p < 0.001$)

with tolterodine ER 4 mg once daily for 6 months, but interestingly also found improved maximum flow rate ($+1.9$ ml/s, $p < 0.001$) and PVR (-22.0 ml, $p < 0.03$). All of these improvements were seen after only 1 month of treatment, but showed little change thereafter. Each of the seven individual AUA symptom score indices was significantly reduced at 6 months. When comparing the combined storage symptom domains against the combined voiding domains, there was no difference evident, with a decrease of about 35% for each of the combined domains. Voiding diary data showed significant reductions in nocturia (4.1 to 2.9 voids per night) and frequency (9.8 to 6.3 voids per day).

It should be noted, particularly with regard to symptom scores, that this was an open-label study, although the symptomatic results are largely consistent with other studies, and with more objective parameters. Patients were not tested urodynamically other than by flow rates, so neither BOO nor DO was confirmed in these patients. To that extent, the findings may be easier to generalize to routine urological practice, where urodynamic results will tend not to be available except when a patient is being considered for invasive therapy. The other strength of this study is that it offers the longest follow-up of any of the studies reported, albeit with a small number of patients.

SHOULD ANTIMUSCARINICS BE USED IN CONJUNCTION WITH TREATMENT TO REDUCE BLADDER OUTLET OBSTRUCTION?

As the possible role of antimuscarinics in men with LUTS suggestive of BOO has come to be recognized, a consensus seems to have evolved that bladder outlet resistance should be reduced by drug treatment (normally alpha-blockers) before adding anticholinergics.[16] Is this justified? Current evidence is insufficient to prove the contrary, but recent work suggests that concomitant treatment to reduce BOO may be unnecessary.

Recently published work from Abrams et al. provides more evidence.[15] It appears that tolterodine is relatively safe as monotherapy in patients with mild to severe obstruction over a period 3 months. However, patients with PVR over 200 ml were excluded. Safety has not been established for patients with high residual urine, or

for longer periods of treatment. Kaplan's study provides additional evidence that antimuscarinics can be used safely in isolation, with no retention over 6 months of follow-up.[6] In all of the remaining studies, all patients were on alpha-blockers, and therefore they are of no use in answering this question.

OTHER TREATMENT OPTIONS

Although the pharmacotherapy of OAB is centered on antimuscarinics, it is worth noting that alpha-blockers may have an effect on OAB itself, rather than simply an effect on OAB symptoms due to relief of obstruction. Several potential sites of action, other than bladder outlet smooth muscle, have been suggested for alpha-blockers.[17] Thus there may be an additive effect on OAB symptoms when patients are treated with a combination of alpha-blockers and antimuscarinics, in addition to an effect on the outlet.

A wide variety of other targets have been identified for possible future treatment of overactive bladder.[18–20] There is an increasing realization of the importance of the urothelium in detrusor overactivity, which may yield further new targets.[21] However, at present, the only pharmacotherapeutic options for treatment of DO in routine clinical practice are those aimed at muscarinic receptors, and there are no data to support the use of any other agents in men with probable BOO.

While there is a growing body of evidence on the efficacy of botulinum toxin injections as a treatment for DO refractory to antimuscarinics,[22] there are no data on its use in men with LUTS suggestive of BOO. It seems likely that such patients would be at a significant risk of retention after treatment. Also the cost-effectiveness of such treatment seems doubtful. Suitable patients may well be limited to a very small group with severe OAB symptoms who are able and willing to perform intermittent catheterization but are too unfit for outlet surgery. There may also be a role for botulinum toxin for the small number of men with severe, refractory OAB after surgical treatment of BOO.

FUTURE RESEARCH

The current literature consists of short studies, some of which have other limitations such as lack of blinding and/or randomization, small sample size, and so on. Pharmaceutical companies may well see a potential for expanding the use of antimuscarinics, and may be prepared to invest in longer, large scale studies to address some of the limitations of the existing literature. Several questions need to be answered:

1. Are antimuscarinics safe over longer follow-up?
2. Is monitoring of residual urine or other follow-up required, with associated additional costs?
3. If there are any doubts about the risk of retention in the longer term, does the addition of alpha-blockers or 5α-reductase inhibitors reduce the risk?
4. Is efficacy maintained over the long term?
5. Are all antimuscarinics equally effective?
6. Are antimuscarinics equivalent to, or even superior to, alpha-blockers as primary therapy for LUTS, particularly where OAB symptoms are predominant? A direct head-to-head comparison of alpha-blockers against antimuscarinics is needed.
7. Are antimuscarinics cost-effective in reducing symptoms over the longer term, particularly if combined treatment or additional follow-up is required?

CONCLUSIONS

Recent evidence suggests that, despite clinicians' natural concerns about the safety of antimuscarinics in men with probable BOO, the incidence of acute retention is low or zero in the short term, even in studies including patients with severe obstruction. However, it has not been established that antimuscarinics are safe in patients with larger residuals, or that they are safe in long-term use. While there is now good evidence for both safety and efficacy in patients with LUTS suggestive of BOO, the precise place of antimuscarinics amongst the various drug treatment options remains to be defined.

REFERENCES

1. Berry SJ, Coffey DS, Walsh PC, Ewing LL. The development of human benign prostatic hyperpllasia with age. J Urol 1984; 132: 474–9.

2. Peters TJ, Donovan JL, Kay HE et al. The International Continence Society Benign Prostatic Hyperplasia study: the bothersomeness of urinary symptoms. J Urol 1997; 157: 885–9.

3. de Nunzio C, Franco G, Rocchegiani A et al. The evolution of detrusor overactivity after watchful waiting, medical therapy and surgery in patients with bladder outlet obstruction. J Urol 2003; 169: 535–9.

4. Fusco F, Groutz A, Blaivas J G, Chaikin DC, Weiss JP. Videourodynamic studies in men with lower urinary tract symptoms: a comparison of community based versus referral urological practices. J Urol 2001; 166: 910–13.

5. Knutson T, Edlund C, Fall M, Dahlstrand C. BPH with coexisting overactive bladder dysfunction – an everyday urological dilemma. Neurourol Urodyn 2001; 20: 237–47.

6. Kaplan SA, Walmsley K, Te AE. Tolterodine extended release attenuates lower urinary tract symptoms in men with benign prostatic hyperplasia. J Urol 2005; 174: 2273–5.

7. Haab F, Cardozo L, Chapple C, Ridder AM. Long-term open label solifenacin treatment associated with persistence with therapy in patients with overactive bladder syndrome. Eur Urol 2005; 47: 376–84.

8. Kreder KJ, Brubaker L, Makar AA. Tolterodine is equally effective in patients with mixed incontinence and those with urge incontinence alone. BJU Int 2003; 92: 418–21.

9. Athanasopoulos A, Gyftopoulos K, Giannitsas K et al. Combination treatment with an alpha-blocker plus an anticholinergic for bladder outlet obstruction: prospective randomized controlled study. J Urol 2003; 169: 2253–6.

10. Lee K-S, Choo M-S, Kim D-Y et al. Combination treatment with propiverine hydrochloride plus doxazosin controlled release gastrointestinal therapeutic system formulation for overactive bladder and coexisting benign prostatic obstruction: a prospective, randomized, controlled multicenter study. J Urol 2005; 174: 1334–8.

11. Abrams P. Bladder outlet obstruction index, bladder contractility index and bladder voiding efficiency: three simple indices to define bladder voiding function. BJU Int 1999; 84: 14–15.

12. Malone-Lee J, Henshaw DJ, Cummings K. Urodynamic verification of an overactive bladder is not a prerequisite for antimuscarinic treatment response. BJU Int 2003; 92: 415–17.

13. Lee JY, Kim HW, Lee SJ et al. Comparison of dox-azosin with or without tolterodine in men with symptomatic bladder outlet obstruction and an overactive bladder. BJU Int 2004; 94: 817–20.

14. Okada H, Shirakawa T, Muto S et al. Propiverine hydrochloride relieves irritative symptoms of benign prostatic hyperplasia. J Urol 2004; 171 (4 Suppl): 357–8 (abstr).

15. Abrams P, Kaplan SA, De Koning Gans HJ, Miller EM. Safety and tolerability of tolterodine for the treatment of overactive bladder in men with bladder outlet obstruction. J Urol 2006; 175: 999–1004.

16. Gonzalez RR, Te AE. Overactive bladder and men: indications for anticholinergics. Curr Urol Rep 2003; 4: 429–35.

17. Ruggieri MR, Braverman AS, Pontari MA. Combined use of alpha-adrenergic and muscarinic antagonists for the treatment of voiding dysfunction. J Urol 2005; 174: 1743–8.

18. Andersson K-E, Pehrson R. CNS involvement in overactive bladder: pathophysiology and opportunities for pharmacological intervention. Drugs 2003; 63: 2595–611.

19. Chess-Williams R. Potential therapeutic targets for the treatment of detrusor overactivity. Expert Opin Therapeutic Targets 2004; 8: 95–106.

20. Andersson K-E, Wein AJ. Pharmacology of the lower urinary tract: basis for current and future treatments of urinary incontinence. Pharmacol Rev 2004; 56: 581–631.

21. Kumar V, Templeman L, Chapple CR, Chess-Williams R. Recent developments in the management of detrusor overactivity. Curr Opin Urol 2003; 13: 285–91.

22. Sahai A, Khan M, Fowler CJ, Dasgupta P. Botulinum toxin for the treatment of lower urinary tract symptoms: a review. Neurourol Urodyn 2005; 24: 2–12.

22

Botulinum toxin (Botox®)

Christopher P Smith and George T Somogyi

Introduction • Materials and methods • Background and pathophysiology • Clinical applications
• Mechanism of action • Clinical results • Injection techniques • Adverse events
• Resistance to toxin effects • Conclusion

INTRODUCTION

Botulinum toxin (BTX), first isolated by van Ermengem in 1895, is the most potent biological agent known to man.[1] BTX's mechanism of action has been traditionally described as inhibiting acetylcholine release at the presynaptic cholinergic junction. However, in later sections we will present evidence that BTX could inhibit other transmitter systems and cellular processes also thought to play an important role in the development of bladder overactivity. Clinically, the urologic community's initial experience with botulinum toxin A (BTX-A) was to treat bladder overactivity resulting from neurologic insult (i.e. spinal cord injury, etc.). Over the past few years, however, use of BTX-A has been expanded to treat patients with non-neurogenic overactive bladder (OAB). The rapid expansion in the use of BTX to treat OAB is due, in large part, to the inadequacy of current standard pharmacologic treatment (i.e. antimuscarinic agents) as well as to the demonstration of BTX's efficacy, durability, and tolerability in early clinical series. However, at the time of this writing, use of BTX in the bladder is Food and Drug Administration (FDA) off-label, and caution should be exercised until randomized clinical trials are completed. The purpose of this chapter is to review the mechanisms underlying the effects of botulinum toxin treatment and to summarize the current off-label usage of this agent to treat OAB, including clinical results, injection techniques, and adverse events.

MATERIALS AND METHODS

A Medline search from 1966 to 2006 was performed using the word "bladder" combined with the words "botulinum toxin". A total of 176 records were obtained and cross-referenced and demonstrated an exponential growth in the number of articles using these keywords as well as the number of patients treated with bladder BTX injection (Figures 22.1 and 22.2). We used only full manuscripts in this review from 2000 to the present, limiting the extent of our search to the year in which BTX was first described to treat OAB symptoms. Information was collected regarding indications for usage, study design, type of botulinum toxin, site of injection, dosage, efficacy, and adverse effects (local and systemic).

BACKGROUND AND PATHOPHYSIOLOGY

Botulinum poisoning was first described in cases of sausage intoxication in the late 1700s in Germany. A local medical officer collected data on 230 cases of botulism, and the illness became known as "Kerner's disease".[2] It was not until 1895 that van Ermengem isolated the spore-forming obligate anaerobic bacteria, *Clostridium botulinum*.[1]

Botulinum toxins are synthesized as single chain polypeptides with a molecular weight of around 150 kilodaltons (kDa).[3] Initially, the parent chain is cleaved into its active, dichain polypeptide form, consisting of a heavy chain

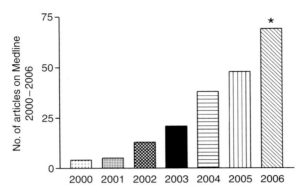

Figure 22.1 Bar graph demonstrating number of Medline citations using the keywords "botulinum toxin and bladder" between 2000 and 2006. *Signifies estimated number of citations for year 2006 at time of chapter submission.

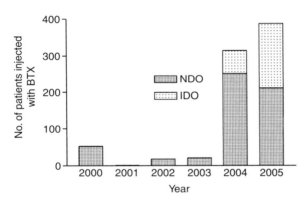

Figure 22.2 Bar graph depicting the actual number of patients treated with botulinum toxin (BTX) bladder injections between the years 2000 and 2005. NDO, neurogenic detrusor overactivity; IDO, idiopathic detrusor overactivity.

(approximately 100 kDa) connected by a disulfide bond to a light chain (approximately 50 kDa) with an associated zinc atom.[4] Four steps are required for toxin-induced paralysis: (1) binding of the toxin heavy chain to a specific nerve terminal receptor; (2) internalization of the toxin within the nerve terminal; (3) translocation of the light chain into the cytosol; and (4) inhibition of neurotransmitter release.

Structural studies have demonstrated that BTX-A's structure is characterized by three domains which directly guide its actions on target tissues.[5] For example, the heavy chain contains a

binding domain at its C-terminus that mediates BTX-A binding to neuronal cell membranes, and a translocation domain at its N-terminal end that is responsible for the creation of ion channels within the endocytosed vesicle. The vesicle channels allow BTX-A light chain passage into the neuronal cytosol.[6-8] The light chain contains a zinc-dependent endopeptidase catalytic domain that inhibits neurotransmitter exocytosis by cleaving specific proteins within presynaptic nerve terminals.[4,9]

Neurotransmitter release involves the adenosine triphosphate (ATP)-dependent transport of the vesicle from the cytosol to the plasma membrane.[10] Vesicle docking requires the interaction of various cytoplasmic, vesicle, and target membrane (i.e. SNARE: soluble N-ethylmaleimide-sensitive fusion attachment protein receptor) proteins, some of which are specifically targeted with clostridial neurotoxins. BTX-A, for example, cleaves the cytosolic translocation protein SNAP-25, thus preventing vesicle fusion with the plasma membrane (Figure 22.3).[9]

BTX-A treatment is a durable, yet reversible, treatment option as nerves eventually recover their original function. However, although the clinical effects of BTX-A in skeletal muscle spasticity typically last 3–4 months, longer durations have been observed following BTX-A injection in bladder smooth muscle (6 months). Similar clinical responses from BTX-A treatment in other autonomic disorders (e.g. axillary/palmar hyperhidrosis, gustatory sweating, sialorrhea) have been described (range 4–36 months), suggesting that differences in toxin effect or reinnervation may account for the more prolonged clinical responses observed in autonomic versus somatically innervated tissues.[11-13]

Recent studies have identified the binding site for the BTX-A heavy chain C-terminus to be a synaptic vesicle protein called SV2.[14] Because SV2 is a synaptic vesicle protein, its exposure on the surface of nerve terminals increases when more neurotransmitter is released. In this regard, BTX-A preferentially targets nerves that are more active. Similarly, the expression of SV2 is also inhibited by BTX-A intoxication, which ingeniously allows remaining extracellular toxin to bind to and inhibit unoccupied nerve terminals to induce a greater paralytic effect.

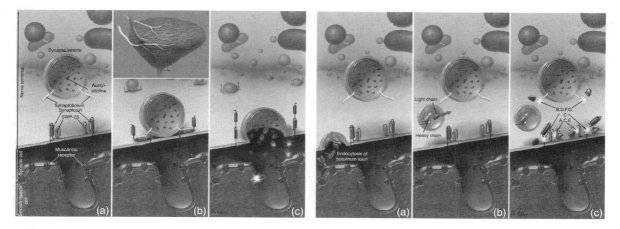

Figure 22.3 Schematic diagram demonstrating: (1) normal fusion and release of acetylcholine from nerve terminals via interaction of SNARE (soluble *N*-ethylmaleimide-sensitive fusion attachment receptor) proteins (left panel, a–c) and (2) binding, internalization, and cleavage of specific SNARE proteins by botulinum neurotoxins A–G (right panel, a–c). (See also color plate section).

CLINICAL APPLICATIONS

Seven immunologically distinct neurotoxins are known: types A, B, C, D, E, F, and G. Only botulinum toxin types A and B are commercially available worldwide. Currently, two types of botulinum toxin are available in the United States: type A (Botox®; Allergan, Irvine, CA) and type B (Myobloc®; Elan Pharmaceuticals, Inc., San Francisco, CA). Two other formulations of botulinum toxin A are available in Europe (Dysport®; Ipsen Ltd, Slough, United Kingdom; and Xeomin®; Merz Pharma GmbH, Frankfurt am Main, Germany). The potency of each toxin is expressed in units of activity.

Botox® is supplied as a vacuum dried powder and stored at or below −5°C. The vial contains 100 international units (IU) that are diluted with preservative-free normal saline to the desired final concentration. Manufacturer's instructions state that care must be taken to avoid agitation of the toxin while mixing to avoid foaming and possible loss of potency (Botox® product insert, Allergan, Inc., Irvine, CA). In addition, one is instructed to utilize the toxin within 4 hours of mixing, and one should never refreeze but should refrigerate unused portions of toxin. However, recent clinical studies have brought into question these recommendations. A recent multicenter, double blind study demonstrated no deterioration in clinical efficacy of Botox® when applied up to 6 weeks after reconstitution with saline.[15] In addition, a small study suggests that foam produced during agitated reconstitution does not affect the potency of botulinum toxin type A.[16] However, until larger or more sensitive studies more clearly identify the loss of toxicity with reconstitution, it is recommended that one mixes BTX-A solution with as little agitation and foaming as possible. Proper mixing includes limiting the rapid descent of the syringe plunger to the vacuum pull of the diluent and, once diluted, gently rotating and swirling the vial.[17,18] In contrast to BTX-A preparations, Myobloc® is already premixed in liquid form, and therefore does not have to be reconstituted with saline.

Botox® dosage is expressed in terms of international units, 1 IU representing the lethal dose (LD$_{50}$) to kill 50% of a colony of 10–20 Swiss Webster mice by intraperitoneal injection. However, preparations of BTX from different companies or different batches within a company may have variable potencies even if the same number of units is used, because lethal potency depends not only on the amount of toxin but also other biological factors that do not always correlate to therapeutic potency. For example, Botox® is comprised of 900-kDa neurotoxin complexes, whereas Dysport® is a mixture of 500–900-kDa neurotoxin complexes. Clinical observations reporting that Botox® is associated with a lower rate of adverse events than is Dysport®[19–21] are consistent with preclinical evidence suggesting that the larger, more uniform size of the Botox® neurotoxin complex protein (i.e. 900 kDa) minimizes unwanted migration and the development of adverse events.[22]

Thus, while Botox® has been reported to be three times as potent therapeutically as an equal amount of Dysport® and 50–100 times as potent as Myobloc (in LD_{50} units), differences in systemic effects versus muscle weakening ratios between these agents make it difficult to use a strict dose ratio when comparing these preparations.[23,24]

MECHANISM OF ACTION

Efferent effect

Smith and colleagues found significant decreases in the release of labeled acetylcholine (ACh) in BTX-A injected normal rat bladders, suggesting that BTX-A could reduce cholinergic nerve transmission.[25] Although BTX-A is known to exhibit cholinergic specificity, the release of other transmitters can be inhibited, particularly if adequate concentrations are utilized.[26–29] For example, contractile data suggest that BTX-A may impair ATP release in addition to acetylcholine (ACh) release from isolated bladder tissue.[30] These results have clinical significance in lieu of recent investigations into alterations in P2X receptor expression and increased purinergic bladder response in patients with idiopathic detrusor instability. In fact, O'Reilly and colleagues found that approximately 50% of the nerve-mediated contractions in bladder tissues extracted from patients with idiopathic detrusor overactivity were purinergic in origin.[31]

Afferent effect

BTX-A's efficacy in conditions of detrusor overactivity not only may result from an inhibitory effect on detrusor muscle, but some effects of the drug may be mediated by altering afferent (sensory) input. Urothelium possesses muscarinic receptor populations with a density twice as high as in detrusor smooth muscle, and dorsal root ganglionectomy experiments demonstrating the persistence of acetylcholinesterase staining nerves near the urothelium suggest that parasympathetic nerves supply some innervation to the urothelium.[32–34] Besides receiving cholinergic innervation, human urothelium has also been shown to release the neurotransmitter ACh at rest.[35] Thus, ACh, released from urothelium and acting on nearby muscarinic receptor populations (i.e. urothelium or afferent nerves) or neuronal sources of ACh binding to muscarinic receptors within urothelium or afferent nerves, could have a significant impact on bladder sensory input to the central nervous system and may be impacted by BTX treatment.

In addition, recent basic and clinical evidence suggests that BTX-A may have sensory inhibitory effects unrelated to its actions on ACh release. For example, an in vitro model of mechanoreceptor-stimulated urothelial ATP release was tested in spinal cord injured rat bladders to determine whether intravesical botulinum toxin A administration would inhibit urothelial ATP release, a measure of sensory nerve activation.[36] The results demonstrated that hypo-osmotic stimulation of bladder urothelium evoked a significant release of ATP that was markedly inhibited by BTX-A (e.g. 53%), suggesting that impairment of urothelial ATP release may be one mechanism by which BTX-A reduces detrusor overactivity. BTX-A has also been shown to inhibit release of neuropeptides such as calcitonin gene related peptide (CGRP), substances thought to play a role in OAB conditions such as sensory urgency or chronic bladder inflammation (i.e. interstitial cystitis).[37,38]

Inhibition of growth factor release and receptor expression

BTX-A's effects are not limited solely to inhibiting neurotransmitter release. In fact, any process that involves SNARE proteins and, in particular, SNAP-25, could be impacted by BTX-A treatment. For example, laboratory studies have shown that TRPV1 (i.e. capsaicin-sensitive) receptors and nerve growth factor are released by SNARE-dependent processes and can be inhibited by BTX-A treatment.[39,40] Clinically, studies in spinal cord injured human patients found that bladder hyperactivity as well as bladder nerve growth factor (NGF) tissue level was significantly reduced by bladder BTX-A

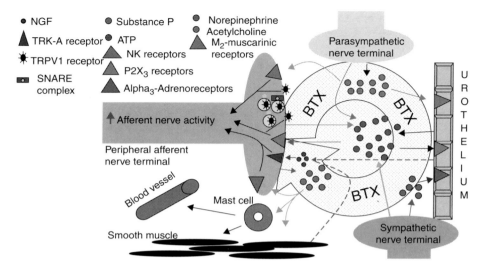

Figure 22.4 Illustration of mechanisms of action of botulinum toxin (BTX) in suppressing detrusor overactivity that include: (1) inhibiting acetylcholine or adenosine triphosphate (ATP) or norepinephrine release from parasympathetic nerves, sympathetic nerves, afferent nerves, or bladder urothelium; (2) blocking neuropeptide release such as calcitonin gene related peptide (CGRP) or substance P from afferent nerves; (3) diminishing nerve growth factor release from urothelium or smooth muscle; and (4) reducing expression of TRPV1 or P2X3 receptors on sensory nerve terminals. NGF, nerve growth factor. (See also color plate section).

treatment.[41] In addition, Apostolidis and colleagues demonstrated that the density of TRPV1 and P2X$_3$ sensory receptors was decreased significantly in bladder biopsies of patients with neurogenic or idiopathic detrusor overactivity treated with BTX-A injections.[42] In summary, BTX-A's beneficial effects in patients with refractory overactive bladder symptoms are probably multifactorial and may account, in part, for the slow onset and prolonged duration of action of bladder BTX-A injections compared to skeletal muscle injections (Figure 22.4).

CLINICAL RESULTS

Neurogenic detrusor overactivity

The use of BTX-A in the urinary bladder was first described in manuscript form by Schurch and colleagues who demonstrated a significant increase in mean maximum bladder capacity (296 to 480 ml, $p < 0.016$) and a significant decrease in mean maximum detrusor voiding pressure (65 to 35 cmH$_2$O, $p < 0.016$) in 21 patients with detrusor hyperreflexia (DH) who were injected with BTX-A.[43] Seventeen of 19 patients were completely continent at 6 weeks' follow-up, and were very

satisfied with the procedure. Interestingly, baseline improvement in urodynamic parameters and incontinence persisted at 36 weeks in their follow-up of 11 patients. In the largest clinical series presented to date, a multicenter retrospective study examined 200 patients with neurogenic bladder treated with intravesical BTX-A injections.[44] At both 3- and 6-month follow-up, mean cystometric bladder capacity and mean voiding pressure decreased significantly.

A strong impetus driving clinical trials examining the effects of BTX-A on detrusor overactivity was provided by the only randomized, placebo-controlled trial investigating the effects of two doses of Botox® (i.e. 200 or 300 units) versus saline injection on various parameters including urodynamic measurements, urinary incontinence episodes, and quality of life questionnaires.[45] Significant decreases in incontinent episodes (approximately 50%), significant increases in maximal cystometric capacity (approximately 170–215 ml), and significant improvements in quality of life scores were demonstrated in both BTX-A treatment groups compared to controls. Beneficial effects lasted the duration of the study (6 weeks). The study was not powered to detect statistical differences between the two BTX-A doses injected. Importantly, no safety concerns related to adverse events from BTX-A treatment were reported.

Ruffion and colleagues utilized the Dysport® preparation of BTX-A to compare the effect of 500 U or 1000 U in 45 patients with neurogenic detrusor overactivity.[46] While maximal bladder capacity and median duration of response (4.83 vs. 10.45 months, respectively) were increased with the higher Dysport® dose, one patient complained of generalized muscle weakness for 1 month following injection that prevented her from performing her normal transfer functions. The authors postulated that 750 U would be the most suitable dose to maximize efficacy while minimizing adverse events.

Mixed neurogenic and idiopathic detrusor overactivity

Popat and colleagues prospectively examined the effects of BTX-A detrusor injection in 44 patients with neurogenic and 31 patients with non-neurogenic detrusor overactivity proven by preoperative urodynamic studies.[47] The benefits of treatment in both patient populations included significant increases in maximal cystometric capacity and significant reductions in incontinence episodes and urinary urgency. Impressively, 60.3% of all patients achieved complete continence. Their results are supported by smaller comparative studies demonstrating the efficacy of BTX-A in neurogenic and non-neurogenic populations.[48–50] What is most meaningful from all of these studies of BTX-A treatment of bladder overactivity is that many patients successfully treated were either poorly responsive or refractory to antimuscarinic therapy. This finding supports basic research described earlier that BTX-A works through other mechanisms in addition to the inhibition of ACh release from parasympathetic nerve terminals.

Ghei and colleagues investigated the effectiveness of BTX-B in 20 patients with either neurogenic or non-neurogenic detrusor overactivity.[51] The study was a randomized, double-blind crossover trial, and demonstrated significant reductions in urinary frequency and episodes of incontinence between active treatment and placebo. However, the low durability of BTX-B's effects was evidenced by the minimal carryover effect

noted upon crossing over after a short-time period (i.e. 6 weeks).

Idiopathic detrusor overactivity

Rapp and colleagues initially presented a series of 35 patients with refractory overactive bladder symptoms treated with 300 units of BTX-A detrusor injections. Patient response to treatment was assessed using the Incontinence Impact Questionnaire (IIQ-7) and Urogenital Distress Inventory (UDI-6) questionnaire.[52] At the 3-week follow-up, mean IIQ and UDI symptom scores decreased significantly by 28% and 24%, respectively. Symptom improvement persisted in 14 patients followed up to 6 months after treatment, and pad usage per day decreased from a mean of 3.9 to 1.8. Beneficial effects of BTX-A injection were also demonstrated in several smaller series, including one series of patients who presented with overactive bladder symptoms but in whom urodynamic examination excluded detrusor overactivity.

Schmid and colleagues recently presented a prospective, non-randomized study of 100 patients with idiopathic overactive bladder resistant to antimuscarinic treatment.[53] Patients were injected with 100 units of BTX-A at 30 sites within the detrusor muscle. Urgency resolved completely in 72% and incontinence disappeared in 74% of patients, 4 weeks following injections. Mean maximal bladder capacity increased by 56%, and the beneficial effects of BTX-A lasted approximately 6 months. Poor response was noted in 8% of patients treated, and was thought to result from decreased bladder compliance secondary to bladder wall fibrosis.

Botulinum toxin A in pediatric patients

Investigators have also successfully utilized intravesical BTX-A to treat neurogenic bladders in pediatric myelomeningocele patients. Within this patient population, BTX-A treatment could function as an alternative to bladder augmentation in the 8–12% of patients who fail conservative treatment (e.g. clean intermittent catheterization (CIC) and anticholinergic medications).[54,55] Schulte-Baukloh and colleagues presented data on 17 myelomeningocele children (mean age 10.8 years) with detrusor hyperreflexia and intravesical pressures exceeding 40 cmH$_2$O, who were either resistant to high-dose anticholinergic medication or who developed unacceptable anticholinergic side effects.[56] Patients were injected with 85–300 units of Botox® in 30–40 sites of the bladder. Urodynamic follow-up was performed 2–4 weeks after injection. BTX-A treatment induced significant increases in maximal bladder capacity (56.5%) and compliance (121.6%), and a significant decrease in maximal detrusor pressure (32.6%).

Botulinum toxin A versus resiniferatoxin

A prospective study that compared the effects of intravesical resiniferatoxin (RTX) versus BTX-A was conducted in 25 patients with detrusor hyperreflexia.[57] At 18 months' follow-up, BTX-A injections led to significantly greater reductions in the frequency of daily incontinence episodes (e.g. 4.8 to 0.7 following BTX-A vs. 5.4 to 2.0 following RTX treatment) and to significantly greater increases in maximal bladder capacity (e.g. 212 ml to 451 ml vs. 223 ml to 328 ml, respectively). Moreover, the response to BTX-A was more durable than that to RTX (mean duration of response following BTX-A injection of 6.8 months compared to 51.6 days following RTX instillation).

Botulinum toxin A in spinal cord injured patients with poor detrusor compliance

While BTX-A has been shown to reduce detrusor overactivity in patients with neurogenic bladders, earlier studies did not investigate whether BTX-A treatment could improve bladder compliance, and, possibly, reduce the need for invasive surgery. Klaphajone and colleagues examined the effects of injecting 300 units of Botox® into the detrusor muscle of 10 spinal cord injured patients with detrusor compliance ≤20 ml/cmH$_2$O.[58] Significant improvements were noted in mean bladder compliance (6.5 ± 5.0 to 13.2 ± 5.2 ml/cmH$_2$O) and mean functional bladder capacity (mean increase of 156 ml). In addition, 70% of patients were completely continent at 6 weeks' follow-up, and continence was maintained in 50% of patients 9 months after injection. These results are in stark contrast to the poor results achieved in eight patients with idiopathic bladder overactivity and decreased detrusor compliance.[53] However,

beneficial effects of BTX-A in patients with poor detrusor compliance should only be expected if the decreased compliance is a result of increased neurogenic tone of the detrusor muscle and not secondary to bladder wall fibrosis.

Repeat botulinum toxin A injections

Grosse and colleagues evaluated the effectiveness of repeated detrusor injections of BTX-A.[59] A total of 49 patients with refractory neurogenic detrusor overactivity received between 2–5 injections of BTX-A. The authors found significant and similar reductions in detrusor overactivity and in the use of anticholinergic medication, in addition to significant increases in bladder capacity and compliance after both the first and second injections with BTX-A. The average interval between injections was 11 months. As more patients are repeatedly treated with BTX-A injections into the lower urinary tract, urologists will gain better insight into patients' risk of developing antibodies and becoming clinically non-responsive. Similar to studies in adults, investigators have also found that children respond favorably to repeated injections with BTX-A.[60,61]

Histologic changes after botulinum toxin A injection

Recent articles have examined the histologic and ultrastructural effects of BTX-A injection into the detrusor. While prior work in skeletal muscle demonstrated significant axonal sprouting following BTX-A injection that eventually regressed,[62] Haferkamp and colleagues found little evidence of axonal sprouting in bladder biopsies obtained from 24 patients with neurogenic detrusor overactivity following detrusor BTX-A injection.[63] Understanding the differences in recovery of bladder parasympathetic versus somatic nerves may provide a better insight into the mechanisms behind clinical differences in BTX-A's duration of action. Not only does BTX-A appear to have little effect on neuronal architecture within the bladder, but investigators have also shown that BTX-A does not induce bladder inflammation, edema, or fibrosis.[64] These findings should alleviate concerns from urologists that repeated detrusor injections with BTX-A will induce bladder wall fibrosis and lead patients more rapidly to surgical options.

INJECTION TECHNIQUES

For adult patients, Botox® doses have ranged from 200 to 300 units with a Dysport® dose equivalence of approximately 3 Dysport® : 1 Botox® unit. However, no controlled studies have been performed to determine the optimum dose or toxin dilution in neurogenic and OAB patient populations. In children, Schulte-Baukloh et al. utilized 12 units/kg of Botox®, similar to doses given in other neuropediatric populations.[56]

We perform intravesical BTX-A injections by first diluting 100–300 units of Botox® into 10–30 ml of preservative-free saline (i.e. 10 units/ml). Patients are treated after local anesthetization with intraurethral 2% lidocaine jelly and 30 ml of intravesical 2% lidocaine for 15–20 minutes. Using a 25-gauge Cook® Williams collagen injection needle with a rigid cystoscope, or, alternatively, using a 27-gauge disposable injection needle and a non-disposable injection needle sheath (Olympus, Inc.) with a flexible cystoscope, BTX-A is injected into 10–40 sites within the detrusor muscle targeting the trigone, base of the bladder, and lateral walls, while avoiding the dome and posterior walls to prevent inadvertent perforation and bowel injection (Figure 22.5). The 10-site injection technique is utilized for patients with idiopathic overactive bladders and is a modification of our 30–40-site injection technique previously described in treating patients with neurogenic or severe idiopathic overactive bladder.[65] We target trigonal injections because of the rich sensory innervation in this area that may play a role in the symptoms of bladder overactivity and could be impacted by BTX treatment. Although other investigators avoid trigonal injections, none of our patients have experienced clinical signs of vesico-ureteral reflux (e.g. pyelonephritis). All patients receive perioperative oral antibiotics and are followed up subjectively by either phone or office interview in addition to post-void residual measurement with bladder ultrasound during clinic visits.

As BTX-A is becoming more widespread within the urologic community and non-neurogenic populations are offered this treatment, future studies need to identify the minimal effective treatment to achieve efficacy while diminishing local side effects. Issues to be investigated more fully include total toxin dosage, toxin dilution

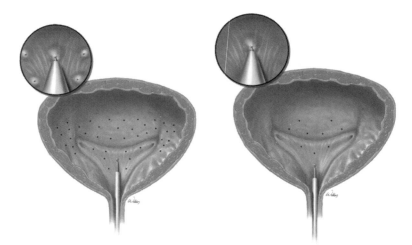

Figure 22. 5 Diagram depicting botulinum toxin injection sites within the detrusor muscle of the bladder. In contrast to other investigators, we target the trigone because of its rich sensory innervation. However, we avoid injecting the posterior wall and dome of the bladder to prevent inadvertent bowel perforation. The panel on the left depicts our 30–40 injection template utilized for neurogenic or severe idiopathic overactive bladder patients and typically 200–300 units of Botox® injection. In contrast, the right panel describes the paradigm we use in mild to moderate idiopathic overactive bladder patients or patients with interstitial cystitis using 100–200 units of Botox®.

volume, and number and location of injection sites. In our hands, 10 injections of a total of 100 units of BTX-A into the bladder trigone and base may effectively suppress irritative symptoms in patients with refractory OAB without inducing elevations in PVR.

ADVERSE EVENTS

Systemic side effects

The lethal dose of BTX-A in primates is 39–40 IU/kg.[66] If one extrapolated primate data to humans, a lethal dose in humans would range from 2000 to 3000 units. Rare systemic cases have been reported including a case of fatal heart block, although no direct causal link was established.[67] In general, weakness is a rare event following BTX therapy, although it has been reported as an adverse event in 2.3% of patients following treatment with Dysport® (1000 units), as well as in seven patients with detrusor hyperreflexia following bladder injection with 1000 units of Dysport® or 300 units of Botox®.[68–72] For the most part, upper extremity weakness resolved within a couple of weeks following bladder injection with BTX-A, although Wyndaele and Van Dromme noted that muscle weakness in their bladder-injected patients lasted 3 months.[71] Surprisingly, generalized weakness developed in one patient who showed no local benefit in the bladder, and in another patient, the generalized muscle weakness outlasted the localized improvement in bladder function. Autonomic side effects including detrusor areflexia, urinary retention, increased residual urine volume, and transient erectile dysfunction have been reported in association with a case of wound botulism and following BTX treatment of achalasia and spastic leg muscles.[73–76] In many cases, the dosage of toxin, toxin dilution, or the specific toxin formulation may have contributed to the development of systemic toxicity. For example, while studies have shown that increasing toxin dilution maximizes the local paralytic effect of BTX, increasing toxin dilution may also increase the risk of systemic absorption and lead to generalized weakness, particularly in susceptible patient populations.[77]

Absolute contraindications to BTX injection include sensitivity to any agent in the toxin preparation and infection at the injection site. Relative contraindications of BTX treatment include pregnant patients and patients with motor neuropathies (e.g. amyotrophic lateral sclerosis) or neuromuscular junction disorders (e.g. myasthenia gravis or Lambert–Eaton syndrome), or patients receiving aminoglycosides or other agents interfering with neuromuscular transmission (e.g. curare-like compounds). Typical doses in these patients may increase the risk of clinically significant systemic side effects including severe dysphagia and respiratory compromise.

Local side effects

Most patients would refuse to choose BTX-A treatment if there was a significant risk of long-term catheterization. Interestingly, Popat and colleagues described de novo self-catheterization rates of as high as 69% in neurogenic and 19% in idiopathic patients after injection of 300 units and 200 units of BTX-A, respectively.[47] In addition, Kessler et al. described de novo catheterization rates of 45% in idiopathic and neurogenic overactive bladder patients following detrusor injection of 300 units of BTX-A.[49] The high rates of self-catheterization observed in some series might be explained by differences in what each study defines as a clinically relevant post-void residual (PVR; e.g. > 100 ml in the study by Popat et al.[47] vs. > 150 ml in the study by Kessler et al.[49]) However, two other series reported low post-injection PVRs, of 15 ml[78] and 42 ml[48] after injection of 300 units and 100–300 units of BTX-A, respectively. Table 22.1 summarizes incidence of idiopathic detrusor overactive (IDO) and neurogenic detrusor overactive (NDO) patients requiring clean intermittent catheterization (CIC) following BTX-A injection. While the efficacy of BTX-A treatment has been demonstrated in all the studies currently cited, the impact of toxin dosage and delivery (i.e. toxin dose and dilution, and the site and depth of injections) on the development of adverse events remains to be established.

RESISTANCE TO TOXIN EFFECTS

Under certain conditions, humans may form antibodies to the botulinum neurotoxin itself, associated non-toxin proteins, or both. Approximately

Table 22.1 Risk of clean intermittent catheterization (CIC) after bladder botulinum toxin A (BTX-A) injection

Lead author	Year	Condition	No. of patients	Units of BTX-A injected	Trigone injected	Urethral sphincter injected	PVR (ml) criteria to start CIC	CIC (% of patients)
Rapp[52]	2006	IDO	35	300	Yes	No	NA	0
Flynn[79]	2004	IDO	7	150	No	No	NA	0
Werner[80]	2005	IDO	26	100	No	No	> 100	8
Kuo[50]	2005	IDO	20	200	No	No	> 250	30–50
Schulte-Baukloh[81]	2005	IDO	44	200–300	Yes	If pre-injection PVR > 15 ml	NA (post-injection PVR < 90 ml)	0
Schulte-Baukloh[78]	2005	IDO	7	300	Yes	Yes	NA (post-injection PVR < 15 ml)	0
Schmid[53]	2006	IDO	100	100	No	No	> 400	4 (15/100 patients with PVR 150–200 ml)
Kuo[82]	2004	IDO + NDO	30	200	No	No	NA	20
Smith[48]	2005	IDO + NDO	42	100–300	Yes	No	NA (post-injection PVR 47 ml)	0
Popat[47]	2005	IDO + NDO	44	200–300	No	No	> 100	69 (NDO) / 19 (IDO)
Kessler[49]	2005	IDO + NDO	22	300	No	No	> 150	45 (NDO) / 36 (IDO)

The main objective of this table is to demonstrate the risk defined by each author of clean intermittent catheterization (CIC) following bladder botulinum toxin A (BTX-A) injection in idiopathic (IDO) or mixed idiopathic and neurogenic (IDO + NDO) detrusor overactive patients. Post-void residual (PVR) data, unless otherwise stated, represent values determined by each investigator as warranting initiation of CIC. In many cases, these criteria or actual post-injection PVR data were not available, represented by NA

5–17% of cervical dystonia patients treated with the original formulation of BTX-A developed neutralizing antibodies.[83–85] However, whereas the original BTX-A preparation contained 25 ng of neurotoxin complex protein per 100 units, the current Botox® formulation contains only 5 ng of complex protein per 100 units. Jankovic and colleagues recently found a six-fold reduction in the risk of developing neutralizing antibodies in cervical dystonia patients treated with the newer formulation of Botox®.[86] While Botox® preparations contain 20 units/ng of neurotoxin complex protein, Dysport® and Myobloc® contain 40 units/ng and 100 units/ng of neurotoxin complex protein, respectively. Given that effective doses of Dysport® and Myobloc® are, in general, 3–4 and 50–100 times, respectively, the doses given with Botox®, one would expect to find the highest incidence of neutralizing antibodies with Myobloc® followed by Dysport® and then Botox®. Studies have shown that higher doses as well as shorter intervals between doses contribute to the development of clinical resistance.[84,85] Therefore, most investigators currently recommend waiting at least 3 months between treatments, avoiding the use of booster injections, and using the smallest dose that will achieve the desired clinical effect.[23,84]

What options are available if a patient becomes clinically non-responsive to BTX-A? Studies have demonstrated the clinical efficacy of BTX-B (Myobloc®) in both type A-responsive and type A-resistant patients.[87,88] Case reports within urological literature also support a role for bladder injection with BTX-B in type A resistant patients.[89,90] However, in vitro studies have also found that approximately one-third of patients treated with BTX-A demonstrate cross-reactive antibodies against BTX-B despite never having been treated with BTX-B.[91] If these in vitro studies are clinically significant, it may mean that some patients who develop antibodies to BTX-A may also be non-responsive to BTX-B or may not respond after only a few injections. Thus, it is paramount that clinicians take steps to minimize the potential for antibody formation in order to preserve long-term clinical responsiveness to BTX.

CONCLUSION

Obviously, more basic research studies are needed to better define BTX's role in autonomic and somatic nervous pathways innervating the lower urinary tract as well as to identify new possible avenues of clinical benefit to pursue. Since the use of BTX is currently FDA off-label, and, in support of evidence based medicine practices, caution should be applied until current randomized clinical studies are completed that will guide physicians in making decisions about the use of BTX in patients with OAB symptoms.

REFERENCES

1. van Ermengem E. Ueber einen neuen anaeroben Bacillus und seine Beziehungen zum Botulisms. Ztsch Hyg Infekt 1897; 26: 1.
2. Dickson EC. Botulism. A clinical and experimental study. Rockefeller Inst Med Res Monogr 1918; 8: 1.
3. Dasgupta BR. Structures of botulinum neurotoxin, its functional domains, and perspectives on the crystalline type A toxin. In: Jankovic J, Hallett M, eds. Therapy with Botulinum Toxin. New York: Marcel Dekker, 1994: 15–39.
4. Schiavo G, Rossetto O, Santucci A, Dasgupta BR, Montecucco C. Botulinum neurotoxins are zinc proteins. J Biol Chem 1992; 267: 23479–83.
5. Segelke B, Knapp M, Kadkhodayan S, Balhorn R, Rupp B. Crystal structure of *Clostridium botulinum* neurotoxin protease in a product-bound state: evidence for noncanonical zinc protease activity. Proc Natl Acad Sci USA 2004; 101: 6888–93.
6. Kozaki S, Miki A, Kamata Y, Ogasawara J, Sakaguchi G. Immunological characterization of papain-induced fragments of *Clostridium botulinum* type A neurotoxin and interaction of the fragments with brain synaptosomes. Infect Immun 1989; 57: 2634–9.
7. Blaustein RO, Germann WJ, Finkelstein A, DasGupta BR. The N-terminal half of the heavy chain of botulinum type A neurotoxin forms channels in planar phospholipid bilayers. FEBS Lett 1987; 226: 115–20.
8. Turton K, Chaddock JA, Acharya KR. Botulinum and tetanus neurotoxins: structure, function and therapeutic utility. Trends Biochem Sci 2002; 27: 552–8.
9. Schiavo G, Santucci A, DasGupta BR et al. Botulinum neurotoxins serotypes A and E cleave SNAP-25 at distinct COOH-terminal peptide bonds. FEBS Lett 1993; 335: 99–103.
10. Barinaga M. Secrets of secretion revealed. Science 1993; 260: 487–9.

11. Heckmann M, Ceballos-Baumann AO, Plewig G. Hyperhidrosis Study Group: Botulinum toxin A for axillary hyperhidrosis (excessive sweating). N Engl J Med 2001; 344: 488–93.

12. Porta M, Gamba M, Bertacchi G, Vaj P. Treatment of sialorrhoea with ultrasound guided botulinum toxin type A injection in patients with neurological disorders. J Neurol Neurosurg Psychiatry 2001; 70: 538–40.

13. von Lindern JJ, Niederhagen B, Berge S, Hagler G, Reich RH. Frey syndrome: treatment with type A botulinum toxin. Cancer 2000; 89: 1659–63.

14. Dong M, Yeh F, Tepp WH et al. SV2 is the protein receptor for botulinum neurotoxin A. Science 2006; 312: 592–6.

15. Hexsel DM, De Almeida AT, Rutowitsch M et al. Multicenter, double-blind study of the efficacy of injections with botulinum toxin type A reconstituted up to six consecutive weeks before application. Dermatol Surg 2003; 29 (5): 523–9.

16. De Almeida ART, Kadunc BV, Di Chiacchio ND, Neto DR. Foam during reconstitution does not affect the potency of botulinum toxin type A. Dermatol Surg 2003; 29 (5): 530–1.

17. Flynn TC, Carruthers JA, Carruthers JA. Botulinum A toxin treatment of the lower eyelid improves infraorbital rhytides and widens the eye. Dermatol Surg 2001; 27: 703–8.

18. Fulton JE. Botulinum toxin: the Newport Beach experience. Dermatol Surg 1998; 24: 1219–24.

19. Sampaio C, Ferreira JJ, Simoes F et al. DYSBOT: a single-blind, randomized parallel study to determine whether any differences can be detected in the efficacy and tolerability of two formulations of botulinum toxin type A—Dysport and Botox—assuming a ratio of 4:1. Mov Disord 1997; 12: 1013–18.

20. Marchetti A, Magar R, Findley L et al. Retrospective evaluation of the dose of Dysport and BOTOX in the management of cervical dystonia and blepharospasm: the REAL DOSE study. Mov Disord 2005; 20: 937–44.

21. Ranoux D, Gury C, Fondarai J, Mas JL, Zuber M. Respective potencies of Botox and Dysport: a double blind, randomised, crossover study in cervical dystonia. J Neurol Neurosurg Psychiatry 2002; 72: 459–62.

22. Borodic GE, Joseph M, Fay L, Cozzolino D, Ferrante RJ. Botulinum A toxin for the treatment of spasmodic torticollis: dysphagia and regional toxin spread. Head Neck 1990; 12: 392–9.

23. Brin MF. Botulinum toxin: chemistry, pharmacology, toxicity, and immunology. Muscle Nerve Suppl 1997; 6: S146–68.

24. Aoki KR. Immunologic and other properties of therapeutic botulinum toxin serotypes. In: Brin MF, Jankovic J, Hallet M, eds. Scientific and Therapeutic Aspects of Botulinum Toxin. Philadelphia: Lippincott Williams & Wilkins, 2002; 9: 103.

25. Smith CP, Franks ME, McNeil BK et al. Effect of botulinum toxin A on the autonomic nervous system of the rat lower urinary tract. J Urol 2003; 169: 1896–900.

26. Mackenzie I, Burnstock G, Dolly JO. The effects of purified botulinum neurotoxin type A on cholinergic, adrenergic and non-adrenergic, atropine-resistant autonomic neuromuscular transmission. Neuroscience 1982; 7: 997–1006.

27. Kim HJ, Seo K, Yum KW et al. Effects of botulinum toxin type A on the superior cervical ganglia in rabbits. Auton Neurosci 2002; 102: 8–12.

28. Morris JL, Jobling P, Gibbins IL. Differential inhibition by botulinum neurotoxin A of cotransmitters released from autonomic vasodilator neurons. Am J Physiol Heart Circ Physiol 2001; 281: H2124–32.

29. Ishikawa H, Mitsui Y, Yoshitomi T et al. Presynaptic effects of botulinum toxin type A on the neuronally evoked response of albino and pigmented rabbit iris sphincter and dilator muscles. Nippon Ganka Gakkai Zasshi 2001; 105: 218–22.

30. Smith CP, Boone TB, de Groat WC, Chancellor MB, Somogyi GT. Effect of stimulation intensity and botulinum toxin isoform on rat bladder strip contractions. Brain Res Bull 2003; 61: 165–71.

31. O'Reilly BA, Kosaka AH, Knight GF et al. P2X receptors and their role in female idiopathic detrusor instability. J Urol 2002; 167: 157–64.

32. Hawthorn MH, Chapple CR, Cock M, Chess-Williams R. Urothelium-derived inhibitory factor(s) influence detrusor muscle contractility in vitro. Br J Pharmacol 2000; 129: 416–19.

33. Wakabayashi Y, Kojima Y, Makiura Y et al. Free terminal fibers of autonomic nerves in the mucosa of the cat urinary bladder. In: Wegmann RJ, Wegmann MA, eds. Recent Advances in Cellular and Molecular Biology, Vol 3. Leuven, Belgium: Peeters Press, 2000: 109–17.

34. Wakabayashi Y, Kojima Y, Makiura Y et al. Acetylcholinesterase positive axons in the mucosa of urinary bladder of adult cats: retrograde tracing

and degeneration studies. Histol Histopathol 1995; 10: 523–30.

35. Andersson KE, Yoshida M. Antimuscarinics and the overactive detrusor—which is the main mechanism of action. Eur Urol 2003; 43: 1–5.

36. Khera M, Somogyi GT, Kiss S, Boone TB, Smith CP. Botulinum toxin A inhibits ATP release from bladder urothelium after chronic spinal cord injury. Neurochem Int 2004; 45: 987–93.

37. Rapp DE, Turk KW, Bales GT, Cook SP. Botulinum toxin type A inhibits calcitonin gene-related peptide release from isolated rat bladder. J Urol 2006; 175: 1138–42.

38. Chuang YC, Yoshimura N, Huang CC, Chiang PH, Chancellor MB. Intravesical botulinum toxin A administration produces analgesia against acetic acid induced bladder pain responses in rats. J Urol 2004; 172: 1529–32.

39. Morenilla-Palao C, Planells-Cases R, Garcia-Sanz N, Ferrer-Montiel A. Regulated exocytosis contributes to protein kinase C potentiation of vanilloid receptor activity. J Biol Chem 2004; 279: 25665–72.

40. Blochl A. SNAP-25 and syntaxin, but not synaptobrevin 2, cooperate in the regulated release of nerve growth factor. Neuroreport 1998; 9: 1701–5.

41. Giannantoni A, Di Stasi SM, Nardicchi V et al. Botulinum-A toxin injections into the detrusor muscle decrease nerve growth factor bladder tissue levels in patients with neurogenic detrusor overactivity. J Urol 2006; 175: 2341–4.

42. Apostolidis A, Popat R, Yiangou Y et al. Decreased sensory receptors P2X3 and TRPV1 in suburothelial nerve fibers following intradetrusor injections of botulinum toxin for human detrusor overactivity. J Urol 2005; 174: 977–82; discussion 982–3.

43. Schurch B, Stohrer M, Kramer G et al. Botulinum-A toxin for treating detrusor hyperreflexia in spinal cord injured patients: a new alternative to anticholinergic drugs? Preliminary results. J Urol 2000; 164: 692–7.

44. Reitz A, Stohrer M, Kramer G et al. European experience of 200 cases treated with botulinum-A toxin injections into the detrusor muscle for neurogenic incontinence due to neurogenic detrusor overactivity. Eur Urol 2004; 45: 510–15.

45. Schurch B, de Seze M, Denys P et al. Botox Detrusor Hyperreflexia Study Team. Botulinum toxin type a is a safe and effective treatment for neurogenic urinary incontinence: results of a single treatment, randomized, placebo controlled 6-month study. J Urol 2005; 174: 196–200.

46. Ruffion A, Capelle O, Paparel P et al. What is the optimum dose of type A botulinum toxin for treating neurogenic bladder overactivity? BJU Int 2006; 97: 1030–4.

47. Popat R, Apostolidis A, Kalsi V et al. A comparison between the response of patients with idiopathic detrusor overactivity and neurogenic detrusor overactivity to the first intradetrusor injection of botulinum-A toxin. J Urol 2005; 174: 984–9.

48. Smith CP, Nishiguchi J, O'Leary M, Yoshimura N, Chancellor MB. Single-institution experience in 110 patients with botulinum toxin A injection into bladder or urethra. Urology 2005; 65: 37–41.

49. Kessler TM, Danuser H, Schumacher M, Studer UE, Burkhard FC. Botulinum A toxin injections into the detrusor: an effective treatment in idiopathic and neurogenic detrusor overactivity? Neurourol Urodyn 2005; 24: 231–6.

50. Kuo HC. Clinical effects of suburothelial injection of botulinum A toxin on patients with nonneurogenic detrusor overactivity refractory to anticholinergics. Urology 2005; 66: 94–8.

51. Ghei M, Maraj BH, Miller R et al. Effects of botulinum toxin B on refractory detrusor overactivity: a randomized, double-blind, placebo controlled, crossover trial. J Urol 2005; 174: 1873–7.

52. Rapp DE, Lucioni A, Katz EE, O'Connor RC, Gerber GS, Bales GT. Use of botulinum-A toxin for the treatment of refractory overactive bladder symptoms: an initial experience. Urology 2004; 63(6): 1071–5.

53. Schmid DM, Sauermann P, Werner M et al. Experience with 100 cases treated with botulinum-A toxin injections in the detrusor muscle for idiopathic overactive bladder syndrome refractory to anticholinergics. J Urol 2006; 176: 177–85.

54. Hernandez RD, Hurwitz RS, Foote JE et al. Non-surgical management of threatened upper urinary tracts and incontinence in children with myelomeningocele. J Urol 1994; 152: 1582–5.

55. Skobejko-Wlodarska L, Strulak K, Nachulewicz P et al. Bladder autoaugmentation in myelodysplastic children. Br J Urol 1998; 81 (Suppl 3): 114–16.

56. Schulte-Baukloh H, Michael T, Schobert J, Stolze T, Knispel HH. Efficacy of botulinum-A toxin in children with detrusor hyperreflexia due to myelomeningocele: preliminary results. Urology 2002; 59: 325–7.

57. Giannantoni A, Di Stasi SM, Stephen RL et al. Intravesical resiniferatoxin versus botulinum-A toxin injections for neurogenic detrusor overactivity: a prospective randomized study. J Urol 2004; 172: 240–3.

58. Klaphajone J, Kitisomprayoonkul W, Sriplakit S. Botulinum toxin type A injections for treating neurogenic detrusor overactivity combined with low-compliance bladder in patients with spinal cord lesions. Arch Phys Med Rehabil 2005; 86: 2114–18.

59. Grosse J, Kramer G, Stohrer M. Success of repeat detrusor injections of botulinum A toxin in patients with severe neurogenic detrusor overactivity and incontinence. Eur Urol 2005; 47: 653–9.

60. Altaweel W, Jednack R, Bilodeau C, Corcos J. Repeated intradetrusor botulinum toxin type A in children with neurogenic bladder due to myelomeningocele. J Urol 2006; 175: 1102–5.

61. Schulte-Baukloh H, Knispel HH, Stolze T et al. Repeated botulinum-A toxin injections in treatment of children with neurogenic detrusor overactivity. Urology 2005; 66: 865–70; discussion 870.

62. Meunier FA, Schiavo G, Molgo J. Botulinum neurotoxins: from paralysis to recovery of functional neuromuscular transmission. J Physiol Paris 2002; 96: 105–13.

63. Haferkamp A, Schurch B, Reitz A et al. Lack of ultrastructural detrusor changes following endoscopic injection of botulinum toxin type A in overactive neurogenic bladder. Eur Urol 2004; 46: 784–91.

64. Comperat E, Reitz A, Delcourt A et al. Histologic features in the urinary bladder wall affected from neurogenic overactivity – a comparison of inflammation, oedema and fibrosis with and without injection of botulinum toxin type A. Eur Urol 2006; 50: 1058–64.

65. Smith CP, Chancellor MB. Simplified bladder botulinum-toxin delivery technique using flexible cystoscope and 10 sites of injection. J Endourol 2005; 19: 880–2.

66. Scott AB, Suzuki D. Systemic toxicity of botulinum toxin by intramuscular injection in the monkey. Mov Disord 1988; 3: 333–5.

67. Malnick SD, Metchnik L, Somin M, Bergman N, Attali M. Fatal heart block following treatment with botulinum toxin for achalasia. Am J Gastroenterol 2000; 95: 3333–4.

68. Bakheit AMO, Ward CD, McLellian DL. Generalized botulism-like syndrome after intramuscular injections of botulinum toxin type A: a report of two cases. J Neurol Neurosurg Psychiatry 1997; 62: 198.

69. Bhatia KP, Munchau A, Thompson PD et al. Generalised muscular weakness after botulinum toxin injection for dystonia: a report of three cases. J Neurol Neurosurg Psychiatry 1999; 67: 90–3.

70. Kessler KR, Skutta M, Benecke R. Long-term treatment of cervical dystonia with botulinum toxin A: efficacy, safety, and antibody frequency. German Dystonia Study Group. J Neurol 1999; 246: 265–74.

71. Wyndaele JJ, Van Dromme SA. Muscular weakness as side effect of botulinum toxin injection for neurogenic detrusor overactivity. Spinal Cord 2002; 40: 599–600.

72. Del Popolo G. Botulinum-A toxin in the treatment of detrusor hyperreflexia. Neurourol Urodyn 2001; 20: 522–4 (abstr).

73. Sautter T, Herzog A, Hauri D, Schurch B. Transient paralysis of the bladder due to wound botulism. Eur Urol 2001; 39 (5): 610–12.

74. Papadonikolakis AS, Vekris MD, Kostas JP, Korompilias AV, Soucacos PN. Transient erectile dysfunction associated with intramuscular injection of botulinum toxin type A. J South Orthop Assoc 2002; 11 (2): 116–18.

75. Schnider P, Berger T, Schmied M, Fertl L, Auff E. Increased residual urine volume after local injection of botulinum A toxin. Nervenarzt, [in German] 1995; 66: 465–7.

76. Khurana V, Nehme O, Hurana R, Barkin JS. Urinary retention secondary to detrusor muscle hypofunction after botulinum toxin injection for achalasia. Am J Gastroenterol 2001; 96: 3211–12.

77. Kim HS, Hwang JH, Jeong ST et al. Effect of muscle activity and botulinum toxin dilution volume on muscle paralysis. Dev Med Child Neurol 2003; 45: 200–6.

78. Schulte-Baukloh H, Weiss C, Stolze T, Sturzebecher B, Knispel HH. Botulinum-A toxin for treatment of overactive bladder without detrusor overactivity: urodynamic outcome and patient satisfaction. Urology 2005; 66: 82–7.

79. Flynn MK, Webster GD, Amundsen CL. The effect of botulinum-A toxin on patients with

severe urge urinary incontinence. J Urol 2004; 172: 2316–20.

80. Werner M, Schmid DM, Schussler B. Efficacy of botulinum-A toxin in the treatment of detrusor overactivity incontinence: a prospective nonrandomized study. Am J Obstet Gynecol 2005; 192: 1735–40.

81. Schulte-Baukloh H, Weiss C, Stolze T et al. Botulinum-A toxin detrusor and sphincter injection in treatment of overactive bladder syndrome: objective outcome and patient satisfaction. Eur Urol 2005; 48: 984–90.

82. Kuo HC. Urodynamic evidence of effectiveness of botulinum A toxin injection in treatment of detrusor overactivity refractory to anticholinergic agents. Urology 2004; 63: 868–72.

83. Hatheway CL, Dang C. Immunogenicity of neurotoxins of Clostridium botulinum. In: Jankovic J, Hallet M, eds. Therapy with Botulinum Toxin. New York: Marcel Dekker, 1994; 93–107.

84. Greene P, Fahn S, Diamond B. Development of resistance to botulinum toxin type A in patients with torticollis. Mov Disord 1994; 9: 213–17.

85. Jankovic J, Schwartz K. Response and immunoresistance to botulinum toxin injections. Neurology 1995; 45: 1743–6.

86. Jankovic J, Vuong KD, Ahsan J. Comparison of efficacy and immunogenicity of original versus current botulinum toxin in cervical dystonia. Neurology 2003; 60: 1186–8.

87. Brashear A, Lew MF, Dykstra DD et al. Safety and efficacy of NeuroBloc (botulinum toxin type B) in type A-responsive cervical dystonia. Neurology 1999; 53: 1439–46.

88. Brin MF, Lew MF, Adler CH et al. Safety and efficacy of NeuroBloc (botulinum toxin type B) in type A-resistant cervical dystonia. Neurology 1999; 53: 1431–8.

89. Reitz A, Schurch B. Botulinum toxin type B injection for management of type A resistant neurogenic detrusor overactivity. J Urol 2004; 171: 804.

90. Pistolesi D, Selli C, Rossi B, Stampacchia G. Botulinum toxin type B for type A resistant bladder spasticity. J Urol 2004; 171: 802–3.

91. Doellgast GJ, Brown JE, Koufman JA et al. Sensitive assay for measurement of antibodies to Clostridium botulinum neurotoxins A, B, and E: use of hapten-labeled antibody elution to isolate specific complexes. J Clin Microbiol 1997; 35: 578–83.

23

Acupuncture for treatment of overactive bladder

Mary P FitzGerald

Acupuncture mechanism of action • Incontinence in traditional Chinese medicine • Acupuncture treatments • Acupuncture for overactive bladder, incontinence • Conclusion

For many of us, it is difficult to believe that one might place acupuncture needles at favored locations on the body wall and expect to bring about meaningful improvements in bladder symptoms. Nonetheless, acupuncture has been used for the treatment of overactive bladder (OAB) symptoms for about 5000 years. This chapter will provide an overview of acupuncture therapy and of some evidence supporting the opinion that acupuncture can be an effective OAB treatment.

ACUPUNCTURE MECHANISM OF ACTION

Debate continues about the mechanism of any acupuncture effects that are seen. The interested reader is referred to an authoritative text[1] for detailed descriptions of several theories and their supporting evidence. Much of the evidence supporting acupuncture theories arises from studies that can be easily criticized as suffering from poor research methodology, and most results have not been reproduced. Despite these reservations, there is a body of evidence suggesting that acupuncture points have certain characteristics. Acupuncture points have higher electrical conductance, higher temperature, and higher metabolic rate than non-acupuncture points,[2] and electrical resistance between two acupuncture points on an acupuncture channel is less than the electrical resistance between two nearby control points.[3] Acupuncture points are

often, but not always, located at nerve endings or bifurcations, and sites where cutaneous nerves pierce fascia or bone foramina.[4]

The location of acupuncture points and suggestions of reasonable neurological mechanisms have convinced many that acupuncture effects are primarily mediated through the nervous system. For example, analgesic effects of acupuncture are blocked by local anesthetics, suggesting that actions of the peripheral nervous system are crucial. It has also been demonstrated that endorphin production is induced by acupuncture analgesia, and that acupuncture analgesia can be blocked by naloxone.[5] Others reject the idea that acupuncture is primarily neurologically based, noting for example that some of the most commonly used acupuncture points (e.g. in the auricle of the ear) have no demonstrably important nerves or vessels nearby.

Physicians are comfortable with the notion that diseased organs can refer pain to somatic tissues via *viscerocutaneous effects* (referred pain and sensitivity) along dermatomal and myotomal distributions. For example, urologists may be familiar with studies that demonstrate persistently increased sensitivity of the ipsilateral body wall long after an episode of ureteric colic.[6] Neurologically mediated acupuncture treatments are theorized by some authors to similarly occur through activation of *cutaneovisceral effects* that affect viscera through stimulation of the skin and subcutaneous tissues. Such somatovisceral effects may underlie the effectiveness of the Stoller afferent nerve stimulator (SANS) device for treatment of urge incontinence.[7] The SANS device is actually placed over an acupuncture point (SP-6) along the path of the posterior tibial nerve, which has the same segmental innervation as the bladder.

The idea that acupuncture acts through cutaneovisceral effects is supported by evidence from animal experiments. The presence of somatovisceral reflexes involving the autonomic nervous system in general and the lower urinary tract in particular has been well established. For example, reflex inhibition of detrusor contractions by perineal stimulation has been reported,[8] and specific animal studies of acupuncture suggest that cutaneous acupuncture stimuli have real effects on urethral activity. In anesthetized rats, when acupuncture stimuli were applied to the skin and underlying tissues with the same segmental innervation as the bladder, there was activation or inhibition of periurethral electromyogram (EMG) activity.[9]

Contemporary physicians can rationalize acupuncture by referral to neuroanatomic effects, and indeed the school of *neuroanatomic acupuncture* relies heavily on the choice of acupuncture treatment points that is rooted in an understanding of the anatomy and physiology of peripheral and central nerves. Traditional acupuncturists obviously did not have access to this knowledge, and are likely to have discovered the effects of acupuncture entirely through experience, i.e. traditional acupuncture has an empiric basis.

INCONTINENCE IN TRADITIONAL CHINESE MEDICINE

The ancient Chinese understanding of the nature of the life-force ("Qi") and the functions of the organs was based on millennia of observations of the ways in which environmental factors (e.g. wet, cold, damp), foods, and herbs interacted with persons of various constitutions to bring about health or disease. This understanding developed into an elegant model of the functioning of the human body which is markedly different from the allopathic model. In some instances, the functions of the human organs overlap when viewed from the traditional Chinese medicine (TCM) and the allopathic

perspective – for example, in both traditions the kidney produces fluid that is passed from the bladder, and the heart regulates the movement of blood in the arteries. However, other attributes are also ascribed to the organs, such as the notion that the liver rules the tendons, ligaments, and muscles and is manifest in the eyes. Such attributes arose because of observations that patients with liver problems also tend to have problems such as muscle tremors and poor vision.

In TCM, the functions of the kidneys include: "to govern water, to open into the ears, to manifest in the hair, to house willpower, govern birth, growth, reproduction and development".[10] The kidney is also considered to be the "controller of the two lower orifices", i.e. the anus and urethra. If kidney Qi is deficient, urine leakage may occur, and the prevalence of kidney Qi deficiency is known to rise with aging. Disorders of the bladder itself are also manifest in urinary incontinence. For example, bladder deficiency and cold can arise from kidney deficiency (since the bladder derives its Qi from the kidney), and results in frequent, pale, and abundant urine, urinary incontinence, and nocturnal enuresis. "Bladder deficiency and cold" is sometimes attributed to living in cold and/or damp places, and women are supposedly particularly vulnerable during their menses.[10] Treatment is by tonification (increasing) of the bladder and kidney Qi. This can be accomplished either through the use of acupuncture needles or administration of herbs, or through manual body treatments (Tui Na) that are focused upon relevant channels through which the Qi flows.

ACUPUNCTURE TREATMENTS

Acupuncture treatments involve needling one or more points along acupuncture meridians, which are favored channels along which Qi is thought to flow. An agreed-upon international nomenclature permits some standardization of acupuncture treatments. For example, BL-10 denotes the 10th point on the bladder meridian, whose location is known to all acupuncturists (Figure 23.1). There are 12 principal meridians, namely bladder (BL), heart (HT), small intestine (SI), kidney (KI), liver (LR), master of the heart (MH), triple heater (TH), gall bladder (GB),

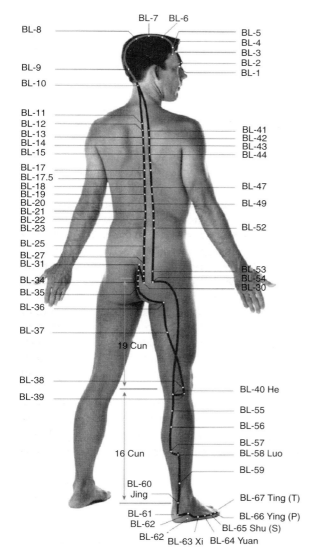

BL-8
BL-7   BL-6
BL-5
BL-4
BL-3
BL-2
BL-1
BL-9
BL-10
BL-11
BL-12
BL-13
BL-14
BL-15
BL-41
BL-42
BL-43
BL-44
BL-17
BL-17.5
BL-18
BL-19
BL-20
BL-21
BL-22
BL-23
BL-47
BL-49
BL-52
BL-25
BL-27
BL-31
BL-34
BL-35
BL-36
BL-53
BL-54
BL-30
BL-37
19 Cun
BL-38
BL-39
BL-40 He
BL-55
BL-56
BL-57
BL-58 Luo
BL-59
16 Cun
BL-60
Jing
BL-67 Ting (T)
BL-61
BL-62
BL-66 Ying (P)
BL-65 Shu (S)
BL-62   BL-63 Xi   BL-64 Yuan

Figure 23.1 Acupuncture points related to the bladder.

spleen (SP), lung (LU), large intestine (LI), and stomach (ST). Points are chosen for acupuncture treatments according to their observed effects (or "attributes") and are usually needled bilaterally. There are two midline meridians: governor vessel (GV) and conception vessel (CV).

During acupuncture treatments, the efficacy of needling is thought to be enhanced by heating the needles by the application of moxibustion and electrical stimulation of the needles. Moxibustion involves lighting a smokeless herbal cigar (moxa), made from compressed *Artemesia*

vulgaris (mugwort). Once enough warmth is produced from the cigar, it is brought near to the needles to warm them. In the United States, the acupuncturist places one of their own fingers between the moxa and the patient, to ensure that patient burns do not occur. In other countries, moxa is burned directly on acupuncture points with the express purpose of burning the skin and producing a scar.

In general, acupuncture treatments can be described as either based upon a standardized "formula" or based upon the underlying diagnosis. The use of formula acupuncture grew during the Chinese Cultural Revolution, when "barefoot doctors" were trained to utilize acupuncture based on the symptoms that patients presented. The equivalent in allopathic terms would be to treat all headaches similarly, even though some will be due to migraine while others arise secondary to the presence of a brain tumor. Most acupuncture practitioners prefer the sophistication of treatments based on the underlying diagnosis, which will presumably yield higher success rates. No studies have published differential response rates, however.

ACUPUNCTURE FOR OVERACTIVE BLADDER, INCONTINENCE

With one exception,[11] the acupuncture literature concerning urinary incontinence is characterized by case reports and uncontrolled case series with undefined outcome measures. This is typified by a case series[12] describing acupuncture treatment of 76 patients of mean age 63 years. Patients received acupuncture five times weekly for 1 or 2 weeks. After one or two treatment courses, 38 patients were "cured", and had no leakage with the sound of running water. Another 20 patients achieved "basic control" of urination, but still had leakage with the sound of running water.

There are three published case series of reasonable quality. One case series from Sweden[13] described results when 15 patients with urge or mixed incontinence, whose symptoms were not satisfactorily relieved after at least 2 months' treatment with pelvic floor training and medication, received 12 acupuncture treatments during a 6-week period. Three months after the end of treatment, eight of the 15 women (53%) rated their symptoms as being "Much improved" overall. The magnitude of leakage on a pad test was also significantly reduced from a median of 123 g before treatment, to a median of 12 g 3 months after treatment. There were no adverse effects of acupuncture.

Another non-randomized study[14] without well-defined outcomes sought to examine the effect of acupuncture treatment on lower urinary tract function in a group of 52 women with frequency, urgency, and dysuria. The women received acupuncture to either SP-6 or a control acupuncture point not expected to be beneficial for urinary symptoms. The acupuncture treatment was repeated an undisclosed number of times if initial response was seen. Clinically, 22 of the 26 (85%) patients who had acupuncture at SP-6 had subjective symptom improvement (not well defined), with 17 patients experiencing no further symptoms. Just six of the 26 (23%) patients treated with control acupuncture experienced symptomatic improvement.

Finally, another case series[15] describes results of acupuncture in patients with "symptoms associated with a urodynamic diagnosis of bladder instability" who were treated with weekly acupuncture for 10–12 weeks. Considering the 13 patients with diurnal symptoms, 10 (77%) noted significant symptomatic improvement. Incontinence was abolished in eight (62%), with effects lasting for up to 2 years after treatment.

There has been one randomized trial of the effect of acupuncture on symptoms of OAB with urge incontinence.[11] In that study, 85 women with a clinical diagnosis of OAB with urge incontinence were randomly assigned to receive an acupuncture treatment expected to improve their bladder symptoms, or a comparison acupuncture treatment designed to promote overall relaxation. Patients had cystometry, and completed a urinary diary and urinary questionnaires before and after 4 weekly treatments. Among the 74 women completing the study, those in the active acupuncture group had statistically significantly greater improvements in bladder capacity (12% increase vs. 4% increase in volume), urgency (30% vs. 3% decrease in urgency episodes), frequency (14% vs. 4% decrease), and urinary quality of life scores compared with women who received the comparison acupuncture treatment. The treatment effect in the active

treatment group was a 59% reduction in incontinence episode frequency, compared to a 40% decrease in the control group ($p > 0.05$). There were no adverse effects of acupuncture.

CONCLUSION

Acupuncture is an ancient treatment for OAB symptoms, with several studies suggesting that it results in real symptom improvements without adverse events or side effects. The use of acupuncture is probably limited by lack of awareness and acceptance of the treatment modality among both physicians and patients, and by lack of insurance coverage for treatments. As acupuncture becomes a more mainstream medical treatment, OAB patients made aware of the possible efficacy of acupuncture may be eager to explore this treatment modality. It is clear that further high-quality study of acupuncture in this setting is needed before acupuncture can be widely accepted as a worthwhile first-line therapy.

REFERENCES

1. Helms JM. Acupuncture Energetics. A Clinical Approach for Physicians. Berkeley: Medical Acupuncture Publishers, 1995.
2. Shang C. Mechanism of acupuncture – beyond neurohumoral theory. Med Acupunct 1999; 11: 36–42.
3. Reichmanis M, Marino AA, Becker RO. DC skin conductance variation at acupuncture loci. Am J Chin Med 1976; 4: 69–72.
4. Dung HC. Anatomical features contributing to the formation of acupuncture points. Am J Acupunct 1984; 12: 139–43.
5. Mayer DJ, Price DD, Rafii A. Antagonism of acupuncture analgesia in man by the narcotic antagonist naloxone. Brain Res 1977; 121: 368–72.
6. Vecchiet L, Giamberardino M, de Bigontina P. Referred pain from viscera: when the pain persists despite the extinction of the visceral focus. Adv Pain Res Ther 1992; 20: 101–10.
7. Karademir K, Baykal K, Sen B et al. A peripheral neuromodulation technique for curing detrusor overactivity: Stoller afferent neurostimulation. Scand J Urol Nephrol 2005; 39: 230–3.
8. deGroat WC. Inhibition and excitation of sacral parasympathetic neurons by visceral and cutaneous stimuli in the cat. Brain Res 1971; 33: 499–503.

9. Morrison JF, Sato A, Sato Y, Suzuki A. Long-lasting facilitation and depression of periurethral skeletal muscle following acupuncture-like stimulation in anesthetized rats. Neurosci Res 1995; 23: 159–69.

10. Maciocia G. The Foundations of Chinese Medicine. New York: Churchill Livingstone, 1989.

11. Emmons SL, Otto L. Acupuncture for overactive bladder. Obstet Gynecol 2005; 106: 138–41.

12. Hong S. Scalp acupuncture plus body acupuncture for senile urinary incontinence. Int J Clin Acupunct 1999; 10: 101–3.

13. Bergstrom K, Carlsson CP, Lindholm C, Widengren R. Improvement of urge- and mixed-incontinence after acupuncture treatment among elderly women – a pilot study. J Auton Nerv Syst 2000; 79: 173–80.

14. Chang PL. Urodynamic studies in acupuncture for women with frequency, urgency and dysuria. J Urol 1988; 140: 563–6.

15. Philp T, Shah PJR, Worth PHL. Acupuncture in the treatment of bladder instability. Br J Urol 1988; 61: 490–3.

24

Fesoterodine

Roger R Dmochowski and Karl J Kreder

Pharmacodynamic profiling of fesoterodine • Phase III analysis • Conclusion

Fesoterodine is a newly identified selective muscarinic M_3 receptor antagonist which is currently being considered for regulatory approval in the treatment of overactive bladder. The chemical name of fesoterodine is 2-methylpropionic acid 2-[3-(N, N-diisopropylamino)-1(R)-phenylpropyl]-4-(hydroxymethyl)phenyl ester. The molecular formula is $C_{26}H_{37}NO_3$. Fesoterodine is extensively and rapidly hydrolyzed in both humans and rodents to its primary active metabolite, SPM 7605 (Figure 24.1). The conversion of fesoterodine to its primary metabolite is by hepatic hydrolysis. The active metabolite has demonstrated potent-specific and non-subtype selective antimuscarinic activity in both *in vitro* and *in vivo* preclinical studies. *In vitro* studies have shown tissue selectivity three times greater for the bladder than for the salivary gland for SPM 7605.

PHARMACODYNAMIC PROFILING OF FESOTERODINE

Extensive preclinical evaluation of fesoterodine has been undertaken. Fesoterodine, SPM 7605, oxybutynin, and atropine were studied in rodent bladder strips either under carbachol-induced or electrical field stimulation conditions.[1] The potencies of fesoterodine and SPM 7605 for the inhibition of carbachol-induced contractions were similar to those of oxybutynin and atropine. Both fesoterodine and SPM 7605 showed a concentration-dependent shift of induced bladder contraction curves. Similarly, the reduction of electrical field-induced contractions was of similar

magnitude with both fesoterodine and SPM 7605, and the degree of reduction associated with these compounds was matched only at higher concentrations of oxybutynin and atropine.

In the same study, fesoterodine and SPM 7605 doses of 0.01, 0.1, and 1 mg/kg were administered intravenously to female Sprague–Dawley rats to assess the *in vivo* cystometric effect. After intravenous administration of both compounds, potent increases in bladder capacity and bladder inter-contraction intervals were seen with both of the active agents at low doses (0.01 mg/kg). Both active agents also reduced the micturition pressure significantly at doses as low as 0.01 mg/kg, and these effects were similar to those seen with oxybutynin and atropine, yet at higher doses of the comparator compounds. The authors concluded that both fesoterodine and SPM 7605 showed significant smooth-muscle relaxation at lower concentrations than either oxybutynin or atropine, with corresponding increases in bladder capacity and inter-contraction intervals.

In another rodent study, gastrointestinal transit was evaluated with both non-selective and selective antimuscarinic agents. In comparison to drugs such as solifenacin and darifenacin, in this study model, the intestinal transit time was less inhibited by non-selective agents such as fesoterodine and tolterodine. Receptor binding assays in this study demonstrated that fesoterodine, tolterodine, and SPM 7605 showed a slightly higher affinity for the M_2 as compared to the M_3 receptor in this particular model.[2]

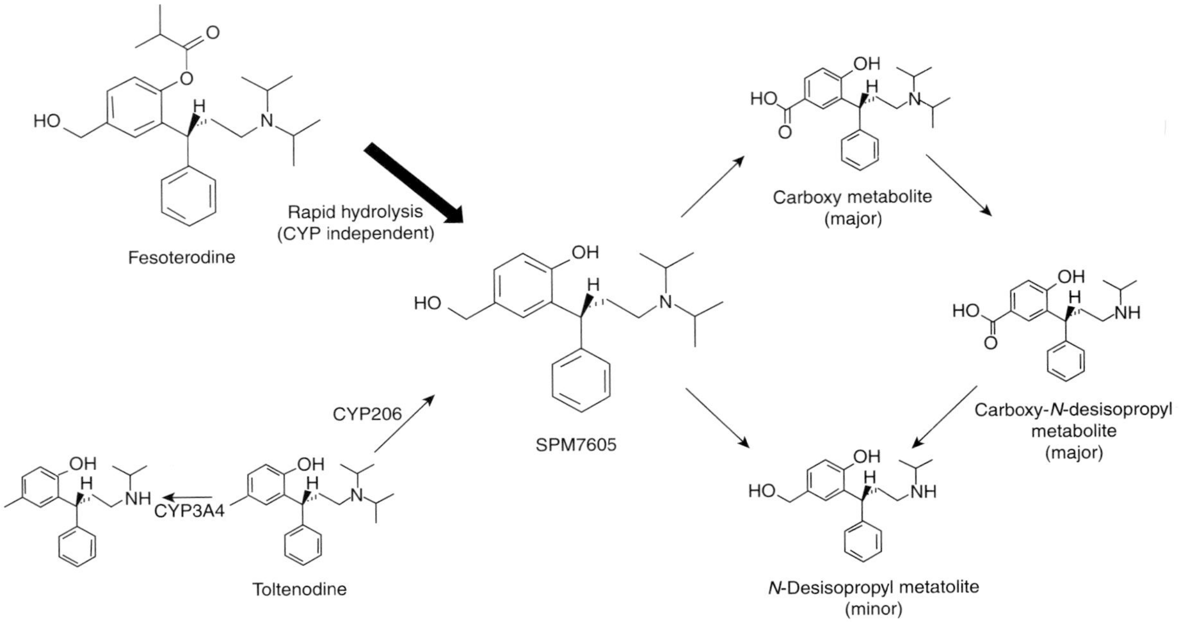

Figure 24.1 Metabolic pathway of fesoterodine: SPM 7605 is the main active principle of fesoterodine.

Using *in vitro* analysis of human bladder detrusor musculature and mucosa, several antimuscarinic agents were assessed for their radioligand binding characteristics. Fesoterodine was demonstrated to have binding characteristics in bladder mucosa and detrusor musculature similar to the affinities noted for oxybutynin. Other drugs in the class were noted to have different binding affinities.[3]

In initial human safety studies, using a randomized, double-blind, placebo-controlled design, ascending oral doses of 4, 8, 12, 20, and 28 mg of fesoterodine administered once daily versus placebo were studied in eight healthy male volunteers. Six subjects received active drug and two received placebo.[4] The intent of the study was to investigate the safety and tolerability of ascending oral doses of fesoterodine and also investigate the pharmacodynamic effects of the drug, using residual urinary volume (PVR) and salivary volume output as endpoints. Secondary safety parameter evaluations including laboratory parameters, electrocardiography (ECG), vital signs, and general well-being were also assessed. Residual urinary volume was determined at baseline and 9 and 24 hours after administration.

Salivary volume was monitored at baseline and 5 and 9 hours after first administration; 1, 5, and 9 hours after the second administration; and 1, 5, 9, and 24 hours after the last administration. Pharmacodynamic effects also included monitoring of subjective and objective evidence of xerostomia in subject patients.

Heart rate response was noted to parallel dosing, with increasing oral doses producing heart rate increases. Urinary residual volume also increased with fesoterodine dose increase, with an initial effect noted at the 12-mg dose. Increasing residual volumes were noted with higher doses, with one subject experiencing a PVR of 400 cm^3 at the 28-mg dose. Salivary production was noted to demonstrate a variable pattern. Decreases in salivary flow were noted with the 12-, 20-, and 28-mg doses. No dry mouth or salivary flow reduction was noted with placebo ingestion. However, all subjects experienced dry mouth at the highest dose of 28 mg, and four of these patients experienced dysuria as well (dysuria not defined).

In the same population, pharmacokinetic parameters were evaluated for the ascending dose regimen.[5] Samples were collected at baseline and 2, 4, 5, 6, 8, 12, and 24 hours post-dose on each day, with urine samples being collected at 6-hour intervals at 0, 6, and 12 hours post-dose on each day. Peak drug concentration (C_{max}), time to C_{max} (t_{max}), terminal half-life ($t_{1/2}$), area under the curve (AUC), mean residence time (MRT), total body clearance (Cl_{tot}), urinary amount excreted (A_e), and renal clearance (Cl_{ren}) were also evaluated. Fesoterodine could not be detected in any blood samples due to presumed rapid metabolism to SPM 7605. SPM 7605 plasma profiles showed increasing maximal values according to dosing. Mean maximal concentration values were noted between 4 and 6 hours after administration of any single dose, with a terminal half-life of 5–7 hours. Mean residence time of the active metabolite was 11–13 hours, with other pharmacokinetic parameters showing linear pharmacokinetics according to the dose ranging tested. High reproducibility of plasma concentration values was also noted. At 4 mg dosing, the mean C_{max} (ng/ml) was 2.2 (standard deviation (SD) 1.28), and at 8 mg the mean C_{max} was 5.15 (SD 2.02). Half-life (hours) at the 4-mg dose was 4.17 (SD 2.04) and at 8 mg was 5.0 (SD 0); $t_{1/2}$ at 4 mg was 5.83 (SD 2.62) and at 8 mg was 6.61 (SD 1.99).

In another safety and tolerability trial, three groups of 16 subjects each (12 receiving active drug and four receiving placebo) were studied. One of these three groups was composed of healthy male subjects age 40 and under, a second group was healthy males greater than 65 years of age, and the third group was healthy females greater than 65 years of age. The study protocol called for subjects to receive a single oral dose of 8 mg or placebo, with safety and pharmacokinetic parameters assessed. Forty-eight total subjects were randomized and completed the trial. No safety differences were noted between subjects based upon either age or gender. Adverse event occurrence patterns were similar in the three populations, with no serious adverse events being experienced by any subject. SPM 7605 concentrations were noted to peak at 5 hours post-administration. All three populations showed similar C_{max} and AUC values. All three populations also demonstrated similar residence times (11 hours). Renal clearance was slightly lower in the elderly group, and this was attributed to decreased glomerular filtration rate in this subgroup. Adverse events included dry mouth, headache,

and dysuria. The authors concluded that fesoterodine showed similar pK parameters between various populations, and that the compound could be safely administered to elderly patients.[6]

In yet another study the pharmacokinetics and the pharmacodynamic effects of fesoterodine on heart rate, saliva volume, and residual urine volume were evaluated. The safety and tolerability of ascending doses of fesoterodine were assessed in a randomized, double-blind, placebo-controlled group comparison. Healthy males, aged 18–45, received escalating doses of fesoterodine, with eight subjects per study group, six receiving fesoterodine and two receiving placebo. Multiple oral doses ranging from 4 to 28 mg or placebo were received once daily for 3 days, with pharmacodynamic parameters assessed, including heart rate, saliva volume, and residual urine volume. Laboratory and ECG parameters were also monitored, as were pharmacokinetic parameters.[7]

Results indicated that no safety parameters were influenced by the study drug. The most frequent adverse events were dry mouth and voiding difficulties at higher doses. Ascending doses of fesoterodine caused mild to moderate increases in heart rate. At 12-mg or above dosing regimens, residual volumes were noted to increase in some subjects. Salivary volume again demonstrated significant circadian variability, with decreased salivary production being noticed at 12-mg and higher doses. Pharmacokinetic evaluation demonstrated maximal plasma levels occurring approximately 5 hours after administration, with a dose-proportionate pharmacokinetic range between 4 and 28 mg. Importantly, no accumulation of the metabolite was noted with once-daily dosing. The authors concluded that fesoterodine offered a broad safety margin with characteristic pharmacologic effects using a once-daily dosing paradigm.

Given the similarity of this compound to other antimuscarinics, an investigation was promulgated in patients with CYP2D6 genotype deficiency.[8] In this study, 24 healthy males, 16 of whom were extensive CYP2D6 metabolizers and eight of whom were poor metabolizers, received single doses of 4, 8, and 12 mg fesoterodine, and pharmacokinetic parameters were assessed. As in prior studies, maximal levels of the primary metabolite were noted 5 hours after oral administration. Dose-proportional increases in both C_{max} and AUC were noted between 4 and 12 mg in both poor and extensive metabolizers. However, poor metabolizers demonstrated 1.7–2 times higher concentrations than the extensive metabolizers. Despite these concentration increases, terminal half-life was similar in both poor and extensive metabolizers. The overall exposure to SPM 7605 was considered to be less than two-fold in the poor metabolizers compared to the extensive metabolizer cohort, and the CYP2D6-deficient genotype was concluded not to influence terminal half-life.[6]

To evaluate the possible effect of ethnicity on the metabolism of fesoterodine, active drug at an 8-mg dose versus placebo was administered to 16 healthy Caucasian subjects under 45 years of age and 16 black African subjects. Pharmacodynamic (salivary production) and pharmacokinetic parameters were evaluated, as were safety parameters. No significant safety concerns were noted.

There were two adverse events noted in the Caucasian population which were not considered significant (asymptomatic tachycardia and facial carbuncle). Salivary volume showed significant variability, but a decrease in salivary production was noted in both active groups at approximately 5 hours post-treatment, which was not associated with complaints of xerostomia.

Pharmacokinetic analysis revealed that maximal serum levels were obtained 6 hours after administration in both groups, and that pharmacokinetic profiles were similar in both groups. The authors concluded that ethnicity did not affect pharmacodynamic or pharmacokinetic activity of the drug.[9]

The effect of ketoconazole inhibition of cytochrome CYP3A4 was examined in a group of healthy males.[10] Ketoconazole administration resulted in a 1.5–2.2-fold increase of maximum SPM 7605 plasma levels in poor versus extensive metabolizers. However, the half-life was not affected by cotreatment with ketoconazole. Patients with moderate liver impairment (Child–Pugh stage B) manifested a 1.4-fold increase in serum levels of SPM 7605.[10] Based upon these findings, it was concluded that dose adjustment may not be necessary in poor CYP2D6 metabolizers with concomitant cytochrome 3A4 blockade or in patients with moderate liver impairment.

Further evaluation of fesoterodine administration in fasting versus high-fat, high-caloric dietary conditions has also been undertaken.[11] Sixteen healthy males, 18–45 years of age, received a single dose of 8 mg of fesoterodine in either the fasted or a high-caloric state. Safety and pharmacokinetic parameters were evaluated. No safety concerns were noted; however, 14 mild adverse events were identified (headache, dry mouth, and dysuria). There was no difference in the plasma concentration profile of SPM 7605 in the fasted or the fed state. The pharmacokinetic parameters increased slightly after a high-fat, high-caloric meal (C_{max}, AUC), and terminal half-life was shortened from 8.7 ± 3 hours in the fasted state to 6.6 ± 2.2 hours in the fed state; however, time to reach C_{max} was comparable for both conditions. The conclusion of this trial was that fesoterodine may be taken without regard to meals in patients with overactive bladder symptomatology, and that similar pharmacokinetic profiles were obtained after the administration of drug in either state. The small difference in half-life, C_{max}, and AUC (19%) was not felt to be clinically significant.

An expanded evaluation of patients with hepatic impairment has also been accomplished.[12] Eight patients with moderate hepatic impairment (Child–Pugh stage B) were evaluated for safety and pharmacokinetic parameters after acute fesoterodine administration. No significant safety events were noted. All adverse events were related to dry mouth. In subjects with moderate hepatic impairment, maximum plasma concentrations increased by 39% as compared to healthy subjects (C_{max}). t_{max} was approximately 2 hours longer (7.4 versus 5.4) in affected patients. Terminal half-life, however, was unchanged. The authors concluded that terminal half-life calculations suggested no serum accumulation, and that dose adjustment was not necessary for administration of this drug in patients with moderate liver impairment.[12]

In a larger study of CYP2D6 poor metabolizers, a group of six patients were compared to 12 extensive metabolizers for the effect of ketoconazole (CYP3A450 inhibitor).[13] All patients underwent safety and pharmacokinetic parameter evaluation. No serious adverse events were noted in this population. Tolerability was similar in both poor and extensive metabolizers. Bioavailability of SPM 7605 as expressed by the AUC was approximately doubled in poor and extensive metabolizers with treatment with ketoconazole. Plasma concentration (C_{max}) of SPM 7605 increased approximately 1.5-fold in poor and 2.2-fold in extensive metabolizers, respectively. The mean terminal half-life of 7.4 hours was similar in both groups after the administration of fesoterodine alone or after coadministration of ketoconazole and fesoterodine. Time to reach C_{max} was not significantly different between the two populations. The authors concluded that there did not appear to be significant changes in fesoterodine pharmacokinetics in patients who are poor versus extensive metabolizers, and that dose adjustment is probably not necessary in patients ingesting fesoterodine when administered with potent cytochrome A4 inhibitors.

Based upon these data, expanded clinical evaluation of fesoterodine was begun. A phase II analysis of fesoterodine 4, 8, and 12 mg was completed in 728 subjects with overactive bladder.[14] Trial design was randomized and placebo-controlled. In this trial, no safety issues arose and no significant adverse events occurred. Drop-out rates due to adverse events occurred in 4% of the placebo group, 6% of the 4-mg group, 2% of the 8-mg group, and 12% of the 12-mg fesoterodine group. The most common adverse event was dry mouth, occurring in 9% (placebo), 25% (4 mg), 26% (8 mg), and 34% (12 mg) of study subjects. Dry mouth was mild to moderate in severity. In this study, 728 patients were randomized and treated; 698 patients were evaluated for primary efficacy analysis. Mean age was 56 and ranged from 18 to 79 years, with 84% of the subjects being female. The primary efficacy outcomes were reduction in frequency (over 24 hours) and urge incontinence episodes (per week). These were reported as mean changes. Overall reductions in micturition for 24 hours were: 1.42 (placebo), 2.2 (4 mg), 2.37 (8 mg), and 2.41 (12 mg) (all statistically significant). For urge incontinence episodes, reductions were: 10.18 (placebo), 12.79 (fesoterodine 4 mg), 11.79 (8 mg), and 13.43 (12 mg). Rapid improvement occurred within the first 2 weeks of double-blind treatment as compared to placebo, with increases in both efficacy endpoints occurring with time. The use of visual analog scales to assess xerostomia demonstrated that dry mouth was mild to moderate in most cases. Drop-out rates were 4% in the placebo group, 6% in the 4-mg group, 2% in the 8-mg group, and 12% in the 12-mg group. Twenty-five per cent of subjects experienced dry mouth at the 4-mg dose, 26% at the 8-mg dose, and 34% at the 12-mg dose. Constipation occurred in 3% of placebo patients, 2% of the 4-mg patients, 3% of the patients receiving 8 mg, and 6% of the patients receiving 12 mg. Visual disturbances were similar across all groups (approximately 1%). Headache occurred in 16% of placebo patients, 17% of the 4-mg subjects, 16% of the 8-mg subjects, and 15% of the 12-mg subjects. No clinically relevant changes in vital signs or ECG parameters were noted. The authors concluded that fesoterodine was a potent and well tolerated muscarinic.

In another trial,[15] 173 patients were randomized to receive an 8-week double-blind treatment course of placebo versus fesoterodine doses of 4, 8, and 12 mg, respectively (43 patients received placebo; and 4 mg (44 patients), 8 mg (47 patients), and 12 mg (39 patients)). Patients were assigned to one of two strata based upon urodynamic findings. Stratum A had greater than or equal to one overactive detrusor contraction on urodynamic tracing, whereas stratum B had normal filling cystometry without evidence of detrusor overactivity. Primary efficacy outcomes were changes in number of micturitions for 24 hours and urge incontinent episode reduction. After 2 weeks of active therapy, patients receiving fesoterodine at all doses manifested reductions in micturitions for 24 hours ($p = 0.049$) in both patient strata. A linear dose–response relationship was noted. Similar improvement was noted in mean urgent incontinent episodes per week with fesoterodine using multiple regression analysis, indicating a slope of 0.72 ($p = 0.0022$), again denoting a linear dose–response relationship. The authors concluded that the results suggested that treatment response to antimuscarinic agents in urge incontinent patients was independent of urodynamic detrusor overactivity. They also concluded that fesoterodine fumarate demonstrated efficacy and tolerability in patients with overactive bladder (OAB) symptomatology and which was not influenced by urodynamic characterization.

In a second analysis of this population, analysis of covariance (ANCOVA) for the number of urge incontinent episodes per week demonstrated fesoterodine to be significantly superior to placebo ($p = 0.0396$ for 4 mg, 0.0010 for 8 mg, and 0.0067 for 12 mg). Significant reductions in micturitions for 24 hours were seen for all doses of fesoterodine as compared to placebo, with 4 mg producing a 0.996 ($p = 0.0446$) reduction, 8 mg 1.815 ($p = 0.0003$), and 12 mg 1.784 ($p = 0.007$). Dry mouth, headache, and gastrointestinal symptoms were the most common adverse events. Ten patients discontinued medication due to adverse events, two in the placebo group, one at the 4-mg dose, two at the 8-mg dose, and five at the 12-mg dose. Dry mouth was mild to moderate in the majority of cases, with three cases of severe dry mouth being noted at 8 mg and two dry mouth cases being noted at 12 mg. Sixteen patients at 4 mg, 20 patients at 8 mg, and 14 patients at 12 mg noted dry mouth. There were five cases of dry mouth with placebo ingestion. The authors concluded that all three doses of fesoterodine produced significant and clinically meaningful reductions in urinary frequency and incontinence episodes, with improvements noted as early as 2 weeks after randomization, and that fesoterodine was relatively well tolerated.[16]

PHASE III ANALYSIS

In an expanded phase III trial of fesoterodine at 4 and 8 mg dosing versus placebo and tolterodine at the 4-mg dose,[17] 1135 subjects were evaluated. A total of 1103 patients were available for intent to treat analysis and 988 completed the trial. The population of this trial was predominantly female (81%), with a mean age of 56.6 years.

Patients were evaluated for co-primary efficacy variables: mean frequency change for 24 hours and mean urge incontinence change for 24 hours on a 3-day micturition diary. Other outcomes included self-assessment of treatment benefit using a treatment benefit scale, and safety analysis.

Drop-out rates due to adverse events were low in all treatment groups: placebo (2%), fesoterodine 4 mg (3%), fesoterodine 8 mg (5%), and tolterodine 4 mg extended-release (3%). The most frequent adverse event occurring in all groups was dry mouth in 7% (placebo), 22% (4 mg fesoterodine), 34% (8 mg fesoterodine), and 17% (4 mg extended-release tolterodine). Intensity was mild to moderate in most cases. Other than dry mouth, no significant adverse event occurred in greater than 5% of the study population. There were no significant relevant changes in vital signs, laboratory or ECG parameters, or post-void residual volume. Overall reductions in micturitions

per 24 hours and urge incontinent episodes were significantly greater than with placebo for all active treatment groups. Treatment response indicated statistically significant improvement over placebo for the active treatment groups. Treatment response was more pronounced with fesoterodine in the 4- or 8-mg dose than for tolterodine 4 mg. Treatment response also correlated well with a reduction in OAB symptoms.

The authors concluded that all active agents showed clinically significant and clinically relevant improvements over placebo, and the improvements were more significant with fesoterodine 4 and 8 mg as compared to those with tolterodine 4 mg in regard to reduction of urge incontinent episodes. Treatment response as judged by treatment assessment was well correlated with improvement in OAB symptoms and with onset of action occurring within 2 weeks.

Nitti et al.[18] recently reported results of the second phase III placebo-controlled trial conducted in North America. This study utilized a similar double-blind, randomized, placebo-controlled trial design, with patients having standard inclusion criteria of greater than or equal to eight micturitions in 24 hours, with greater than or equal to six urinary urgency episodes during that time frame and greater than or equal to three incontinence episodes per day over a 3-day diary run-in period. Patients received either placebo or fesoterodine at 4- or 8-mg doses.

Primary outcome measures assessed were micturitions per 24 hours, change in average number of urge incontinent episodes per 24 hours, and treatment response derived from a treatment benefit scale. Statistical analysis was utilized using ANCOVA. A total of 836 patients were randomized, of whom 681 completed the 12-week treatment criteria. Both 4 and 8 mg of fesoterodine were found to be clinically statistically significant in terms of results over placebo, with mean changes from baseline being 1.02 (placebo), 1.86 (fesoterodine 4 mg), and 1.94 (fesoterodine 8 mg), respectively.

Decreases in urge and urinary incontinence episodes for 24 hours were 1.0 (placebo), 1.77 (fesoterodine 4 mg), and 2.42 (fesoterodine 8 mg), respectively. Patients perceived treatment response to be significantly improved also with the 4- and 8-mg doses, at 64 and 74% ($p < 0.001$), as compared to placebo (45%). Dry mouth was the most common adverse event reported in 7% (placebo),

16% (4 mg fesoterodine), and 36% (8 mg fesoterodine). The authors concluded that both doses of fesoterodine led to substantial improvement in efficacy parameters as well as improvements in urinary frequency, urgency incontinence, and perception of treatment response. Treatment results were seen as early as 2 weeks, and fesoterodine was generally well tolerated.

CONCLUSION

Fesoterodine is the newest member of the antimuscarinic class of drugs to undergo clinical evaluation. It is currently awaiting Food and Drug Administration (FDA) approval. Clinical trials have shown that the compound is generally well tolerated and has efficacy which demonstrates a dose responsiveness.

REFERENCES

1. Breidenbach A, Pandita R, Selve N, Andersson K-E. Pharmacodynamic profiling of the novel antimuscarinic drug fesoterodine on rat bladder. Proc Int Continence Soc 2002; 32: 449.
2. Ney P, Stoehr T. M3 selective antimuscarinics affect gastrointestinal transit in the mouse more potently than nonselective drugs. Naunyn Schmiedebergs Arch Pharmacol 2002; 365 (Suppl 1): 413.
3. Mansfield KJ, Vaux K, Millard RJ, Burcher E. Comparison of receptor binding characteristics of commonly used muscarinic antagonists in human bladder detrusor and mucosa. Proc Int Continence Soc 2002; 32: 449.
4. Sachse R, Cawello W, Auer S, Horstmann R. Pharmacodynamics of multiple dose treatment with the novel antimuscarinic drug fesoterodine. Naunyn Schmiedebergs Arch Pharmacol 2002; 365 (Suppl 1): 413.
5. Cawello W, Auer S, Hammes W, Sachse R, Horstmann R. Multiple dose pharmacokinetics of fesoterodine in human subjects. Naunyn Schmiedebergs Arch Pharmacol 2002; 365 (Suppl 1): 428.
6. Sachse R, Cawello W, Hammes W, Horstmann R. Safety and pharmacokinetics of the novel antimuscarinic drug fesoterodine in populations of different age or gender. Proc Int Continence Soc 2002; 32: 441.
7. Sachse R, Cawello W, Haag C, Horstmann R. Pharmacodynamics and pharmacokinetics of ascending multiple oral doses of novel bladder-selective antimuscarinic fesoterodine. Eur Urol Suppl 2003; 2: 30.
8. Sachse R, Cawello W, Haag C, Horstmann R. Dose-proportional pharmacokinetics of the new antimuscarinic fesoterodine. Naunyn Schmiedebergs Arch Pharmacol 2003; 367 (Suppl 1): 446.
9. Sachse R, Cawello W, Hammes W, Horstmann R. Safety and pharmacokinetics of the novel bladder-selective antimuscarinic fesoterodine in populations of different ethnic origin. Proc Int Continence Soc 2003; 33: 377.
10. Sachse R, Cawello W, Horstmann R. Clinical pharmacological aspects of the novel bladder-selective antimuscarinic fesoterodine. Prog Urol 2004; 14 (Suppl 3): 58.
11. Sachse R, Cawello W, Hammes W, Horstmann R. Concomitant food intake does not significantly influence the pharmacokinetics of the novel, bladder-selective antimuscarinic fesoterodine. Proc Int Continence Soc 2004; 34: 580.
12. Sachse R, Krastev Z, Mateva L et al. Safety, tolerability and pharmacokinetics of fesoterodine in patients with hepatic impairment. Proc Int Continence Soc 2004; 34: 585.
13. Sachse R, Cawello W, Horstmann R. Safety, tolerability and pharmacokinetics of fesoterodine after co-treatment with the potent cytochrome P450 3A4 inhibitor ketoconazole. Proc Int Continence Soc 2004; 34: 586.
14. Chapple C. Fesoterodine: a new effective and well-tolerated antimuscarinic for the treatment of urgency-frequency syndrome: results of a phase 2 controlled study. Presented at European Association of Urology, Paris, France, March, 2004.
15. Nitti V, Wiatrak M, Kreitman L, Lipsitz D. Fesoterodine is an effective antimuscarinic for patients with overactive bladder (OAB): results of a phase 2 trial.
16. Rovner E, Payne C, Yalla S, Nitti V. Response to fesoterodine in overactive bladder (OAB) patients is independent of the urodynamic finding of detrusor overactivity.
17. Chapple C, Van Kerrebroeck P, Tubaro A, Millard R. Fesoterodine in non-neurogenic voiding dysfunction – results on efficacy and safety in a phase 3 trial. Presented at Annual Meeting of the European Association of Urology, Paris, France, 5–8 April, 2006.
18. Nitti V W, Dmochowski R R, Willliams T, Alvarez-Jacinto O R. Efficacy, safety, and tolerability of fesoterodine in patients with overactive bladder: a phase 3 placebo controlled trial in the United States. J Urol 2006; 175 (4 Suppl):

Neuromodulation

25

Neuromodulation: mechanisms of action

Tomas L Griebling

Normal voiding • **Pathophysiology of voiding dysfunction** • **Neuromodulation** • **Urodynamic and neurologic effects of neuromodulation** • **Future directions**

Once considered unusual and experimental, neuromodulation has become a widely accepted tool in the therapeutic armamentarium for some forms of voiding dysfunction. The technology has evolved from the ancient practices of acupuncture to incorporate computerized equipment and sophisticated electrical stimulation methods. One of the most interesting paradoxes is that the therapy appears to work for both bladder over-activity and some forms of idiopathic urinary retention (Figure 25.1). Although the exact mechanisms of neuromodulation for the treatment of voiding dysfunction are still not entirely under-stood, recent research in the field has advanced the various hypotheses regarding the neurophysiology of these complex processes. This chapter reviews the current state of knowledge regarding neuromodulation for disorders of the lower urinary tract.

NORMAL VOIDING

The physiological processes of normal urine storage and voiding require a series of highly coordinated interactions between the central and peripheral nervous systems, the neuro-muscular interface, and the organs of the lower urinary tract. The overall system must coordinate both effective bladder storage of urine at low pressures, and efficient evacuation of urine during a micturition event. Innervation to the detrusor muscle is under the control of the autonomic nervous system. This occurs via a combination of interactions from the sympathetic and para-sympathetic components. Although a complete review of voiding neurophysiology is beyond the scope of this chapter, a brief overview will be useful to help understand the purported mechanistic theories of neuromodulation[1] (Figure 25.2).

The spinal micturition center is located in the sacral region of the spinal cord (S_2–S_4). The nerve roots at this level give rise to the pelvic nerves (parasympathetic). These provide the major afferent pathway for the normal micturition reflex. There are two distinct types of bladder afferents. The small, myelinated Aδ fibers communicate the sensations of filling via the mechanoreceptors and tension receptors in the bladder. In contrast, the larger, unmyelinated C fibers transmit noxious stimuli from the nociceptors in the bladder and produce sensations of pain and temperature. Stimulation of the C fibers may also trigger reflex voiding events.

Efferent sympathetic innervation is provided via the hypogastric nerves (T_{10}–L_2). The pudendal nerves provide somatic innervation (S_2–S_4), including input to the external striated sphincter. Signals from the sacral spinal micturition center are communicated via the spinal cord to the pontine micturition center and the cerebral cortex of the brain. The suprapontine regions of the brain typically produce inhibitory signals which facilitate urine storage. The stretch receptors in the bladder trigger increased afferent activity which is conducted to the brain via the posterior roots of the sacral spinal cord and the lateral

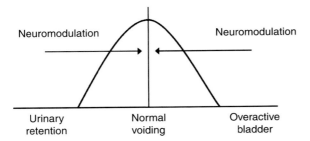

Figure 25.1 The functional goal of neuromodulation is to restore a more normal voiding pattern. This may include improvement in storage and/or micturition parameters.

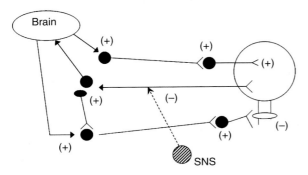

Figure 25.2 The voiding reflex. Detrusor contractility is mediated by parasympathetic efferent nerves. The urethra is controlled by afferent innervation. Sacral nerve stimulation (SNS) at the S_3 nerve root helps improve urinary urgency, frequency, and urge incontinence by inhibiting these reflexes.

spinothalamic tracts. With continued filling, a threshold signal is reached which leads to a sensation of bladder fullness and a subsequent desire to void.

Initiation of micturition is influenced by input from the pontine micturition center and a complex series of reflexes between the bladder and brain stem. Urethral relaxation occurs, and is rapidly followed by relaxation of the pelvic floor muscles, funneling of the bladder neck, and detrusor contraction. This portion of the process is under parasympathetic control.

Three groups of nerves innervate the detrusor muscle. Cholinergic nerves release acetylcholine (ACh) and provide much of the motor control during contraction of the detrusor muscles. Noradrenergic neurons provide sympathetic innervation, and are most concentrated in the base of the bladder. Non-adrenergic non-cholinergic sensorimotor nerves innervating the detrusor produce an array of peptide neurotransmitters. The specific functions of each of these various neuropeptides are not yet well understood.

In addition, the urothelium itself likely represents an important control mechanism in the process of normal micturition. This tissue releases acetylcholine which can affect detrusor contractility. Other local factors may impact on the viscoelastic properties of the bladder which can in turn alter filling sensation.

The guarding reflex is caused by sympathetic efferent input from the pudendal nerves, which leads to urethral smooth muscle contraction[2] (Figure 25.3). This reflex is most active during events which may trigger stress incontinence such as coughing or sneezing. The reflex is absent during normal micturition.

PATHOPHYSIOLOGY OF VOIDING DYSFUNCTION

Physiologic disorders of bladder function generally fall into two broad categories. Overactive bladder (OAB) refers to the conditions that produce a sense of urinary urgency, frequency, and in

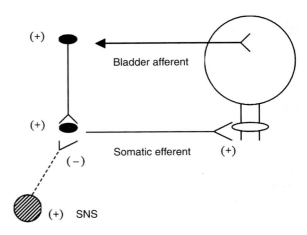

Figure 25.3 The guarding reflex. Sympathetic efferent input via the pudendal nerves causes urethral smooth muscle contraction during stress events such as coughing and sneezing. Sacral nerve stimulation (SNS) at the S_3 nerve root leads to inhibition of the guarding reflex and a reduction in sphincteric overactivity in cases of idiopathic urinary retention.

some cases urge urinary incontinence. In contrast, urinary retention is often caused by detrusor underactivity or chronic pelvic floor hypertonicity with incomplete urinary evacuation. Urinary retention caused by obstruction will not be discussed in this chapter because neuromodulation is not indicated for these situations.

Overactive bladder

There are several proposed mechanisms which may lead to overactive bladder.[3] A decrease in suprapontine inhibition of the micturition reflexes may lead to an increase in unopposed afferent neural activity with loss of inhibition at the peripheral level. This can cause an increase in excitatory impulse transmission and lead to contraction of the detrusor muscles. This type of problem is commonly seen in cases of multiple sclerosis and stroke. Partial denervation of the bladder smooth muscle may cause "micromotions" of the muscle fibers, leading to the typical OAB sensations of urinary urgency and frequency. Newer hypotheses include possible excess production of acetylcholine from the urothelium, or hypersensitivity of the ACh receptors. This could lead to increased bladder contractility and subsequent symptoms. Alternatively, there may be a leak of ACh from efferent nerve fibers which could cause "micromotions" of bladder smooth muscle fibers. This activity could trigger central pathways causing a sensation of urinary urgency typical of OAB.

Urinary retention

Decreased afferent activity can lead to impairment of detrusor muscle contractility with subsequent urinary retention. If the degree of hypocontractility is sufficient, the bladder may no longer be able to overcome the inherent urethral and bladder neck resistance needed to empty. This may be true even if the external urethral sphincter is completely relaxed.

Conversely, urinary retention may be caused by a chronic increased tonicity of the pelvic floor and urethra. A hyperactive guarding reflex may be present. This may also be associated with chronic excitation and contraction of the striated sphincter, a condition referred to as the "Fowler syndrome".[4] This also leads to an inability to

overcome the outlet resistance and a functional rather than true anatomic obstruction.

NEUROMODULATION

Historical perspectives

Numerous investigators have searched for methods of neuromodulation to improve urinary control. However, it is only in the recent past that this research has come to significant fruition. In 1982, Tanagho and Schmidt were the first to present the results of sacral root stimulation in paraplegic dogs.[5] Subsequent work has led to the evolution of modern neurostimulation methodology including minimally invasive electrical leads and implantable programmable pulse generators.

Neural pathways

Although this chapter focuses on sacral nerve stimulation (SNS) with implantable neuroelectrodes, a number of other anatomic sites and neural pathways have been tested with varying degrees of success. Transcutaneous electrical nerve stimulation (TENS) has been associated with short-term improvement in detrusor overactivity and urinary urgency and frequency. Bower and her colleagues conducted a sham-controlled trial of TENS of the suprapubic and sacral skin in a series of 47 women.[6] They found that TENS produced a significant reduction in the mean maximum height of detrusor contractions compared to the sham control. Improvement was better in those subjects who had a demonstrable component of motor urgency compared to those with sensory urgency alone. Similarly, in a sham-controlled trial of antidromic TENS applied to the third sacral nerve (S_3), Walsh et al. found that stimulation led to a significant increase in bladder storage capacity without an associated increase in detrusor pressure.[7] This urodynamic finding was not observed in the control subjects. The disadvantage of TENS is that it must be applied frequently, and is therefore less convenient than an implantable programmable device.

TENS technology has also been applied to the thigh muscles for the treatment of detrusor overactivity. Okada et al. examined this technique in a series of 19 patients with either detrusor hyperreflexia or idiopathic detrusor instability.[8]

Surface electrodes were applied to the quadriceps or hamstring muscles of one or both legs for 20 minutes daily over a period of 2 weeks. Follow-up urodynamic evaluation revealed a greater than 50% increase in maximum cystometric capacity compared to pretreatment values in 58% of the subjects. Symptomatic improvement was seen in about half of these patients, and the result was sustained for up to 3 months. The authors hypothesized that the effect was caused by reflex-mediated stimulation of pudendal afferents which can lead to a centrally induced inhibition of pelvic efferent activity. In addition, they postulated that modulation of cholinergic and β-adrenergic neurotransmission may be involved in the process.

Inserted vaginal and anal electrodes have also been used for pelvic floor rehabilitation, and these may work by a similar neurophysiologic mechanism. In two small series, Nakamura and colleagues reported successful temporary inhibition of bladder overactivity using transcutaneous perianal or penile electrodes.[9,10] Wheeler et al. also reported success in two patients treated with penile stimulation after spinal cord injury.[11]

Treatment of urinary retention caused by more complete spinal cord injury using various methods of neuromodulation has proven more problematic. Walter et al. demonstrated that direct bladder stimulation was more effective than sacral nerve stimulation in producing an effective voiding pattern in a feline model.[12] Indeed, the currently approved sacral nerve stimulator devices are not approved for use in cases of urinary retention due to complete spinal cord lesions. This supports the contention that interaction between the peripheral and central nervous systems is facilitated by sacral neuromodulation.

Transcutaneous posterior tibial nerve stimulation has also been used with some clinical success.[13] The posterior tibial nerve is a mixed motor and sensory nerve that projects to the sacral spinal cord in the areas of the sacral micturition center and Onuf's nucleus. It is hypothesized that electrical stimulation of this nerve leads to reflex stimulation of the sacral micturition center with subsequent excitation of pudendal afferents. This in turn may lead to a reduction of detrusor contractility and OAB symptoms. The effect appears to be sustained, although only for short periods of time (< 2 weeks).[14,15]

Percutaneous sacral neuromodulation

Sacral neuromodulation is currently the most widely used technique for the treatment of voiding dysfunction. A multipolar electrode is placed percutaneously into the foramen of the third sacral nerve root (S_3) (Figure 25.4). This is connected to a programmable pulse generator and battery unit (Figure 25.5). Electrical stimulation

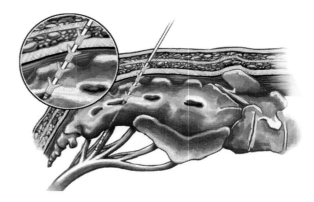

Figure 25.4 The quadripolar electrode in position in the S_3 foramen. The lead is secured in position by the tines at the level of the lumbodorsal fascia (inset). (Reprinted with the permission of Medtronic, Inc. © 2006). (See also color plate section).

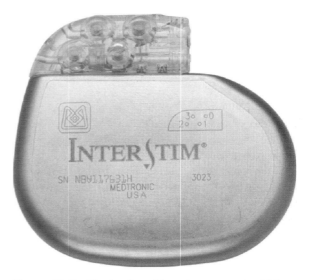

Figure 25.5 The implantable pulse generator. This unit contains the programmable components which attach to the lead shown in Figure 25.4 and the battery. (Reprinted with the permission of Medtronic, Inc. © 2006).

of this nerve causes a reflex contraction of the levator ani, coccygeus, and external anal sphincter muscles via the pudendal nerve. This produces a "bellows" response which is elicited during the implantation procedure. A reflex arc through the tibial branch of the sciatic nerve causes flexion of the ipsilateral great toe. The typical sensory responses are conducted by two nerves. Stimulation of the perineal branch of the pudendal nerve and the posterior femoral cutaneous nerve leads to a vibratory sensation in the urethra, penis, and scrotum in men, and in the labia majora and vagina in women. Stimulation of the inferior rectal nerve leads to a vibratory sensation in the rectum.[16]

In ideal cases, the patient experiences both sensory and motor responses during test stimulation and lead implantation. However, in some cases this does not occur. There are data to suggest that the motor response may be the stronger predictor of a successful clinical outcome. In a series of 35 patients who underwent lead implantation for refractory urinary urgency or urge incontinence, Cohen et al. reported that an isolated sensory response was associated with only a 4.7% chance of a successful test stimulation.[17] In contrast, 95% of patients with a successful test stimulation had a positive motor response during implantation, compared to only 21.4% of those with unsuccessful test implants.

Several theories have been proposed to explain the efficacy of sacral neuromodulation in disparate conditions including OAB and urinary retention (Table 25.1). The mechanisms of action of sacral neuromodulation are most likely multifactorial, and they probably impact on the neuroaxis at several different levels[2,18,19] (Figure 25.6).

One popular theory of neuromodulation for OAB suggests that stimulation of the sacral nerve leads to indirect stimulation of the pudendal nerve and direct inhibition of bladder preganglionic neurons. This in turn leads to a suppression of detrusor overactivity and subsequent improvement in clinical symptoms. The fact that effective electrical intensities do not activate striated muscle contraction supports this hypothesis. These frequencies are also under the threshold required to activate autonomic nerve fibers, which prevents a concomitant bladder contraction. This suggests that somatic afferents are involved in this process.[3]

An alternative explanation is that sacral neuromodulation may inhibit involuntary reflex voiding by altering the transmission of sensory input from the bladder to the pontine micturition center. This is mediated by inhibition of the ascending afferent pathway and spinal tract neurons. However, the descending efferent parasympathetic pathways are not inhibited. This may

---

Table 25.1 Theoretical mechanisms of neuromodulation by sacral nerve stimulation (SNS)

Overactive bladder
SNS causes stimulation of the pudendal nerve which inhibits bladder preganglionic neurons
SNS causes inhibition of the ascending afferent signals which alters sensory input at the pontine micturition center
SNS leads to stimulation of $A\delta$ fibers which excite central inhibitory pathways

Urinary retention
SNS inhibits the guarding reflex with subsequent relaxation of the pelvic floor
SNS causes a "rebound" phenomenon which results in improved detrusor contraction

---

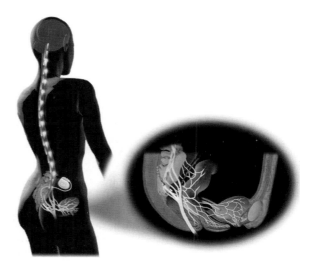

Figure 25.6 Sacral neuromodulation influences both the central and peripheral nervous systems through a variety of pathways. (Reprinted with the permission of Medtronic, Inc. © 2006). (See also color plate section).

explain why reflex micturition is suppressed while volitional voiding is preserved.[2,18,19] It is also possible that stimulation of the Aδ fibers in the sacral nerve root may excite central inhibitory pathways. This may modulate the external urethral sphincter and pelvic floor muscles via somatic input through the pelvic nerve.

In the case of non-obstructive urinary retention, neuromodulation most likely causes an inhibition of the guarding reflex.[2,18,19] This leads to a reduction in sphincteric overactivity which reduces functional outlet resistance at the bladder neck and urethra. Sacral nerve root stimulation may also improve relaxation of the pelvic floor musculature, which could in turn decrease outlet resistance. A "rebound" phenomenon has also been described. In this scenario, prolonged stimulation induces bladder inhibition and hypocontractility. Cessation of this stimulation, modulated by the sacral nerve stimulator, results in an improvement in bladder wall contractility during volitional voiding attempts.[20] A long-latency afferent mediated reflex has been described which is associated with prolonged latency of the anal wink response. This may be part of why sacral neuromodulation has shown efficacy for some patients with fecal urgency and fecal incontinence in addition to voiding dysfunction.[21]

URODYNAMIC AND NEUROLOGIC EFFECTS OF NEUROMODULATION

A variety of recent studies have examined the physiologic effects caused by neuromodulation both at the central and peripheral levels. These studies help to provide support for the theoretical framework regarding the mechanisms of action of neuromodulation.

Urodynamic effects

There is urodynamic evidence that neurostimulation leads to peripheral effects at the level of the bladder during both the storage and voiding phases. Groen and colleagues performed cystometric analysis on 26 consecutive patients (22 women and four men) who were treated with sacral neuromodulation for urinary urgency and urge incontinence.[22] They measured multiple cystometric parameters including cystometric capacity, time to instability during filling,

and contraction pressures. Overall, they found that all variables responded favorably to neuromodulation. However, only the amplitude of the initial and maximum unstable contractions, the maximum detrusor pressure, and the mean active pressures during unstable episodes reached statistical significance.

This group also examined urodynamic variables during micturition.[23] Urodynamic assessments were performed at baseline and at 6 months after neurostimulator implantation in a series of 33 women treated for urge incontinence. In general, the observed effects included an increase in voided volume, an increase in maximum flow rate, a decrease in urethral resistance, and an increase in the bladder contractility index. However, none of these parameters were statistically significant when only the 26 clinical responders were considered. This suggests that neuromodulation may lead to a reduction in bladder overactivity without significant alteration in either urethral resistance or detrusor contraction strength.

These findings imply that clinical success may rely on physiologic changes other than just standard urodynamic factors. Future research on the urodynamic effects of neuromodulation may help to better explain these complex interactions.

Neurologic effects

Advances in the technology for brain imaging have allowed researchers to study the direct effects of neuromodulation in the central nervous system. Dasgupta and colleagues examined changes in brain activity in eight women with urinary retention treated with sacral neuromodulation, and eight control subjects.[24] Positron emission tomography (PET) scanning was performed on each subject with the bladder both empty and full. Multiple scans were obtained for each subject in each state to help minimize variations. Subjects with a history of urinary retention were tested with the neurostimulator in both the activated and deactivated modes. In control subjects, a full bladder was associated with increased activity in the anterior midbrain near the substantia nigra and at the junction of the pons and medulla. A full bladder also prompted increased activity in the anterior and posterior portions of the cingulate cortex. In contrast, subjects with a history of urinary retention did not demonstrate enhanced midbrain activity with bladder filling when the neurostimulator was in the "off" position. However, they did demonstrate activity in the anterior and posterior cingulate cortex. When the neurostimulator was activated, these subjects demonstrated increased activity in the midbrain and pons at levels similar to that seen in the control subjects. The urinary retention subjects also had an attenuation of activity in the anterior and posterior cingulate cortex during activation of the neurostimulator. This suggests that the limbic activity may be inhibiting the voiding mechanism through descending pathways.

Braun et al. utilized electroencephalography (EEG) to examine the effects of neuromodulation of the S_3 nerve root on the central nervous system.[25] Ten subjects were studied, including two with urinary retention and eight with various forms of overactive bladder. The neurostimulation was set in an on–off cycling mode with 1.5 seconds "on" followed by 10 seconds "off". All subjects displayed similar EEG changes. The initial response was an electronegative cortical potential complex (50 milliseconds at a mean amplitude of 23 microvolts). This was followed by a late potential complex (253 milliseconds at a mean amplitude of 5 microvolts). The maximum activity for both of these complexes was at the "Cz" focus, which corresponds to the postcentral gyrus. Some subjects were able to feel the stimulator when it was turned on and off, but other subjects did not have these sensations. It is interesting that the EEG findings were consistent and independent of the sensory input status of the subjects.

Sacral neuromodulation also appears to influence the somatosensory evoked potentials (SEPs) for the pudendal and posterior tibial nerves. Malaguti et al. studied 24 female subjects, including 16 with urinary retention and eight with either urinary urgency/frequency or urge incontinence, who underwent unilateral sacral neuromodulation.[26] SEP patterns were examined both prior to and 1 month after neurostimulator implantation. Post-implantation tests were performed with pulse rates of both 21 Hz and 40 Hz. Sixteen subjects had a good clinical response to the initial test stimulation with at least a 50% reduction in residual urinary (urinary retention) or number of incontinent or urgent voiding episodes

(urge incontinence or urgency/frequency). In this group of clinical responders, activation of the neurostimulator led to a significant reduction in pudendal SEP latency for the first positive deflection (P40). This finding was observed both ipsilateral and contralateral to the neuromodulator lead. These changes in SEP were not consistently observed in the group of clinical non-responders. Five subjects had no alteration of pudendal SEP compared to baseline, and three subjects had a decrease in P40 latency that was not statistically significantly different from baseline. These findings provide additional evidence that the afferent pathway from the spinal nerves to the cortical sensory area is involved in the regulation of micturition and the response to neuromodulation.

Stimulation of the S_3 nerve root also produces peripheral neurologic effects. Wyndaele et al. examined the effect of neurostimulation on the electrosensory thresholds in the lower urinary tract in a group of ten subjects (seven women and three men).[27] Six subjects had detrusor hypocontractility with urinary retention, and four had detrusor overactivity with urgency and urge incontinence. After a mean of 5 days of neuromodulation, the electrosensory threshold was measured in the bladder and urethra using catheter-mounted electrodes. An electrode placed on the skin of the forearm was used as a control. Neurostimulation impulses were standardized for all subjects. Neurostimulation resulted in a decrease in bladder electrosensory thresholds. Four subjects underwent bilateral neurostimulation and six had unilateral neurostimulation. In the subjects with unilateral stimulation, these findings were observed in the ipsilateral side of the bladder. There were no observed effects on the forearm or in the urethra. The findings were consistent regardless of the clinical success of neurostimulation for the underlying voiding symptoms. These results support the premise that S_3 neurostimulation works via the afferent nervous system in the pelvic nerves.

There is some evidence that sacral neuromodulation may also lead to alterations in autonomic nerve function. Kenefick et al. examined the effects of sacral neuromodulation on rectal blood flow.[28] This physiological parameter can be used as a measure of autonomic nerve function. Sixteen subjects who underwent successful sacral neuromodulation for the treatment of fecal incontinence were examined. Rectal laser Doppler flowmetry was performed at the level of chronic stimulation for each patient. This testing was subsequently repeated without neurostimulation, and then with progressive voltage increments. Activation of the neurostimulator led to a marked increase in blood flux compared to baseline. The increase was most notable between baseline and 1.0 volts. Additional increases in stimulation amplitude (up to a maximum of 5.0 volts) resulted in only subtle increases in blood flux which were not statistically significant. The initial changes were rapid and reached a steady state within seconds. These findings suggest that sacral neurostimulation leads to modulation of autonomic neural activity.

The data from these various studies support the hypothesis that supraspinal micturition centers and various peripheral mechanisms are involved in the physiologic response to neuromodulation for voiding dysfunction. Additional research will help to better define these complex interactions.

Neurochemistry and neuromodulation

There is growing evidence that neuromodulation may influence various neurotransmitters and growth factors which could have an impact on urinary physiology (Table 25.2). In a rat model of cystitis, blockade of the N-methyl-D-aspartate (NMDA) receptors did not appear to influence the effect of neuromodulation on bladder contractility.[29] In contrast, blockade of the non-NMDA receptors and blockade of nitric oxide (NO) synthase did influence the observed effects. Wang and Hassouna have demonstrated that sacral neuromodulation reduces c-fos gene expression and associated bladder hyperreflexia in a rat

---

Table 25.2 Neurotransmitters and growth factors associated with sacral nerve stimulation (SNS)

Non-NMDA receptors
Nitric oxide (NO) synthase
c-fos
Vanilloids
Nerve growth factor (NGF)

*NMDA, N-methyl-D-aspartate

---

model of spinal injury.[30] This effect is thought to be modulated through the afferent C fibers.[31]

It is hypothesized that vanilloids may be involved in the conduction of noxious stimuli. Using a rat model, Zhou et al. have demonstrated that vanilloid receptor 1 (VR_1) expression in the spinal cord is upregulated after spinal cord injury.[32] Sacral nerve root modulation led to decreased staining for VR_1 on immunohistochemical analysis. Anecdotal reports suggest that neuromodulation might be beneficial in some patients with chronic pelvic pain due to inflammatory conditions such as interstitial cystitis.[33,34] It is possible that the observed improvements may be mediated by changes in vanilloid receptor expression.

Nerve growth factor (NGF) is a trophic protein that facilitates interaction between peripheral tissues and innervating neurons.[31] Bladder and vascular smooth muscle both produce NGF. The expression of NGF is altered in various pathologic conditions, and it may play a role as an endogenous mediator of persistent pain. The effects of neuromodulation on NGF expression are not well understood, but may be a valuable focus for future research.

FUTURE DIRECTIONS

Sacral neuromodulation has become an important treatment option for select patients with urinary urgency and frequency, urge urinary incontinence, and some forms of idiopathic urinary retention. As our understanding of the mechanisms of action for this therapy evolve, it is likely that the clinical indications and therapeutic techniques will also expand. The role of bilateral stimulation is controversial and deserves additional research.[35,36] Neuromodulation has shown promise for the treatment of refractory fecal urgency and fecal incontinence, and it may be helpful for some forms of chronic constipation.[21,28,37] Additional research is needed to define the role of neuromodulation for urinary disorders associated with specific neurologic and other clinical conditions such as multiple sclerosis, Parkinson's disease, stroke, interstitial cystitis, and chronic genitourinary pain syndromes.[37,38]

Ongoing research will likely lead to miniaturization of neuromodulation equipment. Medtronic, Inc. has recently introduced a second generation implantable pulse generator for the InterStim® device which is smaller and may help improve patient comfort. Direct pudendal nerve stimulation using an implantable ministimulator is one of the newest techniques in the field of neuromodulation. Early data suggest that this may be a viable alternative to sacral neuromodulation for the treatment of refractory voiding dysfunction.[39,40]

Neuromodulation is one of the most rapidly evolving tools in the area of voiding dysfunction. Future research will help to increase our understanding of the underlying physiologic principles and mechanisms of action for this therapy. This information will also help to validate the various theories of both normal and altered bladder neurophysiology.

REFERENCES

1. de Groat WC. Central nervous system control of micturition. In: O'Donnell PD, ed. Urinary Incontinence. St Louis: Mosby 1997: 33–47.
2. Leng WW, Chancellor MB. How sacral nerve stimulation neuromodulation works. Urol Clin North Am 2005; 32: 11–18.
3. Wein AJ, Rackley RR. Overactive bladder: a better understanding of pathophysiology, diagnosis and management. J Urol 2006; 175: S5–10.
4. Fowler CJ, Christmas TJ, Chapple CR. Abnormal electromyographic activity of the urethral sphincter, voiding dysfunction, and polycystic ovaries: a new syndrome? BMJ 1988; 297: 1436–8.
5. Tanagho EA, Schmidt RA. Bladder pacemaker: scientific basis and clinical future. Urology 1982; 20: 614–19.
6. Bower WF, Moore KH, Adams RD, Shepherd R. A urodynamic study of surface neuromodulation versus sham in detrusor instability and sensory urgency. J Urol 1998; 160: 2133–6.
7. Walsh IK, Thompson T, Loughridge WG et al. Non-invasive antidromic neurostimulation: a simple effective method for improving bladder storage. Neurourol Urodyn 2001; 20: 73–84.
8. Okada N, Igawa Y, Ogawa A, Nishizawa O. Transcutaneous electrical stimulation of thigh muscles in the treatment of detrusor overactivity. Br J Urol 1998; 81: 560–4.
9. Nakamura M, Sakurai T, Tsujimoto Y, Tada Y. Bladder inhibition by electrical stimulation of the perianal skin. Urol Int 1986; 41: 62–3.
10. Nakamura M, Sakurai T. Bladder inhibition by penile electrical stimulation. Br J Urol 1984; 56: 413–15.
11. Wheeler JS Jr, Walter JS, Sibley P. Management of incontinent SCI patients with penile stimulation: preliminary results. J Am Paraplegia Soc 1994; 17: 55–9.
12. Walter JS, Sidarous R, Robinson CJ, Wheeler JS, Wurster RD. Comparison of direct bladder and sacral nerve stimulation in spinal cats. J Rehab Res Dev 1992; 29: 13–22.
13. Vandoninck V, van Balken MR, Finazzi Agro E et al. Posterior tibial nerve stimulation in the treatment of urge incontinence. Neurourol Urodyn 2003; 22: 17–23.
14. van der Pal F, van Balken MR, Heesakkers JP, Debruyne FM, Bemelmans BL. Percutaneous tibial nerve stimulation in the treatment of refractory overactive bladder syndrome: is maintenance treatment necessary? BJU Int 2006; 97: 547–50.
15. Amarenco G, Ismael SS, Even-Schneider A et al. Urodynamic effect of acute transcutaneous posterior tibial nerve stimulation in overactive bladder. J Urol 2003; 169: 2210–15.
16. Mamo GA. Anatomy of the sacral region. In: Jonas U, Grunewald V, eds. New Perspectives in Sacral Nerve Stimulation for Control of Lower Urinary Tract Dysfunction. London: Martin Dunitz, 2002: 9–15.
17. Cohen BL, Tunuguntla HSGR, Gousse A. Predictors of success for first stage neuromodulation: motor versus sensory response. J Urol 2006; 175: 2178–81.
18. Chancellor MB, Leng W. The mechanism of action of sacral nerve stimulation in the treatment of detrusor overactivity and urinary retention. In: Jonas U, Grunewald V, eds. New Perspectives in Sacral Nerve Stimulation for Control of Lower Urinary Tract Dysfunction. London: Martin Dunitz, 2002: 17–28.
19. Chancellor MB, Chartier-Kastler EJ. Principles of sacral nerve stimulation (SNS) for the treatment of bladder and urethral sphincter dysfunctions. Neuromodulation 2000; 3: 15–26.
20. Schultz-Lampel D, Jiang C, Lindstrom S, Thüroff JW. Experimental results on mechanisms of action of electrical neuromodulation in chronic urinary retention. World J Urol 1998; 16: 301–4.
21. Jarrett MED. Neuromodulation for constipation and fecal incontinence. Urol Clin North Am 2005; 32: 79–87.

22. Groen J, van Mastrigt R, Bosch JL. Computerized assessment of detrusor instability in patients treated with sacral neuromodulation. J Urol 2001; 165: 169–73.

23. Groen J, Ruud Bosch JL, van Mastrigt R. Sacral neuromodulation in women with idiopathic detrusor overactivity incontinence: decreased overactivity but unchanged bladder contraction strength and urethral resistance during voiding. J Urol 2006; 175: 1005–9.

24. Dasgupta R, Critchley HD, Dolan RF, Fowler CJ. Changes in brain activity following sacral neuromodulation for urinary retention. J Urol 2005; 174: 2268–72.

25. Braun PM, Baezner H, Seif C et al. Alterations of cortical electrical activity in patients with sacral neuromodulation. Eur Urol 2002; 41: 562–6.

26. Malaguti S, Spinelli M, Giardiello G, Lazzeri M, VanDenHombergh U. Neurophysiological evidence may predict the outcome of sacral neuromodulation. J Urol 2003; 170: 2323–6.

27. Wyndaele JJ, Michielsen D, Van Dromme S. Influence of sacral neuromodulation of electrosensation of the lower urinary tract. J Urol 2000; 163: 221–4.

28. Kenefick NJ, Emmanuel A, Nicholls RJ, Kamm MA. Effect of sacral nerve stimulation on autonomic nerve function. Br J Surg 2003; 90: 1256–60.

29. Riazimand SH, Mense S. A rat model for studying effects of sacral neuromodulation on the contractile activity of a chronically inflamed bladder. BJU Int 2004; 94: 158–63.

30. Wang Y, Hassouna MM. Neuromodulation reduces c-fos gene expression in spinalized rats: a double-blind randomized study. J Urol 2000; 163: 1966–70.

31. Hassouna MM. Neuromodulation and growth factors in the lower urinary tract. In: Jonas U, Grunewald V, eds. New Perspectives in Sacral Nerve Stimulation for Control of Lower Urinary Tract Dysfunction. London: Martin Dunitz, 2002: 55–67.

32. Zhou Y, Wang Y, Abdelhady M, Mourad MS, Hassouna MM. Change of vanilloid receptor 1 following neuromodulation in rats with spinal cord injury. J Surg Res 2002; 107: 104–44.

33. Aló KM, McKay E. Selective nerve root stimulation (SNRS) for the treatment of intractable pelvic pain and motor dysfunction: a case report. Neuromodulation 2001; 4: 19–23.

34. Feler CA, Whitworth LA, Brookoff D, Powell R. Recent advances: sacral nerve root stimulation using a retrograde method of lead insertion for the treatment of pelvic pain due to interstitial cystitis. Neuromodulation 1999; 2: 211–16.

35. Scheepens WA, de Bie RA, Weil EH, van Kerrebroeck PE. Unilateral versus bilateral sacral neuromodulation in patients with chronic voiding dysfunction. J Urol 2002; 168: 2046–50.

36. Seif C, Eckermann J, Bross S et al. Findings with bilateral sacral neurostimulation: sixty-two PNE-tests in patients with neurogenic and idiopathic bladder dysfunctions. Neuromodulation 2004; 7: 141–5.

37. Bernstein AJ, Peters KM. Expanding indications for neuromodulation. Urol Clin North Am 2005; 32: 59–63.

38. Minardi D, Muzzonigro G. Lower urinary tract and bowel disorders and multiple sclerosis: role of sacral neuromodulation: a preliminary report. Neuromodulation 2005; 8: 176–81.

39. Groen J, Amiel C, Ruud Bosch JLH. Chronic pudendal nerve neuromodulation in women with idiopathic refractory detrusor overactivity incontinence: results of a pilot study with a novel minimally invasive implantable mini-stimulator. Neurourol Urodyn 2005; 24: 226–30.

40. Bosch JLHR. The Bion device: a minimally invasive implantable ministimulator for pudendal nerve neuromodulation in patients with detrusor overactivity incontinence. Urol Clin North Am 2005; 32: 109–12.

26

Sacral nerve stimulation for overactive bladder symptoms

Suzette E Sutherland and Steven W Siegel

Introduction • Brief background of sacral nerve stimulation • Basic theory: how sacral nerve stimulation works • Basic procedure: how it is done • Patient selection • Reported sacral nerve stimulation experience with overactive bladder • Expanding indications • Troubleshooting with tips and tricks • Summary

INTRODUCTION

The urinary symptom complex known as overactive bladder (OAB) is a condition which affects millions of Americans[1] by negatively impacting on their quality of life and contributing to millions in healthcare costs.[2,3] Conventional treatments for this disease include pharmacologic therapy (primarily anticholinergics), behavioral modifications, pelvic floor biofeedback, and neuromuscular rehabilitation. When these treatment modalities prove insufficient for the relief of urinary symptoms, interventions such as sacral nerve stimulation (SNS) and detrusor botulinum toxin injections are available. While the use of Botox® in the bladder is new and not yet Food and Drug Administration (FDA)-approved, sacral neuromodulation for voiding dysfunction has been utilized for several decades, and is an FDA-approved form of therapy for certain types of voiding dysfunction: urge incontinence, urgency–frequency syndrome, OAB, and idiopathic non-obstructive urinary retention. SNS is now considered the standard of care for the treatment of overactive bladder when conventional therapies fail,[4] with tens of thousands of implants performed worldwide.[5]

BRIEF BACKGROUND OF SACRAL NERVE STIMULATION

Brindley, Schmidt, and Tanagho were some of the first to describe the use of chronic electrical stimulation to treat voiding dysfunction in humans. Brindley et al. treated paraplegic subjects with sacral anterior root stimulation as early as 1976, with 60% of the 50 patients treated reporting complete continence.[6] Interestingly, 93% of the 28 male patients were also able to achieve penile erections through sacral root stimulation. In 1988, Schmidt reported a three-step technique for evaluation and placement of an electrode for stimulation at the S_3 nerve root or pudendal nerve.[7] His first procedures were performed in an attempt to treat chronic pelvic pain, with a greater than 50% decrease in perceived pain reported in almost half of the patients.[8] In 1990, Tanagho reported that almost 70% of patients with urinary urge incontinence appreciated subjective improvements of at least 50% following SNS, as noted by their self-rated symptom score.[9] And in 1998, Shaker and Hassouna attempted SNS therapy in patients with idiopathic non-obstructive urinary retention, and reported significant improvements in both voided and post-void residual volumes, as well as pelvic pain.[10] Since that time, there have been significant refinements in the test stimulation, lead design, and surgical technique that have improved therapeutic outcomes for patients with voiding dysfunction. SNS was first FDA-approved for use in the United States for intractable urinary urge incontinence in 1997, for urinary urgency–frequency syndrome and non-obstructive urinary retention in 1999, and for the symptom complex of OAB in 2003. Patients from these groups are appropriate candidates for SNS when, after trials of other more conservative treatment options, their chronic symptoms continue to significantly affect their quality of life.[4,11]

BASIC THEORY: HOW SACRAL NERVE STIMULATION WORKS

Many theories exist as to the possible mechanism of action of SNS (Table 26.1). Although the exact mechanism is not yet fully understood, significant evidence suggests that the most important factor is somatic afferent stimulation of the pelvic and pudendal nerves via the sacral nerve roots, which ultimately results in modulation of voiding and continence reflex pathways in the central nervous system (CNS).[12–15] A recent study involving positron emission tomography (PET) scanning of the brain during sacral neuromodulation identified the interaction of several brain centers (cingulated cortex, midbrain, and pons) as being important for proper urinary control.[16] Restoration of activity associated with brain stem autoregulation and attenuation of cingulated activity seems to be associated with the therapeutic effect seen during sacral neuromodulation. Additional evidence supporting the afferent pathways as the main target includes the finding that beneficial effects of SNS occur at low electrical stimulation intensities, which are insufficient for activation of striated muscle movements.[17,18] Inhibition of detrusor hyperreflexia can occur: (1) by direct inhibition of sacral interneuronal transmission in the afferent limb and (2) by inhibition of the bladder preganglionic neurons of the efferent limb of the micturition reflex. In patients with idiopathic, non-obstructive urinary retention, sacral afferent stimulation can suppress the overly excitatory outflow to the urethral outlet associated with an overactive guarding reflex, facilitating voiding reflexes that promote normal bladder emptying.[19,20]

Table 26.1 Theoretical mechanisms of action for sacral nerve stimulation
Inhibits postganglionic nerve terminals
Inhibits primary afferents presynaptically
Modulates pudendal afferents that transmit somatic and visceral neurochemical signaling
Inhibits spinal tract neurons of the micturition reflex
Inhibits interneurons involved in spinal segmental reflexes
Indirectly suppresses overactive guarding reflexes by turning off bladder afferent input to internal sphincter sympathetic or external sphincter interneurons
Activates bladder postganglionic efferents to stimulate voiding, while simultaneously suppressing urethral excitatory pathways through afferent-interneuronal transmission

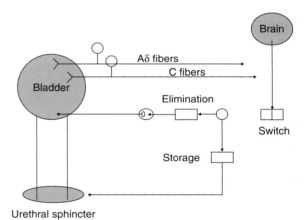

Figure 26.1 Micturition reflex pathways (modified from reference 21). As the bladder fills, Aδ fibers and C fibers provide afferent sensory signaling to the brain. The brain, in turn, signals spinal pathways that lead to a "turning off" of the guarding reflex, resulting in relaxation of the external urethral sphincter, contraction of the detrusor, and voluntary voiding of urine.

A simpler concept is that certain pathologic voiding states represent an imbalance between the reflexes of the bladder, urethral sphincter, and pelvic floor muscles. By modulating the CNS at the level where reflex signals responsible for switching between bladder emptying and storage are located (the pons or dorsal horn), SNS restores the appropriate balance between the reflexes for normal bladder function (Figure 26.1).[21]

This explains how SNS can paradoxically be beneficial for abnormal voiding states that seem to be pathological opposites: OAB and urinary retention. Pudendal afferent stimulation seems to serve as a common crossroads in the neurological wiring of the urinary system for correction of both OAB and urinary retention. Symptoms of voiding dysfunction may represent an alteration of the pelvic neuromuscular environment that changes pelvic organ function, as opposed to a disorder of the organs themselves. Neuromodulation is a method of altering or regulating that environment to promote normal voiding function.

BASIC PROCEDURE: HOW IT IS DONE

Initially, SNS trials were done via percutaneous neuromodulatory evaluation (PNE), utilizing a small temporary wire placed percutaneously through the S_3 foramen.[22] It was typically performed in the office, with local anesthetic, and without fluoroscopic guidance. Proper localization of S_3 was performed by palpation of bony landmarks and assessment of the patient's motor and sensory responses to stimulation. The temporary wire was secured to the patient with tape, and a 3–4 day stimulation trial with an external stimulator ensued, to assess efficacy of the therapy on the patient's symptoms. A > 50% improvement in symptoms was required (such as voiding frequency, number of incontinence episodes, number of pads required, or number of self-catheterizations performed) before proceeding to the next step. After removal of the temporary lead, simultaneous surgical placement of both a permanent S_3 lead and an implantable pulse generator (IPG) was performed. This surgical step was usually done under general anesthesia, and there was no reliable way to ensure that the placement of the permanent implantable lead replicated the exact location – and the same efficacy – as the temporary lead. Several techniques were used for implanting and securing the permanent lead, all requiring a significant incision: (1) fixation of the lead to the dorsal sacral periosteum,[17] (2) anchoring the lead to lumbosacral fascia,[23] or (3) sacral laminectomy to directly expose the S_3 nerve roots.[24] Changing the patient's position from prone to lateral or supine, the IPG was then implanted in the anterior abdominal wall, connected to the sacral lead by a long lead extension.

Over the years, significant refinements to the test stimulation, lead design, and surgical technique have led to the development of the two-staged implantation method.[25] It is our preference to perform such a staged implant procedure, utilizing a permanent lead for the initial therapeutic trial. The first stage involves percutaneous placement of a permanent tined lead through the S_3 foramen using fluoroscopic assistance (Figure 26.2). The percutaneous procedure utilizes a special introducer and the Seldinger technique to insert a permanent lead with tined plastic hooks into the S_3 foramen (Figure 26.3).

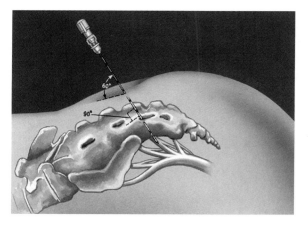

Figure 26.2 Needle placement through S_3 sacral foramen.

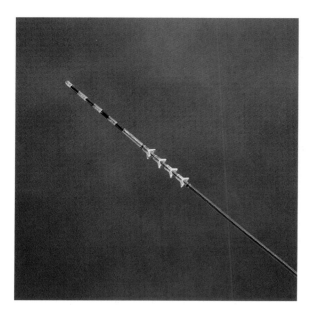

Figure 26.3 Tined lead, placed with an introducer (Seldinger technique).

Anterior–posterior (AP) imaging allows for easy localization of the S_3 foramen for starting the percutaneous access, while lateral imaging helps to determine the depth required for final placement of the S_3 lead (Figure 26.4). The addition of fluoroscopy certainly assisted greatly with the transition from an open lead implantation procedure to a minimally invasive, percutaneous approach. Performed in the operating room with local anesthesia (0.25% bupivacaine (Marcaine®)) and fast-acting intravenous (IV) sedation (propofal (Diprivan®), fentanyl (Sublimaze®), midazolam hydrochloride (Versed®)), both sensory and motor feedback during positioning of the lead are obtainable. These factors serve to increase the accuracy of lead site selection, thereby increasing the likelihood of clinical success, and decreasing the risk of uncomfortable sensations during chronic stimulation. Once implanted, the lead is attached to an extension wire, which is tunneled under the skin in the back and ultimately externalized for stimulation by a temporary external generator (Figure 26.5). A trial of chronic stimulation ensues. With this method of patient testing using a permanent tined lead, the chance for lead migration is less – almost 12% of lead migration seen with PNE[11] – and longer testing trials are therefore possible; subsequently, a better ability to predict clinical efficacy and long-term success is seen. We typically conduct a 3–4-week trial, and feel that this two-staged technique and length of trial decreases false positive rates, which may occur if previously successful PNE location is not exactly duplicated, or if sufficient time to gauge the response is not allotted. If > 50% improvement in patient symptoms is appreciated after the trial, the patient returns to the operating room for the second stage of the procedure. If sufficient change in symptoms is not appreciated, the tined lead is easily removed through a small incision. During the second phase for completion of the implant, using local anesthesia and IV sedation, a subcutaneous pocket for the IPG is created in the upper buttock, and the previously placed lead is then connected to the device using a short lead extension. Once the IPG incision has been closed, removal of the temporary external wires

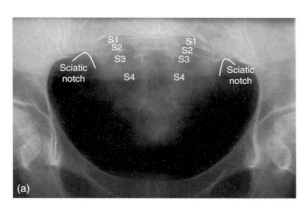

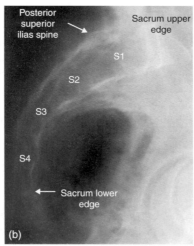

Figure 26.4 Anterior–posterior (a) and lateral (b) views of the sacrum with appropriate landmarks noted.

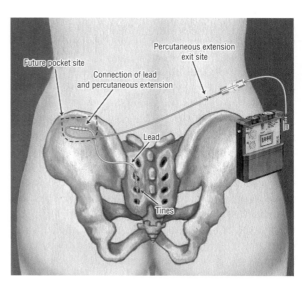

Figure 26.5 Test stimulation with chronic lead. (Reprinted with the permission of Medtronic, Inc. © 2006). (See also color plate section).

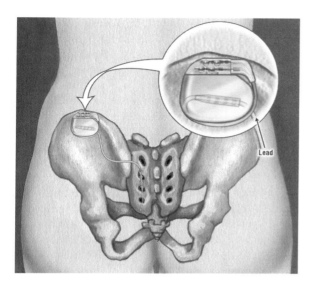

Figure 26.6 Implanted lead, extension connector, and implantable pulse generator (IPG). (Reprinted with the permission of Medtronic, Inc. © 2006). (See also color plate section).

is accomplished (Figure 26.6). Placement of the IPG in the upper buttocks[26] solved a variety of problems that were associated with the original placement of the devices in the anterior abdominal wall.[11]

We prefer to program the newly implanted IPG in the postoperative recovery area prior to the patient's discharge. The settings deemed most successful during the trial phase are those that are chosen during this initial programming session. Our experience shows that typical programming parameters for successful sacral neuromodulation include a frequency or rate of stimulation between 10 and 20 Hz, and a pulse width between 180 and 240 ms. Stimulation frequencies > 30 Hz are felt to be potentially harmful to peripheral nerves.[27] The stimulation amplitude can be highly variable, and depends most on the proximity of the lead to the nerve during lead placement. It is selected by the patient based on comfort. Ideally, patients should feel stimulatory sensation at thresholds < 4 volts. High intensity stimulation will deplete the battery prematurely. Under ideal circumstances, the devices have a battery life of 6–10 years. Patients have the ability to increase and decrease the signaling intensity as needed using the handheld programming device (Figure 26.7). Reprogramming in a unipolar (IPG case POSITIVE) or bipolar (IPG case OFF)

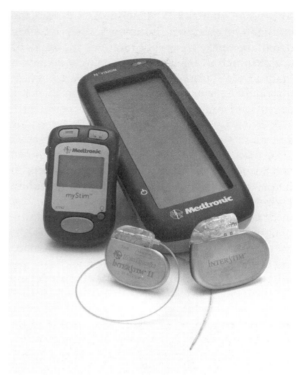

Figure 26.7 Patient programmer with control magnet. Physician programmer also viewed. (Reprinted with the permission of Medtronic, Inc. © 2006). (See also color plate section).

fashion is performed if uncomfortable stimulation or decreased efficacy is experienced.

A new, smaller IPG (InterStim® II) was recently FDA-approved for use in July 2006. It is 50% smaller and lighter, and ideally suited for smaller adults and pediatric patients, as well as those with lower stimulation intensity requirements (as determined during the test stimulation trial). With its new patient and physician programmers, and upgraded software, this newer system provides additional patient programming and data tracking opportunities. Due to its smaller size, a shorter battery life of approximately 5 years is expected.

PATIENT SELECTION

Although SNS is an accepted form of treatment for certain types of refractory voiding dysfunction – urge incontinence, urgency–frequency syndrome, OAB, and idiopathic non-obstructive urinary retention – proper patient selection remains somewhat empiric. It is helpful to define the patient's problem in terms of their voiding behaviors, pelvic symptoms, and pelvic floor muscle function, instead of using diagnostic labels that are often organ-based.[28] We now recognize that pelvic floor muscle dysfunction plays a key role in common pelvic-oriented disorders.[29] Hypertonicity of the pelvic floor can be a unifying feature in symptoms associated with overactive or *over-facilitated states* such as (1) voiding dysfunction (e.g. OAB, urethral syndrome); (2) incontinence (e.g. detrusor/rectal instability, urethral/anal sphincter instability); (3) pelvic pain (e.g. interstitial cystitis, "endometriosis", prostadynia, orchalgia); (4) bowel function (e.g. irritable bowel, anal fissures, proctalgia fulgax, hemorrhoids); (5) neuropathic voiding (e.g. multiple sclerosis, transverse myelitis, spinal trauma syndromes, peripheral neuropathies, "RSD" (reflex sympathetic dystrophy) syndromes). Manifestation of *over-inhibited states* can also be seen, such as in urinary retention and chronic constipation.[30] Recent reports on the effect of SNS on idiopathic urinary retention also noted improved success among patients with notable spasticity and hyperactivity of the pelvic floor musculature.[19,31] While isolated symptoms of pelvic floor muscle dysfunction, pelvic pain, and/or bowel dysfunction are not FDA-approved indications for sacral neuromodulation, they are commonly present in patients who are otherwise candidates for SNS, and frequently improve along with the urinary complaints if the therapy is otherwise successful.[32–37]

Pelvic floor muscle behavior can be easily assessed on pelvic examination with direct transvaginal and/or transrectal palpation of the levator ani muscles. Assessments can also be made during urodynamic studies with concomitant use of pelvic floor muscle electromyography (EMG). Patients who are unable to identify their pelvic floor muscles, and who do not have a normal range of motion from coordinated relaxation to efficient contraction, are usually unable to find their voluntary "on–off" switch to the bladder, and are therefore prone to voiding dysfunction and/or other pelvic disorders. These patients are excellent candidates for SNS when conservative treatment modalities including pelvic floor rehabilitation with EMG biofeedback prove unsuccessful.

Previously, SNS therapy has been reserved as a final treatment option – before radical surgery such as augmentation cystoplasty or cystectomy with urinary diversion – after prolonged trials of all other possible treatment modalities have failed. This usually means that, upon presentation for SNS therapy, patients are older, and have numerous comorbidities. Both of these factors may contribute to their refractory response to more conservative treatment modalities.[38,39] In a recent review of our own institution's 11-year experience with SNS,[40] mean duration of voiding symptoms prior to initiation of, or referral for, SNS therapy was 116 ± 130 months (range 9–600 months). The average age at implantation in this series was 50 ± 13.4 years (range 20–80 years), and shows a bias towards adopting this treatment option early in the algorithm of refractory cases. A recent study by Amundsen et al. noted significantly greater clinical success with SNS for intractable urge incontinence in patients who were younger (< 55 years old) and healthier (fewer comorbidities).[41] They hypothesized that age-related changes in the bladder, pelvic floor, and neural control systems for the micturition reflex decrease the chance of success with SNS therapy. Intervening before such irreversible age-related changes occur may be one key to success.

Finally, whenever SNS is being considered for an individual patient, it is helpful to view the trial phase as a low risk and reversible diagnostic procedure. A trial of stimulation still remains the best indicator for patient success.

REPORTED SACRAL NERVE STIMULATION EXPERIENCE WITH OVERACTIVE BLADDER

Initial reports on the efficacy of SNS therapy for refractory urinary urge incontinence formed part of the work of the Sacral Nerve Stimulation Study Group, which was published in 1999.[42] This was a multicenter study involving 16 sites worldwide and 76 patients. Randomized to immediate implantation (study group) or delayed implantation (control group) and followed for 6 months, significant differences between the two groups were seen in the number of incontinence episodes/day, the severity of incontinence episodes/day, and the number of protective pads used/day. Following SNS therapy, 47% were completely dry, with an additional 29% noting $> 50\%$

improvement in symptoms at 6 months. In order to address the potential placebo effect, a therapy evaluation test was performed by deactivating the devices after 6 months, and virtually all treated patients returned to their baseline pre-implant symptoms.

SNS for urgency–frequency syndrome was similarly evaluated in 51 patients via a multicenter, randomized study with a control arm (delayed implantation), and with evaluation points at 1, 3, 6, 12, 18, and 24 months.[43] At 6 months, significant improvements in the stimulation group were noted, including average number of voids/day (16.9 ± 9.7 to 9.3 ± 5.1), measured volume/void (118 ± 74 to 226 ± 124 ml), and degree of urgency (rank 2.2 ± 0.6 to 1.6 ± 0.9); patients in the control group showed no significant changes in voiding parameters. Quality of life (QoL) was also significantly improved in the SNS group, as noted by changes in the short form health survey questionnaire (SF-36). Again, when the neurostimulators were turned off in the stimulation group at 6 months, urinary symptoms promptly returned to baseline. Following reactivation, SNS was again shown to be effective up through the 24 months studied.

In 2000, a follow-up report of some of these patients was published, showing interval results in urinary symptoms over 3 years.[11] At 2 years, 56% of urgency–frequency patients showed > 50% improvement in the number of voids/day. At 3 years, 59% of patients with urge incontinence noted > 50% reduction in wetting episodes, with 46% completely dry.

Published in 2002, the experience noted from the United States sacral neuromodulation patient registry showed a > 50% improvement in urinary symptoms in 63% of those with urge incontinence and 53% of those with urgency–frequency syndrome.[44]

Post FDA-approval studies supported by Medtronic were conducted, which continued to follow the original patients from the previous aforementioned multicenter trials.[45] New patients were also enrolled to this population to ensure adequate sample size and to account for the evolution of techniques. Assessment of long-term efficacy and safety was the goal, with patients followed to 5 years. In patients with urgency, statistically significant improvements were seen in number of leaks/day, number of heavy

leaks/day, the severity of leaks overall, and the number of pads/day. Excellent durability of this response to SNS therapy was also seen, with significant differences noted in the above-mentioned parameters at every annual visit up to 5 years. At 5 years, the average number of leaks/ day decreased from 9.6 to 3.9, with 59% of patients classified as clinically successful; the average number of heavy leaks/day decreased from 2.6 to 0.8, with 71% of patients classified as clinically successful; the average number of pads used/day decreased from 5.3 to 1.8, with 67% of patients classified as clinically successful. In patients with urgency–frequency syndrome, the average number of voids/day decreased significantly from 19.3 to 14.8, with a 50% and 39% clinical success rate at 4 and 5 years, respectively. Volume voided/void also improved from 93.9 ml to 202.4 ml at 5 years, with clinical success rate reported as 59% and 56% at 4 and 5 years, respectively. The clinical success rates in perceived degree of urgency were 74% at 3 years, 64% at 4 years, and 56% at 5 years. An important finding in this study is the high correlation between the 1- and 5-year success rates for treated patients, indicating a good durability of response with SNS therapy. Of patients who were successfully treated at the 1-year follow-up, 84% with urinary incontinence and 71% with urinary frequency continued to have a successful outcome at 5 years.

Several key differences between available pharmacological therapy for OAB and SNS should be noted. While anticholinergic medications address the motor component of urinary control by blocking bladder muscarinic receptors associated with efferent neural pathways,[46] SNS also addresses the sensory component, as it modulates afferent pathways that influence micturition.[15] In a recent survey of anticholinergic prescription refill patterns over a 12-month period, 56% of patients chose not to refill their prescription for a second time, while only 15% of patients continued to acquire refills at 12 months (Figure 26.8).[47] In another large California Medi-Cal study (n = 2496), nearly 67% of patients discontinued their therapy after 3 months, with approximately 78% unable to remain on their prescription after 5 months. The median time for discontinuation of therapy was a mere 1.5 months.[48] In those who stopped their anticholinergic therapy, the two main reasons for drug discontinuation was

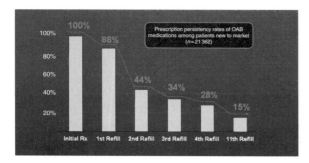

Figure 26.8 How likely are patients to continue with anticholinergic therapy?[47] 56% of patients chose *not* to refill their prescription a second time. Only 15% of patients continued with their therapy through the first year. OAB, overactive bladder. (Reprinted with the permission of Medtronic, Inc. © 2006).

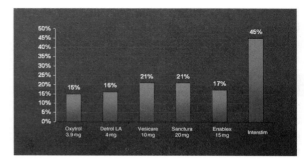

Figure 26.9 Food and Drug Administration (FDA)-approval study results: comparing anticholinergics to sacral nerve stimulation (SNS). Percentage reduction in urinary frequency. Efficacy data points were measured at 12 weeks for all drugs and at 6 months for Inter-Stim® therapy.[43,49–54] Reprinted with the permission of Medtronic, Inc. © 2006.

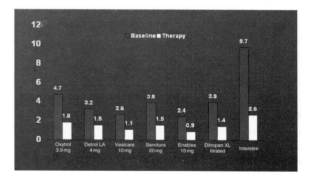

Figure 26.10 Food and Drug Administration (FDA)-approval study results: comparing anticholinergics to sacral nerve stimulation (SNS). Reduction in number of incontinent episodes. Efficacy data points were measured at 12 weeks for all drugs except Ditropan® (dosage titrated then maintained for 2 weeks) and at 6 months for InterStim® therapy.[42,49–54] Reprinted with the permission of Medtronic, Inc. © 2006.

insufficient efficacy (43%) and drug intolerability (21%), with reports of dry mouth and constipation in these patients reaching 65% and 25%, respectively.[47] In the FDA-approval studies performed for the various anticholinergic medications available today,[49–57] dry mouth rates among all study participants were noted at between 15 and 30% overall. Required duration by the FDA for assessment of efficacy and safety for each of these studies was only 12 weeks. With so many patients discontinuing drug therapy within the first few months due to lack of efficacy and drug intolerability, is 12 weeks sufficient? In comparison, FDA-approval requirements for SNS therapy was of 6 months duration. With these study endpoints in mind (12 weeks versus 6 months), those patients on anticholinergic trials had a baseline urinary frequency of 10.1–12.9 voids/day, which decreased to 8.4–10.5 voids/day, while those in the SNS trials had baseline urinary frequency of 16.9 voids/day, which decreased to 9.3 voids/day. The percentage reduction in urinary frequency for the anticholinergic trials ranged from 15 to 20%, while that for SNS was 45% (Figure 26.9). With respect to urge incontinent episodes/day, those on anticholinergics noted a range from 2.4 to 4.7 leaks/day at baseline, which decreased to 0.9–1.8 leaks/day at 12 weeks, while those in the SNS studies started with an average of 9.7 leaks/day, which reduced to 2.6 leaks/day at 6 months (Figure 26.10). In the SNS-approval studies, the severity of urinary symptoms at baseline, the degree of clinical improvement with therapy, and the duration of

the response were all greater when compared to approval studies for contemporary anticholinergic medications. In the right patient, anticholinergic medications prove beneficial for the treatment of OAB symptoms, but if satisfactory efficacy is not appreciated, or if drug therapy proves intolerable, a trial of SNS is certainly warranted.

EXPANDING INDICATIONS

Since its inception, widespread use of SNS for approved urinary conditions has led to incidental improvements in many other pelvic-related symptoms. It has been noted that a significant number of patients with refractory urinary symptoms also harbor other chronic symptoms within the pelvis. Favorable improvements in other such symptoms following neuromodulatory trials include chronic pelvic pain syndromes (i.e. interstitial cystitis, vulvodynia, prostadynia, epididymo-orchalgia),[32–34,37,58,59] a variety of lower gastrointestinal disorders (i.e. fecal incontinence, chronic constipation, irritable bowel syndrome),[60,61] and sexual dysfunction (i.e. dyspareunia, vaginismus, erectile dysfunction).[62–64] Again, in our own institution's 11-year experience with SNS, 46%, 59%, and 51% of patients reported concomitant pelvic pain, bowel complaints, and sexual difficulties, respectively.[40] A better understanding of the effects of pelvic floor muscle dysfunction on the disruption of normal sensory afferent signaling and reflex pathways with respect to bladder and bowel functioning, as well as the sensation of chronic pain, has added to our understanding of SNS treatment for these other types of pelvic symptoms. Some promise has also been seen in the area of neurogenic-related bladder disorders (i.e. spinal cord injury, multiple sclerosis),[65,66] as well as in children with voiding dysfunction.[67,68] Research is ongoing in each of these areas in an attempt to expand the approved indications for sacral neuromodulatory therapy.[69]

TROUBLESHOOTING WITH TIPS AND TRICKS

Lack of efficacy during test stimulation trial

Clinical improvement during the test stimulation trial should not be subtle; at least 50% improvement is desired before proceeding with IPG placement. If a marginal or equivocal response is noted, it is best to reevaluate with another test stimulation trial, performed on the opposite S_3 site, or perhaps at another level (S_2 or S_4). To date, there is no definitive evidence that bilateral stimulation results in a summation effect and is reliably superior to unilateral stimulation.[70]

Persistence during lead placement to ensure optimal response is important. Care should be taken to make every effort to identify the course of the nerve and place all four lead contact points in close proximity to, and in line with, the nerve. Proper lead alignment should yield typical responses at low thresholds (< 4 volts). This also allows for maximal flexibility during subsequent programming, when all lead contact points are usable. In order to achieve a parallel position of the lead with respect to the nerve, the examiner must continue testing the site during needle advancement in increments along the relevant length of the permanent electrode (2 cm). If the response is lost upon needle advancement, it has clearly traveled away from the nerve. In this case, the needle should be pulled back to the skin and another insertion angle should be attempted.

Motor and sensory feedback is certainly important during lead placement to ensure adequate location and tolerability of the stimulation during chronic SNS therapy. Our experience has been that sensory feedback is more important than motor responses; however, assessing both is preferred. Optimal placement of the lead is therefore determined by three factors: the sensory distribution, the motor reflex, and the thresholds for sensation and muscle contraction. Stimulation of the S_3 root should produce a strong contraction of the pelvic floor muscles, drawing up the anus and perineal body, causing a visible inward motion of the intergluteal fold. This is known as a "bellows" response. Contraction of the small muscles of the feet or dorsiflexion of the toes can also be seen with increasing S_3 stimulation intensity, as the stimulation travels down the sciatic and sural branches. Sensation in the anterior perineum, vagina, scrotum, or urethra is optimal. If stimulation results in leg or hip rotation, calf contraction and/or total foot flexion, placement is likely to be too cephalad in S_2 rather than S_3. If sensation is limited to the posterior perineum, anus, or gluteal region, placement is likely to be too caudal in S_4 (Table 26.2).

Fluoroscopy is indispensable to assure optimal lead placement. In the lateral view, the lead should be deployed beneath the bone table, with sites 2 and 3 straddling the anterior bony surface of the sacrum. Once deployed, the tined lead should always have a cephalocaudal orientation. It should also be directed in a slight lateral position from the medial aspect of the S_3 foramen, as seen best in the AR view. To the astute observer, this lateral projection of the lead can be appreciated in the lateral fluoroscopic view, as the spaces between the lead contact points (0–1–2–3) appear closer together between the

Table 26.2 Expected motor and sensory responses to S_2, S_3 and S_4 stimulation

Level	Motor	Sensory
S_2	Bellows (inward motion of intergluteal fold)	Genital
	Clamp (anterior–posterior pinching of perineum/coccyx)	
	Dorsiflexion of foot, heel rotation, calf cramping, leg/hip rotation	
S_3	Bellows (inward motion of intergluteal fold)	Genital, perineal, anal
	Dorsiflexion of great toe, bottom of foot	
S_4	Bellows (inward motion of intergluteal fold)	Anal

more distal sites, indicating that the lead is pointing away as it separates from the anterior surface of the bone.

In rare cases, a mechanical problem can be found. Interrogation of the device by checking circuit impedance measurements assesses the integrity of the system, and usually proves beneficial with diagnosing the problem. Normal impedance is between 400 and 1500 ohms. High impedance (> 4000 ohms) indicates an opening in the circuit that impedes the flow of the electrical current, and is generally associated with a lack of stimulation sensation by the patient. This can occur from a frayed subcutaneous extension wire during the test period, or a loose connection site. During lead interrogation, impedance measurements in unipolar mode, one lead site at a time, can help to identify the exact location of the problem. In the case of a frayed extension wire, if the trial period was already sufficient to determine the patient's clinical response to SNS therapy, the extension wire can be cut at the skin and left until surgical intervention is planned (proceeding with IPG implantation, or lead explantation). If the trial was insufficient, the frayed wire can be exchanged for a new extension wire, and the test trial continued.

Low impedance (< 50 ohms) indicates a short circuit, which amplifies the flow of electrons.[71]

Stimulation may or may not be felt by the patient, but if it is felt, it is often in the wrong location and/or is associated with an uncomfortable sensation (i.e. shocking sensation at the IPG pocket site). In this case, it is best to measure impedance in bipolar mode to identify the short circuit between two wires. Short circuits occur when fluid penetrates a connector site, or when crushed wires come into direct contact with one another. In the case of fluid leakage into the connector, reprogramming around the affected site by using different electrode combinations may solve the problem. Otherwise, intraoperative revision can be attempted by disconnecting the lead from the extension to the IPG and thoroughly irrigating and drying the connection (with sterile water and a small air suction device) before reconnecting and testing. If abnormal impedance persists, the short extension wire can be revised and retested. Seldom is there a problem with the IPG connections, or the IPG itself. If abnormal impedance does not resolve, lead revision is inevitable.

Loss of efficacy over time

If all combinations of unipolar and bipolar stimulation configurations have been tested and a problem still exists, device impedance should be assessed. See the discussion above for details of impedance interrogation. Patient should also be queried about local trauma that could result in device damage and malfunction. Lead migration is also a possibility, especially after a traumatic event. AP and lateral X-rays may be helpful in defining lead displacement, especially when comparisons to prior films from the original lead placement procedure can be made.

A patient's perception of symptoms has also been known to change over time, making residual symptoms during SNS now intolerable. The patient then questions the continued benefit of the therapy. Turning the device off to see if the patient reexperiences the severity of their original symptoms can help to elucidate this issue. This step often demonstrates that the symptoms have been significantly improved by the therapy, albeit incompletely so. If, following this step, the patient still deems the therapy to be insufficient, a repeat staged trial at another site (usually the opposite S_3 site) can be tried. If this proves successful, the new lead can be connected to the existing IPG. If this too is unsuccessful, a trial of pudendal nerve stimulation (currently not FDA-approved) may serve as a salvage neuromodulatory maneuver.[72]

If sudden loss of clinical efficacy is noted, the battery life can be assessed with the programmer. The life expectancy for the InterStim® battery is usually 6–10 years. Although rare, a few cases of early battery depletion (< 5 years) have been noted.[73] The life of the battery depends on the intensity of the stimulation (amplitude) necessary to achieve adequate clinical response, the number of electrodes turned on, the pulse width and rate, and the use of continuous versus cycling mode. The higher that any of these parameters are, the lower is the expected battery life. Most important of these is stimulation amplitude, which depends on the proximity of the lead to the nerve. Ideal amplitudes are < 4 volts; higher amplitudes (6–10 volts) will deplete the battery more quickly.

Infection

As with any surgery, infection prevention is key. We pay particular attention to sterile patient preparation in the operating room, using alcohol, Duraprep™ (3M™), and an Ioban™ (3M™) adhesive covering, before placement of standard sterile drapes.

A preoperative dose of cephazolin (Ancef®) – or vancomycin (Vancocin®), if penicillin allergic – is administered, followed by a week of oral cephalexin (Keflex®). Copious antibiotic irrigation is also used throughout the surgical procedure. Incision depth about the percutaneous lead site must be sufficient to prevent the lead wire from becoming trapped in the skin during tunneling. This could result in lead wire movement, fracture, or exposure over time. Tunnel depth and length must also be adequate to decrease the risk of unpreventable colonization at the exit site from affecting any of the permanent hardware during the testing trial. Tunneling the wires 2 cm deep to the skin through the fatty subcutaneous tissue is recommended: (1) first tunneling the lead wire from the presacral percutaneous site over to the opposite upper buttock incision (site of future permanent IPG) and then, after proper connection to the extension wire, (2) tunneling the extension wire from the upper buttock incision to the opposite lower lateral back to the preplanned exit site.

This amount of tunneling assists in infection prevention. If tunneling remains in the fatty subcutaneous tissue, there is little sensation or discomfort, and only the entrance and exit sites require local anesthesia. We also use staples for the final subcuticular closure (proceeded by a subcutaneous Vicryl® closure), especially for the incision over the anticipated IPG site during the stage I procedure. Previous experience at our institution demonstrated that the surgical knot from a running subcuticular closure is generally still present after 4 weeks, and therefore provides a potential source of contamination during IPG implantation. Staples are removed after 1 week. During the stage II procedure, proper IPG pocket size and depth are important, as is insuring strict pocket hemostasis prior to closure.

In case of infection, all implanted components must be removed. We are unaware of any successful attempts at component salvage. In a recent series of infectious complications reported by the Cleveland Clinic Foundation,[71] five salvage attempts were made by relocating the IPG into either a deeper or another pocket on the contralateral side. Unfortunately, all patients underwent eventual device explantation due to persistent infection. If the presacral incision is not fluctuant, removing the lead from the IPG site incision is usually possible, eliminating the need for a counter-incision over the presacral area. If a capsule has formed around the IPG site, it too should be excised to promote efficient healing. Infected wounds are packed open and left to heal by secondary intent. Quicker resolution of both wound infection and healing can be experienced using a closed suction wound system provided by most enterostomal/wound therapy services.

Following infected device removal, sufficient healing time should be allotted (3–4 months) before reimplantation is considered. We typically proceed with a single stage implant of both tined lead and IPG, provided that sufficient clinical benefit was experienced from the previous lead, and good test stimulation responses were duplicated during new lead placement.

Pain at implanted pulse generator site

Pain at the IPG site is usually either pocket site-related or stimulation-related. The first step should be to turn off the stimulation to see whether the pain or uncomfortable sensation persists. If it persists, pocket site factors should be evaluated. Ideal IPG location is lateral to the sacral margin and below the posterior superior iliac crest. Subcutaneous pocket depth (approximately 2 cm) and size (just big enough to accommodate the IPG without placing the incision on tension) are important. The smooth (no writing), insulated side of the IPG should be facing down, away from the skin, with the connection and wiring placed below. If the pocket dimensions are not appropriate (either too tight or too loose), or if the device is too superficial, or located over a bony prominence, it may eventually need to be repositioned. When repositioning is done, the fibrous capsule from the original IPG should be excised to minimize seroma formation and promote healing. In rare cases, anesthetic patches over the symptomatic pocket, or trigger point injections with local anesthetic, have provided relief.

Pain related to the stimulation is often associated with unipolar programming, in which the IPG case acts as the positive pole. Switching to bipolar programming removes the IPG case from the loop of electrical current. As mentioned previously, short circuits from fluid in the connection site or touching crushed wires can also cause uncomfortable sensations, most often in the IPG pocket site. Device interrogation will reveal low impedance in this situation.

Future magnetic resonance imaging

At this time, Medtronic lists the need for future magnetic resonance imaging (MRI) as a contraindication to InterStim® placement. As more patients try this form of therapy, including those with underlying neurological disorders, the likelihood of needing a future MRI in an implanted patient increases. Although the company is medicolegally bound to declare it unsafe, due to lack of sufficient evidence to the contrary, a recent series noted that MRI was safely used in some patients with InterStim® devices.[74] In these cases the site of imaging was remote from the InterStim® device (such as the head or upper spine), a smaller magnet was used (1.5 tesla), and the device was turned off during imaging. The patient must be able to signal to the imaging technician at the first sign of discomfort about the device site, suggesting overheating of the hardware. The radiologist may also require the patient to sign a waiver releasing them and their staff from responsibility in the case of subsequent device malfunction or other related complications.

Pregnancy

To date, only five cases of pregnancy after InterStim® placement have been reported in the literature.[75] Recommendations to such patients include turning off the stimulator while trying to conceive, or as soon as pregnancy is discovered. If implant deactivation leads to urinary-related complications that can jeopardize the pregnancy – such as urinary retention and recurrent urinary tract infections and/or pyelonephritis – then reactivation should be considered. In this situation, the lowest possible stimulatory settings should be used. Even in those who continued with stimulation throughout their pregnancy, no teratogenic fetal effects were noted. A concern for possible lead displacement during vaginal delivery was noted, as 50% of the women who delivered vaginally, and still required neuromodulatory therapy to control their symptoms in the postpartum setting, experienced a loss of clinical efficacy with reactivation of the lead. This concern needs to be discussed with any patient in her child-bearing years who is contemplating InterStim® therapy, and the potential benefits of elective Cesarean section should be considered.

SUMMARY

Sacral nerve stimulation has emerged as a standard of care for the treatment of intractable symptoms of OAB. It should be considered as an appropriate next step when a combination of pharmacological therapy, behavioral interventions, and pelvic floor biofeedback and rehabilitation do not provide sufficient symptom relief. It certainly should be considered before any major destructive–reconstructive surgery is undertaken. The exact mechanism of action remains unknown, but modulation of sacral afferent nerves and manipulation of the guarding reflex are key elements in restoring a more normal balance of reflexes between the bladder, sphincter, and pelvic floor muscles. The therapy is most appropriate for OAB patients without underlying neuropathology, but has been successful for a range of problems including a variety of pelvic pain syndromes, idiopathic non-obstructive urinary retention, neurogenic voiding dysfunction, chronic constipation and fecal incontinence. A key finding on preoperative assessment which is a good predictor of success is evidence of hypertonicity of the pelvic floor musculature. It is also helpful to think of certain conditions of voiding dysfunction in terms of their behaviors, instead of organ-based labels, and to view the first phase or application of sacral neuromodulation as a reversible diagnostic test. Urinary diaries are essential for objectively documenting the target symptoms before, during, and after a therapeutic trial. We prefer to go directly to a staged tined lead implant as the initial trial phase, eliminating the PNE, since it has been associated with less lead migration and allows for a sufficient length of time (3–4 weeks) to evaluate the therapy for any given patient. The results of the trial using the potentially permanent electrode will also most closely predict the long-term outcome once the IPG is implanted. Keys to successful lead implantation include performance of the procedure with local anesthesia and IV sedation, which allows for sensory feedback during lead placement. Care using fluoroscopy is essential for identifying the level and course of the appropriate sacral nerve root. It is ideal to have as many lead contact points as possible yielding the same responses at low thresholds to give the most flexibility in future programming of the device.

The long-term effectiveness of SNS for intractable OAB has been well documented. This therapy continues to undergo further refinements with the hope of improved ease of use and suitability for a host of urologic disorders. Now that the role of SNS for chronic voiding dysfunction is established, new devices and alternative stimulation targets will emerge, which will need to be compared to sacral nerve stimulation as the gold standard for pelvic neuromodulatory therapy. Large-scale randomized studies or a national pelvic neuromodulatory registry are needed to reveal the true potential of neuromodulation for other pelvic-oriented applications.

REFERENCES

1. Stewart WF, Van Rooyen JB, Cundiff GW et al. Prevalence and burden of overactive bladder in the United States. World J Urol 2003; 20: 327–36.
2. Hu TW, Wagner TH. Health-related consequences of overactive bladder: an economic perspective. BJU Int 2005; 96 (Suppl 1): 43–5.
3. Hu TW, Wagner TH, Bentkover JD et al. Cost of urinary incontinence and overactive bladder in the United States: a comparative study. Urology 2004; 63: 461–5.
4. Abrams P, Blavais JG, Fowler CJ et al. The role of neuromodulation in the management of urinary urge incontinence. BJU Int 2003; 91: 355–9.
5. Data on file. Minneapolis, MN: Medtronic, Inc., 2006.
6. Brindley GS, Polkey CE, Rushton DN et al. Sacral anterior root stimulators for bladder control in paraplegia: the first 50 cases. J Neurol Neurosurg Psychiatry 1986; 49: 1104–14.
7. Schmidt RA. Application of neurostimulation in urology. Neurourol Urodyn 1988; 7: 585–92.
8. Schmidt RA. Treatment of pelvic pain with neuroprosthesis. J Urol 1988; 129: 227A.
9. Tanagho EA. Electrical stimulation. J Am Geriatr Soc 1990; 38: 352–5.
10. Shaker HS, Hassouna M. Sacral root neuromodulation in idiopathic nonobstructive chronic urinary retention. J Urol 1998; 159: 1476–8.
11. Siegel SW, Catanzaro F, Dijkema HE et al. Long-term results of a multi-center study on sacral nerve stimulation for treatment of urinary urge incontinence, urgency-frequency, and retention. Urology 2000; 56 (6 Suppl 1): 87–91.
12. Leng WW, Chancellor MB. How sacral nerve stimulation neuromodulation works. Urol Clin North Am 2005; 32: 11–18.
13. Chancellor MB, Leng WW. The mechanism of action of sacral nerve stimulation in the treatment of detrusor overactivity and urinary retention. In: Jonas U, Grunewald V, eds. New Perspectives in Sacral Nerve Stimulation for Control of Lower Urinary Tract Dysfunction. London: Martin Dunitz 2002: 17–28.
14. Lycklama a Nijeholt AAB, Groenendijk PM, den Boon J. Clinical and urodynamic assessments of the mode of action of sacral nerve stimulation. In: Jonas U, Grunewald V, eds. New Perspectives in Sacral Nerve Stimulation For Control of Lower

Urinary Tract Dysfunction. London: Martin Dunitz 2002: 43–52.

15. Chancellor MB, Chartier-Kastler EJ. Principles of sacral nerve stimulation (SNS) for the treatment of bladder and urethral sphincter dysfunctions. Neuromodulation 2000; 3: 15–26.

16. DasGupta R, Critchley HD, Dolan RJ, Fowler CJ. Changes in brain activity following sacral neuromodulation for urinary retention. J Urol 2005; 174: 2268–72.

17. Thon WF, Baskin LS, Jonas U et al. Surgical principles of sacral foramen electrode implantation. World J Urol 1991; 9: 133–7.

18. de Groat WC, Kruse MN, Vizzard MA et al. Modification of urinary bladder function after neural injury. In: Seil F, ed. Neuronal Regeneration, Reorganization, and Repair. Advances in Neurology, Vol 72. New York: Lippincott-Raven Publishers; 1997: 347–64.

19. Dasgupta R, Wiseman OJ, Kitchen N, Fowler CJ. Long-term results of sacral neuromodulation for women with urinary retention. BJU Int 2004; 94: 335–7.

20. Dasgupta R, Fowler CJ. The management of female voiding dysfunction: Fowler's syndrome – a contemporary update. Curr Opin Urol 2003; 13: 293–9.

21. de Groat WC. Neuroanatomy and neurophysiology: innervation of the lower urinary tract. In: Raz S, ed. Female Urology, 2nd edn. Philadelphia, PA: WB Saunders Company, 1996; 2: 28–42.

22. Siegel SW. Management of voiding dysfunction with an implantable neuroprosthesis. Urol Clinics North Am 1992; 19: 163–70.

23. Chai TC, Mamo GJ. Modified technique of S3 foramen localization and lead implantation in S3 neuromodulation. Urology 2001; 58: 786–90.

24. Hohenfellner M, Schultz-Lampel D, Dahms S et al. Bilateral chronic sacral neuromodulation for treatment of lower urinary tract dysfunction. J Urol 1998; 160: 821–4.

25. Spinelli M, Giardiello G, Gerber M et al. New sacral neuromodulation lead for percutaneous implantation using local anesthesia: description and first experience. J Urol 2003; 170: 1905–7.

26. Scheepens WA, Weil EH, van Koeveringe GA et al. Buttock placement of the implantable pulse generator: a new implantation technique for sacral neuromodulation. A multicenter study. Eur Urol 2001; 40: 434–8.

27. McCreer DB, Agnew WF, Yuen TG, BuUara LA. Relationship between stimulus amplitude, stimulus frequency and neural damage during electrical stimulation of sciatic nerve of cat. Med Biol Eng Comput 1995; 33: 426–9.

28. Siegel SW. Selecting patients for sacral nerve stimulation. Urol Clin North Am 2005; 32: 19–26.

29. Schmidt RA, Doggweiler R. Neurostimulation and neuromodulation: a guide to selecting the right urologic patient. Eur Urol 1998; 34 (Suppl 1): 23–6.

30. Koldewijn EL, Rosier PFWM, Meuleman EJH et al. Predictors of success with neuromodulation in lower urinary tract dysfunction: results of trial stimulation in 100 patients. J Urol 1994; 152: 2071–5.

31. Swinn MJ, Kitchen ND, Goodwin RJ, Fowler CJ. Sacral neuromodulation for women with Fowler's syndrome. Eur Urol 2000; 38: 439–43.

32. Comiter CV. Sacral neuromodulation for the symptomatic treatment of refractory interstitial cystitis: a prospective study. J Urol 2003; 169: 1369–73.

33. Peters KM, Carey JM, Konstandt DB. Sacral neuromodulation for the treatment of refractory interstitial cystitis: outcomes based on technique. Int Urogynecol J Pelvic Floor Dysfunct 2003; 14: 223–8; discussion 228.

34. Peters KM, Konstadt D. Sacral neuromodulation decreases narcotic requirements in refractory interstitial cystitis. BJU Int 2004; 93: 777–9.

35. Lukban JC, Whitmore KE, Sant GR. Current management of interstitial cystitis. Urol Clin North Am 2002; 29: 649–60.

36. Everaert K, Devulder J, De Mynck M et al. The pain cycle: implications for the diagnosis and treatment of pelvic pain syndromes. Int Urogynecol J Pelvic Floor Dysfunct 2001; 12: 9–14.

37. Siegel S, Paszkiewicz E, Kirkpatrick C, Hinkel B, Oleson K. Sacral nerve stimulation in patients with chronic intractable pelvic pain. J Urol 2001; 166: 1742–5.

38. Griffiths D. Clinical studies of cerebral and urinary tract function in elderly people with urinary incontinence. Behav Brain Res 1998; 92: 151–5.

39. Kolta MG, Wallace LJ, Gerald MC. Age-related changes in sensitivity in rat urinary bladder to autonomic agents. Mech Aging Dev 1984; 27: 183–8.

40. Sutherland SE, Lavers A, Carlson A et al. Sacral nerve stimulation for voiding dysfunction: one institution's 11 year experience. Neurourol Urodyn 2007; 26(1): 19–28, discussion 36.

41. Amundsen CL, Romero AA, Jamison MG, Webster GD. Sacral neuromodulation for intractable urge incontinence: are there factors associated with cure? Urology 2005; 66: 746–50.

42. Schmidt RA, Jonas U, Oleson KA et al. Sacral nerve stimulation for treatment of refractory urinary urge incontinence. Sacral Nerve Stimulation Study Group. J Urol 1999; 162: 352–7.

43. Hassouna MM, Siegel SW, Nyeholt AA et al. Sacral neuromodulation in the treatment of urgency-frequency symptoms: a multicenter study on efficacy and safety. J Urol 2000; 163: 1849–54.

44. Pettit PD, Thompson JR, Chen AH. Sacral neuromodulation: new applications in the treatment of female pelvic floor dysfunction. Curr Opin Obstet Gynecol 2002; 14: 521–5.

45. van Kerrebroeck PEV, van Voskuilen AC, Bemelmans B et al. Five-year results of sacral neuromodulation therapy for urinary voiding dysfunction: outcomes of a prospective, worldwide clinical study. J Urol 2004; 171 (Suppl 4): 328 (abs 1246).

46. Yoshima N, Chancellor MB. Current and future pharmacological treatment for overactive bladder. J Urol 2002; 168: 1897–913.

47. The 2002 Gallup Study of the market for prescription incontinence medication. Princeton, NJ: Multi-Sponsor Surveys, 2002.

48. Yu YF, Nichol MB, Yu AP, Ahn J. Persistence and adherence of medications for chronic overactive bladder/urinary incontinence in the California Medicaid population. Value Health 2005; 8: 495–505.

49. Oxytrol® package insert. Corona, CA. Watson Pharma, 2003.

50. Ditropan XL® package insert. Mountain View, CA: AZA Corporation, 2004.

51. Detrol LA® package insert. New York, NY: Pfizer, 2005.

52. Vesicare® package insert. Norman, OK: Yamanouchi Pharma Technologies, 2004.

53. Sanctura® package insert. Lexington, MA: Indevus Pharmaceuticals, 2004.

54. Enablex® package insert. Basel, Switzerland: Novartis Pharmaceuticals Corporation, 2004.

55. Van Kerrebroeck PEV, Kreder K, Jonas U, Zinner N, Wein A. Tolterodine Study Group. Tolterodine once daily: superior efficacy and tolerability in the treatment of the overactive bladder. Urology 2001; 57: 414–21.

56. Diokno A, Appell RA, Sand PK et al. OPERA Study Group. Prospective, randomized, double blind study of the efficacy and tolerability of the extended-release formulations of oxybutynin and tolterodine for overactive bladder: results of the OPERA trial. Mayo Clin Proc 2003; 78: 687–95.

57. Chapple CR, Martinez-Garcia R, Selvaggi L et al. STAR Study Group. A comparison of the efficacy and tolerability of solifenacin succinate and extended release tolterodine at treating overactive bladder syndrome: results of the STAR trial. Eur Urol 2005; 48: 464–70.

58. Everaert K, Kerckhaert W, Caluwaerts H et al. A prospective randomized trial comparing the 1-stage with the 2-stage implantation of a pulse generator in patients with pelvic floor dysfunction selected for sacral nerve stimulation. Eur Urol 2004; 45: 649–54.

59. Feler CA, Whitworth LA, Fernandez J. Sacral neuromodulation for chronic pain conditions. Anesthesiol Clin North Am 2003; 21: 785–95.

60. Jarrett ME. Neuromodulation for constipation and fecal incontinence. Urol Clin North Am 2005; 32: 79–87.

61. Kenefick NJ, Christiansen J. A review of sacral nerve stimulation for the treatment of faecal incontinence. Colorectal Dis 2004; 6: 75–80.

62. Lue TF, Schmidt RA, Tanagho EA. Electrostimulation and penile erection. Urol Int 1985; 40: 60–4.

63. Itano N, Whitmore C. Abstract presented at International Society of Pelvic Neuromodulation 2003, Scottsdale, AZ, USA.

64. van Balken MR, Verguns H, Bemelmans BL. Sexual functioning in patients with lower urinary tract dysfunction improves after percutaneous tibial nerve stimulation. Int J Impot Res 2006; 18: 470–5; discussion 476.

65. Vastenholt JM, Snoek GJ, Buschman HP et al. A 7-year follow-up of sacral anterior root stimulation for bladder control in patients with a spinal cord injury: quality of life and users' experiences. Spinal Cord 2003; 41: 397–402.

66. Bosch JL, Groen J. Sacral nerve neuromodulation in the treatment of patients with refractory motor urge incontinence: long-term results of a prospective longitudinal study. J Urol 2000; 163: 1219–21.

67. Bani-Hani AH, Vandersteen DR, Reinberg YE. Neuromodulation in pediatrics. Urol Clin North Am 2005; 32: 101–7.

68. Humphreys M, Smith C, Smith J et al. Sacral neuromodulation in children: preliminary results in 16 patients [Abstract]. J Urol 2004; 17 (Suppl): 56–7.

69. Bernstein AJ, Peters KM. Expanding indications for neuromodulation. Urol Clin North Am 2005; 32: 59–63.

70. van Kerrebroeck PEV, Scheepens WA, de Bie RA, Weil EHJ. European experience with bilateral sacral neuromodulation in patients with chronic lower urinary tract dysfunction. Urol Clin North Am 2005; 32: 51–7.

71. Hijaz A, Vasavada S. Complications and troubleshooting of sacral neuromodulation therapy. Urol Clin North Am 2005; 32: 65–9.

72. Peters KM, Feber KM, Bennett RC. Sacral versus pudendal nerve stimulation for voiding dysfunction: a prospective, single-blinded, randomized, crossover trial. Neurourol Urodyn 2005; 24: 643–7.

73. Data on file. Minneapolis, MN: Medtronic, Inc., 2006.

74. Elkelini MS, Hassouna MM. Safety of MRI at 1.5 Tesla in patients with implanted sacral nerve neurostimulator. Eur Urol 2006; 50: 311–16.

75. Wiseman OJ, Hombergh U, Kildewijn EL et al. Sacral neuromoduation and pregnancy. J Urol 2002; 167: 165–8.

27

The bion® microstimulator

Jerome L Buller and Kenneth M Peters

Introduction • Pudendal nerve anatomy • RF-bion™ microstimulator • Battery-powered bion® microstimulator • Conclusion

INTRODUCTION

Electrical stimulation methods have been developed as non-destructive and reversible interventions for patients with refractory lower urinary tract dysfunction. The aim of this treatment is to achieve therapeutic effects by chronic, electrical stimulation of afferent somatic sacral nerve fibers. This allows for the application of electrical stimuli at one site to alter present neurotransmission processes at a different site such as the lower urinary tract, a process referred to as neuromodulation. The rationale for these interventions is based on the findings that voiding function can be modulated by somatic afferent pathways in the pudendal nerve that transmit sensory information from the genital organs, urethra, prostate, vagina, anal canal, and perineal skin.[1-3] Various stimulation methods have been evaluated including surface, percutaneous, and implanted electrodes to activate these nerves. Stimulation locations have included sacral dermatomes of S_2–S_4 via surface electrodes, anal and vaginal plug electrodes,[4-6] dorsal penile and clitoral electrodes,[7-10] and implanted electrodes in the pelvic floor.[11-13] Though encouraging, the positive results with these treatments lack durability and in some cases practicality. Plug electrodes are cumbersome and limit daily activity. The use of connecting wires and attachment of electrodes or the need for clinic visits will limit patient participation with these devices. These factors have resulted in limited clinical applicability.

Neuromodulation techniques using implanted electrodes, particularly on the S_3 sacral nerve root, have also produced effective, durable results.[14-22] Limitations of this implanted technology have included concerns about selectivity for bladder inhibition, invasive implantation procedures, relatively high reoperation rates, and failures in some patients. Additionally, sacral nerve stimulation produces afferent stimulation along one of three branches of the pudendal nerve. Direct pudendal nerve stimulation would theoretically allow for afferent stimulation along S_2, S_3, and S_4, and could potentially result in a more robust neuromodulatory effect.

Vodusek et al. were the first to use direct pudendal nerve stimulation.[23] Three patients with hyperreflexic and neurogenic bladders due to multiple sclerosis and cerebral vascular disease were enrolled. Two Teflon®-coated bare-tip electrodes were introduced ipsilaterally into the proximity of the pudendal nerve (at the ischial spine) through the perineum, and were placed approximately 2–3 cm apart. Selective electrical pudendal nerve stimulation calibrated to achieve a "maximal motor response" as recorded electromyographically in the periurethral sphincter was found to increase the micturition threshold in all three patients. Effective stimulation was 200 μs, 5 pulses per second (pps), with currents up to 2 mA. The authors concluded that "the consistent elevation of micturition threshold by direct pudendal nerve stimulation makes it possible to consider an implanted stimulator for the purpose of achieving detrusor inhibition. Inhibition of detrusor contractions, higher bladder capacities, and therefore longer periods in between micturitions, could be 'physiologically' achieved in patients with hyperreflexic detrusors, opening a quite new therapeutic approach for this difficult clinical problem."

Ishigooka et al.[11–13,24] conducted chronic stimulation of the pudendal nerve and adjacent areas in patients having refractory urinary incontinence. They used percutaneous electrodes implanted with a needle adjacent and into the pelvic floor. Ten patients with neuropathic detrusors (mostly spinal cord injury) and overactive bladder conditions were enrolled. Electrodes were implanted bilaterally and maintained for an average of 12 weeks. Four patients had electrodes implanted adjacent to the pudendal nerve and six patients received intramuscular implantation into the levator ani muscle. Stimulation parameters consisted of six stimulation periods of 30 minutes each day using 20 pulses per second. The stimulation voltage was usually 15 V. However, lower stimulating voltages were used if the patient experienced any pain. At the end of the 12-week stimulation period, urinary incontinence was cured in two of the patients; six patients used fewer diapers associated with their incontinence and two patients were not improved by the stimulation. However, the volume at the first unstable contraction improved in all 10 subjects, with an average increase of 90% above control values. Follow-up periods after cessation of treatment ranged from 8 to 96 weeks. Urinary incontinence returned to the pretreatment level in three of the patients by 8–24 weeks. In the other five patients, the improvement was maintained. There were no adverse events associated with the electrode location next to the pudendal nerve or in the levator ani muscles. One electrode migrated from its insertion site as determined by X-ray.

By stimulating the pudendal nerve close to the ischial spine using bipolar electrodes, Vodusek et al.[23] later reported that electrical stimulation with 0.2-ms pulses at a frequency of 5 Hz increased the micturition threshold and inhibited detrusor activity in three patients suffering from neurological diseases, including multiple sclerosis and cerebral vascular disease, who exhibited urinary urgency and frequency. Longer-term effects have also been reported by stimulating pudendal nerves electrically. Ohlsson et al.[25] supplemented transcutaneous electrical stimulation of the perineal region with direct stimulation of the pudendal nerve once a week for a period of 4 weeks in patients with unsatisfactory responses to cutaneous stimulation alone. They showed that such stimulation led to a decrease in frequency of urination and an increase in bladder capacity in the majority of patients. These studies suggest that peripheral electrical stimulation of somatic afferents of the pudendal nerve could have a beneficial effect for the treatment of urge urinary incontinence. However, surgical access for placement of previously available implantable, leaded stimulators was not practical. Consequently, microstimulators have been introduced to address some of the limitations of currently available implantable devices.[26–30] In particular, these small devices allow for minimally invasive implantation procedures. Limitations of radio frequency (RF) devices have included the need for large external generators for the RF field and antennas for transmission. The inclusion of batteries into microstimulators opens up new opportunities for implanted devices that do not require external equipment for long-term stimulation. Such small, implantable microstimulators may be more easily placed directly near peripheral nerves, including the pudendal nerve.

PUDENDAL NERVE ANATOMY

The pudendal nerve provides primary sensory and motor innervation to the external anal sphincter, external urethral sphincter, genitalia, and perineal musculature and skin. It originates from the ventral rami of sacral nerves S2, S3, and S4 on the surface of the piriformis muscle (Figure 27.1). The pudendal nerve, accompanied by the internal pudendal artery and vein, then exits the pelvis via the greater sciatic foramen. In this extrapelvic location, posterior to the sacrotuberous ligament, Gustafson et al.[31] found this branch-free length of pudendal nerve to be 26 ± 7.7 mm with a diameter of 3.2 ± 0.56 mm, with the nerve lying medial to the vasculature. The pudendal neurovascular bundle then immediately reenters the pelvis through the lesser sciatic foramen by coursing around the ischial spine and sacrospinous ligament. The nerve trunk then courses in a

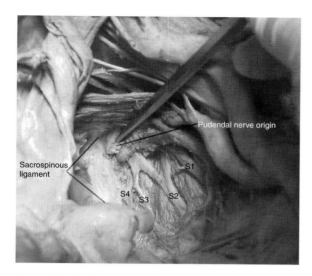

Figure 27.1 Origin of pudendal nerve.

ventrocaudal direction toward the perineal area. The nerve then enters the pudendal (Alcock's) canal, which is formed by a thickening or splitting of the fascia of the obturator internus muscle. There is inconsistency in how and where the branches of the pudendal nerve are given off; [31–38] however, the relationship of the pudendal nerve relative to the ischial spine is much more reliable.[34]

As a site for electrical stimulation, the pudendal nerve provides a wider sacral somatic innervation than could be obtained from a single sacral nerve. Pudendal nerve stimulation activates somatic afferent fibers from three sacral nerves. In contrast, sacral nerve stimulation only activates one sacral nerve, usually S_3. Thus, pudendal nerve stimulation will activate more somatic afferent fibers for potentially improved neuromodulation and bladder inhibition.

RF-BION™ MICROSTIMULATOR

The use of microstimulators is expected to resolve many of the problems of current implantable stimulators. One such stimulator, named the RF-Bion™ microstimulator (Advanced Bionics Corp., Valencia, CA), is also a radio frequency coupled device. This microstimulator has a maximum stimulating current of 12 mA and 225-μs pulse duration.[11,26]

Buller et al. evaluated the RF-bion implanted adjacent to the pudendal nerve at Alcock's canal in women with refractory urge urinary incontinence.[26] The screening test or percutaneous stimulation trial (PST) compared cystometrogram (CMG) parameters with and without pudendal nerve stimulation. After a baseline CMG, a percutaneous needle electrode was inserted adjacent to the pudendal nerve. After 10 minutes of pudendal nerve stimulation with an external pulse generator, a successful trial was indicated by a $\geq 50\%$ increase in cystometric capacity. Six of seven patients passed the percutaneous trial. Five of the subjects with a positive PST underwent placement of the RF-bion, a radio frequency powered, leadless microstimulator, adjacent to the pudendal nerve at Alcock's canal. The procedure was performed under local anesthesia with intravenous sedation in an outpatient surgical setting. Follow-up observations included cystometrogram and 72-hour voiding diaries completed prior to each visit at 15, 30, and 45 days after device activation and again after a minimum of 7 days without stimulation.

Six of the seven subjects (85.7%) had a positive response to the PST. Maximum cystometric capacity was increased from 325.0 ± 150.5 cm^3 to 609.8 ± 167.8 cm^3 ($p = 0.04$) (Figure 27.2). Five subjects with mean age 52.4 ± 13.2 years were implanted. The RF-bion was easily placed in all subjects. Verification of pudendal nerve stimulation was done through clinical palpation and electromyography testing. All cystometrogram volumes improved after stimulation. The mean percentage change in maximum cystometric capacity was 50% after 15 days of stimulation and continued to

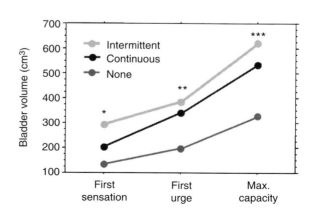

Figure 27.2 Percutaneous stimulation trial data.
*$p = 0.005$; **$p = 0.01$; ***$p = 0.01$
(Kruskal–Wallis). (See also color plate section).

improve thereafter. There was a 64% decrease in incontinence episodes ($p = 0.25$) (Figure 27.3). Though this result did not reach statistical significance due to the small sample size, all patients improved. There was a similar downward trend for daytime voids, night-time voids, and pad usage. This change was maintained over time. There were no perioperative complications reported. The RF-Bion was activated an average of 8–12 hours per day. Data assessed during the period of stimulation only showed even more improvement from baseline voiding diary parameters (see Figure 27.4).

This pilot study demonstrated that chronic pudendal nerve stimulation with the RF-Bion was feasible and had a favorable impact on lower urinary tract symptoms in patients with refractory urge urinary incontinence. The external devices necessary for operation of the RF-Bion device were quite cumbersome for patients (Figure 27.5). Limitations of this and other RF devices have included the need for large external generators for the RF field and antennas for transmission. The inclusion of batteries into microstimulators opens up new opportunities for implanted devices that do not require external equipment for long-term stimulation.

BATTERY-POWERED BION® MICROSTIMULATOR

The bion® device (Advanced Bionics Corp., Valencia, CA) is a fully integrated, programmable, battery-powered microstimulator used for the treatment of refractory voiding dysfunction. This device has a CE Mark in Europe and is in clinical trials in the United States. It is designed to provide chronic pudendal nerve stimulation in a minimally invasive fashion. The bion® is a self-contained, fully programmable, single channel stimulator with two electrodes and a rechargeable battery. It is 27.5 mm long by 3.2 mm wide and it weighs less than 0.7 grams. The bion is placed adjacent to the pudendal nerve at Alcock's canal in a minimally invasive fashion through a small incision in the perineum. A physician programmer allows the adjustment of all stimulation parameters while the patient has her/his own remote control to allow for adjustment of the amplitude of stimulation. The battery is recharged by sitting on a charging pad typically for 20–60 minutes per day, and the battery may last up to 20 years. The components of the bion® microstimulator system are shown in Figure 27.6.

Patient selection

Chronic pudendal neuromodulation is not yet approved by the Food and Drug Administration (FDA) for the treatment of voiding dysfunction. However, two FDA-approved multicenter studies are being conducted in the USA. With appropriate informed consent, patients suffering from refractory voiding dysfunction, including urinary urgency–frequency and urge incontinence, may be candidates for these studies of pudendal

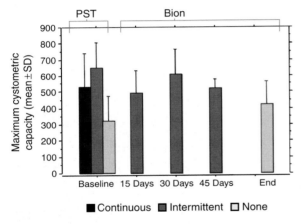

Figure 27.3 RF-Bion™ microstimulator data. PST, percutaneous stimulation trial. (See also color plate section).

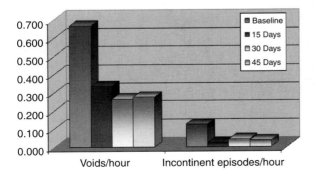

Figure 27.4 RF-Bion™ microstimulator stimulation only data: mean voiding diaries, stimulation for 8–12 hours daily. (See also color plate section).

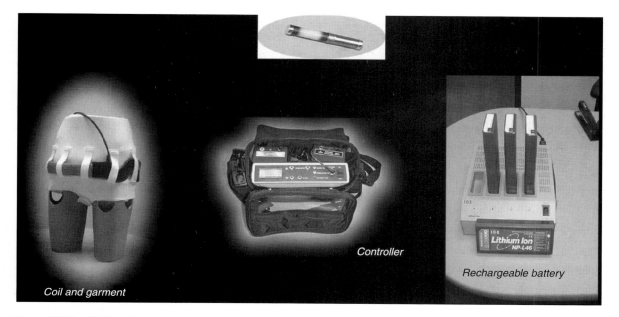

Figure 27.5 RF-Bion™ microstimulator system. (See also color plate section).

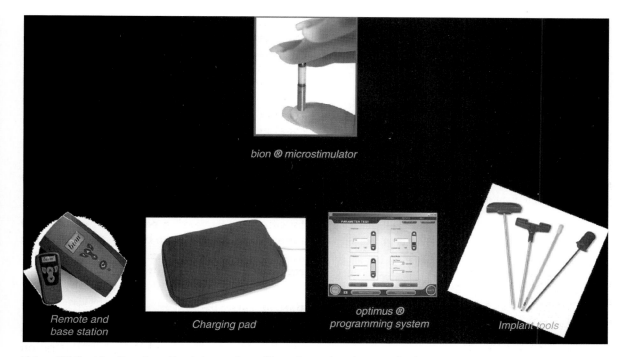

Figure 27.6 bion® microstimulator system. (See also color plate section).

neuromodulation with bion®. In addition, patients who failed sacral nerve stimulation may still benefit from pudendal nerve stimulation.[39] If pudendal nerve stimulation demonstrates clinical efficacy in the ongoing trials, other disease states that may be considered include non-obstructive urinary retention, interstitial cystitis, and neurogenic bladder, which includes partial spinal cord injury, multiple sclerosis, Parkinson's disease, and other neurologic disorders.

A complete voiding diary is paramount in the evaluation of the patient considering neuromodulation. The voiding diary evaluates: time of voids, voided volumes, incontinent episodes, urge scores, pain scores, bowel function, and catheterized volumes if in retention. This baseline information allows accurate postoperative evaluation of patient progress. Since at present these procedures can only be done "on protocol", appropriate Human Investigation Committee approval is required with signature of an informed consent form.

Percutaneous stimulation trial

Prior to implantation of a permanent bion®, a percutaneous stimulation trial is performed in the office. The patient is placed in the lithotomy position at a 45-degree angle; the vagina and perineum are prepped and draped in the normal sterile fashion. Surface electromyography (EMG) electrodes are placed at the anal sphincter. A cystometrogram (CMG) is performed at a fill rate of 50 ml/minute while measuring the volume at first sensation, first urge, maximum cystometric capacity, and volume at first unstable contraction. Next, the ischial tuberosity is palpated and its medial border is traced on the surface of the skin with a marking pen. The ischial spine is palpated through the vagina or rectum as a consistent landmark where the pudendal reenters the pelvis to pass through Alcock's canal. The skin is anesthetized approximately 1.5 cm medial to the ischial tuberosity at a point just posterior to the midpoint of the bituberous plane. With a finger in the vagina or rectum, palpating the ischial spine as an internal point of reference, the stimulating needle is advanced through the fat of the ischiorectal fossa toward the pudendal nerve (Figures 27.7 and 27.8). Confirmation of pudendal nerve stimulation is made both clinically and by electrodiagnostic testing. Clinically, muscle contractions of the bulbocavernosus and external anal sphincter are assessed by direct vision and palpation. The patient's perception of stimulation along the distribution of the pudendal nerve further confirms pudendal stimulation. Sensory response is determined and a pulsating or tingling sensation in the vaginal, vulvar, or anal region is optimum. Leg or buttock pain is undesirable and can usually be easily avoided.

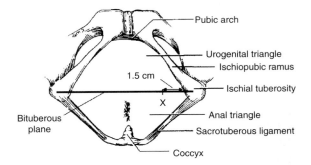

Figure 27.7   bion® microstimulator insertion site.

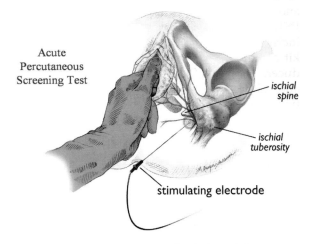

Figure 27.8   Percutaneous stimulation trial.

Measurement of compound muscle action potentials (CMAPs) from surface electrodes over the external anal sphincter is confirmatory of pudendal stimulation. Poor response includes contraction of the obturator internus, leg adductors, or lower extremity muscles, which is usually caused by collateral stimulation of either the levator ani muscles or obturator internus muscles directly, or rarely from stimulation of the obturator nerve.

Once correct needle placement is confirmed, the pudendal nerve is stimulated for 15 minutes at a pulse frequency of 20 Hz, pulse width of 200 μs, 50% duty cycle (5 seconds on/5 seconds off) and amplitude of up to 10.0 mA based on the patient's tolerance. The bladder is emptied with a catheter and the urodynamic catheter is replaced. The CMG is repeated while stimulation continues. A 50% increase in the volume of first urge, cystometric capacity, or volume at unstable bladder contraction constitutes a positive trial supporting implantation of the permanent bion® device.

Implantation of the bion® microstimulator

The implant procedure is done in an outpatient surgical setting utilizing local anesthesia and light sedation. Preoperative broad-spectrum antibiotics are administered intravenously. The patient is lightly sedated and placed in the lithotomy position. The perineal area and vagina are prepped and draped in the normal sterile fashion. Surface EMG electrodes are placed on the anal sphincter approximately 1 cm from the anal verge and connected to an electrodiagnostic monitor. The medial aspect of the ischial tuberosity is marked, and the skin at the insertion site, similar to the PST, is infiltrated with 1% lidocaine. A 2–3 mm incision is made at this site. The bion® implant kit contains a blunt dissector/stimulator, introducer, bion® holder (with preloaded bion®), and placement device (Figure 27.9). With a finger palpating the ischial spine through the vagina or rectum, the blunt dissector/stimulator and introducer are inserted together toward the target (Figure 27.10). Clinical and electrophysiological responses facilitate placement as described above. Once pudendal nerve stimulation is confirmed, the blunt dissector is removed, leaving the introducer in place. The bion® in its holder is advanced through the introducer and the placement tool is advanced through the bion® holder and locked in place by rotating clockwise until it "clicks" into place. For the current application, the bion® is activated with a remote control at a frequency of 20 Hz and pulse width 200 µs, and the amplitude is slowly increased until appropriate responses are again obtained. Sensory, motor, and electrodiagnostic responses are assessed. Once the location is optimized, the bion® is delivered by retracting the bion® holder with

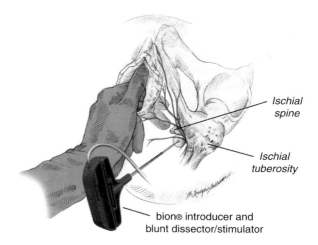

Figure 27.10 bion® microstimulator implant technique.

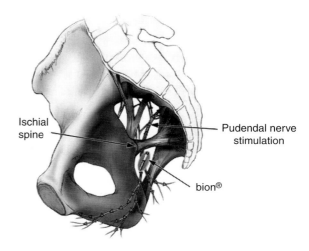

Figure 27.11 Implanted bion® microstimulator. (See also color plate section).

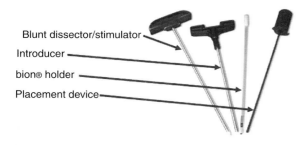

Figure 27.9 bion® microstimulator implant tools.

the placement tool by turning the thumbscrew clockwise until it stops. This deposits the bion® at the site of stimulation (Figures 27.11 and 27.12.) The bion® introducer is removed and a Steri-Strip™ is placed over the skin incision site.

Postoperative follow-up

One week following the implant the patient returns to the office for activation and programming of the bion®, as well as for education

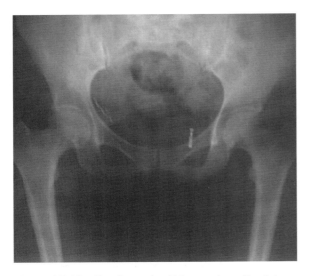

Figure 27.12 X-radiograph of bion® microstimulator.

regarding the system components. The clinician has a programmer that communicates with the bion® and allows the stimulator to be activated, adjustment of the frequency, pulse width, and burst mode, and limits to the stimulation to be set. The patients have their own home kit consisting of a remote control, base station/charger, and chair pad used to charge the bion®. The bion® may last up to 20 years, and can be recharged even if the battery is allowed to completely deplete.

Explantation

Reasons for explantation of the bion® include lack of efficacy, migration, or malposition, device failure, or patient desire. Removing the bion® may be more challenging than placing the device. It is important to remember that one end of the bion® is composed of titanium and the other end is ceramic. On fluoroscopy, the ceramic side appears more radio dense. Given its small size and lead-less design, the position of the bion® must be positively identified. Using fluoroscopy in the lateral and anterior–posterior modes, a spinal needle can be directed through the perineum to localize the device. This will give the direction of approach. Usually, a 2–3-cm perineal incision, large enough to accommodate an index finger and right angle retractors, is sufficient. An index finger in the

vagina directed laterally toward the bion® can help stabilize the device. The fat in the ischial/rectal fossa can be bluntly dissected and, ultimately, the bion® can be palpated in its capsule. Next, with the bion® stabilized, the tissue attachments are bluntly "stripped" off the capsule to help decrease the likelihood of injuring the pudendal nerve. A clamp can be placed on the titanium side of the bion® and the capsule cut with a knife. The device then should slide out easily.

CONCLUSION

Neuromodulation has been shown to treat underlying voiding dysfunction such as urinary urgency, frequency, urge incontinence, and urinary retention. It is also being studied for the treatment of fecal incontinence, chronic constipation, pelvic pain, and other disease states. With new technology such as the tined lead (Medtronic) or smaller implantable stimulators such as the bion® microstimulator (Advanced Bionics), neuromodulation has become minimally invasive, and physicians should be familiar with these procedures to improve the quality of life of their patients with refractory lower urinary tract symptoms. Chronic pudendal stimulation with the bion® provides an attractive, alternative form of neuromodulation. The results of clinical trials will determine its future in treating voiding dysfunction.

REFERENCES

1. Yoshimura N, de Groat WC. Neural control of the lower urinary tract. Int J Urol 1997; 4: 111–25.
2. de Groat WC. Urinary Incontinence. St Louis: Mosby, 1997.
3. de Groat WC, Araki I, Vizzard MA et al. Developmental and injury induced plasticity in the micturition reflex pathway. Behav Brain Res 1998; 92: 127–40.
4. Fall M, Ahlstrom K, Carlsson CA et al. Contelle: pelvic floor stimulator for female stress-urge incontinence. A multicenter study. Urology 1986; 27: 282–7.
5. Janez J, Plevnik S, Suhel P. Urethral and bladder responses to anal electrical stimulation. J Urol 1979; 122: 192–4.
6. Ohlsson B, Lindstrom S, Erlandson BE, Fall M. Effects of some different pulse parameters on

bladder inhibition and urethral closure during intravaginal electrical stimulation: an experimental study in the cat. Med Biol Eng Comput 1986; 24: 27–33.

7. Walter JS, Wheeler JS, Robinson CJ, Wurster RD. Inhibiting the hyperreflexic bladder with electrical stimulation in a spinal animal model. Neurourol Urodyn 1993; 12: 241–52; discussion 253.

8. Wheeler JS Jr, Walter JS, Zaszczurynski PJ. Bladder inhibition by penile nerve stimulation in spinal cord injury patients. J Urol 1992; 147: 100–3.

9. Sundin T, Carlsson CA, Kock NG. Detrusor inhibition induced from mechanical stimulation of the anal region and from electrical stimulation of pudendal nerve afferents. An experimental study in cats. Invest Urol 1974; 11: 374–8.

10. Vodusek DB, Light JK, Libby JM. Detrusor inhibition induced by stimulation of pudendal nerve afferents. Neurourol Urodyn 1986; 5: 381–9.

11. Ishigooka M, Hashimoto T, Sasagawa I, Nakada T, Handa Y. Electrical pelvic floor stimulation by percutaneous implantable electrode. Br J Urol 1994; 74: 191–4.

12. Ishigooka M, Hashimoto T, Sasagawa I, Nakada T, Handa Y. Technique of percutaneous electrode implantation for electrical pelvic floor stimulation. Eur Urol 1993; 23: 413–16.

13. Ishigooka M, Ishii N, Hashimoto T et al. Electrical stimulation of pelvic floor musculature by percutaneous implantable electrodes: a case report. Int Urol Nephrol 1992; 24: 277–82.

14. Schmidt RA, Tanagho EA. Feasibility of controlled micturition through electric stimulation. Urol Int 1979; 34: 199–230.

15. Tanagho EA, Schmidt RA. Electrical stimulation in the clinical management of the neurogenic bladder. J Urol 1988; 140: 1331–9.

16. Schmidt RA, Senn E, Tanagho EA. Functional evaluation of sacral nerve root integrity. Report of a technique. Urology 1990; 35: 388–92.

17. Schmidt RA, Jonas U, Oleson KA et al. Sacral nerve stimulation for treatment of refractory urinary urge incontinence. Sacral Nerve Stimulation Study Group. J Urol 1999; 162: 352–7.

18. Chartier-Kastler EJ, Ruud Bosch JL, Perrigot M et al. Long-term results of sacral nerve stimulation (S3) for the treatment of neurogenic refractory urge incontinence related to detrusor hyperreflexia. J Urol 2000; 164: 1476–80.

19. Janknegt RA, Hassouna MM, Siegel SW et al. Long-term effectiveness of sacral nerve stimulation for refractory urge incontinence. Eur Urol 2001; 39: 101–6.

20. Wein AJ, Rackley RR. Overactive bladder: a better understanding of pathophysiology, diagnosis and management. J Urol 2006; 175: S5–10.

21. van Voskuilen AC, Oerlemans DJ, Weil EH, de Bie RA, van Kerrebroeck PE. Long term results of neuromodulation by sacral nerve stimulation for lower urinary tract symptoms: a retrospective single center study. Eur Urol 2006; 49: 366–72.

22. Peters KM, Carey JM, Konstandt DB. Sacral neuromodulation for the treatment of refractory interstitial cystitis: outcomes based on technique. Int Urogynecol J Pelvic Floor Dysfunct 2003; 14: 223–8; discussion 228.

23. Vodusek DB, Plevnik S, Vrtacnik P, Janez J. Detrusor inhibition on selective pudendal nerve stimulation in the perineum. Neurourol Urodyn 1988; 6: 389–93.

24. Ishigooka M, Hashimoto T, Izumiya K et al. Electrical pelvic floor stimulation in the management of urinary incontinence due to neuropathic overactive bladder. Front Med Biol Eng 1993; 5: 1–10.

25. Ohlsson BL, Fall M, Frankenberg-Sommar S. Effects of external and direct pudendal nerve maximal electrical stimulation in the treatment of the uninhibited overactive bladder. Br J Urol 1989; 64: 374–80.

26. Grill WM, Craggs MD, Foreman RD, Ludlow CL, Buller JL. Emerging clinical applications of electrical stimulation: opportunities for restoration of function. J Rehabil Res Dev 2001; 38: 641–53.

27. Walter JS, Riedy L, King W et al. Short-term bladder-wall response to implantation of microstimulators. J Spinal Cord Med 1997; 20: 319–23.

28. Rijkhoff NJ, Wijkstra H, van Kerrebroeck PE, Debruyne FM. Urinary bladder control by electrical stimulation: review of electrical stimulation techniques in spinal cord injury. Neurourol Urodyn 1997; 16: 39–53.

29. Cameron T, Loeb GE, Peck RA et al. Micromodular implants to provide electrical stimulation of paralyzed muscles and limbs. IEEE Trans Biomed Eng 1997; 44: 781–90.

30. Zealear DL, Garren KC, Rodriguez RJ et al. The biocompatibility, integrity, and positional stability of an injectable microstimulator for reanimation of the paralyzed larynx. IEEE Trans Biomed Eng 2001; 48: 890–7.

31. Gustafson KJ, Zelkovic PF, Feng AH et al. Fascicular anatomy and surgical access of the human pudendal nerve. World J Urol 2005; 23: 411–18.

32. Gruber H, Kovacs P, Piegger J, Brenner E. New, simple, ultrasound-guided infiltration of the pudendal nerve: topographic basics. Dis Colon Rectum 2001; 44: 1376–80.

33. Hollabaugh RS Jr, Steiner MS, Sellers KD, Samm BJ, Dmochowski RR. Neuroanatomy of the pelvis: implications for colonic and rectal resection. Dis Colon Rectum 2000; 43: 1390–7.

34. Kovacs P, Gruber H, Piegger J, Bodner G. New, simple, ultrasound-guided infiltration of the pudendal nerve: ultrasonographic technique. Dis Colon Rectum 2001; 44: 1381–5.

35. Loukas M, Louis RG Jr, Hallner B, Gupta AA, White D. Anatomical and surgical considerations of the sacrotuberous ligament and its relevance in pudendal nerve entrapment syndrome. Surg Radiol Anat 2006; 28: 163–9.

36. O'Bichere A, Green C, Phillips RK. New, simple approach for maximal pudendal nerve exposure: anomalies and prospects for functional reconstruction. Dis Colon Rectum 2000; 43: 956–60.

37. Schraffordt SE, Tjandra JJ, Eizenberg N, Dwyer PL. Anatomy of the pudendal nerve and its terminal branches: a cadaver study. ANZ J Surg 2004; 74: 23–6.

38. Shafik A, Doss S. Surgical anatomy of the somatic terminal innervation to the anal and urethral sphincters: role in anal and urethral surgery. J Urol 1999; 161: 85–9.

39. Bosch JL. The bion device: a minimally invasive implantable ministimulator for pudendal nerve neuromodulation in patients with detrusor overactivity incontinence. Urol Clin North Am 2005; 32: 109–12.

28

The Miniaturo™-I device: a new implantable electrostimulation system for the treatment of voiding dysfunction

Ruud Bosch

Introduction • Device description • Screening test • Implantation procedure • Post-implantation management • Practical experience with the miniaturo™-I device • Safety assessment of the Miniaturo™-I system • Discussion

INTRODUCTION

In 1963, Caldwell[1] was the first to use chronic electrical stimulation for the treatment of urinary incontinence. He implanted electrodes close to the urethral musculature and coupled these to an implantable radio-linked stimulator. Patients with stress as well as urge incontinence were treated with this method, and the treatment was successful in about 50% of cases. Caldwell attributed successful treatment to direct stimulation of the pelvic floor and sphincter musculature. In a dog model, Alexander and Rowan[2] showed that the beneficial effect was mainly due to stimulation of the pudendal nerve and not to direct muscle stimulation. Animal experimental research later showed that bladder inhibition occurred due to pudendal to pelvic nerve reflex action.[3] Detrusor inhibition was obtained due to stimulation of afferent somatic nerve fibers.[4] After this initial experience with an implantable system, the trend shifted towards non-invasive electrical stimulation of the pelvic floor with vaginal and anal plug electrodes, because of the relatively low initial success rate and because of the risks and complications of implantation. Various forms of electrical stimulation have been used in the treatment of female stress and urge urinary incontinence, such as: transvaginal, transanal, and transcutaneous stimulation of various dermatomes.[5]

In the last decade of the 20th century the attention shifted back to implantable systems, since it was recognized that a close spatial relationship of the electrode to the nerve was important for a good effect and that chronic stimulation was more effective than intermittent stimulation.[6] These considerations, together with technological advances in pacemaker technology and electrode design, led to the success of the InterStim® system, making use of sacral spinal nerve stimulation in the treatment of overactive bladder and of non-obstructive urinary retention.[5] Since then, direct electrical stimulation with implantable electrodes has been delivered to the sacral spinal nerves and to the pudendal nerve.[7] The Miniaturo™-I system, using paraurethral stimulation of the sphincter urethrae and pelvic floor muscles is the latest addition to the armamentarium. The rationale behind this approach is based on the finding that, in human volunteers, contraction of the external urethral sphincter induced by electrical stimulation is able to inhibit detrusor contraction.[8]

DEVICE DESCRIPTION

The Miniaturo™-I system (BioControl) is a new implantable system for the treatment of painful bladder syndrome and urinary voiding dysfunction.[9] It consists of a battery-powered electrostimulator and a stimulation lead (Figure 28.1). The non-implantable components include a physician programmer and a safety magnet. The stimulation lead is placed paraurethrally in the pelvic floor. The location of the stimulating electrode is comparable to the original position described by Caldwell.[1] Anatomically this approach is more straightforward than that of other systems that are currently in use (Figure 28.2).

The electrostimulator is capable of delivering electrical pulses, which stimulate the urethral sphincter and pelvic floor. Stimulation parameters are: frequency of up to 12 Hz; average current of up to 40 mA; amplitude of up to 3 V; pulse width of 0.5 μs–2 ms. The device lifetime is calculated at 3–5 years (dependent on the intermittent stimulation intensity level). The stimulation lead is a 35-cm long bipolar lead with a diameter of 1.4 mm.

The physician programmer is used in conjunction with the electrostimulator to non-invasively adjust the stimulation parameters of the electrostimulator to optimize the therapy outcome for each patient. The programmer system consists of a laptop personal computer (PC) running the Miniaturo™ programming software, communication interface, and a programming wand. Parameter adjustments and information transmission are made with the programming wand

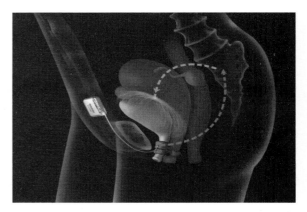

Figure 28.2 Schematic drawing of the implanted Miniaturo™-I system showing the electrode in a paraurethral position and indicating the inhibitory effect of stimulated external urethral sphincter contraction on the detrusor vesicae muscle. (See also color plate section).

placed over the electrostimulator using wireless communication. The programmer is capable of providing telemetry data transmission such as serial number identification, stimulation parameters, manufacturing year and battery status, in addition to the setting of pulse parameters. The patient safety magnet is used to manually turn the electrostimulator on or off.

SCREENING TEST

Test stimulation is performed to assess the patient's suitability for permanent implantation. The Miniaturo™ Test System-I (MTS-I) consists of an external unit and a stimulation lead. The external unit comprises an electrostimulator that is worn on a belt, while the stimulation-lead tip is placed in the pelvic floor. Electrical pulses are transmitted from the MTS-I electrostimulator to the pelvic floor via the lead. The optimal stimulation parameters are determined by the physician for each patient according to their individual sensations. Stimulus output is adjusted to deliver intermittent stimulation with this mode of treatment. Typically, patients were asked to wear the test system for 6–48 hours in the pilot studies, and to keep voiding and/or pain diaries during that period.

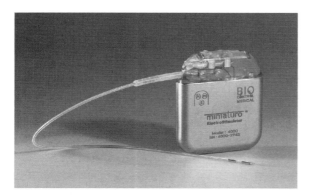

Figure 28.1 The Miniaturo™-I electrostimulator (4 × 5 × 0.8 cm) with electrode connected.

IMPLANTATION PROCEDURE

Implantation can be performed under local anesthesia. A 4-cm long skin incision is made approximately 4 cm cephalad to the pubic bone to create a subcutaneous "pocket". The electrostimulator will later be placed in this "pocket".

Following the suprapubic incision, a second 0.5–1-cm long incision is made in the vaginal mucosa down to the subcutaneous tissue, approximately 1–2 cm lateral to the urethral meatus, at the 2 or 10 o'clock position. A suture is used to anchor the lead to the fascia in order to prevent migration. The long stimulation lead introducer is slightly bent and passed through the paraurethral incision towards the suprapubic incision, to create a subcutaneous tunnel. The introducer guide is then removed. The stimulation lead (with the electrodes first), starting at the suprapubic end, is passed through the introducer until the stimulation lead electrode tip exits at the proximal end of the introducer and the lead connector is near the suprapubic incision. The long introducer is removed, leaving the stimulation lead tip outside the paraurethral incision. A finger is put in the vagina and used to direct the short stimulation lead introducer to its position. The introducer should be felt while inserting it fully into the paraurethral incision for a distance of approximately 3 cm, directed towards the urethral sphincter. A Foley catheter is used as reference to its location in relation to the bladder neck. The lead stylet is withdrawn and the lead tip is then inserted into the introducer until the lead's blue marking is no longer seen (this will indicate that the stimulation lead is about 3–3.5 cm deep in the body). The short introducer is then split and withdrawn. Subsequently, a suture anchors the lead. The free electrode lead is buried subcutaneously (by pulling the lead towards the suprapubic incision), and the paraurethral incision is closed. The device is now secured to the fascia within the pocket. The electrostimulator is placed in the pocket with the engraved side facing outward. The implantation is now complete (Figure 28.3).

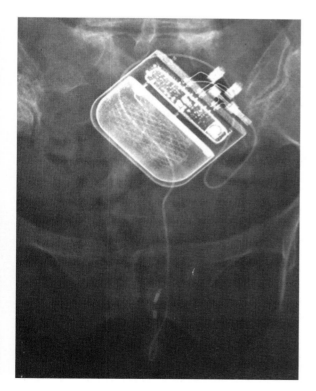

Figure 28.3 Plain X-radiograph of the implanted Miniaturo™-I system, with the electrostimulator in a suprapubic subcutaneous pocket and the electrode tip in a paraurethral position.

POST-IMPLANTATION MANAGEMENT

The Miniaturo™-I is programmed by the external programmer, after implantation (at least 2 weeks). Setting of the optimal electrical stimulation parameters is done on an individual basis. The stimulation output can be adjusted to deliver intermittent stimulation with a frequency of 12 Hz, an average current of up to 40 mA, amplitude of 3 V, and a pulse width of up to 2 ms.

The safety magnet enables the patient to inhibit Miniaturo™-Is stimulations. Once the patient applies the safety magnet over the implanted electrostimulator it will cause the output to turn off. The electrostimulator will not stimulate while the magnet is in place, but will start when the safety magnet is removed.

The safety magnet does not affect programmed parameters; when the stimulator is switched on again, the system resumes previous parameter settings. Patients can stop the electrostimulation for an extended period of time by taping the magnet over the implant device using surgical tape or elastic, wrap-around bandage.

PRACTICAL EXPERIENCE WITH THE MINIATURO™-I DEVICE

Interstitial cystitis

Interstitial cystitis (IC) is a chronic syndrome characterized by a constellation of lower urinary tract irritative symptoms and pain.[10] The broad clinical definition of IC includes patients who complain of urinary urgency, frequency, and/or pelvic/perineal pain in the absence of any identifiable cause, such as bacterial infection or tumor. The etiology is unknown, but may involve microbiologic, immunologic, mucosal, neurogenic, and/or other as yet unidentified factors.

In the mid-1980s the National Institutes of Arthritis, Diabetes, Digestive and Kidney Diseases (NIDDK) developed clinical and cystoscopic diagnostic criteria for research studies of IC.[10] These criteria, including exclusions and cystoscopic findings of ulcers and glomerulations, were then widely adopted for both clinical and research purposes. However, many patients who would be clinically considered to have IC do not fulfill all the NIDDK criteria. The Interstitial Cystitis Database (ICDB) study concluded that the NIDDK criteria were too restrictive for clinical use, because more than 60% of patients regarded by experienced clinicians as suffering from IC fail to meet the criteria.[10]

Several authors performed permanent implantations of the InterStim® device for treatment of patients with IC. Mixed results have been reported with S_3 sacral nerve stimulation. Some investigators report good results, with up to 75% improvement in symptoms,[11,12] whereas others could not demonstrate a significant beneficial effect.[13]

The feasibility study of the Miniaturo™-I in IC patients was planned to determine the safety and objective and subjective efficacy of electrical stimulation of the paraurethral pelvic floor for the treatment of interstitial cystitis. It was initiated in April 2002, and 13 centers worldwide participated in the study.[14]

The inclusion criteria were formulated to reflect the new, clinically based, definition of IC, i.e. the presence of Hunner's ulcers and glomerulations is not obligatory, and either pain or voiding symptoms are inclusion criteria; patients who suffer from stress incontinence are not eligible for the study.

Seventy-three patients were enrolled in the study[14] (mean age of 55.5 years; range 21–80 years). The patients were asked to use the system (external electrostimulator and stimulation lead placed in the pelvic floor) for 6–48 hours during the test phase. Sixteen of the 73 patients (22%) did not pass the MTS-I procedure; 57 patients were implanted with the Miniaturo™-I system. Of these patients, 23% withdrew their consent to participate in the study, 1–25 months postimplantation, mainly due to self-perceived lack of efficacy.

Clinical study results were analyzed for safety and efficacy of the Miniaturo™-I system. Safety was assessed based on the severe adverse event rate and efficacy was based on pain relief and micturition variables (voiding diary) and subjective symptoms (patient symptom and quality of life questionnaires).

Forty-five of 57 patients completed an average follow-up of 18 months (range 1–40 months) and demonstrated an improvement in symptoms. Urinary frequency improved from 24.4 ± 15.1 per day before the implantation to 18.2 ± 12.2 at a mean follow-up of 18 months ($p = 0.02$). Pain score on the Visual Analog Scale (range from 0 to 10) improved from 6 ± 1.9 to 3.1 ± 2.2. The pain score on the Short Form McGill Pain Questionnaire (SF-MPQ)[15] improved from 36.6 ± 10.7 to 17.4 ± 11.2 ($p < 0.0001$). The SF-MPQ is recognized as a valid, useful, and acceptable instrument for moderate to severe chronic or acute pain in all sorts of painful health problems. The O'Leary–Sant IC index[16] improved from 31.4 ± 3.9 to 20.3 ± 9.7, representing a major improvement in quality of life. In summary, pain symptoms and voiding frequency are significantly reduced in these patients who have suffered from severe interstitial cystitis symptoms for years, and have failed or could not tolerate conservative treatments prior to enrollment in the study.

Overactive bladder syndrome

Several studies have evaluated the efficacy and the long-term results of sacral nerve stimulation with an implantable device (InterStim® therapy) for the treatment of urinary urge incontinence and urgency–frequency. Some investigators report good results, with more than 50% reduction in leaking episodes per day in more than 50% of the implanted patients after 3 and 5 years of follow-up,[17,18] whereas one group has reported less good results.[19]

A feasibility study of the Miniaturo™-I in urgency–frequency patients was initiated in August 2002. The purpose of this study was to determine the objective and subjective efficacy of paraurethral electrical stimulation for the treatment of urgency–frequency symptoms and urge incontinence. Urgency and frequency symptoms were calculated based on a micturition diary during all study phases. In addition, patients were asked to complete quality of life questionnaires at baseline and on every follow-up visit. Based on International Continence Society (ICS) terminology, urgency–frequency syndrome and urge incontinence are now termed overactive bladder (OAB) syndrome.

The clinical study results were analyzed for safety and preliminary efficacy. Efficacy was based on micturition variables (voiding diary) and subjective urinary symptoms (patient questionnaires). Patient physical and clinical evaluation, system interrogation, and stimulation parameter adjustments (if necessary) were done 1, 3, 6, and 12 months post-implantation. Prior to each follow-up visit, patients were asked to fill in a 3-day voiding diary. During these visits, patients were asked also to complete quality of life questionnaires. Each patient was asked about urinary symptoms, discomfort, and other problems that might have arisen (adverse events). Patients who completed 12 months of follow-up have been evaluated every 6 months for a total period of 5 years post-implantation.

The results obtained in the first seven patients have been reported.[9] Patients completed an average follow-up of 14.5 months (range 13–17 months) post-implantation. In one patient the device had to be explanted because of infection after 10 months of follow-up. At the last follow-up visit, five women were completely dry and two reported a reduction in the number of leaking episodes from 15 to 6.7 and from 12 to 4 per 24 hours, respectively. The degree of urgency, on a scale from 0 (no urgency) to 3 (severe urgency), significantly improved from 2.0 at baseline to 1.4 at last follow-up. Patient quality of life as measured by the King's Health Questionnaire improved significantly.

SAFETY ASSESSMENT OF THE MINIATURO™-I SYSTEM

Safety assessment for the post-implantation phase included 60 IC and 19 implanted OAB patients, respectively.[20] These patients were evaluated for adverse events in the chronic implant stage of the clinical investigation.

Of the 79 implanted patients, 34 experienced 77 device- or therapy-related adverse events. Twenty-nine patients needed surgical intervention (i.e. repositioning or replacement); this yields a patient surgical revision rate of 36.7%. The number of post implantation events that required surgical intervention is 46. All events were resolved without sequellae. Nevertheless, technical problems such as premature depletion of the battery or implantation of a non-functioning device are less likely to occur in future trials, inasmuch as they have been addressed and corrected. These data compare favorably with adverse events reported for 219 InterStim® implanted patients.[17] The majority of events observed with the InterStim® system were: pain at stimulator site (15.3%), new pain (9%), suspected lead migration (8.4%), infection (6.1%), transient electric shock (5.5%), pain at lead site (5.4%), and adverse changes in bowel function (3%). The investigators noted that the potential for revision surgery did not appear to affect the overall degree of patient satisfaction with that therapy.

DISCUSSION

The initial results of treatment of interstitial cystitis and overactive bladder patients with the implantable Miniaturo™-I system are encouraging. The implantation procedure is straightforward. The potential risk and adverse events are the well-known side effects of surgery, anesthesia, electrical stimulation and technical system defects (battery depletion, system movements). Most of these side effects can be solved without surgical intervention. Due to the nature of the pilot studies, and the "learning curve" associated with the procedure, the number of surgical corrections and adjustments seem acceptable. The Miniaturo™-I treatment is completely reversible and it can be turned off and completely removed at any time.

In the group of patients with interstitial cystitis, improvement was shown in more than 70% of the implanted patients.[14] These results are at least comparable with those achieved with the InterStim® system. Several authors performed permanent implantations of the InterStim® device. Caraballo et al.[11] reported 17 implanted patients with a mean follow-up of 13.4 months. These authors achieved a 20% cure rate. Cure was defined as a more than 75% improvement in symptoms. Comiter[12] also reported 17 implanted patients, with an average follow-up of 14 months. The voided volume per void increased by 58%, the voiding frequency decreased by 49%, and the pain score on a 0–10 scale decreased by more than 70% from 5.8 to 1.6. In the Miniaturo study an improvement from 6 ± 1.9 to 3.1 ± 2.2 was noted.[12] Berman et al. could not confirm these results, however.[13] In 13 patients who were implanted with the InterStim® device, five (38%) underwent removal of the device for lack of efficacy. Of the remaining eight patients, two (25%) were pleased or delighted with the surgical results, four patients (50%) reported improvement in their frequency and urgency symptoms, and only two patients reported that their pain was resolved following the treatment. The conclusion from this study was that InterStim® for frequency, urgency, and pain syndrome does not demonstrate great efficacy.

The long-term results of treatment with the Miniaturo™-I device in interstitial cystitis patients remain to be determined.

Several studies evaluated the efficacy and the long-term results of sacral nerve stimulation with an implantable device (InterStim® therapy) for the treatment of urinary urge incontinence and urgency–frequency. Siegel et al.[17] reported that 3 years post-implantation, 59% of 41 urinary urge incontinent patients showed $\geq 50\%$ reduction in leaking episodes per day, with 46% of patients being completely dry. After 2 years, 56% of urgency–frequency patients showed a more than 50% reduction in voiding frequency. Bosch and Groen[18] reported complete 5-year follow-up data in a group of 36 consecutive patients with refractory detrusor overactivity incontinence implanted with the InterStim® device. These authors found a more than 50% decrease in leaking episodes in 52.8% of the patients; 22.2% even showed a more than 90% decrease in leaking episodes.

A less enthusiastic report of the treatment of OAB patients with the InterStim® device was recently published by Elhilali et al.[19] These authors reported the long-term experience (mean follow-up 6.5 years) in a total of 52 implanted patients, of whom 41 were available for evaluation. Of these, 22, six, and four belonged to the urgency–frequency, urge incontinence, and interstitial cystitis group, respectively. Persistent improvement was found in 10 of 22, one of six, and none of four, respectively. The preliminary and relatively small experience with the Miniaturo™-I device in this indication shows that five out of seven patients no longer used pads and that the other two were significantly improved after a mean follow-up of 14.5 months. Although the numbers are small, it seems that these early results are comparable to the early results achieved with the InterStim device. Confirmation of these results in a larger patient group with longer follow-up is awaited.

REFERENCES

1. Caldwell KP. The electrical control of sphincter incompetence. Lancet 1963; 2: 174–5.
2. Alexander S, Rowan D. Closure of the urinary sphincter mechanism in anaesthetized dogs by means of electrical stimulation of the perineal muscles. Br J Surg 1966; 52: 808–12.
3. Teague CT, Merrill DC. Electric pelvic floor stimulation: mechanism of action. Invest Urol 1977; 15: 65–9.
4. Sundin T, Carlsson CA, Kock NG. Detrusor inhibition induced from mechanical stimulation of the anal region and from electrical stimulation of pudendal nerve afferents. Invest Urol 1974; 11: 374–8.
5. Groen J, Bosch JLHR. Neuromodulation techniques in the treatment of the overactive bladder. BJU Int 2001; 87: 723–31.
6. Bosch JLHR. Sacral neuromodulation: treatment success is not just a matter of optimal electrode position. BJU Int 2000; 85: 20–3.
7. Groen J, Amiel C, Bosch JLHR. Chronic pudendal nerve neuromodulation in women with idiopathic refractory detrusor overactivity incontinence: results of a pilot study with a novel minimally invasive implantable mini-stimulator. Neurourol Urodyn 2005; 24: 226–30.

8. Shafik A. A study of the continence mechanism of the external urethral sphincter with identification of the voluntary urinary inhibition reflex. J Urol 1999; 162: 1967–71.

9. Nissenkorn I, De Jong PR. A novel surgical technique for implanting a new electrostimulation system for treating female overactive bladder: a preliminary report. BJU Int 2005; 95: 1253–8.

10. Hanno PM, Landis JR, Matthews-Cook Y, Kusek J, Nyberg L, and the Interstitial Cystitis Database Study Group. The diagnosis of interstitial cystitis revisited: lessons learned from the National Institutes of Health Interstitial Cystitis Database Study. J Urol 1999; 161: 553–7.

11. Caraballo R, Bologna RA, Lukban J, Whitmore KE. Sacral nerve stimulation as a treatment for urge incontinence and associated pelvic floor disorders at a pelvic floor center: a follow-up study. Urology 2001; 57 (6 Suppl 1): 121.

12. Comiter CV. Sacral neuromodulation for the symptomatic treatment of refractory interstitial cystitis: a prospective study. J Urol 2003; 169: 1369–73.

13. Berman N, Itano J, Gore J, Rodriguez L, Raz S. Poor results using sacral nerve stimulation (Interstim) for treating pelvic pain patients. J Urol 2003; 169 (4 Suppl): 94 (abstr 365).

14. Parsons M, De Jong P, Radziszewski P et al. Analysis of long-term pelvic floor electrostimulation therapy for interstitial cystitis. Eur Urol Suppl 2006; 5: 193 (abstr 683).

15. Melzack R. The Short Form McGill Pain Questionnaire. Pain 1987; 30: 191–7.

16. O'Leary MP, Sant GR, Fowler FJ Jr, Whitmore KE, Spolarich-Kroll J. The interstitial cystitis symptom index and problem index. Urology 1997; 49 (5A Suppl): 58–63.

17. Siegel SW, Catanzaro F, Dijkema H et al. Long-term results of a multicenter study on sacral nerve stimulation for treatment of urinary urge incontinence, urgency-frequency and retention. Urology 2000; 56 (6A Suppl): 87–91.

18. Bosch R, Groen J. Complete 5-year follow-up of sacral (S3) segmental nerve stimulation with an implantable electrode and pulse generator in 36 consecutive patients with refractory detrusor overactivity incontinence. Neurourol Urodyn 2002; 21: 390–1.

19. Elhilali MM, Khaled SM, Kashiwabara T, Elzayat E, Corcos J. Sacral neuromodulation: long-term experience of one center. Urology 2005; 65: 1114–17.

20. Miniaturo-I Investigator Brochure (CU-40-004-RevF). Bellevue, WA: BioControl, December 2005.

Surgical therapy

29

Transvaginal denervation

Jorge Arzola and R Duane Cespedes

Terminology • Epidemiology • Alternative treatments • Historical background • Preoperative evaluation • Surgical technique • Postoperative care • Conclusion • Note

TERMINOLOGY

The most recent definition of *overactive bladder* (OAB) by the International Continence Society is urgency, with or without urge urinary incontinence, usually associated with frequency and nocturia.[1] *Urgency* is the complaint of a sudden compelling desire to pass urine which is difficult to defer, whereas *urge urinary incontinence* (UUI) is a storage phase disorder defined as the complaint of involuntary leakage of urine accompanied by or immediately preceded by a sense of urgency. *Detrusor overactivity* (DO) is a urodynamic observation characterized by involuntary detrusor contractions during the filling phase, which may be spontaneous or provoked. DO may be further classified as *neurogenic* when there is a relevant neurological condition, or *idiopathic* when there is no defined cause. *Detrusor hyperreflexia* denotes a clinical diagnosis in patients with a clearly defined neurologic disorder causing the involuntary bladder contractions, such as Parkinson's disease, multiple sclerosis, and Alzheimer's disease.

EPIDEMIOLOGY

It is estimated that one-third of patients with OAB suffer from UUI.[2] Milsom et al.[3] and Stewart et al.[4] have shown an overall prevalence of OAB in Western Europe and the United States of 16–17%. Two recent summary analyses estimated a median prevalence of UUI between 11 and 13% in women aged 30–60 years and 19–24% in women older than 60.[5,6] As UUI is an embarrassing condition, it is thought to be underreported, and thus prevalence and incidence rates likely grossly underestimate the actual magnitude of this disorder. Clearly, UUI is a well recognized common health problem afflicting women worldwide.

ALTERNATIVE TREATMENTS

Urge urinary incontinence can be difficult to treat, and therefore therapy should be individually tailored for every patient. Uncomplicated and treatment-naive patients can initially be treated by medical and conservative therapies to include behavioral modifications, anticholinergic therapy, and pelvic floor physiotherapy. Urodynamic testing and surgical interventions are typically reserved for patients refractory to conservative measures. Surgical treatment options for patients with refractory UUI include intravesical medications, transvesical botulinim toxin A injections, neuromodulation, central and peripheral denervation, cystolysis, bladder transection, detrusor myectomy and augmentation cystoplasty.[7,8] The benefits and shortcomings of these therapies can be found in detail in other chapters of this book. The emphasis of this chapter will be on the transvaginal modified Ingelman-Sundberg detrusor denervation procedure as a minimally morbid and potentially curative therapy for UUI refractory to conservative measures.

HISTORICAL BACKGROUND

Detrusor denervation was first described by Richer[9] in the treatment of severe pelvic pain by bilateral resection of the hypogastric and lumbar splanchnic nerves along the anterior and posterior aspects of the bladder. Despite modifications by others, this was an extensive operative procedure with significant postoperative morbidity, which quickly fell out of favor. Peripheral, partial detrusor denervation was initially described in the 1950s by Dr Axel Ingelman-Sundberg from Stockholm, Sweden, in a female patient who had incidental postoperative resolution of urge incontinence after a radical hysterectomy for cervical carcinoma.[10,11] Theorizing that the parasympathetic ganglia were situated within the bladder wall itself, Ingleman-Sundberg attempted to denervate the bladder in other patients suffering from urge incontinence by disrupting all neural innervation to the bladder from the inferior hypogastric plexus.[10] Operative candidates were screened by performing urodynamics before and after a subtrigonal injection of 0.25% lidocaine with 0.0005% epinephrine. Patients with increased bladder capacities, improved urgency, and normal cystometry curve following the anesthetic screening test were selected for the procedure. Using a transvaginal approach, this operation consisted of extensive dissection to the cervix and bladder pedicles bilaterally with division of the pelvic nerve branches to the inferior surface of the bladder. This procedure thereby disrupted the majority of the innervation from the inferior hypogastric plexus to the bladder[12] (Figure 29.1).

In 1959, Ingelman-Sundberg[11] reported an initial 88% primary cure rate (30/34 patients), with a short-term follow-up. In 1978, Ingelman-Sundberg reported a 70% long-term cure rate using this procedure.[13] Lower long-term success rates of approximately 50% were reported by Warrell, and by Hodgkinson and Drukker,[12,14] using a similar transvaginal dissection, in 1977. While the procedure benefited some patients, patient selection was difficult and treatment results were unreliable, causing this procedure to rarely be used.

Current understanding of vesical neuroanatomy suggests that selective transection of only the parasympathetic ganglia as originally theorized by Ingelman-Sundberg is highly unlikely. We now know that the ganglia are close to the neuroterminal plexus of the detrusor musculature, and sympathetic preganglionic and postganglionic fibers of the nerves are intertwined. Therefore, selective transection can be made near the bladder, but it would involve fibers of the parasympathetic, sympathetic, preganglionic, and postganglionic types.

Armed with this knowledge and the theory that the majority of the benefit of the procedure stems from decreased sensory input, Wan et al.[15] described a modified Ingelman-Sundberg procedure in 1991, in which the originally extensive vaginal dissection was modified to concentrate dissection to the area below the trigone. They reported a 72% success rate in 62 patients with minimum 1 year of follow-up. Most recently, Cespedes et al.[16] demonstrated a 64% cure rate at a mean follow-up of 14.8 months, in 1996, with a subsequent 68% long-term cure or improved rate reported in 2002,[17] using the modified Ingelman-Sundberg procedure.

PREOPERATIVE EVALUATION

A thorough history, physical examination, urodynamic evaluation, and cystoscopy (to rule out anatomic reasons for urgency) should be performed in all patients who fail conservative medical and behavioral therapy. An anesthetic screening test is then performed via transvaginal subtrigonal infiltration using 10 ml of 0.25% bupivacaine.

Anesthetic block

The bupivacaine block is performed in the office setting with the patient in the dorsolithotomy

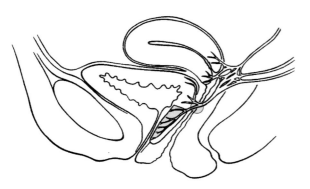

Figure 29.1 Terminal branches of pelvic nerve entering bladder at trigonal level (shaded) and the more proximal nerve fiber (circled and shaded).

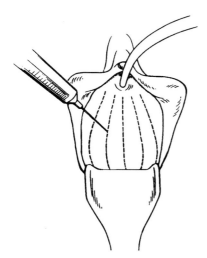

Figure 29.2 Subtrigonal injection of local anesthetic performed in the clinic to test for a potential response to the Ingelman-Sundberg procedure.

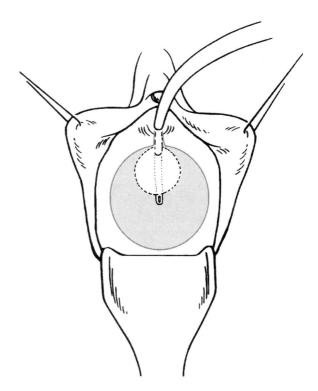

Figure 29.3 The trigone is identified by Foley catheter balloon inflated to 30 ml.

position. The bottom blade of a speculum is used to retract the posterior vaginal wall downward. Local anesthetic (10 ml) is injected subtrigonally using a 22-gauge spinal needle (Figure 29.2). A Foley catheter can be placed temporarily to more accurately identify the trigone. The patients are contacted the following day to determine the efficacy of the injection, the duration of response, and the improvement in urgency and/or urge incontinent episodes. Any commonly used quality of life (QoL) questionnaire can be employed. A positive response is interpreted as 50% or greater decrease in urgency and/or urge incontinent episodes during the duration of action of the local anesthetic (6–24 hours). In our experience, approximately 40–50% of patients will respond positively to the injection.

The presence of urodynamically proven detrusor instability is not used as a selection criterion, because provocative cystometry fails to induce a contraction in as many as 50% of patients with true detrusor contractile incontinence and there is a 15% false positive contraction rate in the elderly.[18]

SURGICAL TECHNIQUE

All procedures are performed using general or regional anesthesia. The patient is positioned in the dorsal lithotomy position using Allen stirrups,

and a Foley catheter is placed. If necessary, saline may be injected just beneath the vaginal mucosa to facilitate dissection. An inverted U-shaped vaginal incision is made in the anterior vaginal wall, centered over the trigone (Figures 29.3 and 29.4). The vaginal epithelium and perivesical fascia are dissected off the trigone (Figures 29.5 and 29.6). The plane of dissection is slightly deeper than that used for an incontinence procedure and is just within the serosal layer of the bladder. Limited lateral (to the endopelvic fascia) and posterior (to the cervix or cuff) sharp dissection is performed to obtain more extensive nerve disruption in the area of the terminal branches of the pelvic nerve. The vaginal mucosa is then reapproximated with 2-0 chromic in running locking or interrupted fashion. An estrogen cream-impregnated vaginal pack is then placed to minimize postoperative bleeding. Operative time is approximately 15–20 minutes, with an average estimated blood loss of approximately 25–50 ml.

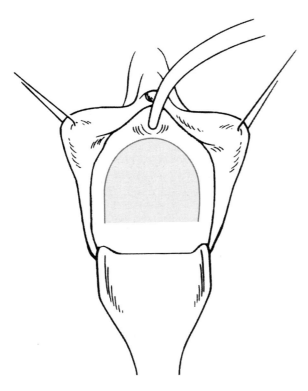

Figure 29.4 The limits of the inverted U-shaped vaginal incision used in this procedure.

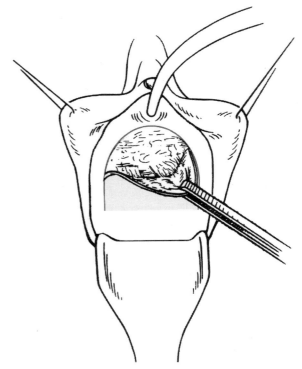

Figure 29.5 Dissection of vaginal epithelium and perivesical fascia from underlying bladder at trigonal level.

POSTOPERATIVE CARE

Patients can be discharged after anesthesia recovery or observed overnight, and the Foley catheter and vaginal pack are removed the morning after surgery. A single post-void residual urine volume is assessed to confirm that the patient is emptying the bladder. The postoperative response should be immediately noticeable as reported by the patient. Vaginal spotting should be expected for about 2 weeks.[8] Follow-up visits are made at 3 weeks, 3 and 6 months postoperatively, and yearly thereafter.

CONCLUSION

The modified Ingelman-Sundberg partial bladder denervation procedure is an excellent surgical option with minimal morbidity and durable cure for intractable urge incontinence. It is a relatively rapid and technically simple operative procedure which should be considered prior to other more extensive and morbid therapies such as autoaugmentation or augmentation

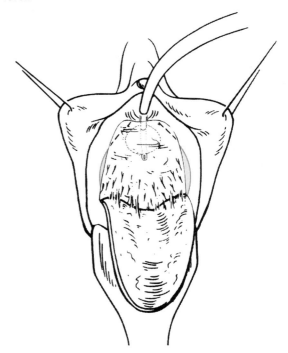

Figure 29.6 Completed Ingelman-Sundberg dissection.

enterocystoplasty. This procedure can easily be combined with other incontinence operations if necessary. If a cure is not achieved with this procedure, alternative options for urge incontinence are not compromised.

NOTE

The views expressed herein are those of the authors and do not reflect the views of the United States Air Force or Department of Defense.

REFERENCES

1. Abrams P, Cardozo L, Fall M et al. The standardisation of terminology of lower urinary tract function: report from the Standardisation Subcommittee of the International Continence Society. Urology 2003; 61: 37–49.
2. Wein AJ, Rackley RR. Overactive bladder: a better understanding of pathophysiology, diagnosis and management. J Urol 2006; 175: S5–10.
3. Milsom I, Abrams P, Cardozo L et al. How widespread are the symptoms of an overactive bladder and how are they managed? A population based prevalence study. BJU Int 2001; 87: 760–6.
4. Stewart W, Herzog AR, Wein AJ et al. Prevalence and impact of overactive bladder in the US: results from the NOBLE program. Neurourol Urodyn 2001; 20: 406.
5. Thom DH. Overactive bladder: epidemiology and impact on quality of life. Contemp Ob/Gyn 2000; 45: 6–13.
6. Brown JS, Grady D, Ouslander JG et al. Prevalence of urinary incontinence and associated risk factors in postmenopausal women. Obstet Gynecol 1999; 94: 66–70.
7. Oyama IA. Advanced procedures for urinary incontinence. J Pelvic Med Surg 2004; 10: 289–304.
8. Westney OL, McGuire EJ. Surgical procedures for the treatment of urge incontinence. Tech Urol 2001; 7: 126–32.
9. Richer V. La resection des nerfs erecteuret des ganglions hypogastriques. J Chir 1935; 45: 54.
10. Ingelman-Sundberg A. Urinary incontinence in women, excluding fistulas. Acta Obstet Gynecol Scand 1952; 31: 266–91.
11. Ingelman-Sundberg A. Partial denervation of the bladder. A new operation for the treatment of urge incontinence and similar conditions in women. Acta Obstet Gynecol Scand 1959; 38: 487–502.
12. Hodgkinson CP, Drukker BH. Infravesical nerve resection for detrussor dyssynergia. The Ingelman-Sundberg operation. Acta Obstet Gynecol Scand 1977; 56: 401–8.
13. Ingelman-Sundberg A. Partial bladder denervation for detrussor dyssynergia. Clin Obstet Gynecol 1978; 21: 797–805.
14. Warrell DW. Vaginal denervation of the bladder nerve supply. Urol Int 1977; 32: 114–16.
15. Wan J, McGuire EJ, Wang S, Cerny JC, Hodgkinson CP. Ingelman-Sundberg bladder denervation for detrusor instability. J Urol 1991; 145: 358A (abstr 581).
16. Cespedes RD, Cross CA, McGuire EJ. Modified Ingelman-Sundberg bladder denervation procedure for refractory urge incontinence. J Urol 1996; 156: 1744–7.
17. Westney OL, Lee JT, McGuire EJ et al. Long-term results of Ingelman-Sundberg denervation procedure for urge incontinence refractory to medical therapy. J Urol 2002; 168: 1044–7.
18. Cespedes RD, Cross CA, McGuire EJ. Re: Modified Ingelman-Sundberg bladder denervation procedure for intractable urge incontinence. J Urol 1997; 158: 888.

30

Autoaugmentation

Jerilyn M Latini

Introduction • Surgical technique • Animal model studies • Human studies
• Modifications of autoaugmentation: seromuscular cystoplasty • Laparoscopic autoaugmentation
• Pregnancy and autoaugmentation • Advantages of autoaugmentation • Potential complications
and morbidity • Concerns • Conclusions

INTRODUCTION

Pharmacologic therapies and neuromodulation have been used for the management of detrusor overactivity, bladder dysfunction with poor compliance, and non-compliant small capacity bladders with or without overactivity due to infectious, inflammatory, neurogenic, congenital, iatrogenic, and idiopathic disorders. When more conservative therapies are ineffective, augmentation cystoplasty is indicated.

Augmentation cystoplasty is an effective treatment for refractory or intractable detrusor overactivity. Goals of augmentation cystoplasty include creation of a low-pressure, capacious urine reservoir. Important principles include attainment of adequate bladder capacity, low storage pressure or normal compliance, urine storage without electrolyte abnormalities, and minimal surgical and postoperative morbidity. Augmentation cystoplasty effectively provides a well functioning reservoir with increased functional bladder capacity and decreased maximal detrusor pressure during bladder filling and at capacity. These effects prevent incontinence, protect the upper urinary tract, and allow for improved quality of life. Clean intermittent catheterization (CIC) is often needed to facilitate complete bladder emptying following augmentation cystoplasty.

Successful augmentation cystoplasty has been performed using stomach, jejunum, ileum, cecum, transverse and descending colon, ureter, and deserosalized gastrointestinal tissue. Alternative techniques have been described to attain the goals of augmentation cystoplasty but avoid inclusion of gastrointestinal mucosa in the urinary tract. Various alloplastic materials, alloplastic or biodegradable scaffolds grafted with autologous urothelial cells, seromuscular augmentation cystoplasty, and autoaugmentation have been described.

Autoaugmentation provides augmentation of the bladder using native urothelial tissue. It avoids the disadvantages associated with augmentation cystoplasty and potential morbidity related to the use of gastrointestinal segments, such as bacteriuria, infection, calculus formation, mucus production, absorption of urine components and electrolyte disturbances, enterohepatic circulation disruption, diarrhea, vitamin B_{12} deficiency, bowel obstruction, intestinal adhesions, metaplastic bone formation, perforation of the augmentation cystoplasty, enteric or urinary fistulization, graft rejection, graft contracture, hematuria–dysuria syndrome, metabolic alkalosis, hypergastrinemia, and malignant potential. The operative time for autoaugmentation is much shorter than augmentation cystoplasty since no anastomoses are required. The primary indications for autoaugmentation are poor bladder compliance and refractory or intractable detrusor overactivity with and without incontinence, due to either idiopathic or neurogenic causes.

Autoaugmentation creates a large, diffuse bulge or bladder diverticulum in the dome of the bladder by partially excising the detrusor muscle while leaving the bladder mucosa intact. This can be thought of as comparable to the naturally occurring, large bladder diverticulum that is seen in patients with long-standing bladder outlet obstruction. The diverticulum allows for storage of increased urine volumes at lower pressures. Also, removal of a portion of the detrusor muscle will decrease the efficiency and magnitude of any residual bladder contractions.

The general technique of technique of autoaugmentation was initially described in 1917 by Neuhof[1] and then Huggins[2] in the 1930s. These authors used autoaugmentation to prevent calcification after fascial repairs of the bladder and other hollow viscera.

Cartwright and Snow described autoaugmentation of the bladder in 1989, and coined the term when they reported their experience with partial vesicomyomectomy in dog model studies.[3] Five of the six operated dogs survived to undergo postoperative urodynamics. Four dogs had an increase in pressure-specific bladder capacity. All dogs had normal bladders preoperatively, so results are difficult to interpret. Cartwright and Snow described the autoaugmentation procedure used to surgically create a large, well draining, wide-mouthed diverticular bulge of the bladder that augmented storage capacity. Autoaugmentation, as they described it, involves surgical removal of the detrusor muscle over the entire dome of the bladder, leaving the underlying bladder mucosa intact. This allows the mucosa to bulge and function as a large, wide-mouth diverticulum, improving bladder compliance and capacity.

In their description (Figure 30.1)[4], Cartwright and Snow made a midline incision through the detrusor muscle via an extraperitoneal approach. With the bladder distended with saline, the mucosa bulged from the detrusor incision as a diverticulum. The detrusor muscle was then mobilized and excised laterally in each direction. To prevent collapse of the bladder diverticulum, the lateral edges of the detrusor muscle were secured to the psoas muscle bilaterally.

SURGICAL TECHNIQUE

The patient should be preoperatively prepared as for any intraabdominal procedure. Patients should be preoperatively counseled, consented, and prepared for augmentation cystoplasty in addition to autoaugmentation, in the event that autoaugmentation is not technically possible at the time of operation. For this reason, patients should have complete antibiotic and mechanical bowel preparation preoperatively.

Preoperative antibiotic is administered. With the patient in the supine position, bilateral sequential compressive devices are placed on the lower extremities. General anesthesia is administered. The patient is frog-legged to allow for sterile urethral catheter placement. The abdomen and genitalia are prepped and draped in sterile fashion. A urethral Foley catheter is placed to allow for bladder filling and emptying during autoaugmentation. The bladder is exposed through a Pfannensteil or low midline abdominal incision. A self-retaining retractor retracts the rectus muscles laterally. The bladder is filled almost to capacity. The anterior wall of the bladder is exposed and the peritoneum is mobilized off of the bladder dome. Electrocautery or a knife is used to create a large midline incision through

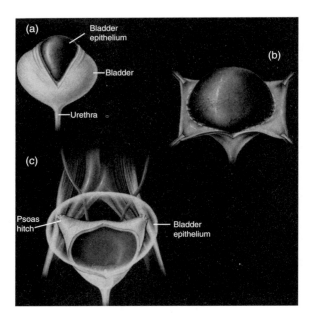

Figure 30.1 Diagram of autoaugmentation: (a) detrusor incised; (b) detrusor stripped from intact bladder epithelium; (c) epithelium bulges with bladder filling. (Reprinted with permission from reference 4).

the detrusor muscle. After the detrusor is divided for three-quarters of its thickness, the remaining detrusor fibers overlying the bladder mucosa are spread with a hemostat and carefully divided sharply, keeping the underlying mucosa intact. Alternatively, a #15 blade can be used to make a transverse incision in the detrusor muscle (Figure 30.2a).[5] In either case, the fibers of the detrusor muscle must be carefully divided layer by layer until the translucent blue-gray bladder mucosa is seen. The bladder mucosa is now visible along the length of the incision in the detrusor muscle over the entire dome. The cut edge of the detrusor muscle is grasped with an Allis clamp. Starting in an area where the bladder mucosa is exposed well, a plane between the detrusor muscle and the intact bladder epithelium is created and continued laterally. Careful sharp dissection of the detrusor muscle from the intact, underlying bladder mucosa is continued until essentially half of the entire detrusor muscle has been stripped off of the bladder (Figure 30.2b). Church scissors or similar like are most useful. Dissection is continued in all directions until a large bladder mucosal diverticulum has been created, from the mid-anterior bladder wall to the peritoneal reflection. The flaps of detrusor muscle are excised (Figure 30.2c). To prevent collapse of the diverticulum and narrowing of the mouth of the mucosal diverticulum, the remaining lateral edges of the detrusor muscle are secured to the ipsilateral psoas muscle as a psoas hitch or fixed to the pelvic sidewall bilaterally. The result is a thin, bulging diverticular patch of bladder mucosa that bulges from the incision with bladder filling.

In patients with markedly thickened, trabeculated, and hypervascular bladders, clean dissection of the detrusor muscle can be difficult. Often, the detrusor muscle is removed "piecemeal", rather than in distinct flaps of detrusor as originally described.

Any inadvertent holes in the bladder mucosa must be carefully oversewn with 4-0 polyglactin or chromic catgut sutures. If an inadvertent cystotomy occurs, a small drain may be placed in the perivesical space via a counterincision. Omentum may be brought down to cover the area. A drain is not routinely placed. The fascia, subcutaneous tissues, and skin are closed in the usual manner. The urethral catheter is placed to gravity drainage postoperatively.

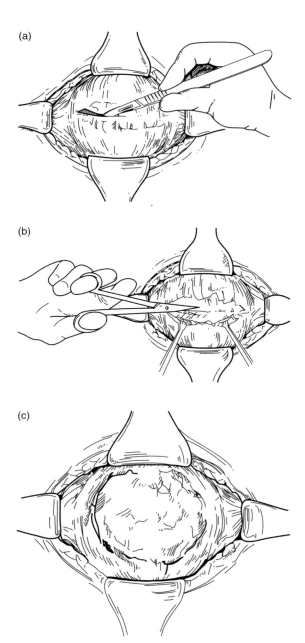

(a)

(b)

(c)

Figure 30.2 Operative technique of detrusor myectomy. (a) Careful division of the detrusor musculature. (b) Sharp dissection of the detrusor musculature from the mucosa. (c) Creation of an anterior mucosal diverticulum. (Reprinted with permission from reference 5).

Usually the urethral catheter is removed on postoperative day 1. Patients without neurogenic bladder dysfunction are allowed to urinate spontaneously and post-void residuals are checked.

Patients with neurogenic bladders are started or continued on CIC. For those who empty by reflex voiding, their post-void residuals are checked and CIC started if their ability to empty has been impacted.

If an inadvertent cystotomy occurs, the urethral catheter is maintained for 2–7 days postoperatively until a cystogram demonstrates no extravasation of contrast material. Patients can be maintained on a prophylactic antibiotic while the catheter is indwelling. In order to prevent contraction of the bladder mucosal diverticulum, repeated cycles of bladder filling and emptying have been advocated.

Autoaugmentation can be accomplished with a short hospital stay. Some perform laparoscopic autoaugmentation as an outpatient procedure. In either case, it does require delicate and meticulous technique to avoid cystotomy while dissecting the detrusor from the mucosa. Some surgeons recommend $2.5 \times$ loupe magnification. If concomitant ureteral reimplantation or bladder neck surgery is indicated with autoaugmentation, any related procedure should be done first and the bladder closed prior to detrusorectomy.[6]

Alternative terms for autoaugmentation include vesicomyomectomy or detrusorectomy, detrusor myomectomy, vesicomyotomy or detrusorotomy, detrusorrhaphy, and autocystoplasty. Autoaugmentation can be performed using various techniques. The dissected detrusor muscle can be partially[3,4,6] or completely used for attachment to a nearby structure such as the psoas or rectus muscles as a hitch,[7,8] or can be partially[3,4,6] or completely removed.[9–11] The detrusor muscle can be partially or completely reflected from the bladder mucosa.[12–18]

ANIMAL MODEL STUDIES

Animal models of autoaugmentation have been developed to investigate techniques to avoid the consequences of direct contact of gastrointestinal mucosa with the urinary tract that can occur in traditional augmentation cystoplasty.

In an effort to determine whether detrusorotomy (incision of the detrusor) or detrusorectomy (excision of the released detrusor) provided better functional results, Johnson et al.[19] performed 16 vesicomyotomies (incision) and 16 vesicomyectomies (excision) in rabbits with previously reduced bladder capacity. There was no statistical difference in functional bladder capacity between techniques; both increased by 43.5%. These results are difficult to interpret because pressure at capacity was not reported.

Even if adequate bladder expansion is achieved initially, there is concern regarding longevity.[14] One animal study showed progressive thickening and contracture of the autoaugmentation site because of collagenous infiltration with a decrease in surface area by 50% at 12 weeks.[19] A study of dogs undergoing detrusorotomy showed better results when a graft (omentum) healed over the exposed bladder mucosa in between the edges of the split detrusor muscle to prevent readhesion of the muscular edges, whereas all other animals had a progressive decrease in postoperative bladder capacity over time.[20]

Garibay et al.[21] showed a statistically significant decrease in capacity after vesicomyomectomy in dogs with talc induced bladder fibrosis. Dewan et al.[22] were unable to demonstrate long-term increases in bladder capacity in lambs after vesicomyomectomy with omental reinforcement. Surer et al.[23] described autoaugmentation where a circular section of the detrusor was excised, creating a large circular diverticulum in a rabbit model. They reported that the circular vesicomyotomy technique produced effective increases in capacity and compliance compared to the vertical (classically described) vesicomyotomy.

HUMAN STUDIES

Following their initial canine studies, Cartwright and Snow[4] performed autoaugmentation in seven children (4–17 years) with urodynamically documented poorly compliant bladders (neurogenic in three, posterior urethral valves in one, idiopathic in three). Although follow-up was short, five showed marked clinical improvement, one gained modest improvement, and one eventually required augmentation cystoplasty. Postoperative urodynamics showed increased bladder capacity of up to 150% in three, no change in one, and a 30% decrease in another. There was improved compliance in four. All were placed on CIC. In a later report,[24] the authors reported their evaluation of 19 patients with follow-up of 3 months to 4 years and found that 80% were completely continent and another 10% had an improvement in continence. They noted that bladder capacity does not consistently increase but most patients continued to store urine at a given volume at lower pressure postoperatively. An increase in bladder capacity of more than 50 ml was documented in 40%, with minimal change in 35% and decreased capacity in 25%. Despite considerable variations in postoperative urodynamics, patients were continent and satisfied. The authors attributed this to a shift in the compliance curve during bladder filling and storage. After autoaugmentation, continence improved and hydronephrosis decreased in most. They reported that 10% had little or no clinical improvement after autoaugmentation. Two patients later underwent augmentation cystoplasty. All patients who voided volitionally preoperatively continued to do so after autoaugmentation. The authors summarized by stating that autoaugmentation, in the early experience, may be effective in achieving continence, decreasing hydronephrosis and improving bladder compliance, but it did not reliably increase bladder capacity.

Vesicomyotomy with no fixation of the detrusor laterally to the psoas (rather than vesicomyectomy) was performed in 12 pediatric patients (4–14 years) with low bladder capacity with detrusor overactivity, 10 of which were neurogenic. They showed a mean increase in bladder capacity of 40% (range 15–70%) and decrease in mean leak point pressure of 33% at 6 months of follow-up. There were no significant complications. The authors concluded that excision holds no advantage over incision.[19]

Kennelly et al.[9] reported their experience with five adults with small, non-compliant bladders due to spinal cord injury ($n=1$), myelomeningocele ($n=2$), and complex postsurgical issues ($n=2$). With follow-up of 12–82 weeks all patients had improved compliance with increased capacity (increased by 75–310 cm^3, or 40–310%) measured at an intravesical pressure of 40 cmH$_2$O. None required augmentation cystoplasty. The authors postulated that the improvement in compliance after autoaugmentation may be due to complete disruption of the detrusor muscle. The bladder may be incapable of contracting in a coordinated manner and generating higher pressures after autoaugmentation because the anterior detrusor muscle has been removed.

Landau and Moorehead[25] reported 12 detrusorectomies, with excellent results in five, acceptable results in two, and one lost to follow-up. Four patients failed autoaugmentation with hydronephrosis ($n=1$), persistent incontinence ($n=2$), and worsening renal insufficiency ($n=1$). Three underwent gastrocystoplasty or ileocystoplasty. Autoaugmentation usually improves compliance, although the increase in capacity may be modest. Snow and Cartwright[26] reported data supporting this, with 52% of patients obtaining a good result after autoaugmentation, whereas 20% had a poor outcome. Future augmentation cystoplasty was not complicated by prior detrusorectomy, but the authors note that the urothelial diverticulum was thick and fibrous, reminiscent of "a leather bag".

Stohrer and colleagues[10,27,28] reported their experience with 29 patients (19 female, 10 male; mean age 35 years, range 14–64) who underwent autoaugmentation. All patients had preoperative urodynamics characterized by low capacity and low compliance. Twenty-four had refractory neurogenic bladder dysfunction. Detrusorectomy was performed but without fixation of the detrusor laterally to the psoas. Twelve of the 29 patients had inadvertent cystotomy (or cystotomies) at the time of autoaugmentation, repaired using chromic catgut. After 7 years of follow-up there had been improved compliance and increased cystometric capacity by 130–600 ml. In the five patients with preoperative reflux, the reflux resolved in two and improved from bilateral to unilateral in two. Half of the patients voided without significant residuals and half required CIC. The authors recommended that autoaugmentation be considered for patients with low capacity, poorly compliant bladders, as the procedure carries low morbidity and a low rate of complications, and is a simple procedure that does not preclude other procedures in the future.

Skobejko-Wlodarska et al.[29] reported long-term outcomes after autoaugmentation in myelodysplastic children with low compliance neurogenic bladders confirmed urodynamically, with vesicoureteral reflux ($n=6$) and dilated upper tracts without reflux ($n=8$) that were refractory to conservative management. Seventeen of the 21 children were assessed urodynamically and followed for 3 months to 8 years (mean 6 years). In 13 children capacity increased by 60 ml, and in

14, intravesical pressure decreased by 65 cmH$_2$O. Fourteen were continent with CIC. Reflux resolved in two, improved in two, and was unchanged in two. Seven of the eight children with dilated, non-refluxing upper tracts improved. Two children required anticholinergic medication after autoaugmentation. Four had no improvement in capacity and three had no improvement in compliance. Two of the 21 children went on to intestinal augmentation cystoplasty.

Leng et al.[5] reported 26 male and 35 female patients (11–81 years), including 11 children (11–15 years) who underwent a total of 37 detrusor myectomies and 32 augmentation cystoplasties using bowel. Diagnoses included intractable detrusor instability ($n=10$), interstitial cystitis ($n=8$), myelodysplasia ($n=16$), radiation cystitis ($n=9$), neurogenic bladder dysfunction ($n=11$), and miscellaneous ($n=7$). Preoperative vesico-ureteral reflux or hydronephrosis was noted in 14 patients. Autoaugmentation offered consistent success in patients with refractory detrusor overactivity, whereas autoaugmentation failure rates were higher in those with interstitial cystitis, neurogenic bladder dysfunction, and myelomeningocele. Interestingly, most patients with preoperative refractory detrusor overactivity were able to urinate spontaneously after autoaugmentation. The authors caution that all patients undergoing autoaugmentation must be willing to perform lifelong CIC postoperatively. They speculate that significant fibrotic changes of the detrusor seen in neurogenic bladders, and with interstitial and radiation cystitis, may affect the ability to effectively resect the detrusor in these patients. Nine (27%) of the 33 primary autoaugmentations failed and went on to augmentation cystoplasty using bowel. The authors stated that autoaugmentation failures identified urodynamically within 4 weeks of surgery should be offered augmentation cystoplasty. Based on their experience, patients with bladder capacities of less than 100 ml would probably be better served by augmentation cystoplasty rather than autoaugmentation. They noted that autoaugmentation did not preclude augmentation cystoplasty using bowel in their series.

Westney and McGuire[30] reviewed 40 patients who underwent autoaugmentation, of whom 30 had pre- and postoperative urodynamics. At a mean follow-up of 42 months, 63% had improvement in compliance and/or resolution of uninhibited bladder contractions. One complication (extraperitoneal bladder leak treated with Foley catheterization for 5 days) was reported in this series.

Perovic et al.[31] reported their initial series of seven children who underwent bladder autoaugmentation with rectus muscle backing or rectus muscle hitch. They updated their patient series in 2003,[32] when they reported their experience with 19 patients (12 girls, seven boys; median age 8 years, range 4–12) with small capacity, poorly compliant neurogenic bladders who underwent autoaugmentation (detrusorectomy) where the detrusor muscle edges were hitched to the rectus muscles bilaterally rather than the psoas. Patients were followed for a median of 21 months (range 6–35). At 1 year, bladder capacity increased in all 19 patients, ranging from 190 to 411 ml (median 313 ml) with improved compliance and clinical status. At 2 years, five patients maintained improved capacity and compliance. Seven voided voluntarily without residual urine while 12 voided and catheterized due to post-void residual urine. The three children who were incontinent before autoaugmentation were continent afterwards.

Stohrer et al.[11] reported their experience with autoaugmentation in 50 patients with neurogenic bladders. Postoperative urodynamics in 36 patients were available, and for those with 6 or more months of follow-up, cystometric capacity increased from 121 to 406 ml and compliance from 6.1 to 29.3 cmH$_2$O. Maximal voiding pressure decreased from 86.4 to 50.9 cmH$_2$O and residual urine increased from 20 to 76 ml. About 60% required CIC after autoaugmentation. Five of the 50 patients were reported to have failed autoaugmentation, and went on to augmentation cystoplasty ($n=2$) or deafferentation ($n=1$). One bladder rupture occurred after autoaugmentation, attributed to an obstructive effect from an artificial sphincter implanted concurrently. This is the only report of bladder rupture after autoaugmentation that we are aware of in the literature. The authors reported longer-term outcomes with continued benefit for their series of patients.[33] They recommend autoaugmentation as an effective procedure for those patients with low-capacity, poorly compliant bladders who are willing to perform CIC; and view autoaugmentation as the treatment of choice before augmentation cystoplasty.

In a review of alternative techniques for augmentation cystoplasty, Duel et al.[34] concluded that the available literature suggested that autoaugmentation techniques had not fulfilled their initial promise of an effective technique for urothelial-lined augmentation cystoplasty. Long-term data at the time were lacking. Unfortunately, late outcomes showed connective tissue proliferation at the autoaugmentation site that appeared to be related to progressive loss of bladder volume and decreased compliance.

Potter and colleagues[35] followed six girls and three boys (mean age 9.3 years, range 5–14) after autoaugmentation (detrusor myotomy) with bilateral psoas muscle hitching. Omentum was placed over the autoaugmentation site in two, and a Mitrofanoff stoma was created concurrently in one. All had neurogenic bladder dysfunction with incontinence: spina bifida ($n=7$), traumatic T_4 paraplegia ($n=1$), and possible bladder dysfunction related to posterior urethral valves versus occult neuropathy ($n=1$). All underwent urodynamics preoperatively. Patients were followed postoperatively for at least 5 years (mean 71 months, range 62–80), until the procedure failed or the patient died. All patients had postoperative urodynamics at 3 months and intermittently thereafter. The authors report no major complication directly related to autoaugmentation. Of the three with preoperative urodynamic bladder overactivity and normal compliance, two had urodynamic improvement and became continent, whereas one had persistent bladder overactivity and incontinence. This patient had low detrusor leak point pressure, and this may at least partially explain the failure of her autoaugmentation. She became continent after bladder neck closure and revision of her Mitrofanoff. Of the six with urodynamic bladder overactivity and abnormal compliance preoperatively, none were continent after autoaugmentation despite significant decreases in filling pressure at capacity, but two were improved. The four with no improvement in continence had low leak point pressures below 40 cmH_2O. Five underwent augmentation cystoplasty with ($n=3$) or without ($n=2$) bladder neck closure and Mitrofanoff creation. The remaining patient died from unrelated causes. Mean time to reoperation was 23 months (range 6–38). The authors summarize by stating that patients most likely to benefit from autoaugmentation are those with bladder overactivity and relatively higher urethral leak point pressures. They suggest that the mechanism of action of autoaugmentation may primarily involve disruption of detrusor contractions rather than in an increase in bladder capacity. Therefore, these authors recommend autoaugmentation for those with bladder overactivity and incontinence, rather than altered bladder compliance where augmentation cystoplasty may be better indicated.

Long-term follow-up of autoaugmentation (detrusor myectomy) in 11 myelodysplastic children was reported by Marte et al.[36] Eight girls and three boys (mean age 12.8 years) were followed for a mean of 6.6 years. Preoperatively, the mean leak point volume was 94 ml and mean leak point pressure was 58 cmH_2O. One year after autoaugmentation, the mean leak point volume was 297 ml and cystometric capacity at 40 cmH_2O was 167 ml. Mean leak point pressure remained stable at 60 cmH_2O. Preoperatively, five with vesicoureteral reflux underwent endoscopic suburethral collagen injection 1–3 weeks before autoaugmentation. Unfortunately, four had recurrent reflux. Ultimately, five children underwent augmentation cystoplasty because of recurrent reflux, urine infection, or incontinence. Overall, with over 6 years of follow-up, autoaugmentation failed in seven of 11 patients in this series. The authors conclude that their results do not justify the routine use of autoaugmentation in patients with poorly compliant, hypertonic neurogenic bladders due to myelomeningocele.

Another series of children with myelodysplasia were followed after autoaugmentation (detrusor myotomy), performed for upper tract deterioration and/or incontinence due to hyperreflexia, poor bladder compliance, or low bladder capacity.[37] Autoaugmentation was performed in 17 children (mean age 10.2 years, range 2.2–13.2) and mean clinical follow-up was 75 months (range 4–126). Twelve of the 17 patients were considered clinical failures based on upper tract deterioration or continued incontinence. Fourteen of 15 patients with urodynamics were considered failures due to persistent poor compliance or less than anticipated improvement in bladder capacity with somatic growth. Progressive hydronephrosis developed in five, and four subsequently required augmentation cystoplasty. Of 13 children, eight remained incontinent. Although promising results were noted earlier in their series, the authors concluded that clinical benefit after autoaugmentation did not appear durable, and that autoaugmentation should not be endorsed for the management of neurogenic bladder dysfunction due to myelodysplasia.

In a series of 10 patients with neurogenic and 17 with idiopathic detrusor overactivity treated with autoaugmentation,[38] 63% patients improved after 1 year of follow-up. Improvement was greater in those with idiopathic detrusor overactivity (12 of 17 improved) compared to those with neurogenic detrusor overactivity (five of 10). Significant urodynamic improvements were seen in both groups, but there was no difference between the idiopathic and neuropathic groups. Volume at first uninhibited bladder contraction increased from a mean of 108 to 177 ml ($p < 0.01$); maximum uninhibited bladder contraction decreased from 65 to 30 cmH$_2$O ($p = 0.004$); capacity increased from a mean of 209 to 271 ml ($p < 0.01$); detrusor pressure at maximum flow decreased from a mean of 83 to 52 cmH$_2$O ($p < 0.001$); and residual urine increased from a mean of 13 to 64 ml ($p < 0.001$).

In 2005, Kumar and Abrams[39] reported longer-term follow-up of the series previously reported by Swami et al. Thirty consecutive patients (median age 33 years, range 10–62) underwent autoaugmentation (detrusor myectomy) for refractory, idiopathic detrusor overactivity (24 patients: 18 females, six males) and neurogenic detrusor overactivity (six patients: two females, four males). All patients had urodynamically documented detrusor overactivity preoperatively, and 26 (86%) had urodynamics after autoaugmentation. Patients were followed for a median of 79 months (range 28–142). Interestingly, 50% of patients had a mucosal breach during autoaugmentation, but the authors found no correlation between this intraoperative event and long-term outcome. Twenty-one (70%) patients (19 idiopathic and two neurogenic) had continued postoperative improvement. Fourteen (67%) had no evidence of detrusor overactivity on cystometry.

Cystometric capacity increased by a mean of 165 ml in 80% of patients ($p < 0.001$). Detrusor pressure at maximum flow decreased in 60% but not significantly. Ten patients intermittently catheterized after autoaugmentation. Eight (five neurogenic, three idiopathic) had secondary procedures for their detrusor overactivity, two others chose no further treatment for their persistent symptoms, and one was lost to follow-up. Patients with neurogenic detrusor overactivity failed autoaugmentation more often than those with idiopathic detrusor overactivity. After autoaugmentation, uninhibited bladder contractions may still occur. In the absence of a functional, competent urethral sphincter, the bladder mucosal diverticulum will not enlarge, because the patient will leak instead. The authors discuss their theory that in patients with idiopathic detrusor overactivity with a competent sphincter and those with neurogenic detrusor overactivity with detrusor sphincter dyssynergia, the uninhibited bladder contractions will be resisted by the sphincter/pelvic muscle contraction and allow the bladder mucosal diverticulum to develop. This will lead to an increase in capacity and compliance. In those with an incompetent sphincter, urine leakage will occur and the diverticulum will not expand. The authors concluded by recommending autoaugmentation for patients with idiopathic detrusor overactivity rather than neurogenic detrusor overactivity.

MODIFICATIONS OF AUTOAUGMENTATION: SEROMUSCULAR CYSTOPLASTY

Although autoaugmentation avoids the problems associated with incorporation of gastrointestinal mucosa into the urinary tract, the resulting improvements in bladder capacity and compliance do not appear to be maintained due to possible progressive fibrosis. To attempt to eliminate this complication, the bladder mucosa has been covered with a variety of tissues and materials including deserosalized segments of stomach, and small and large intestine. These modifications were thought to retain the initial increase in bladder capacity after autoaugmentation by providing a grafted material/tissue between the detrusor muscle edges and preventing collapse and contraction of the autoaugmentation diverticulum.[20] There has been theoretical concern of perforation through the bladder mucosal diverticulum after autoaugmentation, although this has not been realized clinically. Similar modifications to cover the detrusor defect with a number of materials and grafts, specifically to prevent inadvertent perforation during CIC, have been reported.

Autoaugmentation cystoplasty was developed from a combination of principles of autoaugmentation and demucosalized augmentation cystoplasty, and the availability of stomach and intestine for augmentation cystoplasty. Dewan[40] described a series of experiments leading to the development of autoaugmentation gastrocystoplasty and autoaugmentation colocystoplasty techniques. Denuded stomach and denuded colon were used to provide a muscular backing to the bladder mucosa of the autoaugmentation in sheep model studies. Despite the advantages of avoiding gastrointestinal mucosa contact with urine, long operative times and technical difficulty have prevented these techniques from becoming clinically useful compared to traditional augmentation cystoplasty.[41] For more detailed information, the reader is referred to a review of autoaugmentation gastrocystoplasty.[42] Demucosalized augmentation cystoplasty or combinations with other tissues to cover the exposed mucosa have been performed.[12–17]

In animal studies primarily involving dog, sheep, and rat models, autoaugmentation defects have been covered using deepithelialized small intestine, stomach, and lyophilized human dura mater,[43–45] demucosalized reversed seromuscular flaps of ileum, colon, and stomach,[22, 46–50] sigmoid,[16] and rectus abdominus and/or gracilis muscle flaps.[44,51,52] Despite good reepithelialization of the bowel serosa, there was contraction of the patch thought to be due to trauma during mucosal stripping. Contraction and fibrosis of the pedicled rectus muscle flaps occurred, with progressive loss of bladder capacity. Reliable increases in capacity and compliance have, in most animal studies, been inferior to the benefits obtained with conventional augmentation cystoplasty. Recent studies of autoaugmentation gastrocystoplasty in a sheep model of non-neurogenic bladder dysfunction showed improved bladder compliance and capacity compared with prior studies, but at 6 months the improvement in compliance was not significantly higher than that seen in control animals.[53]

Studies in humans have reported reasonable short-term results.[16,17,54,55] Gonzalez et al.[17] reported a series of 16 pediatric patients where reconfigured demucosalized sigmoid was placed over the urothelium after detrusorectomy. Bladder capacity increased in 10, with encouraging short-term results. Oge et al.[56] reported their experience in 13 patients with autoaugmentation covered by a peritoneal flap. Mean bladder capacity increased by 18.6%, and mean compliance at capacity increased from 3.4 to 5.8 cmH$_2$O. Four went on to augmentation cystoplasty and an additional six required anticholinergic therapy after surgery. Given their results, the authors recommend that this autoaugmentation technique be reserved for patients with relatively good initial capacity. Seromuscular cystoplasty has not been accepted into widespread clinical use due to longer operative times, relative technical difficulty, and progressive loss of capacity and compliance, compared with conventional augmentation cystoplasty.

LAPAROSCOPIC AUTOAUGMENTATION

Ehrlich and Gershman[18] first reported laparoscopic detrusor myotomy. Autoaugmentation requires no harvesting of gastrointestinal segments and involves little suturing, and is adaptable to minimally invasive surgical techniques. Laparoscopic autoaugmentation has been performed in animal models,[7] in children,[18,57,58] and both transperitoneally and extraperitoneally.[8,59] Laparoscopic autoaugmentation gastrocystoplasty has been reported in a dog model.[60] Laparoscopic autoaugmentation holds advantages compared to open surgery in terms of smaller incisions, lower pain medication requirements, shorter postoperative hospitalization, faster return to work, etc. Laparoscopic surgeons have reported laser-assisted laparoscopic seromyotomy to prevent excess fibrosis.[7,8,18,61] It appears that laparoscopic autoaugmentation is feasible, and early results are comparable to open autoaugmentation.

PREGNANCY AND AUTOAUGMENTATION

Niknejad and Atala[62] reviewed the available literature pertaining to pregnancy and delivery after augmentation cystoplasty. At the present time, there are no reports of which we are aware on outcomes following pregnancy and delivery in women who have previously undergone autoaugmentation.

ADVANTAGES OF AUTOAUGMENTATION

Native urothelial tissue is used. Advantages of a urothelium-lined bladder include the avoidance of the complications of bowel mucosa in contact with urine (malignant potential, mucus, calculus formation, metabolic acidosis, and reduced linear growth in children) and the complications of gastric mucosa in contact with urine (hematuria–dysuria syndrome, metabolic alkalosis, and hypergastrinemia). Autoaugmentation is compatible with CIC. It is an extraperitoneal surgical procedure, avoiding the morbidity and risks of intestinal surgery and allowing for shorter operative times. It may be a preferred procedure for those patients who have undergone prior abdominal surgery because it is extraperitoneal. Autoaugmentation does not appear to preclude or complicate subsequent augmentation cystoplasty, if it becomes necessary.

POTENTIAL COMPLICATIONS AND MORBIDITY

Autoaugmentation is generally an uncomplicated procedure. Inadvertent holes created in the bladder mucosa during autoaugmentation can create difficulty with subsequent detrusor muscle mobilization and lead to a relative increase in operative time. Accidental cystotomy(s) may contribute to prolonged postoperative extravasation, which usually stops with adequate bladder drainage. However, prolonged postoperative drainage may lead to theoretical collapse of the diverticulum and compromised surgical results.

The rate of bladder perforation after augmentation cystoplasty is reported to be about 10% and thought to be due to high intravesical pressures. It is of concern that patients may be at greater risk for bladder perforation given the relative thinness of the bladder mucosa in the bulging diverticulum after autoaugmentation. In an animal model, Rivas[63] showed that autoaugmentation results in a higher risk of bladder perforation, at lower pressures, than in ileal augmentation cystoplasty. To date there has been no clinical report of bladder perforation following autoaugmentation in the available literature. This may be related to the fibrosis that occurs around the bladder mucosal diverticulum over time. Although seemingly protective, if the fibrosis is progressive, this raises concern regarding the durability of the initial benefits seen with autoaugmentation.[64] Early experimental and clinical results were promising in terms of improvements in bladder capacity and compliance. The limited increase in capacity and improvement in compliance seen in the longer term corresponds to the fibrosis that has been noted in follow-up studies. Late outcomes overall have been somewhat disappointing, presumably related to fibrosis leading to diverticular collapse.[19,25]

CONCERNS

The main concern with autoaugmentation is a limited increase in bladder capacity. As such, preoperative bladder capacity may be the most important predictor of postoperative success.[5,25,56] If the maximum capacity and volume of urine held at $40\,cmH_2O$ are similar, then the patient may be better served by augmentation cystoplasty. Regardless of which particular technique is used, most authors report that if there is concern at the time of autoaugmentation that adequate expansion was not achieved, it is recommended to proceed with augmentation cystoplasty immediately. Therefore, patients and surgical teams should be prepared for this potential event. Many patients experience clinical improvement after autoaugmentation without a significant change in urodynamics. The reasons for this clinical improvement are not completely understood.

CONCLUSIONS

The principle of autoaugmentation – urothelial preservation – is attractive because it creates a compliant urinary reservoir without the associated metabolic disturbances, morbidity, and malignant potential. There are relatively few cases reported in the available literature, especially regarding patients with idiopathic detrusor overactivity. Autoaugmentation should be considered only for adults with reasonable bladder capacity and refractory bladder overactivity with or without incontinence, or those with poor compliance who do not need a large increase in bladder capacity. If a considerable increase in bladder capacity is required, then augmentation cystoplasty is indicated. Review of the available literature supports that the most appropriate patients to be considered for autoaugmentation may be those with idiopathic detrusor overactivity as compared with neurogenic etiologies. Autoaugmentation holds a place in the management algorithm of detrusor overactivity. The use of botulinum toxin, resiniferatoxin, and other pharmacologic therapies, as well as promising innovations in tissue engineering, may facilitate the concept of autoaugmentation to provide further improvements in clinical outcomes for patients with refractory detrusor overactivity.

REFERENCES

1. Neuhof H. Fascia transplantation into visceral defects. Surg Gynecol Obstet 1917; 24: 383–427.
2. Huggins CB. The formation of bone under the influence of epithelium of the urinary tract. Arch Surg 1930; 22: 377–408.
3. Cartwright PC, Snow BW. Bladder autoaugmentation: partial detrusor excision to augment the bladder without the use of bowel. J Urol 1989; 142: 1050–3.
4. Cartwright PC, Snow BW. Bladder autoaugmentation: early clinical experience. J Urol 1989; 142: 505–8; discussion 520–1.
5. Leng WW, Blalock HJ, Fredriksson WH et al. Enterocystoplasty or detrusor myectomy? Comparison of indications and outcomes for bladder augmentation. J Urol 1999; 161: 758–63.
6. Stothers L, Johnson H, Arnold W et al. Bladder autoaugmentation by vesicostomy in pediatric neurogenic bladder. Urology 1994; 44:110–13.
7. Britanisky RG, Poppas DP, Shichman SN et al. Laparoscopic laser-assisted bladder autoaugmentation. Urology 1995; 46: 31–5.
8. McDougall EM, Clayman RV, Figenshau RS, Pearl MS. Laparoscopic retropubic autoaugmentation of the bladder. J Urol 1995; 153: 123–6.
9. Kennelly MJ, Gormley EA, McGuire EJ. Early clinical experience with adult bladder autoaugmentation. J Urol 1994; 152: 303–6.
10. Stohrer M, Kramer A, Goepel M et al. Bladder auto-augmentation – an alternative for enterocystoplasty: preliminary results. Neurourol Urodyn 1995; 14: 11–23.
11. Stohrer M, Kramer G, Goepel M et al. Bladder autoaugmentation in adult patients with neurogenic voiding dysfunction. Spinal Cord 1997; 35: 456–62.
12. Dewan PA, Stefanek W, Lorenz C, Byard RW. Autoaugmentation omentocystoplasty in a sheep model. Urology 1994; 43: 888–91.
13. Dewan PA, Stefanek W. Autoaugmentation gastrocystoplasty: early clinical results. Br J Urol 1994; 74: 460–4.
14. Dewan PA, Lorenz C, Stefanek W, Byard RW. Urothelial lined colocystoplasty in a sheep model. Eur Urol 1994; 26: 240–6.
15. Dewan PA, Owen AJ, Stefanek W, Lorenz C, Byard RW. Late follow-up of autoaugmentation omentocystoplasty in a sheep model. Aust NZ J Surg 1995; 65: 596–9.
16. Lima SV, Araujo LA, Vilar FO, Kummer CL, Lima EC. Nonsecretory sigmoid cystoplasty: experimental and clinical results. J Urol 1995; 153: 1651–4.
17. Gonzalez R, Buson H, Reid C, Reinberg Y. Seromuscular colocystoplasty lined with urothelium: experience with 16 patients. Urology 1995; 45: 124–9.
18. Ehrlich RM, Gershman A. Laparoscopic seromyotomy (auto-augmentation) for non-neurogenic neurogenic bladder in a child: initial case report. Urology 1993; 42: 175–8.
19. Johnson HW, Nigro MK, Stothers L et al. Laboratory variables of autoaugmentation in an animal model. Urology 1994; 44: 260–3.
20. Taneli C, Genc A. Long-term follow-up and evaluation of autoaugmentation cystoplasty (detrusorotomy) in an animal model. Int Urol Nephrol 1999; 31: 55–9.
21. Garibay JT, Manivel JC, Gonzalez R. Effect of seromuscular colocystoplasty lined with urothelium and partial detrusorectomy on a new canine model of reduced bladder capacity. J Urol 1995; 154: 903–6.
22. Dewan PA, Stefanek W, Lorenz C, Owen AJ, Byard RW. Autoaugmentation gastrocystoplasty and demucosalized gastrocystoplasty in a sheep model. Urology 1995; 45: 291–5.
23. Surer I, Elicevik M, Ozturk H, Sakarya MT, Cetinkursun S. An alternative approach to bladder autoaugmentation. Tech Urol 1999; 5: 100–3.

24. Snow BW, Cartwright PC. Autoaugmentation of the bladder. Contemp Urol 1992; 4: 41–51.

25. Landau HM, Moorehead JD. Detrusorectomy. Probl Pediatr Urol 1994; 8: 204–9.

26. Snow BW, Cartwright PC. Bladder autoaugmentation. Urol Clin North Am 1996; 23: 323–31.

27. Stohrer M. Bladder auto-augmentation. In: Colleen S, Mansson W, eds. Reconstructive Surgery of the Lower Genito-urinary Tract in Adults. Oxford: Isis Medical Media, 1995: 32–40.

28. Kramer G, Stohrer M. Neurourology. Curr Opin Urol 1996; 176–83.

29. Skobejko-Wlodarska L, Strulak K, Nachulewicz P, Szymkiewicz C. Bladder autoaugmentation in myelodysplastic children. Br J Urol 1998; 81 (Suppl 3): 114–16.

30. Westney OL, McGuire EJ. Surgical procedures for the treatment of urge incontinence. Tech Urol 2001; 7: 126–32.

31. Perovic SV, Djordjevic MLJ, Kekic ZK, Vukadinovic VM. Bladder autoaugmentation with rectus muscle backing. J Urol 2002; 168: 1877–80.

32. Perovic SV, Djordjevic MLJ, Kekic ZK, Vukadinovic VM. Detrusorectomy with rectus muscle hitch and backing. J Pediatr Surg 2003; 38: 1637–41.

33. Stohrer M, Goepel M, Kramer G et al. Detrusor myectomy (autoaugmentation) in the treatment of hyper-reflexive low compliance bladder. Urologe A 1999; 38: 30–7.

34. Duel BP, Gonzalez R, Barthold JS. Alternative techniques for augmentation cystoplasty. J Urol 1998; 159: 998–1005.

35. Potter JM, Duffy PG, Gordon EM, Malone PR. Detrusor myotomy: a 5-year review in unstable and non-compliant bladders. BJU Int 2002; 89: 932–5.

36. Marte A, DiMeglio D, Cotrufo AM et al. A long-term follow-up of autoaugmentation in myelodysplastic children. BJU Int 2002; 89: 928–31.

37. MacNeily AE, Afshar K, Coleman GU, Johnson HW. Autoaugmentation by detrusor myotomy: its lack of effectiveness in the management of congenital neuropathic bladder. J Urol 2003; 170: 1643–6.

38. Swami KS, Feneley RCL, Hammonds JC, Abrams P. Detrusor myectomy for detrusor overactivity: a minimum 1-year follow-up. Br J Urol 1998; 81: 68–72.

39. Kumar SPV, Abrams PH. Detrusor myectomy: long-term results with a minimum follow-up of 2 years. BJU Int 2005; 96: 341–4.

40. Dewan PA. Autoaugmentation demucosalized enterocystoplasty. World J Urol 1998; 16: 255–61.

41. Cranidis A, Nestoridis G. Bladder augmentation. Int Urogynecol J 2000; 11: 33–40.

42. Close CE, Dewan PA, Ashwood PJ, Byard RJ, Mitchell ME. Autoaugmentation peritoneocystoplasty in a sheep model. BJU Int 2001; 88: 414–17.

43. Cranidis A, Nestoridis G, Delakas D, Lumbakis P, Kanavaros P. Bladder autoaugmentation in the rabbit using de-epithelialized segments of small intestine, stomach and lyophilized human dura mater. Br J Urol 1998; 81: 62–7.

44. Elicevik M, Celayir S, Dervisoglu S, Buyukunal SN. Comparison of different bladder autoaugmentation techniques in a rabbit model. Br J Urol 1998; 81: 49–54.

45. Bleustein CB, Cuomo B, Mingin GC et al. Laser-assisted demucosalized gastrocystoplasty with autoaugmentation in a canine model. Urology 2000; 55: 437–42.

46. Salle JL, Fraga JC, Lucib A et al. Seromuscular enterocystoplasty in dogs. J Urol 1990; 144: 454–6.

47. Cheng E, Rento R, Grayhack JT, Oyasu R, McVary KT. Reversed seromuscular flaps in the urinary tract in dogs. J Urol 1994; 152: 2252–7.

48. Buson H, Manivel JC, Dayang M, Long R, Gonzalez R. Seromuscular colocystoplasty lined with urothelium: experimental study. Urology 1994; 44: 743–8.

49. Frey P, Lutz N, Leuba AL. Augmentation cystoplasty using pedicaled and de-epithelialized gastric patches in the mini-pig model. J Urol 1995; 156: 608–13.

50. Close CE. Autoaugmentation gastrocystoplasty. BJU Int 2001; 88: 757–61.

51. Erol A, Ozgur S, Erol U et al. Partial bladder reconstruction with pedicled rectus and gracilis muscle flaps: an experimental study in dogs. Br J Urol 1994; 74: 775–8.

52. Manzoni C, Grottesi A, D'Urzo C et al. An original technique for bladder autoaugmentation with protective abdominal rectus muscle flaps: an experimental study in rats. J Surg Res 2001; 99: 169–74.

53. Close CE, Anderson PD, Edwards GA, Mitchell ME, Dewan PA. Autoaugmentation gastrocystoplasty: further studies of the sheep model. BJU Int 2004; 94: 658–62.

54. Nguyen DH, Mitchell ME, Horowitz M, Bagli DJ, Carr MC. Demucosalized augmentation gastrocystoplasty with bladder autoaugmentation in pediatric patients. J Urol 1996; 156: 206–9.

55. Donald HN, Mitchell ME, Mark H, Darius JB, Can CG. Demucosalized augmentation gastrocytoplasty with bladder autoaugmentation in paediatric patients. J Urol 1996; 156: 206–9.

56. Oge O, Tekgul S, Ergen A, Kendi S. Urothelium-preserving augmentation cystoplasty covered with a peritoneal flap. BJU Int 2000; 85: 802–5.

57. Poppas DP, Uzzo RG, Britanisky RG, Mininberg DT. Laparoscopic laser assisted auto-augmentation of the pediatric neurogenic bladder: Early experience with urodynamic followup [see Comments]. J Urol 1996; 155: 1057–60.

58. Braren V, Bishop MR. Laparoscopic bladder auto-augmentation in children. Urol Clin North Am 1998; 25: 533–40.

59. Siracusano S, Trombetta C, Liguori G et al. Laparoscopic bladder auto-augmentation in an incomplete traumatic spinal cord injury. Spinal Cord 2000; 38: 59–61.

60. Specht M, Pareek G, Lin DD et al. Hand-assisted laparoscopic autoaugmentation gastrocystoplasty. Surg Endosc 2002; 16: 1538–41.

61. Gonzalez R. Re: Laparoscopic laser assisted auto-augmentation of the pediatric neurogenic bladder: Early experience with urodynamic followup [Letter; Comment]. J Urol 1996; 156: 1783.

62. Niknejad KG, Atala A. Bladder augmentation techniques in women. Int Urogynecol J 2000; 11: 156–69.

63. Rivas DA, Chancellor MB, Huang B, Epple A, Figueroa TE. Comparison of bladder rupture pressure after intestinal bladder augmentation (ileocystoplasty) and myomyotomy (autoaugmentation). Urology 1996; 48: 40–6.

64. Chapple CR, Bryan NP. Surgery for detrusor overactivity. World J Urol 1998; 16: 268–73.

31

Augmentation cystoplasty for overactive bladder

Anthony R Stone and Dana K. Nanigian

Introduction • Definition • Indications • Evaluation • Surgical techniques • Choice of bowel segment • Postoperative care • Complications • Patient outcomes • Interstitial cystitis • Conclusion

INTRODUCTION

Overactive bladder syndrome,[1] defined as a symptom complex suggestive of lower urinary tract dysfunction, specifically urgency, with or without urge incontinence, usually accompanied by frequency and nocturia, affects the quality of life of many people worldwide.[2,3] Patients are managed initially with pharmacologic and behavioral therapy. A small percentage of these patients will fail these conservative measures and require operative intervention. Surgical therapies that are currently offered include botulinum toxin injection, neuromodulation, peripheral bladder denervation, autoaugmentation, augmentation cystoplasty, or urinary diversion. This chapter will focus on augmentation cystoplasty for patients with idiopathic detrusor overactivity and specifically address patient satisfaction and long-term outcomes in this patient population.

DEFINITION

Augmentation cystoplasty refers to a surgical procedure aimed at increasing bladder capacity. This goal may be accomplished without other tissues (autoaugmentation) or with incorporation of other tissues (intestine, ureter, manufactured materials), with or without reconfiguring the intestinal segment, and with or without resection of a portion of the original bladder. Bladder substitution, on the other hand, refers to total replacement of the bladder by an isolated segment of intestinal tissue.

INDICATIONS

During the 1950s, augmentation cystoplasty was performed predominantly in patients with small, contracted bladders secondary to tuberculosis. The popularity of this technique was limited by the high incidence of postoperative urinary retention. A turning point came in 1972 when Lapides et al. introduced the concept of clean intermittent catheterization.[4] This practice soon gained wide acceptance, allowing the indications for bladder augmentation to further expand. Currently, bladder augmentation is most commonly performed in patients with spina bifida and hostile bladders, to increase compliance and capacity and protect the kidneys from damage secondary to high intravesical pressure. Other neurogenic patients with poorly compliant or hyperreflexive bladders who have failed pharmacologic therapy are also undergoing bladder augmentation, with excellent satisfaction rates.[5,6] Indications for bladder augmentation in non-neurogenic patients are less clear, and urinary diversion may be a more viable alternative for these patients. A subset of these patients, however, whose severe symptoms are attributable to small bladder capacity (< 200 ml), may have a better outcome with bladder augmentation. Patients with interstitial cystitis rarely experience improvement in quality of life after bladder augmentation.[7]

EVALUATION

A complete history and physical examination is an essential part of the initial evaluation. Patients with significant hypersensitivity or pain do not improve after bladder augmentation. In general, patients should be informed of the high likelihood that postoperative intermittent self-catheterization will be required. Likewise, they should be aware that an augmented bladder will require lifelong surveillance. On physical examination, it is important to note the presence of suprapubic pain. In neuropathic patients, an assessment of manual dexterity is important, to ensure that they will be able to perform self-catheterization.

Urodynamic evaluation

Urodynamic evaluation allows for a formal, objective assessment of bladder function. The presence of detrusor overactivity can be documented, and diagnosis of associated stress urinary incontinence can be made. Videourodynamic testing provides a means to visually assess the bladder for evidence of reflux and check for intrinsic sphincter deficiency.

Radiological evaluation

A cystogram is necessary to rule out reflux if videourodynamics is not performed. An intravenous pyelogram or renal ultrasound will provide information about upper tract anatomy and the presence of an obstruction. Most patients with storage failure have been followed with serial renal ultrasonograms, and will have a recent one available prior to surgery to act as a baseline reference. If renal function is marginal, a nuclear renal scan will provide information on differential function and the presence of an obstruction. Imaging of the bowel is not recommended unless an underlying bowel disorder is present or the patient has had previous intestinal surgery.

Laboratory evaluation

A complete blood count, coagulation factors, and a chemistry panel, which includes serum creatinine to assess renal function, are obtained in every patient. In patients with chronic renal insufficiency, creatinine clearance measurement allows for an accurate determination of true renal function and serves as a baseline reference in follow-up. A preoperative urine culture is necessary to ensure that the urine is sterilized before surgery.

Endoscopy

Cystoscopy should be performed in any patients with irritative symptoms or a history of hematuria who have not yet undergone lower tract evaluation, to rule out malignancy. It can be used to verify an absence of diverticula and to identify small calculi within the bladder that may be missed by routine X-ray evaluation.

General preoperative considerations

As the patient undergoes evaluation for augmentation cystoplasty, a plan for reconstruction must be developed based on history, physical examination, renal function, metabolic status, urodynamic evaluation, and radiological appearance. Patients with concomitant stress incontinence may undergo a procedure to enhance their outlet, such as a pubovaginal sling or artificial urinary sphincter, during the same operation. The presence of reflux may necessitate ureteral reimplantation at the time of augmentation. If the reflux is secondary to poor bladder compliance, studies have shown that vesicoureteral reflux will resolve with augmentation alone, secondary to the correction of bladder dynamics.[8,9]

In patients who are wheelchair-bound, particularly females, a discussion of the creation of a continent, catheterizable, abdominal stoma should occur. Finally, in the multiple meetings with the patient leading up to the surgery it is important to reinforce the need to remain motivated after surgery, because clean intermittent self-catheterization is required in all neurogenic patients and a large percentage of neurologically intact patients with idiopathic overactivity. In addition, the patient must understand the risks and limitations of the procedure as well as the need for subsequent procedures. A well-informed patient who thoroughly understands the postoperative responsibilities of managing an augmented bladder will most effectively be able to enjoy the benefits that this procedure can provide.

SURGICAL TECHNIQUES

Preoperative bowel preparation is essential. In the neuropathic population, bowel cleansing begins 3 days in advance, consisting of daily enemas and a clear liquid diet if possible. The day before surgery the patient undergoes a bowel preparation with either GoLYTELY® or magnesium citrate, as well as bowel sterilization with neomycin and erythromycin.

In patients with spina bifida, strict latex precautions are enforced even if the patient has had no previous latex reactions. Anaphylactic reactions to latex can occur after repeated exposures and intraoperatively.

Patients are positioned in the low lithotomy position for females and supine for males. The incision is most often made in the lower midline, although we have used a Pfannenstiel incision in women who have an existing scar.

With the patient in the Trendelenburg position, the bowel falls into the upper abdomen and a self-retaining retractor can be used to provide pelvic exposure. The bladder is grasped between Allis clamps, and the lateral peritoneal attachments are taken down with Bovie electrocautery to the vasa deferens in the male and the superior pedicle in the female. Blunt dissection then allows for anterior and lateral mobilization of the bladder.

The bladder is opened at the dome transversely down to the trigone on each side. The incision is extended in front of the ureters on either side to prevent an hourglass deformity. With the bladder bivalved in this way, the greatest volume of augmentation can be achieved with the least amount of material, retaining the spherical orientation of the bladder (Figure 31.1). Criticism of this coronal dissection includes potential interference with the native ureterovesical junctions. An alternative technique is to bivalve the bladder in the sagittal plane. Either way, it is essential to extend the incision down to the trigone.

In the majority of these patients, bladder tissue does not need to be excised. Supratrigonal cystectomy may be carried out in patients with end-stage interstitial cystitis or in neuropathic bladders where disease in the bladder may compromise

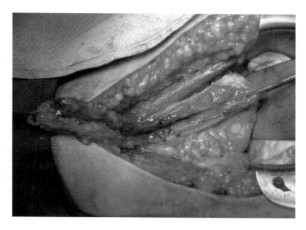

Figure 31.1 Lateral view of open bladder. Bladder split coronally: "clam". A, anterior; P, posterior. (See also color plate section).

the overall result. If supratrigonal cystectomy is required, the bladder is initially opened sagitally. The mucosa is then scored with the Bovie knife just above the ureters, posteriorly and laterally. Each half of the bladder is carefully dissected off the ureters on each side, with vessels being fulgurated as they are identified. A small fringe of bladder is left anteriorly, and just enough is left above the ureters and across the trigone to allow an adequate enterovesical anastamosis to be completed.

CHOICE OF BOWEL SEGMENT

Each bowel segment differs in its availability, compliance, mucus production, and electrolyte permeability. Choice of a bowel segment needs to take these factors into account as well as the patient's preoperative status. When performing augmentation cystoplasty for overactive bladder either ileum or sigmoid is recommended.

Ileum is the most widely used bowel segment; it has been used for ileal conduit urinary diversion for years. A segment of ileum approximately 20–35 cm in length is isolated on its mesentery, commencing approximately 15 cm from the ileocecal valve as this produces the least metabolic disturbance. The length of the ileal segment is dependent on the defect in the bladder; however, precise measurement of the bladder is not necessary as ileum is a highly compliant material. The ileal patch is detubularized to interrupt the circular muscle fibers and help prevent contractions.

A side to side stapled or hand sewn anastamosis is performed to reconstitute bowel continuity. The isolated segment is placed caudally to this anastamosis in a U-shaped configuration, with the curve of the U directed inferiorly. The contiguous borders of this bowel segment are sutured together with a running seromuscular 3-0 polyglycolic acid suture (PGA). The bowel is then opened along this suture line to completely detubularize it. This suture line is then reinforced with another running 3-0 PGA through all layers. Recently this maneuver has been achieved using absorbable staples (Poly GIA™ 75 stapler). This stapling device provides a rapid, two-layer, watertight closure.

The dependent portion of the opened bowel is sutured to the apex of the posterior aspect of the "clammed" bladder. This anastamosis is continued down both sides of the posterior wing of the "clam", with the bowel being sutured down into the open corners of the bladder. Infant feeding tubes, 5 or 8 French, may be placed in the ureters during this portion of the anastamosis to ensure that the ureters are not damaged in any way. Once the suture lines reach the anterior aspect of the opened bladder, the upper aspect of the bowel segment is then folded over and anastamosed to the anterior wing of the "clam". This suture line is then continued until the ileovesical closure is completed. Any redundant bowel may be sutured to itself. Suturing the open bowel segment into the "clammed" bladder in this way rather than reconfiguring the segment into a "cap" first allows the bowel to be easily tailored to any size of opened bladder without complicated measuring techniques being required.

Before closure of the vesicointestinal anastamosis, a Malecot catheter is placed through a stab incision in the bowel portion of the cystoplasty. A purse string suture is placed around this exiting tube to prevent leakage. Suprapubic drainage with a wide bore catheter such as a Malecot is essential to efficiently remove mucus and clots postoperatively.

At this time the ileocecal anastamosis is tested by filling the cystoplasty with saline solution and closing any areas of leakage with interrupted absorbable sutures.

This technique provides a reliable, low pressure, spherical reservoir. However, some authors do not believe it necessary to reconfigure the bowel segment but merely detubularize and suture this open segment to the bladder.

If possible, the omentum is mobilized from the transverse colon and pedicled down either of the pericolic gutters. The omentum is wrapped around the cystoplasty and sutured in place with two or three interrupted absorbable sutures. The omentum is specifically attached to the cystoplasty adherent to the exiting catheter and this is then sutured to the anterior abdominal wall adjacent to the exiting catheter to seal any potential leaks that might occur when this tube is removed.

If ileum is not available secondary to adhesions, short mesentery, or prior small bowel surgery, sigmoid colon is also an excellent bowel segment for augmentation cystoplasty (Figure 31.2). Advantages of sigmoid colon include its large lumen, accessibility, and low pressure characteristics. A segment of approximately 15 cm is usually appropriate. Because of the larger lumen, the sigmoid is not reconfigured into a U-shape, but simply detubularized and sutured into the bladder (Figure 31.3 and 31.4). Disadvantages of sigmoid cystoplasty include more mucus production and theoretical increased risk of long-term malignancy.

Cecum is typically used for bladder substitution when supratrigonal cystectomy is being considered, as it provides a large reservoir. The cecum is mobilized on the ileocolic vascular pedicle and should include the hepatic flexure and transverse colon up to the middle colic artery.

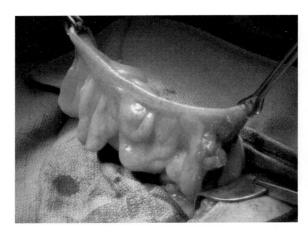

Figure 31.2 Segment of sigmoid colon isolated on mesentery. (See also color plate section).

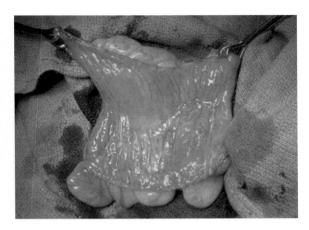

Figure 31.3 Bowel opened on antimesenteric border. (See also color plate section).

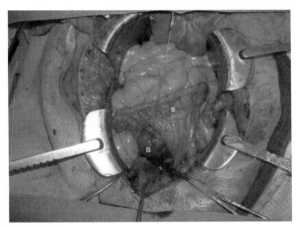

Figure 31.4 Open segment of sigmoid (S) sutured to posterior wing of clammed bladder (B). (See also color plate section).

The segment is opened through the anterior tenia and then folded over on itself. The sides of the segment are sewn to each other to form a pouch. The inferior open portion of the pouch is then sewn into the opened bladder to form the cystoplasty.

A gastrocystoplasty is never the first choice of bowel segment in an adult undergoing bladder augmentation for detrusor overactivity. It is typically only used in children with renal insufficiency or in adults with irradiated bowel.

In a patient with a hydronephrotic, non-functioning kidney, the dilated ureter can be used as the augmentation segment. Advantages of using ureter include lack of mucus production and a segment lined with transitional epithelium.

Practically, however, ureterocystoplasty is rarely applicable.

POSTOPERATIVE CARE

Postoperatively, the newly augmented bladder is irrigated with 30 ml of normal saline every 8 hours to prevent mucus accumulation and plugging. The nasogastric tube is removed upon the return of bowel function and the peritoneal drain is removed when drainage is minimal. Patients begin irrigating their catheter in the hospital under nursing supervision so that they are comfortable doing it twice daily while at home.

A cystogram is performed 2–3 weeks postoperatively through the suprapubic tube. If no extravasation is seen, the suprapubic tube is removed and the patient begins clean intermittent catheterization if they cannot volitionally void. If the ureters were reimplanted at the time of surgery, the stents are removed at this follow-up visit as well. Even in patients able to empty their bladder volitionally, intermittent catheterization is recommended in the first few months postoperatively to allow complete healing of the bladder. The typical catheterization regimen consists of every 2 hour catheterization including one time overnight for the first 2 weeks, which is extended to every 4 hours over the next 4–6 weeks.

Subsequent follow-up includes regular laboratory work at 3-month intervals to monitor renal function and electrolytes. If laboratory tests are normal for the first year postoperatively, this interval is extended to once a year. Treatment of bacteriuria is based on the clinical picture of the patient.

Renal ultrasound is performed at 3, 6, and 12 months postoperatively to evaluate for hydronephrosis, renal parenchymal disease, and stones. Cystoscopy is performed every 3 years to evaluate for small stones and monitor for malignancy.

COMPLICATIONS

Metabolic disturbance

Bowel has an active epithelial layer which is involved in the absorption and secretion of electrolytes across its surface. This electrolyte exchange can cause metabolic derangements, the degree of which varies with the surface area of the bowel patch, the type of bowel used, the time period in which bowel is in contact with urine, and the patient's renal function.

Ileum and colon can both cause a hypokalemic, hyperchloremic metabolic acidosis. The hyperchloremia arises from absorption of urinary ammonium chloride into the blood stream. Ammonium secretion is the kidneys' principal mechanism to excrete the body's acid load. Impairment of this mechanism results in a chronic metabolic acidosis. The body compensates by titrating acid using bone buffers such as calcium carbonate. This phenomenon can cause a reduction in the growth potential of children and osteopenia in older individuals.

Use of the jejunum causes a hypochloremic, hyperkalemic, hyponatremic metabolic acidosis. Jejunum secretes sodium and chloride and absorbs potassium and hydrogen. The loss of sodium results in water loss and dehydration, which leads to the release of aldosterone which only enhances the metabolic derangement.

Stomach, which is rarely used, is the only bowel segment that causes a metabolic alkalosis, and is therefore thought to be a good choice for use in children or renal failure patients.

In a patient with adequate renal function, these electrolyte abnormalities will not be evident, as the kidneys will be able to compensate and establish a new metabolic equilibrium. Patients with impaired renal function need to be monitored more closely. Persistent metabolic acidosis will be corrected by oral bicarbonate in most cases.

Leakage

Despite detubularization and reconfiguration of the bowel segment, continued peristaltic activity may occur and lead to postoperative leakage of urine. Pope et al. reviewed 323 patients who underwent primary enterocystoplasty and found that 5.9% continued to have high pressure bladder contractions and required augmentation of the previously augmented bladder.[10] Sigmoid colon and stomach were shown to be the two most contractile segments. The bladder can also maintain hyperactivity, which may be managed with anticholinergic medication as before surgery.

If conservative attempts at managing continued leakage fail, and poor outlet resistance has been ruled out, an additional patch of bowel may need to be inserted into the cytoplasty.

Renal function

Renal function deterioration can occur in patients after augmentation cystoplasty and is related to baseline renal function. For 80% of patients, the storage of urine in intestinal reservoirs did not change renal function at the 10-year follow-up.[11] Twenty percent of patients had some deterioration in renal function during the 10-year follow-up, usually from identifiable and remediable causes such as inadequate emptying or recurrent infection.

Mucus production

The bowel segment will continue to produce mucus, with average daily production estimated to be approximately 35–40 grams. Despite a time-related villous atrophy of the bowel segment, the mucus production never completely tapers off. Mucus poses problems postoperatively as it can impair adequate catheter drainage, and in the long term can be a nidus for stone formation and infection.[12] Oral ranitidine has been shown to reduce mucus production, and acetylcysteine washouts help to dissolve excess mucus.[13,14]

Stone formation

The development of bladder stones, believed to be caused by chronic bacteriuria, urinary stasis, and mucus, has been reported with an incidence of 10–52%.[12,15–19] Stones are less common in patients who void and empty adequately compared to patients who require clean intermittent catheterization, implicating stasis as an important factor in stone formation. Urinary tract infection also appears to be an independent risk factor for stone formation. Stone formation has been shown to be lower in patients who catheterize via their native urethra rather than an abdominal stoma. Gastrocystoplasty has a significantly lower risk of stone formation than does augmentation with ileum or colon.[20,21] Data suggest that a routine irrigation protocol used postoperatively can significantly reduce the number of reservoir calculi from 43% to 7%.[21] While open cystolithotomy is the gold standard for removal of cystoplasty stones, endoscopic management is safe and effective in the majority of patients.[22]

Bacteriuria

Asymptomatic bacteriuria with mixed flora occurs in most patients with augmentation cystoplasties, but the incidence of clinically relevant urinary tract infection (UTI) is lower. Mucus production, urinary stasis, and catheterization put augmented bladders at higher risk for infection. If recurrent infection becomes an issue, patients can be managed with daily neosporin irrigation.

Risk of carcinoma

The incidence of carcinoma in an augmented bladder is rare. In a review of 45 bladder augmentations with malignancy, 27 malignancies were adenocarcinoma, six were transitional cell carcinoma, and four were signet ring carcinoma. A long latency period between the augmentation and occurrence of cancer was found. However, because most bladder augmentations are now performed in young children, careful surveillance is important. Regular endoscopic surveillance beginning at the third postoperative year is mandatory.[23]

Spontaneous perforation

One of the most morbid and life-threatening complications following enterocystoplasty is spontaneous perforation. Mortality is reported to be as high as 23–25%.[24,25] Ischemia of the bowel segment caused by overdistention is generally the underlying cause. Overall risk is about 13%, with ileum and sigmoid being the most common perforated segments. Patients with neuropathy, recurrent infections, and on clean intermittent catheterization (CIC) are at higher risk.[26]

A major factor contributing to the morbidity of perforation is delay in diagnosis. Many neuropathic patients do not have adequate sensation to feel that their bladder is overdistended, and likewise do not have abdominal pain to signify that they have perforated. Similarly, physical examination findings can be fairly unremarkable, and the physician should have a high index

of suspicion. Patients may often only present in the later stages of perforation, including sepsis, peritonitis, abscess formation, and renal failure. Diagnostic study of choice is a computed tomography (CT) cystogram, which can identify a perforation as well as any other abdominal pathology. If, however, clinical suspicion is high, the patient should be taken directly to the operating room, as contrast cystography has a measurable false negative rate. Because most of these patients have bacteriuria, conservative management with catheter drainage and antibiotics, although it has been reported, is not recommended.[27]

Inadequate emptying/clean intermittent self-catheterization

Bladder augmentation interrupts the typical coordinated contraction of the detrusor muscle. Emptying a bladder augmentation often requires abdominal straining with simultaneous relaxation of the bladder outlet.[28] While patients with a neurogenic bladder are typically dependent on catheterization preoperatively, idiopathic patients are not, and many will have a difficult time with this notion. Review of augmentation cystoplasty in neurologically intact patients with detrusor overactivity shows that 13–89% require clean intermittent self-catheterization (CISC) postoperatively.[29–32] The high likelihood of postoperative need for intermittent catherization should be clearly discussed with patients during the pre-operative evaluation. Dependence on postoperative CISC has been shown to affect patient perception of a good long-term outcome.[6]

Pregnancy

Pregnancy in a patient with an augmented bladder poses some challenges. Increased morbidity can be expected from the increased risk of bladder infection and pyelonephritis. In a review of 15 pregnant women with augmented bladders, urinary tract infection or pyelonephritis complicated nine of the 15 pregnancies (60%), and four patients experienced premature labor. Serum creatinine levels remained stable throughout pregnancy in 14 patients (93%). Delivery was vaginal in 10 patients with an intact native continence mechanism and by Cesarean section in five, all of whom had undergone prior surgical

reconstruction of the vesical neck. No intraoperative or postoperative complications were
reported. In patients with augmentation and
reconstruction of the vesical neck, delivery by
Cesarean section is recommended secondary to
potential for disruption of the continence mechanism.[33,34] If a woman with an augment undergoes Cesarean section, having a urologist as part
of the operative team to identify the unusual
anatomy and assist in dissection of the cystoplasty off the uterus is advisable.

PATIENT OUTCOMES

Augmentation cystoplasty in the neurogenic population carries high satisfaction rates.[5,6] In a retrospective review of spinal injured patients who
had undergone "clam" augmentation ileocystoplasty with a mean follow-up of 6.0 ± 3.6 years,
96.2% of patients reported an improvement in
quality of life parameters.[35]

Success and satisfaction rates for augmentation cystoplasty in the treatment of idiopathic
detrusor overactivity are lower. Hasan et al.
studied the long-term outcomes and quality of
life following enterocystoplasty for both idiopathic detrusor instability and neurogenic bladder dysfunction.[6] In the 48 patient cohort, 35
patients had a diagnosis of idiopathic detrusor
instability. The long-term outcome was good or
moderate in only 19 patients (54%) with idiopathic detrusor instability. Seventy-five patients
required self-catheterization postoperatively in
both groups combined. Complications such as
disturbance of bowel habits and recurrent urinary tract infections impaired the outcome in
the long term in patients with idiopathic detrusor instability despite general improvements in
irritative bladder symptoms.

Awad et al. specifically looked at long-term
results and complications of ileocystoplasty
for idiopathic urge incontinence in women.[31]
They retrospectively reviewed 51 women who
underwent augmentation cystoplasty for non-
neurogenic urge incontinence. Twenty-seven
women had associated interstitial cystitis. All
patients had exhausted conservative measures.
At a mean follow-up of 75.4 months, only 53% of
women were completely continent, 25% had occasional leaks, and 18% continued to have disabling
urge incontinence frequently, requiring pads.

The complication rate postoperatively was high,
with 39% of women requiring self-catheterization.
Twenty-four percent of women still required
additional pharmacotherapy. Two women needed
revisions, and four women needed patch exci-
sions. Two women underwent subsequent urinary diversion. All women on self-catheterization
had recurrent infections. Mucus retention occurred
regularly in 10 patients, six had chronic diarrhea,
four had latent bowel obstruction, one developed
a bladder stone, one had an incisional hernia,
and one developed patch necrosis and perforation.
Overall, 53% of patients were happy with the
outcome and 39% were not. Four patients were
not sure whether the surgery had improved
their quality of life.

Flood et al. also reviewed long-term results
and complications in patients after augmentation
cystoplasty.[32] Of the 122 augmentation cystoplasties performed, 63 were non-neuropathic cases.
Of this group, 21 patients had the diagnosis of
interstitial cystitis, 13 patients had detrusor instability, and 13 had radiation or chronic cystitis.
The mean follow-up was 37 months. Overall,
75% of patients had an excellent outcome with
respect to upper tract function, continence, and
comfort. Eighty-nine percent of men and 67% of
women in the non-neuropathic group required
permanent self-catheterization postoperatively.
Stone formation was the most common long-term
complication, occurring in 21%. Reservoir perforations occurred in seven patients. Five of the
seven perforations were in neuropathic patients.
Of all the patients, 15% required surgical revision. Overall, 48% of patients experienced one
or more complications. There was no significant difference in the incidence of complications
between the neuropathic and non-neuropathic
groups.

Other researchers have reported better success.
Mundy and Stephenson treated 40 patients with
refractory urge incontinence by "clam" ileocystoplasty. Thirty patients were cured of their symptoms and were voiding spontaneously, six were
cured of their symptoms but required clean intermittent self-catheterization, and four had their
symptoms significantly improved by the operation. They concluded that augmentation cystoplasty improves bladder compliance and detrusor
instability, but voiding dysfunction is a common
postoperative problem.[29]

Blaivas et al. retrospectively reviewed 76 patients who underwent augmentation cystoplasty or continent urinary diversion because of benign urological conditions.[36] Twelve percent of patients in this study had refractory detrusor overactivity, nine percent had interstitial cystitis, and four percent had low bladder compliance. One hundred percent of the nine patients with detrusor overactivity felt they were cured or improved by the procedure. All seven of the interstitial cystitis patients failed. This particular study does not specify whether these patients with idiopathic detrusor overactivity ultimately underwent augmentation cystoplasty or urinary diversion, however.

Bramble published data on a small series of 15 adult patients with enuresis and/or severe urge incontinence treated by enterocystoplasty using sigmoid colon or ileum.[30] Thirteen patients were dry both by day and by night. Three patients had slight residual urgency and two patients had voiding difficulties following cystoplasty and required intermittent self-catheterization.

Results for augmentation cystoplasty in patients with severe detrusor overactivity are varied. Surgical treatment should only be considered in patients with refractory symptoms who have failed other treatment modalities. Complication rates are high and postoperatively patient satisfaction is low to moderate.

INTERSTITIAL CYSTITIS

Augmentation cystoplasty in the treatment of interstitial cystitis (IC) has yielded poor results overall, and some authors consider it a contraindication to surgery.[36] In a review of 24 patients who underwent substitution cystoplasty for IC, eight patients experienced failure that was attributable to residual active disease in the remaining bladder.[7] All seven IC patients in the Blaivas et al. series failed augmentation. In the Flood et al. series, patients with IC had the poorest results. Of the five patients in their series who were unhappy due to major ongoing problems, three of these patients had IC and developed recurrent frequency, urgency, and pain. Only 56% of the 21 patients with IC who underwent bladder augmentation reported an "excellent" outcome. Good results have been reported in IC patients with small capacity bladders, with relief of pain

in 63% and improvement in 25%. Poor results were associated with normal capacity bladder under anesthesia and those dependent on catheterization after surgery.[37] Overall, the results of augmentation cystoplasty in IC patients are discouraging, and this procedure is not recommended for this patient population.

CONCLUSION

Augmentation cystoplasty has been performed for over 50 years. With the acceptance and popularization of clean intermittent catheterization, this surgery has had a positive impact on the neurogenic population in preventing renal failure and restoring continence. These benefits make the potential risks of bladder augmentation more acceptable in this population. In the neurologically intact population with overactive bladder syndrome refractory to medical and behavioral management, other minimally invasive treatments with low associated complications and morbidity are currently available. Recent months have seen the release of greater numbers and more selective anticholinergic medications. Endoscopic injection of botulinum toxin, first described in the neurogenic population, is now being studied in idiopathic detrusor overactivity with good success.[38] Neuromodulation of the sacral nerves that control bladder, sphincter, and pelvic floor muscles has also shown promising results.[39] Only patients who have failed these measures should be considered for augmentation cystoplasty. Patients need to be aware of the associated complications, high incidence of postoperative catheterization, and poor satisfaction rates in this population.

REFERENCES

1. Abrams P, Cardozo L, Fall M et al. The standardisation of terminology of lower urinary tract function: report from the Standardisation Subcommittee of the International Continence Society. Am J Obstet Gynecol 2002; 187: 116–26.
2. Wein AJ. Diagnosis and treatment of the overactive bladder. Urology 2003; 62 (5 Suppl 2): 20–7.
3. Rovner ES, Wein AJ. Incidence and prevalence of overactive bladder. Curr Urol Rep 2002; 3: 434–8.
4. Lapides J, Diokno AC, Silber SJ, Lowe BS. Clean, intermittent self-catheterization in the treatment of urinary tract disease. J Urol 1972; 107: 458–61.

5. Herschorn S, Hewitt RJ. Patient perspective of long-term outcome of augmentation cystoplasty for neurogenic bladder. Urology 1998; 52: 672–8.

6. Hasan ST, Marshall C, Robson WA, Neal DE. Clinical outcome and quality of life following enterocystoplasty for idiopathic detrusor instability and neurogenic bladder dysfunction. Br J Urol 1995; 76: 551–7.

7. Nurse DE, Parry JR, Mundy AR. Problems in the surgical treatment of interstitial cystitis. Br J Urol 1991; 68: 153–4.

8. Morioka A, Miyano T, Ando K, Yamataka T, Lane GJ. Management of vesicoureteral reflux secondary to neurogenic bladder. Pediatr Surg Int 1998; 13: 584–6.

9. Simforoosh N, Tabibi A, Basiri A et al. Is ureteral reimplantation necessary during augmentation cystoplasty in patients with neurogenic bladder and vesicoureteral reflux? J Urol 2002; 168: 1439–41.

10. Pope JC 4th, Keating MA, Casale AJ, Rink RC. Augmenting the augmented bladder: treatment of the contractile bowel segment. J Urol 1998; 160: 854–7.

11. Fontaine E, Leaver R, Woodhouse CR. The effect of intestinal urinary reservoirs on renal function: a 10-year follow-up. BJU Int 2000; 86: 195–8.

12. Khoury AE, Salomon M, Doche R et al. Stone formation after augmentation cystoplasty: the role of intestinal mucus. J Urol 1997; 158: 1133–7.

13. Gillon G, Mundy AR. The dissolution of urinary mucus after cystoplasty. Br J Urol 1989; 63: 372–4.

14. George VK, Gee JM, Wortley MI et al. The effect of ranitidine on urine mucus concentration in patients with enterocystoplasty. Br J Urol 1992; 70: 30–2.

15. Hendren WH, Hendren RB. Bladder augmentation: experience with 129 children and young adults. J Urol 1990; 144: 445–53; discussion 60.

16. Blyth B, Ewalt DH, Duckett JW, Snyder HM 3rd. Lithogenic properties of enterocystoplasty. J Urol 1992; 148: 575–7; discussion 578–9.

17. Palmer LS, Franco I, Kogan SJ et al. Urolithiasis in children following augmentation cystoplasty. J Urol 1993; 150: 726–9.

18. Kronner KM, Casale AJ, Cain MP et al. Bladder calculi in the pediatric augmented bladder. J Urol 1998; 160: 1096–8; discussion 1103.

19. Nurse DE, McInerney PD, Thomas PJ, Mundy AR. Stones in enterocystoplasties. Br J Urol 1996; 77: 684–7.

20. DeFoor W, Minevich E, Reddy P et al. Bladder calculi after augmentation cystoplasty: risk factors and prevention strategies. J Urol 2004; 172: 1964–6.

21. Hensle TW, Bingham J, Lam J, Shabsigh A. Preventing reservoir calculi after augmentation cystoplasty and continent urinary diversion: the influence of an irrigation protocol. BJU Int 2004; 93: 585–7.

22. Cain MP, Casale AJ, Kaefer M, Yerkes E, Rink RC. Percutaneous cystolithotomy in the pediatric augmented bladder. J Urol 2002; 168: 1881–2.

23. Austen M, Kalble T. Secondary malignancies in different forms of urinary diversion using isolated gut. J Urol 2004; 172: 831–8.

24. Elder JS, Snyder HM, Hulbert WC, Duckett JW. Perforation of the augmented bladder in patients undergoing clean intermittent catheterization. J Urol 1988; 140: 1159–62.

25. Couillard DR, Vapnek JM, Rentzepis MJ, Stone AR. Fatal perforation of augmentation cystoplasty in an adult. Urology 1993; 42: 585–8.

26. DeFoor W, Tackett L, Minevich E, Wacksman J, Sheldon C. Risk factors for spontaneous bladder perforation after augmentation cystoplasty. Urology 2003; 62: 737–41.

27. Leyland JW, Masters JG. Conservative management of an intraperitoneal rupture of an augmentation cystoplasty and continent urinary diversion in an adult. J Urol 2003; 170: 524.

28. Strawbridge LR, Kramer SA, Castillo OA, Barrett DM. Augmentation cystoplasty and the artificial genitourinary sphincter. J Urol 1989; 142: 297–301.

29. Mundy AR, Stephenson TP. "Clam" ileocystoplasty for the treatment of refractory urge incontinence. Br J Urol 1985; 57: 641–6.

30. Bramble FJ. The treatment of adult enuresis and urge incontinence by enterocystoplasty. Br J Urol 1982; 54: 693–6.

31. Awad SA, Al–Zahrani HM, Gajewski JB, Bourque-Kehoe AA. Long-term results and complications of augmentation ileocystoplasty for idiopathic urge incontinence in women. Br J Urol 1998; 81: 569–73.

32. Flood HD, Malhotra SJ, O'Connell HE et al. Long-term results and complications using augmentation cystoplasty in reconstructive urology. Neurourol Urodyn 1995; 14: 297–309.

33. Hill DE, Chantigian PM, Kramer SA. Pregnancy after augmentation cystoplasty. Surg Gynecol Obstet 1990; 170: 485–7.

34. Hill DE, Kramer SA. Management of pregnancy after augmentation cystoplasty. J Urol 1990; 144: 457–9; discussion 460.

35. Khastgir J, Hamid R, Arya M, Shah N, Shah PJ. Surgical and patient reported outcomes of 'clam' augmentation ileocystoplasty in spinal cord injured patients. Eur Urol 2003; 43: 263–9.

36. Blaivas JG, Weiss JP, Desai P et al. Long-term followup of augmentation enterocystoplasty and continent diversion in patients with benign disease. J Urol 2005; 173: 1631–4.

37. Webster GD, Maggio MI. The management of chronic interstitial cystitis by substitution cystoplasty. J Urol 1989; 141: 287–91.

38. Rajkumar GN, Small DR, Mustafa AW, Conn G. A prospective study to evaluate the safety, tolerability, efficacy and durability of response of intravesical injection of botulinum toxin type A into detrusor muscle in patients with refractory idiopathic detrusor overactivity. BJU Int 2005; 96: 848–52.

39. Abrams P, Blaivas JG, Fowler CJ et al. The role of neuromodulation in the management of urinary urge incontinence. BJU Int 2003; 91: 355–9.

Special considerations

Overactive bladder in children

Kenneth G Nepple and Christopher S Cooper

Background • Diagnosis and evaluation • Treatment options and outcomes • Conservative treatment • Anticholinergic medication treatment

BACKGROUND

Overactive bladder (OAB) is second in prevalence only to isolated nocturnal enuresis as a voiding complaint in children.[1-4] Bladder overactivity and urge incontinence may predispose children to urinary tract infections and renal injury.[5,6] The hallmark symptom of OAB in children is urgency, and children with this symptom can clinically be diagnosed with an OAB based on a definition by the International Children's Continence Society (ICCS).[7] A study of the micturition habits of 3556 normal 7-year-old Swedish children entering school showed that 21% of girls and 18% of boys had moderate to severe urinary urgency, and 10 years later only 5.9% of girls and 0.9% of boys reported urgency, daytime incontinence, emptying difficulties, or enuresis.[2,3] Urge incontinence is often coupled with OAB, and is associated with psychosocial implications. Up to 20% of 4–6-year-old children experience occasional daytime wetting, although only 3% have wetting accidents twice or more weekly.[8] The prevalence of daytime wetting in children appears to decrease with increasing age, and occurs at least once every two weeks in 10% of 5–6 year olds, 5% in those from 6 to 12 years, and only 4% from 12 to 18 years of age.[4] Of symptomatic children evaluated by urodynamic study, detrusor overactivity occurs in 52–58%,[5,9] as opposed to the low incidence of 5–18% in asymptomatic children.[10,11] The challenge to the clinician is to attempt to separate a pathologic pattern of urgency and

incontinence from the natural timing of acquisition of toilet training.

The treatment of daytime wetting typically begins with conservative measures such as timed voiding and treatment of constipation. For children whose symptoms persist, pharmacologic therapy is often added. Pharmacologic therapy typically involves anticholinergic medications such as oxybutynin, which antagonizes muscarinic receptors in the detrusor muscle of the bladder, thereby increasing bladder capacity and the micturition threshold pressure.[12] Other therapeutic interventions include neuromodulation, as well as injection of botulinum toxin. This chapter will review the diagnosis and evaluation of pediatric OAB as well as treatment options for these children.

DIAGNOSIS AND EVALUATION

The study of pediatric lower urinary tract dysfunction is an area with widespread semantic confusion. The ICCS has actively worked to update and standardize the descriptive terminology used in the field, with the most recent update published in 2006.[7] Normal voiding frequency in children (after attainment of bladder control or the age of 5) was defined as 4–7 voids per day. OAB is based primarily on the symptom of urgency in children. Detrusor overactivity, in contrast, is the observation during urodynamics of involuntary detrusor contractions during the filling phase, involving a detrusor pressure increase of more than 15 cmH$_2$O. Children with OAB often have detrusor overactivity, but this label is reserved for those children who have been formally evaluated using urodynamics. The presence of incontinence, uncontrollable leakage of urine, is only applicable to children of at least 5 years of age. Voiding dysfunction is a general term which was previously used to describe any abnormality in filling or emptying of the bladder; although the term has been used often in the pediatric urology literature, its use is now discouraged.[7] Similarly, urge syndrome and unstable bladder are terminology formerly used to describe OAB and urge incontinence.

OAB in children can result from functional, neurologic (myelodysplasia), or anatomic causes (bladder outlet obstruction, posterior urethral valves).[13] "Functional" refers to idiopathic OAB with no known neurologic or anatomic cause, and theories on etiology have included maturation delay, prolongation of infantile bladder behavior, or abnormality of acquired toilet training habits.[7,14,15] In children with myelomeningocele, the incidence of detrusor overactivity in the newborn period is 57%, with a higher percentage in those with upper lumbar or thoracic involvement and a lower percentage with low sacral involvement.[16] This chapter will focus primarily on the non-neurogenic sources, but consideration of a neurogenic source should always be assessed in each child.

Routine evaluation of a child with symptoms of urgency or urge incontinence begins with a detailed history to determine severity, duration, and frequency of wetting symptoms. A detailed bladder diary includes information on voiding frequency, voided volume, nocturia, daytime incontinence, enuresis, other urinary symptoms, fluid intake, bowel movements, and encopresis, while a less detailed frequency–volume chart is often used in clinical practice.[7] A complete history takes into account developmental milestones, school performance, events at the time of toilet training, and psychosocial issues.[13] The history may help to identify behavioral urinary postponers, children who intentionally withhold urination and may develop incontinence as a result of purposeful bladder overdistention.[17] Information should be gathered regarding prior urinary tract infections (UTIs) or febrile illnesses. Children with urinary urgency or urge incontinence may have a

history of holding maneuvers such as standing on tiptoes, crossing of the legs, or a curtsey with squatting with the heel pressed into the perineum.[18] One study in children with OAB showed that the risk of having a UTI if posturing was present was increased 2.3 times, compared to those children without posturing.[1]

Physical examination includes neurologic and urologic investigations. Inspection of the back is performed for signs of occult spinal dysraphism that may include a presacral dimple, hair patch, fat pad, or asymmetric gluteal cleft. The neurologic examination should include an assessment of motor strength, deep tendon reflexes, perineal sensation, gait, and coordination.[13] The urologic examination requires inspection of the urethral meatus and external genitalia. Meatal stenosis may present an obstructive cause of OAB. Signs of physical or sexual abuse should be considered, as a prior study by Ellsworth et al.[19] noted that 6% of patients evaluated for voiding dysfunction were found to have a history of sexual abuse, and 89% of that group were female.

Children are also assessed for constipation based on history, as well as physical examination. Although no absolute definition of constipation has been accepted, constipation can be characterized as a decreased frequency of bowel movements (less than every other day) with additional symptoms of hard, pebble-like, large, or painful bowel movements. Classification of the appearance of bowel movements may be assisted by use of the visual representations on the Bristol Stool Scale; constipated feces based on this scale appear as separate hard lumps, like nuts, or lumpy sausage shaped bowel movements.[20] If indicated, an abdominal radiograph is obtained to evaluate the amount of stool.

Non-invasive uroflowmetry and post-void residual (PVR) urine quantification are frequently used tools in the armamentarium of a clinician evaluating children for lower urinary tract dysfunction. Uroflowmetry provides information regarding the emptying, but not the filling phase of the micturition cycle. Others have suggested that most children who present with voiding symptoms can be successfully managed initially based on clinical evaluation.[1] For the performance of non-invasive uroflowmetry, children are asked to wait until they feel at least a strong desire to void, and if possible to wait until they have an urgency to void. The shape of the uroflow curve is categorized based on ICCS guidelines as either normal (smooth and bell shaped) or abnormal (tower, plateau, staccato, or interrupted).[7] A tower shaped curve with a high amplitude and short duration peak may be produced by the explosive voiding contraction of OAB; however, the flow curve may also appear bell shaped, as OAB is primarily a dysfunction of the filling phase.

In uroflow evaluation, maximum flow rate, average flow rate, voided volume, and PVR are recorded. Electromyography activity (using pads affixed to the skin) is defined as either present or absent during voiding. The PVR is often measured using non-invasive ultrasound bladder scanning, and total bladder capacity is calculated as the sum of the voided volume and the PVR. Total bladder capacity and PVR are compared to estimated bladder capacity (EBC) based on age. Several formulas are available to calculate EBC. The ICCS accepted formula is EBC = [30 + (age in years × 30)] in ml.[7] The formula is used until age 12 years, after which age EBC is level at 390 cm^3. An alternative formula that results in slightly higher EBC is EBC = (age + 2) × (30 ml).[21] Another formula for EBC developed by Kaefer et al.,[22] EBC (ml) = ([2 × age] + 2) × 30, was used for children < 2 years, and EBC (ml) = ([age/2] + 6) × 30 for children > 2 years. Functional capacity may be diminished in children with OAB,[6] and one study found that initial bladder capacity equaled 57% of the average age-predicted bladder capacity.[23]

Additional information is gathered from urinalysis. The concentration of the urine is noted as well as any evidence of an underlying source of voiding problems based on the presence of hematuria, proteinuria, or glucosuria. Urine culture to evaluate for infection is performed if indicated by pyuria or bacteriuria. A UTI may either result from or precipitate an OAB.[13] In the presence of voiding dysfunction, the incidence of UTIs was higher in females (34%) versus males (5%) in a study by Hoebeke et al.,[5] while Schulman and colleagues[9] found recurrent UTIs in 60%. UTIs in children should be evaluated with both a renal ultrasound and a voiding cystourethrogram. These studies help to exclude the presence of anatomic and functional abnormalities such as hydronephrosis, vesicoureteral reflux, or urethral obstruction. Vesicoureteral reflux was identified

on videourodynamics in 16–20% of children with voiding dysfunction.[5,9] Treatment of OAB has been shown to improve the spontaneous reflux resolution rate, suggesting an etiologic component of OAB in the genesis of reflux.[24–27] Consideration is given to the use of prophylactic antibiotics in children with recurrent UTIs, especially in the presence of reflux.

Formal fluorourodynamic testing is rarely done as part of the initial evaluation of OAB in children. Urodynamics is warranted in cases of bladder dysfunction refractory to treatment, history of UTIs, or known or suspected neurologic abnormality. Detrusor–sphincter dyssynergia, the cystometric observation of a detrusor voiding contraction with a concurrent urethral contraction, is suggestive of a neurogenic bladder disturbance.[7] Any child with evidence of neurological dysfunction (cutaneous signs, physical examination findings, severely refractory voiding dysfunction, or urodynamic evidence of neurogenic bladder) should be evaluated with magnetic resonance imaging (MRI) to look for occult neurologic lesions.

A challenge in the diagnosis of OAB in children is to differentiate from separate or concomitant dysfunctional voiding, a common finding upon urodynamics in 32% of children evaluated for voiding dysfunction.[5] Dysfunctional voiding is defined as the involuntary intermittent contraction of the urethral sphincter or pelvic floor during voiding, and may be observed on uroflow measurements as an intermittent and/or fluctuating (staccato) uroflow rate.[7] Although pediatric incontinence resulting from a voiding-phase dysfunction is traditionally classified separately from those with OAB, both conditions may coexist and serve to propagate the other condition.[6,28] The astute clinician must also be mindful of the nonneurogenic neurogenic bladder, a severe form of dysfunctional voiding described by Hinman and Baumann in 1973,[29] that can result in a severe form of incontinence and renal impairment.[14]

TREATMENT OPTIONS AND OUTCOMES

The treatment of OAB in children is directed at improving quality of life. Successful symptomatic outcomes have been stratified for research purposes by the ICCS, and these groups are also useful clinically. Changes in wetting are categorized as non-response, partial response, response, or full response. Non-response is defined as having 0–49% decrease, partial response is a 50–89% decrease, response is a 90–99% decrease, and full response is a 100% decrease or less than one symptom occurrence monthly.[7]

CONSERVATIVE TREATMENT

Behavioral/voiding diary/timed voiding

Recommended treatment of OAB in children typically begins with conservative measures such as behavior modification, timed voiding, increased water intake, and treatment of constipation.[1,6,30,31,32] Management using conservative measures should not be considered a lack of treatment. Despite these recommendations, the clinician and parent often desire rapid resolution of a child's symptoms through a less labor-intensive approach. In an attempt to quickly alleviate a child's stress, reduce workload, or treat an unmotivated patient or family, anticholinergic medications may often be used as the initial treatment prior to a trial of conservative treatment. In examining data at the authors' institution from patients treated for daytime incontinence, as many as 76% of children with daytime incontinence may never have had an adequate trial of preliminary non-pharmacologic measures.[33]

With an initial non-pharmacologic approach to treating OAB in children, frequency–volume charts (bladder diaries) are used to record occurrences of voiding, bowel movements, and incontinence. Parents and children are provided with information about normal bladder function and an understandable explanation of the ways in which the child differs from the typical. With timed voiding, children are asked to try to void during the day every 2–3 hours, "by the clock". This allows the child an opportunity to establish regular voiding habits. Children are encouraged to urinate before they have a sense of urgency, try to empty their bladders completely, and avoid abdominal straining.

Compliance with timed voiding treatment as well as improvement in urinary symptoms is based on the child's and/or parent's report as well as a review of the diary at the follow-up visit. This approach can be labor intensive, and requires a high degree of motivation from both the child and the parents. A study conducted by Heilenkotter

et al.[34] demonstrated a greater success rate with non-pharmacologic methods in children aged 9–12 as compared to children at age 8, and it would make intuitive sense that, as a child matures, they may respond better to instruction. Aside from the bladder diary, additional measures to increase compliance with timed voiding include the use of wristwatch alarms to assist the child in remembering to void every 2–3 hours, and change in daily patterns to facilitate timed voiding. Parents are encouraged to reward the child with praise for keeping to the voiding schedule. For some children, a coin may be placed in a jar each time they go to the bathroom or removed if they do not go when asked, and the money may then be used at a specified time to buy a reward for the child's compliance.

Wiener and colleagues[35] evaluated the long-term efficacy of simple behavioral therapy for daytime wetting in children with a mailed questionnaire, returned by 48 children with a follow-up of 4.7 ± 2.1 years. Improvement was noted in 74% of children during the first year following therapy, with 59% showing improvement in daytime urinary control, 51% in frequency, 46% in urgency, and 56% in decreased frequency of UTIs. In a majority of the children, measures of psychological well-being were also improved. As with many of the studies performed in OAB, there was a lack of a control group in Wiener's study, so it is difficult to determine whether the change was due to treatment effect, spontaneous resolution, or a combination of both.

A study at the authors' institution[33] evaluated 63 children with daytime incontinence initially treated with non-anticholinergic methods, with follow-up more than 3 weeks and less than 4 months. By the second visit, four (6%) patients became dry, 24 (38%) showed significant improvement, 23 (37%) slight improvement, and 12 (19%) were unchanged in wetting symptoms. Comparing the patients with good versus poor compliance, Allen and colleagues[33] demonstrated a statistically significant higher rate of improvement in wetting in those children with good compliance. No predictive factors were identified determining which children would respond more rapidly to non-pharmacologic treatment. This led the authors to conclude that given the success, safety, and low cost of timed voiding, an initial non-anticholinergic approach should be used to treat urinary incontinence in all children with non-neurogenic daytime incontinence.

Care must also be taken in examining the literature with respect to conservative management of OAB. Curran et al.[36] examined resolution of daytime incontinence using conservative measures in 30 children labeled as refractory, who had previously failed to respond to treatment, including limiting fluid intake and timed voiding. Their described conservative measures consisted of the routine use of anticholinergic medication and occasional use of a concurrent second anticholinergic. This study showed an 87% resolution or improvement rate with a lengthy average time to resolution of 2.7 years, and 38% of the children who achieved complete or significant resolution were dependent on the medication at the time of the last follow-up to retain continence.

Constipation treatment

The urinary system and the gastrointestinal system are interdependent, and the relationship between voiding dysfunction and constipation is well recognized.[24,37,38] One study noted constipation in 17% of children who were evaluated for lower urinary tract dysfunction.[5] Concomitant constipation often occurs in children with daytime wetting, a condition referred to as dysfunctional elimination.[24] Though the mechanism is not fully understood, two complementary theories predominate. One proposes that the rectal distention in the constipated child can put direct pressure on the posterior bladder wall that leads to detrusor overactivity. Another theory states that because urethral and anal sphincter neural input is considered as one functional unit, prolonged external anal sphincter contraction in the presence of a large amount of rectal material may lead to inappropriate pelvic floor muscle contraction and secondary detrusor–urinary sphincter dyssynergia. An increase in parasympathetic activity may also occur as a result of the colonic and rectal distention.[39,40]

It has been shown that the treatment of constipation in children with concomitant detrusor instability can markedly improve urinary symptoms.[9,28,37–39,41] By evacuating the rectal vault, it is thought that the pressure on the bladder is relieved and a more coordinated neural input into the area is reestablished.[38]

Treatment for constipation in the past has included enemas, fecal disimpaction, and a variety of oral agents such as mineral oil, milk of magnesia, or sorbitol. Each of these methods may be effective in treating constipation, though each has its own problems with compliance and safety. Various laxatives designed to stimulate bowel contractions may also affect bladder contractility, although this has not been well studied. Such an affect on the bladder may or may not be beneficial for the child with urinary incontinence.

Miralax™ (polyethylene glycol; Braintree Laboratories, Braintree, MA, USA) is a tasteless, odorless, non-addictive powder that can be mixed with any liquid and has been shown to be effective in the treatment of constipation.[37] At the authors' institution, 46 children with urinary incontinence and constipation were treated with Miralax.[37] Children were advised to modify dietary habits by increasing fluid intake, and were prescribed Miralax with an adjustment in the dosage every 3 days to achieve the goal of 1–2 very soft bowel movements per day. The average final dose of Miralax was 0.6 g/kg/day and, at an average follow-up of 6 months, 39% were dry, 56% had improved their wetting, and only 5% were unchanged. The only reported side effect was diarrhea in almost 20%. In addition to the anticipated increase in stool frequency (from 0.42 ± 0.12 stools/day to 1.25 ± 0.42 stools/day; $p = 0.0001$), in those who become either dry or improved, there were significant improvements in uroflow data (Table 32.1). These included a significant increase in voided volume, maximum flow (Q_{max}), and average flow (Q_{ave}), and a decrease in PVR and PVR as a percentage of predicted capacity (PVR%); no significant changes were seen in the uroflow data in the children characterized as unchanged. When comparing the group of patients who were still constipated ($n = 10$) with the group who resolved their constipation ($n = 36$), those with resolution were significantly more likely to become dry or improved (36/36 vs. 8/10, $p = 0.045$), emphasizing the importance of treating the concomitant constipation in children with wetting.

Biofeedback treatment

In children with both OAB and a voiding-phase dysfunction, anticholinergic treatment may

Table 32.1 Initial and final urodynamic parameters in children with resolution of constipation[36]

	Initial	Final	p-Value
Bladder Volume (ml)	140 ± 13	204 ± 16	< 0.0001
Q_{ave} (ml/s)	8.8 ± 0.7	12.7 ± 0.9	< 0.0001
PVR (ml)	83 ± 11	30 ± 7	< 0.0001
PVR as % predicted of capacity	29 ± 3	10 ± 1	< 0.0001

Q_{ave}, average flow; PVR, post-void residual

reduce bladder overactivity and permit a decrease in the pelvic floor muscle overactivity performed by the child in an attempt to remain continent. In those failing to respond to oxybutynin or in patients thought to have primarily a voiding-phase dysfunction, treatment of the overactive pelvic floor muscles with biofeedback is considered.[30] Hoekx et al.[42] reported that 70% of patients with detrusor instability and small capacity bladder with refractory enuresis had complete symptom resolution with biofeedback training. Vijverberg et al.[43] used a 10-day inpatient treatment program of biofeedback for the treatment of urge incontinence in 95 children, and they found that 68% obtained good results, 13% showed average improvement, and 19% did not improve.

Outpatient biofeedback has been shown to be effective for the treatment of dysfunctional voiding and high PVR. In a study of children with dysfunctional voiding performed at the authors' institution, biofeedback was associated with improved urinary continence (30% dry, 49% improved), decreased urinary tract infections (resolution in 78%), improvement in uroflow curves and parameters, and a decreased post-void residual; however, the post-treatment improvements in uroflow curves and parameters did not correlate with an improvement in either continence or urinary tract infections.[30] These results suggest that there may be a lag between improvement of

voiding dynamics and subsequent improvement in bladder overactivity, which may reflect the underlying process of bladder rehabilitation/remodeling following relief of the functional obstruction.

ANTICHOLINERGIC MEDICATION TREATMENT

Oxybutynin

Bladder contractions are mediated primarily by cholinergic activity on muscarinic receptors. The use of oxybutynin for urologic purpose due to its anticholinergic effect was described in 1972,[44] and it is thought to work by decreasing detrusor overactivity. Anticholinergic medication is often utilized in children who have both symptoms of bladder overactivity, such as frequency, urgency, and urge incontinence, and a small bladder capacity, as indicated by uroflowmetry and PVR.[14,45] Oxybutynin has traditionally been the initial drug of choice.[14] The dose is usually titrated to treatment effect and side effect tolerance. Children are routinely followed with uroflowmetry and PVR measurement.[23] Children with a history and uroflowmetry suggesting bladder underactivity (lazy bladder syndrome), interrupted (fractionated) voiding pattern, history of urinary retention, or high post-void residuals are routinely considered as having a contraindication to oxybutynin.

The efficacy of oxybutynin in children with OAB has been questioned. Despite the prevalence and significance of pediatric daytime incontinence, few prospective randomized trials assessing treatments have been published. Of these, most have been too small and have had problems with trial design and reporting, and have not reliably demonstrated proven efficacy. One review of randomized controlled trials found that none of the currently used interventions for daytime wetting, including a combination of biofeedback and oxybutynin, had been demonstrated to be effective in treating daytime incontinence in children.[33]

There are several possible reasons that studies have difficulty demonstrating efficacy compared to placebo for pediatric incontinence. The "placebo" treatment often includes bladder diaries and timed voiding, which are known to be an effective part of most treatment plans. Also, there is thought to be a baseline annual resolution rate (about 15%) for pediatric incontinence.[45] Part of the difficulty in proving benefit of treatment may also be related to poor randomization based on unknown prognostic variables between children. The treatment of pediatric bladder overactivity with anticholinergic medications occurs commonly, yet little is known about the influence of a number of variables on the utilization and efficacy of oxybutynin in children with daytime wetting.[36,47]

Hellerstein and Zguta[1] evaluated 144 children, of whom two-thirds were treated with anticholinergic medication, and follow-up averaged 3.2 years. The outcome of behavioral modification or anticholinergic medication could not be determined due to lack of a control group, but they did note symptom resolution or improvement in 90.5% of children with daytime urinary incontinence. The resolution of daytime urinary incontinence showed the best overall outcome, with moderate improvement in urgency (83%) and frequency (80%). Of children with recurrent UTIs, 56% were no longer having UTIs and 30% were having them less frequently.

In an attempt to define predictive factors affecting the continence outcome in children with daytime wetting, a previous study conducted at the authors' institution evaluated 81 children.[48] On average, oxybutynin had been used for 1.2 years, and at the last visit while taking oxybutynin, 31 children (38%) were dry, 25 (31%) were significantly improved, 19 (24%) were slightly improved, and six (7%) were unchanged in their symptoms. No child's symptoms were worsened after beginning oxybutynin. In this review, the only variable significantly associated with an improvement in daytime wetting with oxybutynin was the frequency of wetting episodes. Those patients who became dry presented with significantly fewer wetting episodes than did patients with only slight or no improvement ($p = 0.002$). These findings seem intuitive, and suggest that any benefit provided by oxybutynin would be more likely to result in complete dryness in those children already having relatively few accidents. Interestingly, patient age, gender, duration of symptoms, and uroflowmetry results were not found to correlate to outcome with oxybutynin treatment. A prior study suggesting that a trend might exist such that bladder capacity is prognostic was not supported by these results.[36]

There are five different muscarinic receptor subtypes, and the M_3 receptor is primarily responsible for detrusor contraction,[49] and blockage at other receptors may produce side effects. Oxybutynin has a high affinity for both the M_1 and M_3 receptor subtypes. Side effects of oxybutynin in children may be more frequent than in adults,[50] and may result in decreased compliance or discontinuation of treatment. Common side effects with oxybutynin include constipation, dry mouth, and flushing. In a recent study, only 47 of 81 children (58%) experienced no side effects from oxybutynin.[23] The most common side effects included worsening constipation (19%), dry mouth (17%), flushing (14%), and heat intolerance (4%). Despite these side effects, only 2% of children discontinued oxybutynin after experiencing side effects, while other studies have reported up to 10% of patients stopping treatment due to bothersome side effects.[6]

Cognitive side effects, including memory dysfunction possibly secondary to the role of the muscarinic receptor in memory consolidation, may develop in elderly patients treated with oxybutynin.[51] Understandably, there has been concern over possible cognitive effects in children; however, central nervous system effects appear to be less frequent or apparent in children.[52,53] Sommer et al.[54] used sensitive neuropsychological testing to evaluate the effect of oxybutynin in children after 4 weeks of treatment, and found no associated cognitive impairment.

Ditropan XL®

In one study, 27 children who were changed from oxybutynin to Ditropan XL® were reviewed.[23] The average duration on oxybutynin preceding change to Ditropan XL was 12 months, and the average duration on Ditropan XL was 20 months. Reasons for changing to Ditropan XL included a complete lack of improvement (52%), convenience (28%), intolerable side effects (10%), and disliking the taste (10%). All patients had persistent incontinence while on regular oxybutynin. Thirteen of 27 (48%) children with persistent wetting became dry or had significant improvement in the frequency of wetting by the next visit after changing to Ditropan XL. In a similar fashion, an objective significant improvement was also noted at the first visit following the change to Ditropan

XL in both the voided volume and total bladder capacity. Based on these findings, a trial of Ditropan XL seems warranted in children with daytime wetting refractory to regular oxybutynin.

Preliminary studies of an extended release formulation of oxybutynin (Ditropan XL) reported fewer side effects.[55] In the Van Arendonk et al. study,[23] although some children resolved side effects with the change to Ditropan XL others developed new side effects, and the incidence of side effects between the two medications appeared equivalent. Reported side effects on oxybutynin and Ditropan XL included flushing (19%, 19%, respectively), dry mouth (15%, 15%), new onset of constipation (15%, 7%), heat intolerance (7%, 4%), fatigue (0%, 4%), and rash (1%, 0%). Twenty two percent of children had resolution of side effects after changing to Ditropan XL, while 26% of children developed a new side effect after switching to Ditropan XL.

Ditropan XL is known to maintain a more constant plasma concentration with a lower maximum plasma concentration.[12] In addition, the package insert available from the Food and Drug Administration (FDA) suggests the bioavailability of the active R-enantiomer is 156% that of the immediate release oxybutynin, suggesting that an equivalent milligram dosing actually results in a greater therapeutic dosage. This alteration in pharmacokinetics may result in an improved therapeutic effect. Alternatively, increased compliance with a once-daily medication may account for the differences seen.

Tolterodine

Although it is not FDA-approved in children, other studies have been performed using the anticholinergic medication tolterodine, a selective competitive muscarinic receptor antagonist. In 2000, Goessl and colleagues[56] published the first report of treatment of detrusor overactivity in children with tolterodine, and noted an improvement in urodynamics parameters including bladder capacity and detrusor compliance in previously untreated patients. Raes et al.[57] retrospectively reviewed a total of 256 children with OAB who were either previously treated with or naive to anticholinergics, and reported an improvement to complete continence (50% and 54%, respectively), reduction in wetting episodes (50% both

groups), and reduction in urgency (39% and 29%). Only 3.5% of patients experienced side effects attributed to medication, which were behavioral and gastrointestinal, with no reported dry mouth or flushing.

Nijman et al.[58] evaluated tolterodine extended release (2 mg) in a randomized, placebo controlled trial of 711 children, 5–10 years old. Parental report of benefit was 62% in the tolterodine group versus 47% in the placebo group ($p < 0.05$). At 12 weeks, there was no statistically significant difference between the two groups in the change in number of incontinence episodes; however, there was a significant effect in children weighing 35 kg or less, which was suggestive of a possible underdosage effect in heavier children. In addition, timed voiding instructions were not given, and the follow-up time may have been inadequate to establish a clinically significant effect. Tolterodine was safe and well tolerated, with dry mouth and constipation occurring infrequently. Tolterodine may have a more favorable side effect profile then oxybutynin.

Tolterodine is sometimes used in children who fail oxybutynin treatment or have side effects. Bolduc and coworkers[45] studied 34 children who were changed from ditropan to tolterodine because of side effects, and found at median follow-up of 6 months that reduction in wetting episodes was classified as cured in 68%, improved in 15%, and not improved in 18%, while 24% of children in this selected group discontinued tolterodine because of side effects. Yucel et al.[58] concluded that tolterodine may increase the efficacy of pharmacotherapy in children with daytime urinary incontinence in oxybutynin treatment failures, but their data were not statistically analyzed.

Reinberg et al.[60] retrospectively evaluated the therapeutic efficacy of open-label usage of Ditropan XL and immediate and long-acting tolterodine in 132 children with incontinence and symptoms of overactive bladder, and concluded that Ditropan XL was more effective then either form of tolterodine in the control of daytime incontinence and frequency. The side effects of the three medications in the study were similar, with 82–87% reporting no peripheral anticholinergic side effects. However, the design of the study was limited, secondary to its retrospective nature, non-randomization, and no control group.

New antimuscarinic agents including darifenacin (Enablex®; Novartis, East Hanover, NJ), solifenacin (VESIcare®; Astellas Pharma US, Tokyo, Japan), and trospium (Sanctura®; Esprit Pharmaceuticals, East Brunswick, NJ) have been developed and approved for use in adults in the United States, but have not been studied extensively in the pediatric population.

Neuromodulation

Continence and complete bladder emptying are mediated by a number of neuronal reflex mechanisms. Continence requires a relaxed urinary bladder with closure of the urethra during the collecting phase.[61,62] During micturition, an intravesical pressure above the opening pressure of the simultaneously relaxing urethra is generated. Childhood OAB is commonly attributed to delayed maturation or integration of inhibitory descending inputs from higher centers.[63] Groen and Bosch[61] studied neuromodulation techniques in the treatment of overactive bladder, and theorized mechanisms for activity of electrical stimulation include: reflexogenic stimulation, neuromuscular reeducation, and pain suppression. In the case of bladder overactivity resulting from defective central inhibition, nerve stimulation may help to stimulate inherent spinal inhibitory pathways. Another rationale for nerve stimulation is the production of greater muscle strengthening than with voluntary efforts and recruitment of fast muscle fibers better than with volitional exercises, and, with long term use, muscles assume properties of slow muscle fibers for a more sustained pelvic floor contraction. With electrical stimulation there is thought to be enhancement of β-adrenergic activity (facilitating bladder vault relaxation), reduction of cholinergic activity, and changes in the concentration of selected smooth muscle relaxants (vasoactive intestinal polypeptide (VIP), serotonin) with electrical stimulation. Electric current is also known to stimulate the release of endorphins and encephalins in the cerebrospinal fluid (CSF), and raised opioid levels have been reported to be inhibitory to detrusor overactivity.[61]

The use of neurostimulation with implantable direct sacral nerve stimulation (InterStim®; Medtronic, Minneapolis, MN) to treat adult urge incontinence and urgency–frequency has been well established; however, the practice in children is less common due to its invasiveness.[14,61,64–69] Nevertheless, this changed with the introduction of less invasive surface neuromodulation. Several studies have revealed positive results with the use of surface neuromodulation in children with urgency and/or urge incontinence.[62,64,65,67,70] Gladh et al.[67] reported that in 48 children with therapy-resistant cystometry-proven urge incontinence, treatment with anogenital electrical stimulation resulted in cure in 38% and improvement in 15%. Trsinar and Kralj[62] used anal electrical stimulation in children with symptomatic detrusor overactivity, and 75% were cured or much improved versus 14% in a control group; cystometry after treatment showed a statistically significant decline in the number of uninhibited contractions. The TENS (trancutaneous electrical nerve stimulation) unit allows surface stimulation by placing electrodes on the skin over the sacral region. Hoebeke et al.[70] used TENS (2-hour daily stimulation at the sacral root S_3) to treat 41 children with urge incontinence and confirmed detrusor overactivity that had failed anticholinergic therapy; they noted a 68% response at 1 month and 51% were cured after 1 year. Bower et al.[62] found that dryness improved in 73% and urgency improved after at least 1 month of treatments with transcutaneous neuromodulation. De Gennaro et al.[71] used percutaneous tibial nerve stimulation with a 34-gauge needle in 10 children with overactive bladder; symptoms improved in eight and the procedure was reported as being minimally painful.

Limited data are available regarding the implantable sacral nerve stimulator in children. Humphreys and co-workers[72] reported their experience in 16 children with refractory voiding dysfunction using implantation in a staged fashion. At a mean follow-up of 13 months, incontinence improved or resolved in 75% with parent satisfaction of 66%. Two of 16 devices were explanted.

Botulinum toxin

Botulinum toxin blocks neurotransmitter release from peripheral afferent nerve terminals and inhibits efferent nerve-mediated bladder contractions.[73] The use of botulinum toxin injection for pediatric incontinence has primarily been studied in neurogenic detrusor overactivity. One study evaluated the use of cystoscopic guidance injected botulinum toxin for idiopathic detrusor overactivity in children who had failed medical therapy, and results reported an increase in functional bladder capacity and a reduction in detrusor contractions and urgency symptoms; however, one child required intermittent catheterization for 2 weeks after injection.[74] Further study regarding the invasive use of botulinum toxin in OAB is required before a recommendation can be made.

REFERENCES

1. Hellerstein S, Zguta AA. Outcome of overactive bladder in children. Clin Pediatr (Phila) 2003; 42: 553–6.
2. Hellstrom A, Hanson E, Hansson S, Hjalmas K, Jodal U. Micturition habits and incontinence in 7-year-old Swedish school entrants. Eur J Pediatr 1990; 149: 434–7.
3. Hellstrom A, Hanson E, Hansson S, Hjalmas K, Jodal U. Micturition habits and incontinence at age 17—reinvestigation of a cohort studied at age 7. Br J Urol 1995; 76: 231–4.
4. Robson WL. Diurnal enuresis. Pediatr Rev 1997; 18: 407–12.
5. Hoebeke P, Van Laecke E, Van Camp C et al. One thousand video-urodynamic studies in children with non-neurogenic bladder sphincter dysfunction. BJU Int 2001; 87: 575–80.
6. Nijman RJ: Classification and treatment of functional incontinence in children. BJU Int 2000; 85 (Suppl 3): 37–42.
7. Neveus T, von Gontard A, Hoebeke P et al. The standardization of terminology of lower urinary tract function in children and adolescents: report from the Standardisation Committee of the International Children's Continence Society. J Urol 2006; 176: 314–24.
8. Sureshkumar P, Craig JC, Roy LP, Knight JF. Daytime urinary incontinence in primary school children: a population-based survey. J Pediatr 2000; 137: 814–18.
9. Schulman SL, Quinn CK, Plachter N, Kodman-Jones C. Comprehensive management of dysfunctional voiding. Pediatrics 1999; 103: E31.
10. Yeung CK, Godley ML, Duffy PG, Ransley PG. Natural filling cystometry in infants and children. Br J Urol 1995; 75: 531–7.
11. Wen JG, Tong EC. Cystometry in infants and children with no apparent voiding symptoms. Br J Urol 1998; 81: 468–73.
12. Siddiqui MA, Perry CM, Scott LJ. Oxybutynin extended release: a review of its use in the management of overactive bladder. Drugs 2004; 64: 885–912.
13. Bauer SB. Special considerations of the overactive bladder in children. Urology 2002; 60 (5 Suppl 1): 43–9.
14. Nijman RJ. Role of antimuscarinics in the treatment of nonneurogenic daytime urinary incontinence in children. Urology 2004; 63 (3 Suppl 1): 45–50.
15. Greenfield SP. The overactive bladder in childhood. J Urol 2000; 163: 578–9.
16. Dator DP, Hatchett L, Dyro FM, Shefner JM, Bauer SB. Urodynamic dysfunction in walking myelodysplastic children. J Urol 1992; 148: 362–5.
17. Von Gontard A, Lettgen B, Olbing H et al. Behavioural problems in children with urge incontinence and voiding postponement: a comparison of a paediatric and child psychiatric sample. Br J Urol 1998; 81 (Suppl 3): 100–6.
18. Vincent SA. Postural control of urinary incontinence: the curtsy sign. Lancet 1996; 2: 631–2.
19. Ellsworth PI, Merguerian PA, Copening ME. Sexual abuse: another causative factor in dysfunctional voiding. J Urol 1995; 153: 773–6.
20. Lewis SJ, Heaton KW. Stool form scale as a useful guide to intestinal transit time. Scan J Gastroenterol 1997; 32: 920–4.
21. Koff SA. Estimating bladder capacity in children. Urology 1983; 21: 248.
22. Kaefer M, Zurakowski D, Bauer SB et al. Estimating normal bladder capacity in children. J Urol 1997; 158: 2261–4.
23. Van Arendonk KJ, Knudson MJ, Austin JC, Cooper CS. Improved efficacy of extended release oxybutynin in children with persistent daytime urinary incontinence converted from regular oxybutynin. Urology 2006; 68: 862–5.
24. Koff SA, Wagner TT, Jayanthi VR. The relationship among elimination syndromes, primary vesicoureteral reflux and urinary tract infections in children. J Urol 1998; 160: 1019–22.
25. Koff SA, Murtagh DS. The uninhibited bladder in children: effect of treatment on recurrence of urinary tract infection and vesicoureteral reflux resolution. J Urol 1983; 130: 1138–41.
26. Scholtmeijer RJ, Nijman RJ. Vesicoureteric reflux and videourodynamic studies: results of a

prospective study after three years of follow-up. Urology 1994; 43: 714–18.

27. Willemsen J, Nijman RJ. Vesicoureteral reflux and videourodynamic studies: results of a prospective study. Urology 2000; 55: 939–43.

28. Norgaard JP, van Gool JD, Hjälmås K, Djurhuus JC, Hellstrom AL. Standardization and definitions in lower urinary tract dysfunction in children. International Children's Continence Society. Br J Urol 1998; 81 (Suppl 3): 1–16.

29. Hinman F, Baumann FW. Vesical and ureteral damage from voiding dysfunction in boys without neurologic or obstructive disease. J Urol 1973; 109: 727–32.

30. Nelson JD, Cooper CS, Boyt MA, Hawtrey CE, Austin JC. Improved uroflow parameters and post-void residual following biofeedback therapy in pediatric patients with dysfunctional voiding does not correspond to outcome. J Urol 2004; 172: 1653–6.

31. Schulman SL. Voiding dysfunction in children. Urol Clin North Am 2004; 31: 481–90.

32. Sureshkumar P, Bower W, Craig JC, Knight JF. Treatment of daytime urinary incontinence in children: a systematic review of randomized controlled trials. J Urol 2003; 170: 196–200.

33. Allen HA, Austin JC, Hawtrey CE, Boyt MA, Cooper CS: An initial trial of timed voiding is warranted for all children with daytime incontinence. J Urol 2007, in press.

34. Heilenkotter K, Bachmann C, Janhsen E et al. Prospective evaluation of inpatient and outpatient bladder training in children with functional urinary incontinence. Urology 2006; 67: 176–80.

35. Wiener JS, Scales MT, Hamptom J et al. Long-term efficacy of simple behavioral therapy for daytime wetting in children. J Urol 2000; 164: 786–90.

36. Curran M, Kaefer M, Peters C, Logigian E, Bauer SB. The overactive bladder in childhood: long-term results with conservative treatment. J Urol 2000; 163: 574–7.

37. Erickson BA, Austin JC, Cooper CS, Boyt MA. Polyethylene glycol 3350 for constipation in children with dysfunctional elimination. J Urol 2003; 170: 1518–20.

38. Loening-Baucke V. Urinary incontinence and urinary tract infection and their resolution with treatment of chronic constipation of childhood. Pediatrics 1997; 100: 228–32.

39. O'Regan S, Yazbeck S. Constipation: a cause of enuresis, urinary tract infection and vesico-ureteral reflux in children. Med Hypotheses 1985; 17: 409–13.

40. O'Regan S, Yazbeck S, Schick E. Constipation, bladder instability, urinary tract infection syndrome. Clin Nephrol 1985; 23: 152–4.

41. O'Regan S, Yazbeck S, Hamberger B, Schick E. Constipation: a commonly unrecognized cause of enuresis. Am J Dis Child 1986; 140: 260–1.

42. Hoekx L, Wyndaele JJ, Vermandel A. The role of biofeedback in the treatment of children with refractory nocturnal enuresis associated with idiopathic detrusor instability and small bladder capacity. J Urol 1998; 160: 858–60.

43. Vijverberg MA, Elzinga-Plomp A, Messer AP et al. Bladder rehabilitation, the effect of a cognitive training programme on urge incontinence. Eur Urol 1997; 31: 68–72.

44. Diokno AC, Lapides J. Oxybutynin: a new drug with analgesic and anticholinergic properties. J Urol 1972; 108: 307–9.

45. Bolduc S, Upadhyay J, Payton J et al. The use of tolterodine in children after oxybutynin failure. BJU Int 2003; 91: 398–401.

46. Bloom DA. Overactive bladder: pediatric aspects. BJU Int 2000; 85 (Suppl 3): 43–6.

47. Saedi NA, Schulman SL. Natural history of voiding dysfunction. Pediatr Nephrol 2003; 18: 894–7.

48. Van Arendonk KJ, Austin JC, Boyt MA, Cooper CS. Frequency of wetting is predictive of response to anticholinergic treatment in children with overactive bladder. Urology 2006; 67: 1049–54.

49. Yamanishi T, Chapple CR, Chess-Williams R. Which muscarinic receptor is important in the bladder? World J Urol 2001: 19: 299–306.

50. Jonville AP, Dutertre JP, Berbellion M, Autret E. Adverse effects of oxybutynin chloride (Ditropan) in pediatrics. Arch Fr Pediatr 1993; 50: 27–9.

51. Kay G, Crook T, Rekeda L et al. Differential effects of the antimuscarinic agents Darifenacin and oxybutynin ER on memory in older subjects. Eur Urol 2006; 50: 317–26.

52. Chapple CR, Yamanashi T, Chess-Williams R. Muscarinic receptor subtypes and management of the overactive bladder. Urology 2002; 60 (Suppl 1): 82–9.

53. Pathak AS, Aboseif SR. Overactive bladder: drug therapy versus nerve stimulation. Nat Clin Pract Urol 2005; 2: 310–11.

54. Sommer BR, O'Hara R, Askari N, Kraemer HC, Kennedy WA III. The effect of oxybutynin treatment on cognition in children with diurnal incontinence. J Urol 2005; 173: 2125–7.

55. Youdim K, Kogan BA. Preliminary study of the safety and efficacy of extended-release oxybutynin in children. Urology 2002; 59: 428–32.

56. Goessl C, Sauter T, Michael T et al. Efficacy and tolerability of tolterodine in children with detrusor hyperreflexia. Urology 2000; 55: 414–18.

57. Raes A, Hoebeke P, Segaert I et al. Retrospective analysis of efficacy and tolerability of tolterodine in children with overactive bladder. Eur Urol 2004; 45: 240–4.

58. Nijman RJ, Borgstein NG, Ellsworth P, Djurhuss JC. Tolterodine treatment for children with symptoms of urinary urge incontinence suggestive of detrusor overactivity: results from 2 randomized, placebo controlled trials. J Urol 2005; 173: 1334–9.

59. Yucel S, Akkaya E, Guntekin E et al. Should we switch over to tolterodine in every child with non-neurogenic daytime urinary incontinence in whom oxybutynin failed? Urology 2005; 65: 369–73.

60. Reinberg Y, Crocker J, Wolpert J, Vandersteen D. Therapeutic efficacy of extended release oxybutynin chloride, and immediate release and long acting tolterodine tartrate in children with diurnal urinary incontinence. J Urol 2003; 169: 317–19.

61. Groen J, Bosch JLHR. Neuromodulation techniques in the treatment of the overactive bladder. BJU Int 2001; 87: 723–31.

62. Trsinar B, Kralj B. Maximal electrical stimulation in children with unstable bladder and nocturnal enuresis and/or daytime incontinence. Neurourol Urodyn 1996; 15: 133–42.

63. Homsy YL. Dysfunctional voiding symptoms and vesicoureteric reflux. Pediatr Nephrol 1994; 8: 116–21.

64. Bower WF, Moore KH, Adams RD. A pilot study of the home application of transcutaneous neuromodulation in children with urgency or urge incontinence. J Urol 2001; 166: 2420–2.

65. Bower WF, Yeung CK. A review of non-invasive electroneuromodulation as an intervention for non-neurogenic bladder dysfunction in children. Neurourol Urodyn 2004; 23: 63–7.

66. Bani-Hani AH, Vandersteen DR, Reinberg YE. Neuromodulation in pediatrics. Urol Clin North Am 2005; 32: 101–7.

67. Gladh G, Mattsson S, Lindstrom S. Anogenital electrical stimulation as treatment of urge incontinence in children. BJU Int 2001; 87: 366–71.

68. Hassouna MM, Siegel SW, Nyeholt AA et al. Sacral neuromodulation in the treatment of urgency-frequency symptoms: a multicenter study on efficacy and safety. J Urol 2000; 163: 1849–54.

69. Bernstein AJ, Peters KM. Expanding indications for neuromodulation. Urol Clin North Am 2005; 32: 59–63.

70. Hoebeke P, Van Laecke E, Everaert K et al. Transcutaneous neuromodulation for the treatment of urge syndrome in children: a pilot study. J Urol 2001; 166: 2416–19.

71. De Gennaro M, Capitanucci ML, Mastracci P et al. Percutaneous tibial nerve neuromodulation is well tolerated in children and effective for treating refractory vesical dysfunction. J Urol 2004; 171: 1911–13.

72. Humphreys M, Hollatz P, Smith C et al. Sacral neuromodulation in children: preliminary results in 16 patients. J Urol 2004: 171 (4 Suppl 1): 56–7 (abstr 214).

73. Schurch B, Corcos J. Botulinum toxin injections for paediatric incontinence. Curr Opin Urol 2005; 15: 264–7.

74. Verleyen P, Hoebeke P, Raes P et al. The use of botulinum toxin A in children with a non-neurogenic overactive bladder: a pilot study. BJU Int 2004; 93 (Suppl): 69–72.

33

Geriatric population

Pat D O'Donnell

Economic factors in overactive bladder therapy • **Pathophysiology of overactive bladder in the elderly** • **Pharmacological therapy** • **Behavioral therapy** • **Electrical stimulation** • **Conclusion**

Overactive bladder (OAB) symptoms in older people result in a profound and debilitating loss in quality of life for millions of older people in the United States. The incidence of overactive bladder symptoms increases markedly with each passing decade of life. Symptoms of urinary urgency and urge urinary incontinence are often severe and devastating life events for older people. A self-imposed social isolation occurs in older people who experience OAB symptoms, which markedly reduces their quality of life. At a time in an older person's life when quality of life can be as important to the individual as survival itself, OAB symptoms have the capacity to deprive the older individual of the quality of life that was their greatest aspiration for their later years.

Awareness of the immense impact on quality of life of OAB symptoms among older people as well as among physicians caring for older people continues to be very slow in evolution. The success of behavioral therapies during the 1980s was well known among the scientific community, but has been slow to be integrated into clinical practice. The advent of successful pharmacological therapies for OAB symptoms during the last decade resulted in massive media attention from direct patient marketing that significantly improved public awareness of the problem. Still, the pervasive concepts that OAB symptoms are "part of getting old" and "something you can live with" remain common among millions of older people.

The media attention about OAB symptoms over the past decade has resulted in significant personal insight for older people that "they are not alone", because millions of other older people suffer from OAB symptoms and "something can be done". However, the enormous number of older people with OAB symptoms who have never seen a physician about the problem or have never discussed it with their primary care physician during routine clinic visits remains a perplexing problem to healthcare professionals and a substantial barrier to treatment of OAB symptoms in the elderly. Studies show that less than half of community-dwelling adult women in the United States with symptoms of urinary incontinence have talked with a physician about the problem.[1] Older patients and physicians who care for the elderly have been very reluctant to directly confront the impact of the severe quality of life limitations that OAB symptoms inflict on the elderly.

The magnitude of the cost and despair among older people with OAB symptoms in communities throughout the United States is overwhelming. The incidence of OAB among older people is extremely high, and the limitations imposed by OAB symptoms on the way older people live their lives is profound. Healthcare professionals have been unable to successfully access and educate the elderly population about the problem of OAB and the treatment options that are available.

The "suffering in silence" by millions of older Americans with OAB symptoms will soon become a much more serious medical, social, and economic problem. The older population is on the threshold of an enormous boom. A substantial increase in the number of older people will occur during the 2010–2030 period, after the first "baby boomers" turn 65 in 2011. The older population in 2030 is projected to be twice as large as in 2000, growing from 35 million in 2000 to 72 million in 2030. In 2030, the older population will represent nearly 20% of the total population in the United States.[2]

People in the United States are living longer and healthier lives than ever before. The average life expectancy at birth rose from 47.3 years in 1900 to 76.9 years in 2000. A critical concept for the future of older people and for the welfare of our society is achieving a balance of increased longevity with increased quality of life. A serious concern for the future is a continued increase in longevity due to further medical advances, resulting in large numbers of older survivors who are functionally and cognitively impaired. An intense effort must be made to promote healthier lives that parallel longer survival in the elderly population for the future. Simultaneous progress in prolonging life and improving quality of life is essential for the welfare of older people as well as the integrity of our society. OAB symptoms in older people have an immense debilitating impact on quality of life in this population. Better access, education and treatment options for elderly people with OAB symptoms are an essential part of the health and welfare of millions of older people in the future. Our society cannot experience advances in medicine that prolong survival in older people without making a longer life for the elderly worth living through medical advances that improve quality of life at the same time.

While OAB symptoms in elderly people are debilitating, changes are possible in the future if patient education programs for older people can be implemented and advances in therapeutic programs better utilized by the elderly. Over recent years, disability among the older population is declining. Studies over the past two decades have shown substantial declines in the rates of disability and functional limitations of older people. As the "graying of America" occurs, with a dramatic shift in the population to an aging society, the education of older people can have an impact on the awareness of OAB symptoms, and active patient participation in bladder health programs can change the future quality of life for millions of Americans.

Patient education about OAB symptoms and treatment is essential and possible for the next generation of older people. In 1950, only 17% of the older population had graduated from high school, and only 3% had at least a bachelor's degree. By 2003, 72% of the older population were high school graduates and 17% had at least a bachelor's degree. Patient education is associated with healthier lifestyle choices and a better personal perception of health status among older people. Individual attitudes about aging will be different with the baby boomer generation, which will allow people to grow older astutely and gracefully. The next generation of older people will become active participants in healthier lifestyles. In addition, patient expectations about healthcare for older people will change due to better patient education. One of the most important changes in patient expectations that will occur in the next generation of older people is a requirement for advances in medicine that improve quality of life to occur which will parallel the medical advances that improve longevity. OAB symptoms in older people represent one of the most serious potential compromises in quality of life for the aging baby boomer generation because of the incidence and severity of the problem in the elderly.

One of the greatest fears of the next generation of older people is the possibility that advances in medicine will allow people to live much longer only to suffer devastating losses in quality of life due to functional impairments during the later years. Advances in medicine that affect quality of life must parallel advances that prolong survival in older people. In order to address quality of life, the concept of "active life expectancy" (ALE) is used to measure the number of years that people can expect to live on average without disability.[3-6] The ALE/survival axis in aging is a critical concept for the future of older people, healthcare professionals, and our society. The greatest impact on the cost of healthcare in the United States will be made in achieving a balance in the ALE/survival axis in aging. As people become older, it is essential that they can function independently. When an older person can no longer function independently, quality of life goes down and cost to society goes up. OAB symptoms in older people can limit the ability of an older person to function independently, which results in an immense increase in cost to society.

ECONOMIC FACTORS IN OVERACTIVE BLADDER THERAPY

With national healthcare expenditure totaling an estimated $1.3 trillion in 2000, the United States spent more on healthcare than any other industrialized country in the world.[2] A healthier older population with fewer functional disabilities is critical for the next generation and for our society. The baby boomer generation consists of people born from 1946 to 1964. About 75 million baby boomers were born in the United States. An additional 8 million born in other countries during these years immigrated into the United States. Researchers predict that increased longevity of that generation will have significant implications for the financing of our healthcare systems.[7,8]

By 2008, the first of the baby boomers will turn 62, the earliest age at which an individual can collect Social Security benefits in retirement. A major retirement wave will arrive in 2011, when the first of the baby boomers turn 65. By 2020, the number of adults aged 60–64 is projected to be nearly twice the number in 2000. The annual cost for Social Security funds will exceed tax income starting in 2018, and funds are projected to become exhausted by 2042.[2] Advances in medicine will continue to reduce mortality among older people at a faster rate than was foreseen by the Social Security Administration's forecasts, requiring an increase in the payroll tax rate or a reduction in benefits beyond the Social Security Administration's estimate.[9]

Projections indicate an 18% increase of the total population between 2010 and 2030, but a 78% increase of the older population is projected during that same time frame.[2] This differential growth will result in nearly one in five Americans being aged 65 and older in 2030. Because men are generally older than their spouses and women have higher life expectancy, high proportions of women, particularly the oldest-old women (85 years old and older), will be widows and live alone. Older women are more likely than older men (13% compared with 7%) to live in poverty. Older people are dependent on family, the government, or both for financial, physical, and emotional support. Social Security continues to provide the largest share of income for most older people.

Approximately 19% of the healthcare expenses for older people were paid out-of-pocket and another 12% were paid by private insurance in 2003. The high out-of-pocket expenses for healthcare for older people occur at a time of life when their income level is low. Approximately 65% of healthcare costs for older people were paid by public programs such as Medicare and Medicaid. There were about 40 million Medicare enrollees in 2000, and the Medicare program reported a cost of $222 billion.

An older individual's insurance status has been shown to be associated with his or her likelihood of accessing healthcare. Older people who were uninsured or had Medicare coverage only were more likely to delay or go without medical care than those who had a combination of Medicare and private insurance.[10,11] As stated previously, the older population is projected to double from 35 million in 2000 to 72 million in 2030, which will represent an increase from 12% of the population to 20% of the population in the same time frame. The oldest old population (those aged 85 and older) is also projected to double from 4.7 million in 2003 to 9.6 million in 2030, and to double again to 20.9 million in 2050.

In 2000, the annual estimated cost of urinary incontinence was 19.5 billion dollars, and the estimated cost of overactive bladder was an additional 12.6 billion dollars.[12] The cost of OAB therapies for older people in the future is a serious concern for maintaining a quality of life that parallels survival. New therapeutic interventions for OAB in the elderly must occur that are effective, affordable, and accepted by the elderly population to avoid people living longer lives only to experience debilitating symptoms of OAB in their later years.

PATHOPHYSIOLOGY OF OVERACTIVE BLADDER IN THE ELDERLY

Animal studies and human studies of aging detrusor muscle properties indicate that aging has a minimal effect on the neuromuscular activities of the urinary bladder and that the relationship of changes that have been observed to OAB symptoms in the elderly human population are unclear.[13–16] Clinical observations of

OAB symptoms in older people indicate that the symptoms in the older population seem to differ somewhat from those in younger people. Younger people experience episodes of urinary urgency often having a wide range of intensity for an individual. The intensity of urgency and the warning time before voluntary voiding or urge urinary incontinence occurs often vary among episodes for a younger individual. In contrast, older people often describe urge urinary incontinence with "little or no warning time". Older people may experience relatively normal voiding with occasional episodes of urge incontinence that seem to occur with "no warning". Older people who experience OAB symptoms usually experience nocturia.[17] An urge to void can result in sleep arousal and voluntary voiding without incontinence on one occasion and urge urinary incontinence with "no warning" on another occasion.[18]

In a study of elderly chronic-care men, episodes of urge urinary incontinence were determined to be unrelated to the accumulated volume of urine in the bladder at the time of the episode.[19] In addition, episodes of urge incontinence were not associated with the time interval from the previous incontinence episode.[20,21] In that study, elderly chronic-care men experienced random occurrences of urge incontinence relative to intravesical volume and time between incontinence episodes.[22,23] In most of these patients who experienced random episodes of urge incontinence, voluntary voiding occurred most of the time. The occurrence of urge urinary incontinence in older men appeared to result from abnormal central nervous system (CNS) control of the urinary bladder.[24] It was possible to modify involuntary control of the urinary bladder in that group of elderly men using biofeedback therapy, which suggested that a change in neuromodulation of the CNS control of the urinary bladder had occurred.[25]

Older women who experience OAB symptoms often have coexisting urethral dysfunction and abnormal anterior vaginal wall support. Changes in bladder function of older women associated with aging are influenced by urethral dysfunction and abnormal vaginal support. In studies of age-matched elderly women and men, the American Urological Association symptom scores in older women were found to be the same as in older men.[26] The similarity among older men and older women in voiding symptoms suggests a common etiology related to the aging bladder. Another possible explanation is changes in the CNS control of the bladder that occur with aging which affect bladder function the same way in both older men and older women. Further research on the basic physiology of voiding in older people and the pathophysiology of OAB (both wet and dry) in the elderly will be essential for the evolution of new therapies in the future.

Incontinence in older people is almost always caused by multiple factors, of which not all are directly related to the genitourinary system.[27] Comorbidity is associated with abnormal bladder function in older people. The general health status of the older person is a risk factor for lower urinary tract symptoms. The role of a healthy lifestyle in bladder dysfunctions in older people has not been well studied.

Smoking, excess alcohol, obesity, lack of exercise, and inadequate consumption of fruits and vegetables are some of the risk factors researchers associate with morbidity and mortality at older ages.[2,28] Recent research shows that obesity is a risk factor for coronary artery disease, cancer, diabetes, hypertension, and functional disability.[2,29–32] Functional disability is associated with urinary incontinence in older people. In adults, physical activity has been found to lower the risk of cardiovascular diseases, diabetes, musculoskeletal problems, and cancer, and also to increase strength, physical functioning, and longevity.[2,29,33,34] Aerobic fitness in older people is also found to reduce brain tissue loss.[35] Few older adults achieve the recommended minimum of 30 minutes or more of moderate physical activity on 5 or more days a week.[2] Results show that physical activity decreases with age, with the 65-and-older population about five times more likely never to be physically active than those aged 18–24.[2] The association between a healthy lifestyle and bladder health in older people needs further investigation.

PHARMACOLOGICAL THERAPY

Antimuscarinic drug therapy represents the most common treatment for older patients with overactive bladder. However, antimuscarinic drugs are underutilized in elderly patients with overactive bladder, despite the marked increase in prevalence of overactive bladder symptoms in older people. The underutilization of effective anticholinergic treatment in older people may be related to concerns about the frequency of adverse events such as dry mouth, and the possibility of cognitive impairment and sleep disturbances.[36]

Anticholinergic therapy of OAB symptoms in older people has been shown to be effective in many well conducted studies.[37] Well designed clinical trials demonstrate the clinical efficacy of anticholinergic therapy in the treatment of OAB symptoms in older patients.[38] In reviewing OAB clinical trials it is important to recognize the complexity of the clinical problem being investigated and the many factors that influence the clinical outcome. OAB is a syndrome characterized by urinary urgency. Urinary urgency is a sudden, compelling, and difficult-to-defer desire to void. One-third of OAB patients experience urge urinary incontinence. From a research point of view, when measurement of symptoms with these characteristics is required to determine treatment outcome, the "placebo effect" can be relatively high, as it is in most OAB clinical trials using anticholinergic drugs. This does not necessarily represent a flaw in the research design, but is likely related to the elusive characteristics of the OAB syndrome with regard to clinical investigation.

Anticholinergic medications are not tissue specific, and their use for treatment of OAB has been associated with side effects. However, patients are willing to tolerate certain side effects in exchange for symptom relief.[36] Among the most common side effects of anticholinergic OAB therapy in older people are dry mouth and constipation. Concomitant use of stool softeners in the elderly increases tolerability of constipation, and stool softeners are usually an acceptable alternative to the patient. However, tolerability of dry mouth among older patients is variable.

While anticholinergic therapy for OAB symptoms in older people is widely used in the United States, there is a growing concern about the "anticholinergic load" in the elderly.[39] The anticholinergic load refers to the cumulative effect of taking multiple drugs with anticholinergic activity. It is difficult to evaluate the anticholinergic load in older patients, because many over-the-counter drugs have anticholinergic activity. In addition, older people often take multiple medications that have low anticholinergic activity, but the anticholinergic activity is cumulative.[40]

The cholinergic system is a major neuromodulatory neurotransmitter system interacting with core regions of the brain and affecting learning and memory function. Cholinergic function is severely reduced in patients with pathological conditions such as Alzheimer's disease. The extent to which a particular drug affects the cholinergic system may be determined by its ability to cross the blood–brain barrier. The integrity of the blood–brain barrier decreases with aging. The risk of cognitive impairment in elderly patients with overactive bladder medication may be reduced through use of more selective antagonists and combination therapy using behavioral modification.[39,41]

Cognitive dysfunction due to anticholinergic drug therapy for OAB symptoms needs to be further studied. Relatively sensitive measurement instruments may be required to determine small changes in cognitive function due to anticholinergic medications. Small changes in cognitive function in an older person could have serious implications. For example, the 65-and-over population had the second-highest death rate from motor vehicle accidents in 2000, following those aged 15–24.[2] Maintaining functional status that parallels longevity in older people represents one of the greatest challenges in medicine for the future.

Cardiac adverse events in older people due to anticholinergic therapy for OAB symptoms needs further study. Although millions of elderly patients have received anticholinergic therapy for OAB symptoms and there is no evidence for cardiac risk, the potential for cardiac risk will require further clinical investigation.[42] The M_3 muscarinic receptor subtype appears to be responsible for detrusor smooth muscle contraction.[43,44] The M_2 receptor subtype is primarily responsible for cardiac function. It is a clinical consideration that non-specific anticholinergic activity could prolong cardiac repolarization and prolong the QT interval. Since the QT interval is related to heart rate, a corrected QT interval (QTc interval) is used to evaluate adverse drug effects. Currently, there are multiple formulas for determining the corrected QT interval, including

Bazett, Framingham, Friderica, and Hodges formulas.[45,46] A stronger consensus is needed regarding the definition of an abnormal QTc interval and further clinical investigation regarding the risks and clinical implications of anticholinergic therapy is needed. Clinically, a prolonged QTc interval can result in ventricular arrhythmias that are referred to as torsade de pointes, polymorphic ventricular tachycardia, atypical ventricular tachycardia, proarrhythmia, and drug induced ventricular tachycardia. At this time, the clinical entity appears to be confined to patients receiving cardiovascular drugs that are known to prolong cardiac repolarization.[47]

BEHAVIORAL THERAPY

Despite the proven effectiveness of patient dependent behavioral therapy in older patients, physicians rarely prescribe these interventions for urinary incontinence.[48] Perhaps one of the most perplexing observations in clinical practice patterns of healthcare professionals who manage OAB symptoms in the elderly is the common knowledge of the effectiveness of behavioral therapy in the treatment of OAB symptoms of older people and the rare utilization of the intervention. While behavioral therapy of OAB symptoms in the elderly is effective with minimal side effects, significant barriers to the clinical utilization of behavioral therapy exist. First, the healthcare professional must be committed to the behavioral therapy program. In addition, the patient must be an active participant in the program. Unlike passively taking a pill, behavioral therapy is an active process and requires patient participation.

Of the different behavioral therapies, biofeedback is one of the most effective. Biofeedback therapy in older people requires excellent equipment because some of the older patients will have compromised cortical function. The method of feedback of physiological performance to the patient needs to be engaging so that the patient can actively participate in the biofeedback sessions. The biofeedback therapist needs to be extremely skilled in behavioral therapy techniques as well as skilled in working with older people. Biofeedback therapy of older patients with OAB symptoms requires multiple sessions. Sometimes, it is not feasible for the older patient to travel to the biofeedback laboratory for the

number of therapy sessions that are required for that particular individual. Sometimes, it is not clinically or financially feasible for a healthcare professional to provide biofeedback therapy as a treatment option either in the office or by referral.

Many well designed clinical trials have demonstrated exceptional efficacy using behavioral therapy in older patients who suffer from urinary urgency and urge urinary incontinence. Behavioral therapies present no risk of adverse events for elderly patients. Clinically significant reductions in urinary incontinence are achievable with behavioral therapies in many cognitively intact homebound older adults, despite high levels of comorbidity and functional impairment.[49] Behavioral treatment is a safe and effective conservative intervention that should be made more readily available to patients as a first line treatment for urge and mixed incontinence.[50] Combining drug and behavioral therapy can produce added benefit for patients with urge incontinence.[51] In a study of older community-dwelling women, patients who received both drug treatment and behavioral therapy experienced significant clinical improvement compared with patients receiving monotherapy using either treatment.[52] In a study of older incontinent women, behavioral therapy reduced nocturia significantly more than did drug treatment. Both behavioral training and drug treatment reduced nocturia more than placebo, but behavioral training was the most effective.[53]

ELECTRICAL STIMULATION

Patients implanted with a sacral neuromodulator for refractory urge incontinence showed no daily leakage episodes after permanent implantation in 65% of patients under 55 years old, compared with 37% of patients over 55 years old. Both age and chronic conditions were independent factors associated with failure in patients implanted with a sacral neuromodulator for treatment of refractory urge urinary incontinence.[54] The outcome of sacral nerve stimulation is more unpredictable in the elderly.[55] While results of sacral nerve stimulation in older people have been disappointing, significant improvement in many older patients has occurred. Further clinical investigation using sacral nerve stimulation in older people needs to be done to possibly improve patient selection and to consider combination therapies in the future.

CONCLUSION

OAB is a debilitating condition that affects millions of older Americans. OAB symptoms can be devastating to the quality of life of an older person. Yet, OAB therapies for the elderly remain drastically underutilized. Advances in medicine have resulted in longer life for older people, but quality of life in later years must make the extra years of life meaningful. It is the dawn of an unprecedented era in history that will witness the number of people over 65 years old in the United States double from 35 million in the year 2000 to 72 million in the year 2030. OAB symptoms significantly increase with each passing decade of life. The debilitating symptoms of OAB have the capacity to shatter the hopes and dreams of older people for quality of life in their later years. New OAB therapies need to be available and utilized by the next generation of older people to insure a long and fulfilling life.

REFERENCES

1. Kinchen KS, Burgio K, Diokno AC et al. Factors associated with women's decisions to seek treatment of urinary incontinence. J Womens Health 2003; 12: 687–98.
2. Wan H, Sengupta M, Velkoff VA, DeBarros KA. US Census Bureau, Current Population Reports, P23–209, 65+ in the United States: 2005; Washington, DC: US Government Printing Office, 2005.
3. Manton KG, Stallard E. Health and disability differences among racial and ethnic groups. In: Martin LG, Soldo BJ, eds. Racial and Ethnic Differences in the Health of Older Americans. Washington, DC: National Academy Press 1997: 43–105.
4. Freedman VA. Understanding trends in functional limitations among older Americans. Am J Public Health 1998 10: 1457–62.
5. Manton KG, Gu X. Changes in the prevalence of chronic disability in the United States black and non-black population above age 65, from 1982 to 1999. Proc Natl Acad Sci USA 2001; 98: 6354–9.
6. Freedman VA, Martin LG, Schoeni RF. Recent trends in disability and functioning among older adults in the United States. J Am Med Assoc 2002 288: 3137–46.
7. Spillman BC, Lubitz J. The effect of longevity on spending for acute and long-term care. N Engl J Med 2000; 342: 1409–15.
8. Feder J, Komisar HL, Niefeld M. Long-term care in the United States: an overview. Health Aff 2000; 19: 40–56.
9. Lee R, Tuljapurkar S. Death and taxes: longer life, consumption, and social security. Demography 1997; 34: 67–81.
10. Cohen RA, Bloom B, Simpson G, Parsons PE. Access to health care. Part 3: Older adults. Vital Health Stat 10 1997; 198: 1–32.
11. Landerman LR, Fillenbaum GG, Pieper CF et al. Private health insurance coverage and disability among older Americans. J Gerontol B Psychol Sci Soc Sci 1998; 53: S258–66.
12. Hu TW, Wagner TH, Bentkover JD et al. Costs of urinary incontinence and overactive bladder in the United States: a comparative study. Urology 2004; 63: 461–5.
13. Yoshida M, Miyamae K, Iwashita H et al. Management of detrusor dysfunction in the elderly: changes in acetylcholine and adenosine triphosphate release during aging. Urology 2004; 63: 17–23.
14. Sjuve R, Uvelius B, Arner A. Old age does not affect shortening velocity or content of contractile and cytoskeletal proteins in the rat detrusor smooth muscle. Urol Res 1997; 25: 67–70.
15. Yu JH, Wein JF, Levin RM. Age-related differential susceptibility to calcium channel blocker and low calcium medium in rat detrusor muscle: response to field stimulation. Neurourol Urodyn 1996; 15: 563–76.
16. Wuest M, Morgenstern K, Graf EM et al. Cholinergic and purinergic responses in isolated human detrusor in relation to age. J Urol 2005; 173: 2182–9.
17. Barker JC, Mitteness LS. Nocturia in the elderly. Gerontologist 1988; 28: 99–104.
18. O'Donnell PD. Pathophysiology of incontinence in elderly men. In: O'Donnell PD, ed. Geriatric Urology. Boston: Little Brown: and Co., 1994: 229–38.
19. O'Donnell PD, Walls RC. Residual urine volume following involuntary voiding in elderly inpatient men. Neurourol Urodyn 1990; 9: 35–42.
20. O'Donnell PD, Beck CM, Finkbeiner AE. Incontinence volume measurements in elderly inpatient men. Urology 1990; 35: 499–503.

21. O'Donnell PD. The volume-interval relationship of incontinence episodes in elderly inpatient men. Urology 1993; 41: 334–7.

22. O'Donnell PD, Beck CM. Incontinence volume patterns in elderly inpatient men. Urology 1991; 38: 128–31.

23. O'Donnell PD. The continence interval in elderly incontinent men. Neurourol Urodyn 1989; 8: 1–7.

24. O'Donnell PD. The pathophysiology of urinary incontinence in the elderly. Adv Urol 1991; 4: 129–42.

25. O'Donnell PD, Doyle R. Biofeedback therapy technique for treatment of urinary incontinence. Urology 1991; 37: 432–6.

26. Chancellor MB, Rivas DA. American Urological Association symptom index for women with voiding symptoms: lack of index specificity for benign prostate hyperplasia. J Urol 1993; 150: 1706–8; discussion 1708–9.

27. Dubueau CD. The aging lower urinary tract. J Urol 2006; 175: S11–15.

28. Burns DM. Cigarette smoking among the elderly: disease consequences and the benefits of cessation. Am J Health Promot 2000; 14: 357–61.

29. Blackman DK, Kamimoto LA, Smith SM. Overview: surveillance for selected public health indictors affecting older adults—United States. MMWR Surveill Summ 1999; 48 (SS08): 1–6.

30. Himes CL. Obesity, disease, and functional limitation in later life. Demography 2000; 37: 73–82.

31. Sturum, R. The effects of obesity, smoking, and problem drinking on chronic medical problems and health care costs. Health Affairs 2002; 21: 245–53.

32. RAND Corp. The Health Risks of Obesity: Worse Than Smoking, Drinking, or Poverty. RAND Health Research Highlights 2002: RB–4549.

33. Powell KE. Thompson PD, Caspersen CJ, Kendrick JS. Physical activity and the incidence of coronary heart disease. Annu Rev Public Health 1987; 8: 253–87.

34. Keysor JJ, Jette AM. Have we oversold the benefit of late-life exercise? J Gerontol A Biol Sci Med Sci 2001; 56: M412–23.

35. Colcombe SJ, Erickson KI, Rax N et al. Aerobic fitness reduces brain tissue loss in aging humans. J Gerontol A Biol Sci Med Sci 2003; 58: M176–80.

36. Staskin DR. Overactive bladder in the elderly: a guide to pharmacological management. Drugs Aging 2005; 22: 1013–28.

37. Wagg A, Wyndaele JJ, Sieber P. Efficacy and tolerability of solifenacin in elderly subjects with overactive bladder syndrome: a pooled analysis, Am J Geriatr Pharmacother 2006: 14–24.

38. Foote J, Glavind K, Kralidis G, Wyndaele JJ. Treatment of overactive bladder in the older patient: pooled analysis of three phase III studies of darifenacin, an M3 selective receptor antagonist. Eur Urol 2005; 48: 471–7.

39. Kay G, Pollack BG, Romanzi LJ. Unmasking anticholinergic load: when $1 + 1 = 3$. CNS Spectr 2004; 9: 1–11.

40. Ancelin ML, Artero S, Portet F et al. Non-degenerative mild cognitive impairment in elderly people and use of anticholinergic drugs: longitudinal cohort study. BMJ 2006; 332: 455–9.

41. Lipton RB, Kolodner K, Wesnes K. Assessment of cognitive function of the elderly population: effects of darifenacin. J Urol 2005; 173: 493–8.

42. Garley AD, Burrows L. Benefit-risk assessment of tolterodine in the treatment of overactive bladder in adults. Drug Saf 2004; 27: 1043–57.

43. Scarpero HM, Dmochowski RR. Muscarinic receptors: what we know. Curr Urol Rep 2003; 4: 421–8.

44. Chess-Williams R, Chapple CR, Yamanishi T et al. The minor population of M3-receptors mediate contraction of human detrusor muscle in vitro. J Auton Pharmacol 2001; 21: 243–8.

45. Milic M, Bao X, Rizos D et al. Literature review and pilot studies of the effect of QT correction formulas on reported beta2-agonist-induced CTc prolongation. Clin Ther 2006; 28: 582–90.

46. Luo S, Michler K, Johnston P, Macfarlane PW. A comparison of commonly used QT correction formulae: the effect of heart rate on the QTc of normal ECGs. J Electrocardiol 2004; 37: 81–90.

47. Makkar RR, Fromm BS, Steinman RT et al. Female gender as a risk factor for torsades de pointes associated with cardiovascular drugs. JAMA 1993; 270: 2590–7.

48. Gnanadesigan N, Saliba D, Roth CP et al. The quality of care provided to vulnerable older community-based patients with urinary incontinence. J Am Med Dir Assoc 2004; 5: 141–6.

49. McDowell BJ, Engberg S, Sereika S et al. Effectiveness of behavioral therapy to treat incontinence in homebound older adults. J Am Geriatr Soc 1999; 47: 309–18.

50. Burgio KL, Locher JL, Goode PS et al. Behavioral vs drug treatment for urge urinary incontinence in older women: a randomized controlled trial. JAMA 1998; 280: 1995–2000.

51. Burgio KL, Locher JL, Goode PS. Combined behavioral and drug therapy for urge incontinence in older women. J Am Geriatr Soc 2000; 48: 370–4.

52. Goode PS. Behavioral and drug therapy for urinary incontinence. Urology 2004 63: 58–64.

53. Johnson TM 2nd, Burgio KL, Redden DT et al. Effects of behavioral and drug therapy on nocturia in older incontinent women. J Am Geriatr Soc 2005; 53: 846–50.

54. Amundsen CL, Romero AA, Jamison MG, Webster GD. Sacral neuromodulation for intractable urge incontinence: are there factors associated with cure? Urology 2005; 66: 746–50.

55. Edlund C, Dijkema HE, Hassouna MM et al. Sacral nerve stimulation for refractory urge symptoms in elderly patients. Scand J Urol Nephrol 2004; 38: 131–5.

34

Late breaking information

Jean Jacques Wyndaele

Basic physiology and pathophysiology • **Diagnostic methods** • **Clinical pharmacological data** • **Specific patient groups** • **Neurostimulation** • **Cost**

Recent information about overactive bladder (OAB) is extensive. In PubMed alone, 608 items could be found on a search carried out at the beginning of July 2006 and covering the first 6 months of 2006. This is enough evidence that the topic is still under substantial investigation. The serious impact of the condition on personal, social, and economic life will be one of the reasons for the interest in OAB. The very active involvement of industry is another reason.

We have looked into the newer data concerning OAB, and present here what seems to be the most important. There are findings on basic physiology and pathophysiology, methods to measure the impact of OAB, clinical pharmacological data, specific patient groups such as the elderly and children, and data on neurostimulation.

BASIC PHYSIOLOGY AND PATHOPHYSIOLOGY

A major recent evolution in OAB concepts is the shift from focusing on motor/efferent function to more interest in the sensory/afferent function. Heretofore, attention was given only to the consequences of the OAB condition, the involuntary contractions of the detrusor, and research was almost exclusively directed at postponing, lowering, or abolishing such contractions. More and more it has been appreciated that involuntary contraction of the detrusor can be, and most probably is, the result of altered mechanisms of sensory input from the bladder. Data from animal research have strongly reinforced this idea. Moreover, it has become clear that OAB symptoms

can be present without detrusor overactivity. There has developed a better understanding of how normal bladder activity is regulated, and how changes in these mechanisms may be responsible for the OAB condition. This has led to an ever increasing interest in afferent related physiology and pathophysiology, with applications to diagnosis and treatment.

Neuropeptide Y has an important role in the neural regulation of the lower urinary tract by exerting differential effects on the release of cholinergic and adrenergic transmitters via autoinhibition and heterosynaptic interactions.[1] Haferkamp et al. showed that in detrusor biopsies the number of neuropeptide Y-containing nerves was significantly reduced in patients with neurogenic OAB. They hypothesize that these findings may have been caused by transsynaptic nerve degeneration of the detrusor, as described in patients with spinal cord injury. As neuropeptide Y inhibits the contractile response of the detrusor, the reduction of neuropeptide Y-containing nerves may play a role in the development and persistence of detrusor overactivity (DO).

The role of tachykinins such as neurokinin A (NKA) in regulating bladder function is unclear, but NK_2 receptors seem to mediate contraction in the human bladder, and it has been suggested that these peptides may have a role in the pathophysiology of bladder dysfunction. Sellers et al. investigated neurokinin receptor-mediated contractility of the detrusor muscle in the idiopathic overactive and neurogenic overactive bladder, and investigated the neurokinin receptor subtypes involved.[2] They showed that NKA-induced responses were impaired in detrusor muscle from idiopathic overactive human bladder, but not in detrusor muscle from neurogenic overactive bladder. The NK_2 receptor subtype appears to mediate NKA responses in the normal, idiopathic overactive, and neurogenic overactive detrusor. These findings suggest a difference between the bladder pathophysiology observed in idiopathic versus neurogenic overactive detrusor.

Muscarinic receptor antagonists (antimuscarinics) serve as the cornerstone in the pharmacological management of OAB.[3] They are thought to operate primarily by antagonizing postjunctional excitatory muscarinic receptors (M_2/M_3) in the detrusor. The combination of pharmacological and gene knockout studies has greatly advanced our understanding of the functional role of muscarinic receptors in the bladder. M_3 receptors produce direct smooth muscle contraction by a mechanism that relies on entry of extracellular calcium through L-type channels and activation of a rho kinase. M_2 receptors, which predominate in number, appear to facilitate M_3-mediated contractions. M_2 receptors can also produce bladder contractions indirectly by reversing cyclic adenosine monophosphate (cAMP)-dependent β-adrenoceptor-mediated relaxation, although the physiological role of β-adrenoceptors in detrusor relaxation is controversial. Emerging evidence suggests that muscarinic receptors in the urothelium/suburothelium can modulate the release of certain factors, which in turn may affect bladder function at the efferent or afferent axis.

De Wachter and Wyndaele tested the influence of intravesical oxybutynin on single Aδ and C fibers in the pelvic nerve in rat bladder.[4] They showed that at 15 minutes after oxybutynin was washed out of the bladder, C fiber afferents responded significantly less to intravesical pressure and volume compared with control filling. At 60 minutes, C fibers partly regained mechanosensivity. After 90 minutes, sensitivity still increased, without achieving the response level before oxybutynin. No significant changes were noted in the Aδ fibers during repeat blad-der filling or after oxybutynin instillation. This study showed that intravesical oxybutynin has a direct anesthetic effect within the bladder wall. It temporarily desensitizes C fiber

afferents, which could explain its clinical benefits in decreasing symptoms of bladder overactivity. No measurable effect was found on Aδ fibers after this short exposure time.

De Laet et al. continued this study with systemic administration of oxybutynin.[5] A decrease in afferent activity was noted after systemic administration of oxybutynin for C fibers at 90 and 120 min after drug delivery. After 150 min, the spike rate was still lower compared to the baseline filling, but not significantly. For the Aδ fibers the decrease in afferent spike rate was already significant at 30 min and remained significant during the entire evaluation time. This decrease in afferent spike rate was shown not to be the result of an increased compliance. The findings of this study strongly suggest that oxybutynin directly or indirectly influences bladder sensory nerves, inhibiting the afferent part of the micturition reflex. If confirmed with other, more specific bladder relaxing drugs, this may change our understanding of the action mechanisms with this type of therapy.

Griffiths et al. have, in a pilot study, sought causes of OAB in the supraspinal control system with functional magnetic resonance imaging (fMRI).[6] fMRI detected activation of many brain regions involved in bladder control, including the periaqueductal gray, thalamus, insula, dorsal anterior cingulate, and ventromedial cerebellum. The orbitofrontal cortex, pontine micturition center, and preoptic hypothalamus were visible in subgroup analyses. Activations outweighed deactivations and responses became stronger at larger bladder volumes. Among subjects with good control, this strengthening of response was prominent in the orbitofrontal cortex. Among those with poor control, cortical responses were exaggerated at larger bladder volumes, except in the orbitofrontal cortex, which remained weakly activated. This difference was not due to concurrent detrusor activity. This study suggests a similar neurophysiological basis for poor bladder control in the absence of overt neurological lesion.

Kim et al. investigated changes in urinary nerve growth factor (NGF) and prostaglandins (PGs) in women with OAB.[7] Urinary NGF, PGE_2 and $PGF_{2\alpha}$ were significantly increased in patients with OAB compared with controls. However, urinary PGI_2 was not different between controls and patients with OAB. In patients with OAB, urinary

PGE_2 positively correlated with the volume at first desire to void and maximum cystometric capacity. Urinary NGF, $PGF_{2\alpha}$, and PGI_2 did not correlate with urodynamic parameters in patients with OAB. These findings imply the need to further evaluate the role of urinary levels of NGF and PGs as markers to evaluate OAB symptoms.

DIAGNOSTIC METHODS

Diagnostic methods and criteria for OAB remain controversial. Hashim and Abrams studied the reliability of symptoms for predicting detrusor overactivity using the International Continence Society definitions.[8] They found a better correlation in results between OAB symptoms and the urodynamic diagnosis of DO in men than in women, more so in OAB wet than in OAB dry patients. This finding weakens somewhat the general concept that the bladder is an unreliable witness in all circumstances.

De Wachter and Wyndaele studied frequency–volume charts, and more specifically their importance in assessing bladder sensation and its relationship to urodynamic findings, in healthy volunteers.[9] Bladder sensation can be easily evaluated by scoring the grade of perception of fullness on frequency–volume charts. In non-OAB individuals, voiding usually occurs without a specific desire to void, and this needs to be studied further in patients with OAB. The voided volumes at different sensations of fullness were comparable to the volumes at different sensations of filling during cystometry.

Wyndaele et al. evaluated the differences between patients with overactive bladder (OAB) who felt involuntary detrusor contractions during cystometry (detrusor overactivity, DO) and those who did not feel them.[10] They found that those without DO sensation were more frequently incontinent and had more involuntary detrusor contractions, and these contractions occurred earlier during bladder filling. Those individuals also had the involuntary initiation of voiding more frequently, more pathological sensation of bladder filling, and lower electrical sensory thresholds than the comparator population. The results of drug treatment were better in the group who had sensory aspects attendant with their DO. This study implies that it is likely that different OAB conditions exist with a different neuropathological cause and a different treatment outcome. This study also shows that assessing sensation specifically is clinically important in OAB outcomes reporting.

Evaluation and grading of the OAB condition and its impact on a patient's life has been done in different ways. Patient perception of bladder condition (PPBC) has been extensively studied by Coyne et al.[11] The PPBC, a global patient-reported measure of bladder condition, demonstrated good construct validity and responsiveness to change in post hoc analyses on two 12-week clinical trials for OAB. In a subsequent publication, Coyne et al. established the minimally important difference of the overactive bladder questionnaire.[12] Their findings by multiple methodologies provide strong justification for the recommendation of a 10-point minimally important difference for all overactive bladder questionnaire subscales.

Coyne et al. also validated an overactive bladder awareness tool for use in primary care settings.[13] The participants completed an eight-item questionnaire assessing the amount of "bother" they associated with OAB symptoms. Clinicians then asked the patients four questions regarding urinary frequency, urgency, nocturia, and incontinence. If the screening was positive for symptoms of OAB or if the patient provided positive responses to the urinary symptom questions, the clinician asked additional questions regarding lifestyle and coping behaviors. The clinician then diagnosed the patient, placing him or her in the "no OAB", "possible OAB", or "probable OAB" category. This approach performed well in helping clinicians identify patients with bothersome OAB symptoms in a primary care setting who may benefit from treatment.

Homma and Koyama studied the minimal clinically important change (MCIC) in frequency of incontinence episodes in Japanese patients with OAB, based on the change in domain scores of health-related quality of life (HRQoL).[14] They found that Japanese OAB patients feel that their QoL has improved if their incontinence episodes decrease more than three times/week, suggesting that the reduction of three times/week is an MCIC of incontinence frequency for Japanese OAB patients.

The impact of OAB on quality of life is now becoming better established. A recent study evaluated the effect of OAB on women's QoL during and after the first pregnancy, using self-reported symptom-based QoL questionnaires.[15] The results, in a large population, showed not only that OAB symptoms are common during pregnancy, but also that dry OAB had no effect on QoL, whereas wet OAB compromised QoL both during and after pregnancy, mainly in the "mobility" and "embarrassment" domains. The urge urinary incontinence symptom in wet OAB seems to profoundly compromise QoL. Apparently, in young mothers with wet OAB, limitations in mobility are especially stressful.

The differentiation of neurogenic (NDO) and non-neurogenic (IDO) detrusor overactivity remains an area of active interest. Lemack et al. have recently evaluated the urodynamic characteristics of the two, comparing multiple sclerosis (MS) and idiopathic DO (IDO) in order to determine whether urodynamic distinctions could differentiate the different etiologies of DO.[16] They found the amplitude of the first overactive contraction to be statistically greater in patients with MS and NDO compared with patients with IDO, as was the maximal detrusor contraction. The threshold volume for DO was greater among patients with NDO, likely secondary to the elevated post-void residual urine volume in patients with MS. Using a cutoff value of 30 cmH_2O for amplitude of the first overactive contraction, a positive predictive value of 88% for identifying MS in their data set was noted.

CLINICAL PHARMACOLOGICAL DATA

Placebo response

Van Leeuwen et al. recently reviewed placebo responses in randomized controlled trials (RCTs) for pharmacologic treatment of lower urinary tract symptoms (LUTS), including urinary incontinence, overactive bladder, and benign prostatic hyperplasia. Review papers on placebo effects in non-urologic disorders were assessed, to compare the magnitude of placebo responses in drugs for LUTS with those reported for other diseases.[17] They found that placebo treatment of LUTS yields reductions in incontinence episodes (IEs) ranging from 32% to 65%, whereas prostate or urinary incontinence (UI) symptom scores are reduced by 9–34%. Active pharmacologic agents decrease IEs by 45–77% and symptom scores by 22–45%. Placebo responses are much lower when objective changes in voided volume or peak flow rate are assessed.

Multiple publications have recently summarized results with a variety of agents. Details of the study methods are given in Table 34.1.

Tolterodine

Nitti et al. performed post hoc analysis of data from a 12-week, double-blind study of 850 patients randomized to tolterodine extended release (ER) (4 mg once daily) or placebo, taken within 4 h of going to bed.[18] They described significant improvement in urgency rating (24-h voids were categorized by urgency rating: total (1–5), non-OAB (1–2), OAB (3–4), and severe OAB (4–5) voids) and reduced 24-h OAB, severe OAB, and total voids compared with placebo.

Roehrborn et al. studied the effect of tolterodine ER by post hoc analysis of data collected from men with OAB and urgency incontinence (UI) enrolled in a 12-week, double-blind, placebo-controlled trial.[19] Tolterodine demonstrated a significant reduction in weekly UI episodes, fewer micturitions/24 h (not significant), and significantly higher subjective treatment benefit.

Roberts et al. reported the effect of tolterodine ER on patient- and clinician-reported outcomes in a primary care setting.[20] By week 12, there were statistically significant and clinically meaningful decreases on the OAB questionnaire (OAB-q) and American Urological Association Symptom Index (AUA-SI) total and subscale scores. Seventy-nine percent of patients experienced some improvement in their overall bladder condition. The authors reported that 68% of patients were "much improved" or "very much improved". A separate publication summarized the effect on the most bothersome symptoms of OAB.[21] Among incontinent patients these were daytime frequency, urgency urinary incontinence (UUI), nocturnal frequency, and urgency; among continent patients, these were daytime frequency, nocturnal frequency, and urgency. Sixty-nine percent of patients had one or more comorbid conditions. By week 12, there were significant reductions in patients' most bothersome symptoms: −80% for UUI, −78% for urgency episodes, −40% for nocturnal frequency, and −30% for daytime frequency.

Table 34.1 Literature data of drug studies in OAB published during the last year.

Authors/ trial (ref)	Drug + dose	Type analyse	N patients	Type patients	Duration	Type
Nitti et al (18)	Tolterodine ER 4 mg	Post hoc	513	OAB dry and nocturia	12 w	Double blind placebo controlled
Roerbron et al (19)	Tolterodine ER 4 mg	Post hoc	163	men with OAB and UUI	12 w	Double blind placebo controlled
IMPACT (20–21)	Tolterodine ER 4 mg	prospective	863 ITT intent to treat	OAB	12 w	single
Rackley et al (22)	Tolterodine ER 4 mg night	prospective	850		12 w	Double blind placebo controlled
Abrams et al (23)	Tolterodine 2 × 2mg	prospective	221	Men>40 with outlet obstruction	12 w	RCT with placebo
OPERA (24)	Tolterodine ER versus Oxybutinin ER 10 mg	Post hoc analysis		OAB previous treated or not	12 w	
Staskin and Te (26)	Solifenacin 5 and 10 mg	Prospective	1041 12W 433 40 w	Mixed UI	12 w followed by open 40 weeks	RCT with placebo and extended open label
Millard and Halaska (27)	Solifenacin 5 and 10 mg	Post hoc Pooled	2848	Severe OAB		RCT placebo ,5mg and 10 mg
Cardozo et al (28)	Solifenacin 5 and 10 mg	Posthoc pooled	1873	OAB Incontinence	12 w	RCT's with placebo, 5 mg and 10 mg
Noguchi et al (30)	Propiverine	Prospective	68	Frequency and/ or incontinence	8 w	Open label
Sugiyama et al (31)	Propiverine 10mg, 20 mg qd	prospective	7	Urgency, frequency, incontinence	4 w + 4 w	Cross over
Stohrer et al (32)	Propiverine 15 mg t.i.d versus oxybutynin 5 mg t.i.d	prospective	131	Neurogenic OAB	21 d	RCT, double blind, multicenter between both drugs

Table 34.1 Continued

Authors/ trial (ref)	Drug + dose	Type analyse	N patients	Type patients	Duration	
Rudy et al (33–34)	Trospium 20 mg t.d	prospective	658	OAB	12 w	multicenter, parallel, double-blind, placebo-controlled study
Pannek et al (37)	Oxybutinin, Capsaicin, EMDA intravesical	prospective	52 oxy, 16 capsa, 28 EMDA	DOA	once	Open label
Zinner et al (38)	controlled release darifenacin 15 mg once daily	prospective	445	OAB	12 w	double-blind, randomised placebo-controlled, multicentre
Hill et al (39)	darifenacin controlled-release tablets 7.5 mg, 15 mg or 30 mg qd, or placebo	prospective	439	OAB	12 W	multicenter, double-blind, placebo-controlled dose-ranging study
Wagg et al (40)	Solifenacin 5 mg or 10 mg qd	Retrospective pooled data	1045 12w 509 ext	OAB partients = or > 65	12 w and extended 40 weeks	double-blind, international, multicenter, randomized, parallel-group, fixed-dose, placebo-controlled and open-label, flexible-dose extension
Foote et al (41)	darifenacin 7.5 mg or 15 mg qd or placebo	retrospective pooled data	317	OAB aged = or > 65	12 w	pooled analysis of three phase III, multicentre, randomized, double-blind clinical trials
Kilic et al (44)	Tolterodine or oxybutinin	prospective	30 tolterodine 30 oxybutinin	DOA mean <8 years old	6 m or >	2 treatments outcome
Van Arendonk et al (45)	oxybutinin	retrospective	81	Children daytime UI	Average 1.2 y	Open label

Rackley et al., for the 037 Study Group, studied night-time tolterodine ER (TER) in an RCT.[22] TER reduced the total number of nocturnal micturitions, but, compared with placebo, this difference was not statistically significant. TER significantly reduced OAB-related micturitions during 24-hour, daytime, and night-time intervals. TER did not affect normal (non-OAB) micturitions. Side effects were minimal.

Abrams et al. used pressure flow urodynamics to evaluate safety and tolerability of tolterodine 2 mg twice daily in men with outflow obstruction.[23] Median treatment differences in peak flow (Q_{max}) and detrusor pressure at Q_{max} ($PdetQ_{max}$) were comparable. Tolterodine significantly reduced the bladder outlet obstruction index (BOOI), versus placebo. There were significant treatment differences in volume to first detrusor contraction and maximum cystometric capacity, favoring tolterodine over placebo. Changes in post-void residual (PVR) volume were statistically significantly greater among patients treated with tolterodine. However, the authors speculated that these increases were not clinically significant. Urinary retention was reported by one patient treated with placebo.

Anderson et al. studied the efficacy and the tolerability of extended release oxybutynin chloride, 10 mg daily, and extended release tolterodine tartrate, 4 mg daily, in women with or without prior anticholinergic treatment for OAB (OPERA trial).[24] There results suggest that treatment for OAB may be initiated with extended release oxybutynin, particularly in women presenting with incontinence. Some slight statistical differences between the two groups in efficacy outcomes and safety were noted, which differed between those previously treated for OAB and those who were anticholinergic-naive.

Taylor published a case report about probable interaction between tolterodine and warfarin.[25] When patients are prescribed tolterodine and warfarin concurrently, clinicians should monitor the International Normalized Ratio (INR) carefully, and a reduction in warfarin dosage may be required.

Solifenacin

Staskin and Te studied post hoc data from four studies, and assessed the short- and long-term efficacy of solifenacin in patients with symptoms of mixed urinary incontinence.[26] A 12-week randomized double-blind placebo controlled treatment period followed by an open label period of 40 weeks constituted the study time frame. They concluded that significant reductions in OAB-related frequency, incontinence, and urgency were shown after 12 weeks of solifenacin treatment in patients with a history of mixed urinary incontinence (MUI). Symptom improvement in this subgroup was maintained during long-term treatment.

Millard and Halaska[27] evaluated solifenacin use in patients with severe symptoms of OAB with a pooled analysis. Solifenacin was significantly more effective than placebo for patients with severe symptoms of OAB (as assessed by incontinence episodes and magnitude of urgency). This response was observed for all endpoints with solifenacin 10 mg and for the majority of the endpoints with solifenacin 5 mg.

Cardozo et al. evaluated the effect of solifenacin on OAB-related incontinence.[28] More than 50% of the total population became continent at the study end, with either dose (5 or 10 mg) of solifenacin.

Oki et al. performed a comparative evaluation of exocrine muscarinic receptor binding characteristics and inhibition of salivation with solifenacin in comparison with those of oxybutynin in mice.[29] The results indicate that the weaker suppression of cholinergic salivation by solifenacin compared with oxybutynin may be partially attributed to its relatively fast dissociation from exocrine muscarinic receptors.

Propiverine

Noguchi et al. evaluated how urinary frequency and incontinence affect the patient's subjective quality of life (QoL) and whether an improvement in objective findings by medical treatment is reflected in the subjective QoL assessment. They found that active drug improved subjective QoL and objective findings in Japanese patients with urinary frequency and/or incontinence, and that there was a high correlation between degrees of improvement in subjective and objective measures.[30]

Sugiyama et al. evaluated the clinical benefit of propiverine hydrochloride in OAB, and the relationships between urinary voiding functions and the pharmacokinetics by means of clinical pharmacology (correlative clinical outcomes with pharmacokinetic/pharmacodynamic (PK/PD) values).[31] The volume at first desire to void increased as dosing magnitude increased, while the volume at first involuntary contraction tended to increase according to both dose and drug concentration in plasma. However, no apparent dose–response relationships were observed for maximum urinary flow rate or for detrusor pressure at maximum urinary flow rate. After the administration of propiverine hydrochloride, the concentration in plasma immediately reached levels at which the drug could increase the volume at first involuntary contraction by 50%. Subsequently, the concentration level sustained an effect ranging from 10% to 50% increase in bladder volume. Lower urinary tract obstruction was found to be a predictor of an increase in urinary residual volume.

Stöhrer et al. compared propiverine and oxybutynin in a neurogenic OAB population.[32] They found that propiverine and oxybutynin were equally effective in increasing bladder capacity and lowering bladder pressure in patients with neurogenic detrusor overactivity. The trend for better tolerability with propiverine compared to oxybutynin achieved significance for dryness of the mouth.

Trospium

Rudy et al. studied the efficacy and safety of trospium chloride for OAB in a multicenter, parallel, double-blind, placebo-controlled study.[33] Trospium chloride had significant and sustained effectiveness beginning at the end of week 1 and continuing through 12 weeks of treatment (the average number of daily toilet voids, average urgency severity, urge frequency, and urge urinary incontinence episodes, and increased the average volume per void). Adverse events included dry mouth and constipation.

The same investigators evaluated the time to onset of statistically significant and clinically meaningful effects of trospium chloride in the same patient group.[34] There were clinically meaningful improvements in most endpoints by the end of the first week. The authors concluded that the time to onset of the clinical effect in drug

treatment should be studied more extensively so as to inform patients when they might expect a symptomatically meaningful improvement.

Oxybutinin

Pannek et al. evaluated intravesical treatment with oxybutynin, capsaicin, and EMDA (electromotive drug administration) in patients with detrusor overactivity.[35] Intravesical oxybutynin was successful in 86%, capsaicin in 47%, and EMDA in 78%; however, all sample sizes were small. Two transient ischemic attacks followed EMDA.

Darifenacin

Zinner et al. assessed warning time (time from first sensation of urgency to voiding or involuntary loss of urine) in OAB patients treated with darifenacin amongst other outcome measures.[36] Darifenacin treatment resulted in numerical increases in warning time, but these were not significant compared with placebo, and these changes also were highly variable between individuals. Most other outcome measures (urge incontinence episodes/week, volume voided, QoL, urgency-free time) responded to drug administration.

Hill et al. evaluated darifenacin in a fixed dose study design.[37] Darifenacin significantly reduced the median number of incontinence episodes/week from baseline at 7.5, 15, and 30 mg, and dose-relatedly improved micturition frequency, frequency, and severity of urgency, nocturia, and bladder capacity. The authors conclude that dosing flexibility between 7.5 and 15 mg daily is possible for an optimal result.

Naftopidil

The clinical efficacy of the α-adrenoceptor blocker naftopidil, 50–75 mg/day for 6 weeks, on overactive bladder symptoms in 81 patients with benign prostatic hyperplasia was studied, with frequency–volume charts, by Takahashi et al.[38] They found significant improvement in total International Prostate Symptom Score (IPSS), in both storage and voiding symptom scores, urgency severity scores, daytime and night-time frequency, mean volume/void, and nocturia. Notably, significant improvement in nocturia was observed in patients both with and without nocturnal polyuria.

SPECIFIC PATIENT GROUPS

Elderly

Kay et al. summarized the proceedings of an expert panel meeting convened to review not only the mechanisms by which antimuscarinic agents could affect cognitive function, but also the published literature on cognitive adverse events.[39] A review of the literature shows that the cholinergic system in the central nervous system (CNS) exerts a major influence on cognitive processes, in particular memory, via M_1 cholinergic receptors. In addition, recent evidence suggests a role for M_2 receptors in mediating cognitive function. Thus, cognitive dysfunction (including memory loss) during treatment with non-selective antimuscarinic agents for OAB is of growing concern, particularly in older patients and those with mild cognitive impairment or dementia. Increased blood–brain barrier permeability, which can occur with advanced age and certain comorbidities, may also facilitate CNS access of antimuscarinic agents (regardless of their physiochemical properties), and add to the antimuscarinic burden. On the basis of available evidence, antimuscarinic agents with selectivity for M_3 over M_1 and M_2 receptors, limited CNS penetration, or both, may therefore offer a favorable balance of efficacy in treating OAB with a reduced risk of adverse cognitive events in the older population.

Wagg et al. assessed the efficacy and tolerability of solifenacin 5 and 10 mg once daily for treating elderly subjects (aged $\geq$ 65) with OAB.[40] They found statistically significant improvements in the symptoms of OAB with solifenacin compared with placebo (incontinence episodes/24 hours, number of urgency episodes/24 hours, number of micturitions/24 hours, volume voided/micturition, proportion of subjects with restoration of continence, proportion of subjects with resolution of urgency). Improvements in incontinence, urgency, and micturitions were maintained during the 40-week extension trial. The most common adverse events in both the double-blind and extension trials were dry mouth, constipation, and urinary tract infection.

Foote et al. evaluated darifenacin in a group of older patients (aged $\geq$ 65 years).[41] They noticed a dose-related, significant improvement in all the major symptoms of OAB (median reduction in incontinence episodes/week, micturition frequency, bladder capacity (volume voided), and frequency of urgency episodes). The most common treatment-related adverse events were dry mouth and constipation, which were typically mild or moderate. The use of constipation remedies was low and similar between groups. There were no nervous system or cardiovascular safety concerns.

Children

Fitzgerald et al. evaluated the relationship between childhood urinary symptoms and adult lower urinary tract (LUT) symptoms in women.[42] A population based cohort of 2109 women 40–69 years old who were members of a large health maintenance organization was randomly selected with stratification for age and race. Through self-reported questionnaires, women reported a childhood history of and current LUT symptoms. Current incontinence was also classified as urge or stress incontinence. A significant association was found between childhood daytime frequency and adult urgency; frequent nocturia in childhood and adult nocturia; childhood daytime incontinence and adult urge incontinence; and childhood and adult nocturnal enuresis. A history of more than one childhood urinary tract infection (UTI) was associated with adult UTIs. These results seem to indicate that childhood urinary symptoms and UTIs are significantly associated with adult OAB symptoms.

Kajiwara et al. investigated the prevalence and characteristics of nocturnal enuresis (NE) and examined the prevalence of OAB symptoms in primary schoolchildren.[43] NE (any involuntary loss of urine during sleep, occurring more frequently than once per month) and OAB (increased daytime frequency and/or urge urinary incontinence) were detected in 5.9% and 17.8% of 6917 primary schoolchildren, respectively. Children with a history of cystitis had a significantly higher rate of OAB than children without it.

Kilic et al. compared tolterodine and oxybutynin in children with DO.[44] Reductions in urge urinary incontinence episodes and improvements in urodynamic parameters were similar with tolterodine and oxybutynin. Side effects were more common with oxybutynin.

Van Arendonk et al. examined the variables relative to the response of oxybutynin treatment in children with daytime urinary incontinence.[45] Children with daytime incontinence presenting with the lowest frequency of wetting were most likely to achieve continence. The frequency of wetting should be considered as a prognostic value when assessing the results of therapeutic intervention trials.

Hoebeke et al. determined prospectively the effect of detrusor injection of 100 U botulinum-A toxin, in a cohort of 21 children with therapy resistant non-neurogenic detrusor overactivity.[46] The side effects were 10-day temporary urinary retention in one girl and signs of vesicoureteral reflux with flank pain during voiding in one boy, which disappeared spontaneously after 2 weeks. Two girls experienced one episode of symptomatic lower urinary tract infection. Fifteen children had a minimum follow-up of 6 months: nine patients showed full response (no more urge and dry during the day) and significant increase in bladder capacity, three showed a partial response (50% decrease in urge and incontinence), and three remained unchanged. Eight of the nine full responders were still cured after 12 months, while one had a relapse after 8 months. The three partial responders and the patient with relapse underwent a second injection, with a full response in the former full responder and in one partial responder.

NEUROSTIMULATION

Stoller afferent nerve stimulation

Van Balken et al. attempted to identify prognostic patient characteristics to improve patient selection for neuromodulation.[47] In 132 patients (80 OAB), objective success was seen in 32.6% of patients and subjective success in 51.5%. The only significant negative prognostic factor was impaired mental health as measured with the short form health survey questionnaire (SF-36) mental component summary, and this was independent of symptom severity.

Van der Pal et al. determined the effect of a pause in percutaneous tibial nerve stimulation (PTNS) in 11 successfully treated patients with overactive bladder (OAB), and the reproducibility of successful treatment when restored.[48] They found that continuous neuromodulation therapy is necessary. The efficacy of PTNS can be reproduced in patients formerly treated successfully.

Nuhoglu et al. found in a prospective observational study that Stoller afferent nerve stimulation (SANS) has a short-term positive effect (54%) in patients with resistant overactive bladder. However, it was also established that efficacy was maintained at 1 year in only 23% of subjects.[49]

Sacral nerve stimulation

Brazzelli et al. performed a systematic review of primary studies of sacral nerve stimulation (SNS) for urge incontinence published in English between 1966 and May 2003, and identified four randomized controlled trials and 30 case series.[50] Evidence from the randomized controlled trials, involving approximately 120 patients, showed that about 80% of study subjects achieved either complete continence or at least a greater than 50% improvement in their main incontinence symptoms after SNS, compared with about 3% of controls receiving conservative treatments while waiting for an implant. While case series were larger, they were methodologically less reliable. However, these series showed similar results, with 67% of patients becoming dry or achieving a greater than 50% improvement in symptoms after implantation. Incontinence episodes, leakage severity, voiding frequency, and pad use were significantly lower after implantation. Benefits were reported to persist 3–5 years after implantation. Adverse events were documented in 27 studies. Overall the reoperation rate in implanted cases was 33%. The most common reason for surgical revision was relocation of the generator due to pain or infection. Common complications were pain at the implant or lead site in 25% of patients, lead-related problems such as lead migration in 16%, replacement and repositioning of the implanted pulse generator in 15%, wound problems in 7%, adverse effects on bowel function in 6%, infection in

5%, and generator problems in 5%. Permanent removal of the electrodes was reported in 9% of patients. Technical changes with time have been associated with decreased complication rates.

Groen et al. noted, in a retrospective study, that SNS depressant acitivity on detrusor overactivity occurred in 33 women with OAB (decrease in magnitude and frequency of non-volitional detrusor contractions).[51] No effect on urethral resistance and bladder contraction strength during voiding could be demonstrated using volume independent parameters.

COST

Cost in healthcare is becoming increasingly important. Reeves et al. made an estimate and compared the current and future direct cost of overactive bladder (OAB) for the healthcare systems of five European countries.[52] A health economic model was created to estimate the number of people currently affected by OAB symptoms, the expected number to be affected in the future, and the resultant economic burden on healthcare systems in Germany, Italy, Spain, Sweden, and the United Kingdom. The model estimated that in 2000, 20.2 million people over age 40 in the five countries experienced the symptoms of OAB; 7 million of these had urgency with urge incontinence. This figure is expected to rise to 25.5 million by 2020, including 9 million who will have urgency with urge incontinence. The average annual direct costs of OAB management ranged from 269 euros to 706 euros per patient per year. The largest cost was the use of incontinence pads, accounting for an average of 63% of the annual per patient cost of OAB management. The total cost to healthcare systems across all five countries was estimated at 4.2 billion euros in 2000, and by 2020, the expected total cost was estimated to be 5.2 billion euros, an increase of 1 billion euros (26%). OAB is prevalent, with a substantial direct cost that is anticipated to increase in the future in line with aging populations. The overall burden, including indirect costs, may be considerably larger, and will fall predominantly on the elderly OAB population with urge incontinence. Recommended medical treatments could help to manage those costs and should be evaluated.

REFERENCES

1. Haferkamp A, Freund T, Wagener N. Distribution of neuropeptide Y-containing nerves in the neurogenic and non-neurogenic detrusor. BJU Int 2006; 97: 393–9.
2. Sellers DJ, Chapple CR, W Hay DP, Chess-Williams R. Depressed contractile responses to neurokinin A in idiopathic but not neurogenic overactive human detrusor muscle. Eur Urol 2006; 49: 510–18.
3. Hegde SS. Muscarinic receptors in the bladder: from basic research to therapeutics. Br J Pharmacol 2006; 147 (Suppl 2): S80–7.
4. De Wachter S, Wyndaele JJ. Intravesical oxybutynin: a local anesthetic effect on bladder C afferents. J Urol 2003; 169: 1892–5.
5. De Laet K, De Wachter S, Wyndaele JJ. Systemic oxybutynin decreases afferent activity of the pelvic nerve of the rat: new insights into the working mechanism of antimuscarinics. Neurourol Urodyn 2006; 25: 156–61.
6. Griffiths D, Derbyshire S, Stenger A, Resnick N. Brain control of normal and overactive bladder. J Urol 2005; 174: 1862–7.
7. Kim JC, Park EY, Seo SI, Park YH, Hwang TK. Nerve growth factor and prostaglandins in the urine of female patients with overactive bladder. J Urol 2006; 175: 1773–6.
8. Hashim H, Abrams P. Is the bladder a reliable witness for predicting detrusor overactivity? J Urol 2006; 175: 191–4.
9. De Wachter S, Wyndaele JJ. Frequency-volume charts: a tool to evaluate bladder sensation. Neurourol Urodyn 2003; 22: 638–42.
10. Wyndaele JJ, Van Meel TD, De Wachter S. Detrusor overactivity. Does it represent a difference if patients feel the involuntary contractions? J Urol 2004; 172: 1915–18.
11. Coyne KS, Matza LS, Kopp Z, Abrams P. The validation of the patient perception of bladder condition (PPBC): a single-item global measure for patients with overactive bladder. Eur Urol 2006; 49: 1079–86.
12. Coyne KS, Matza LS, Thompson CL, Kopp ZS, Khullar V. Determining the importance of change in the overactive bladder questionnaire. J Urol 2006; 176: 627–32.
13. Coyne KS, Zyczynski T, Margolis MK, Elinoff V, Roberts RG. Validation of an overactive bladder

awareness tool for use in primary care settings. Adv Ther 2005; 22: 381–94.

14. Homma Y, Koyama N. Minimal clinically important change in urinary incontinence detected by a quality of life assessment tool in overactive bladder syndrome with urge incontinence. Neurourol Urodyn 2006; 25: 228–35.

15. Van Brummen HJ, Bruinse HW, Van de Pol G, Heintz AP, Van der Vaart CH. What is the effect of overactive bladder symptoms on woman's quality of life during and after first pregnancy? BJU Int 2006; 97: 296–300.

16. Lemack GE, Frohman EM, Zimmern PE, Hawker K, Ramnarayan P. Urodynamic distinctions between idiopathic detrusor overactivity and detrusor overactivity secondary to multiple sclerosis. Urology 2006; 67: 960–4.

17. van Leeuwen JH, Castro R, Busse M, Bemelmans BL. The placebo effect in the pharmacologic treatment of patients with lower urinary tract symptoms. Eur Urol 2006; 50: 440–52; discussion 453.

18. Nitti VW, Dmochowski R, Appell RA et al. 037 Study Group. Efficacy and tolerability of tolterodine extended-release in continent patients with overactive bladder and nocturia. BJU Int 2006; 97: 1262–6.

19. Roehrborn CG, Abrams P, Rovner ES et al. Efficacy and tolerability of tolterodine extended-release in men with overactive bladder and urgency urinary incontinence. BJU Int 2006; 97: 1003–6.

20. Roberts R, Bavendam T, Glasser DB et al. Tolterodine extended release improves patient-reported outcomes in overactive bladder: results from the IMPACT trial. Int J Clin Pract 2006; 60: 752–8.

21. Elinoff V, Bavendam T, Glasser DB et al. Symptom-specific efficacy of tolterodine extended release in patients with overactive bladder: the IMPACT trial. Int J Clin Pract 2006; 60: 745–51.

22. Rackley R, Weiss JP, Rovner ES, Wang JT, Guan Z, 037 Study Group. Nighttime dosing with tolterodine reduces overactive bladder-related nocturnal micturitions in patients with overactive bladder and nocturia. Urology 2006; 67: 731–6.

23. Abrams P, Kaplan S, De Koning Gans HJ, Millard R. Safety and tolerability of tolterodine for the treatment of overactive bladder in men with bladder outlet obstruction. J Urol 2006; 175: 999–1004.

24. Anderson RU, MacDiarmid S, Kell S et al. Effectiveness and tolerability of extended-release oxybutynin vs extended-release tolterodine in women with or without prior anticholinergic treatment for overactive bladder. Int Urogynecol J Pelvic Floor Dysfunct 2006; 17: 502–11.

25. Taylor JR. Probable interaction between tolterodine and warfarin. Pharmacotherapy 2006; 26: 719–21.

26. Staskin DR, Te AE. Short- and long-term efficacy of solifenacin treatment in patients with symptoms of mixed urinary incontinence. BJU Int 2006; 97: 1256–61.

27. Millard RJ, Halaska M. Efficacy of solifenacin in patients with severe symptoms of overactive bladder: a pooled analysis. Curr Med Res Opin 2006; 22: 41–8.

28. Cardozo L, Castro-Diaz D, Gittelman M, Ridder A, Huang M. Reductions in overactive bladder-related incontinence from pooled analysis of phase III trials evaluating treatment with solifenacin. Int Urogynecol J Pelvic Floor Dysfunct 2006; 17: 512–19.

29. Oki T, Takeuchi C, Yamada S. Comparative evaluation of exocrine muscarinic receptor binding characteristics and inhibition of salivation of solifenacin in mice. Biol Pharm Bull 2006; 29: 1397–400.

30. Noguchi K, Yamagishi T, Suzuki K et al. Propiverine hydrochloride improved correlatively subjective QOL and objective findings in Japanese patients with urinary frequency and/or incontinence. Hinyokika Kiyo 2006; 52: 343–8.

31. Sugiyama T, Shimizu N, Hashimoto K et al. Pharmacological evaluation of efficacy and safety of propiverine hydrochloride in patients of overactive bladder—relationship between urodynamic observation and propiverine pharmacokinetics. Nippon Hinyokika Gakkai Zasshi 2005; 96: 670–7.

32. Stöhrer M, Murtz G, Kramer G et al. Propiverine compared to oxybutynin in neurogenic detrusor overactivity – results of a randomized, double-blind, multicenter clinical study. Eur Urol 2007; 51: 235–42.

33. Rudy D, Cline K, Harris R, Goldberg K, Dmochowski R. Multicenter phase III trial studying trospium chloride in patients with overactive bladder. Urology 2006; 67: 275–80.

34. Rudy D, Cline K, Harris R, Goldberg K, Dmochowski R. Time to onset of improvement in symptoms of overactive bladder using antimuscarinic treatment. BJU Int 2006; 97: 540–6.

35. Pannek J, Grigoleit U, Wormland R, Goepel M. Intravesical therapy for overactive bladder. Urologe A 2006; 45: 167–8, 170–3.

36. Zinner N, Susset J, Gittelman M et al. Efficacy, tolerability and safety of darifenacin, an M(3) selective receptor antagonist: an investigation of warning time in patients with OAB. Int J Clin Pract 2006; 60: 119–26.

37. Hill S, Khullar V, Wyndaele JJ, Lheritier K, Darifenacin Study Group. Dose response with darifenacin, a novel once-daily M3 selective receptor antagonist for the treatment of overactive bladder: results of a fixed dose study. Int Urogynecol J Pelvic Floor Dysfunct 2006; 17: 239–47.

38. Takahashi S, Tajima A, Matsushima H et al. Clinical efficacy of an alpha-adrenoceptor blocker (naftopidil) on overactive bladder symptoms in patients with benign prostatic hyperplasia. Int J Urol 2006; 13: 15–20.

39. Kay GG, Abou-Donia MB, Messer WS Jr et al. Antimuscarinic drugs for overactive bladder and their potential effects on cognitive function in older patients. J Am Geriatr Soc 2005; 53: 2195-201.

40. Wagg A, Wyndaele JJ, Sieber P. Efficacy and tolerability of solifenacin in elderly subjects with overactive bladder syndrome: a pooled analysis. Am J Geriatr Pharmacother 2006; 4: 14–24.

41. Foote J, Glavind K, Kralidis G, Wyndaele JJ. Treatment of overactive bladder in the older patient: pooled analysis of three phase III studies of darifenacin, an M3 selective receptor antagonist. Eur Urol 2005; 48: 471–7.

42. Fitzgerald MP, Thom DH, Wassel-Fyr C et al. Childhood urinary symptoms predict adult overactive bladder symptoms. J Urol 2006; 175: 989–93.

43. Kajiwara M, Inoue K, Kato M et al. Nocturnal enuresis and overactive bladder in children: an epidemiological study. Int J Urol 2006; 13: 36–41.

44. Kilic N, Balkan E, Akgoz S, Sen N, Dogruyol H. Comparison of the effectiveness and side-effects of tolterodine and oxybutynin in children with detrusor instability. Int J Urol 2006; 13: 105–8.

45. Van Arendonk KJ, Austin JC, Boyt MA, Cooper CS. Frequency of wetting is predictive of response to anticholinergic treatment in children with overactive bladder. Urology 2006; 67: 1049–53.

46. Hoebeke P, De Caestecker K, Vande Walle J et al. The effect of botulinum-A toxin in incontinent children with therapy resistant overactive detrusor. J Urol 2006; 176: 328–30.

47. van Balken MR, Vergunst H, Bemelmans BL. Prognostic factors for successful percutaneous tibial nerve stimulation. Eur Urol 2006; 49: 360–5.

48. van der Pal F, van Balken MR, Heesakkers JP, Debruyne FM, Bemelmans BL. Percutaneous tibial nerve stimulation in the treatment of refractory overactive bladder syndrome: is maintenance treatment necessary? BJU Int 2006; 97: 547–50.

49. Nuhoglu B, Fidan V, Ayyildiz A, Ersoy E, Germiyanoglu C. Stoller afferent nerve stimulation in woman with therapy resistant over active bladder; a 1-year follow up. Int Urogynecol J Pelvic Floor Dysfunct 2006; 17: 204–7.

50. Brazzelli M, Murray A, Fraser C. Efficacy and safety of sacral nerve stimulation for urinary urge incontinence: a systematic review. J Urol 2006; 175: 835–41.

51. Groen J, Bosch RJC, van Mastrigt R. Sacral neuromodulation in women with idiopathic detrusor overactivity incontinence: decreased overactivity but unchanged bladder contraction strength and urethral resistance during voiding. J Urol 2006; 175: 1005–9.

52. Reeves P, Irwin D, Kelleher C et al. The current and future burden and cost of overactive bladder in five European countries. Eur Urol 2006; 50: 1050–7.

Index

Note: Page references in *italics* refer to Figures; those in **bold** refer to Tables

Aδ bladder afferents 12
abdominal leak point pressure (ALPP) 68, *69*
acetylcholine 12, 22
  in neural–urothelial interactions 14–15
active life expectancy (ALE) 386–7
acupuncture 277–80
  cutaneovisceral effects 277
  mechanism of action 277–8
  neuroanatomic acupuncture 278
  for overactive bladder, incontinence 279–80
  treatments 278–9, *278*
  viscerocutaneous effects 277
adenosine triphosphate (ATP) 11, 12
  afferent nerves and 13
  in urothelial-afferent communication 14
adenylyl cyclase 100
adrenergic receptors 11, 99–101
  α-adrenoceptors 12, 99–100
  β-adrenoceptors 12, 100–1
β-adrenoceptor agonists 156
α-blockers 183, 253
Alzheimer's disease 133, 339, 389
amantadine 156
American Urological Association Symptom Index
    (AUA-SI) 183–4, 398
amitriptyline in interstitial cystitis 79–80, 83
amphotericin 119
amyotrophic lateral sclerosis 269
anticholinergics *see* antimuscarinic drugs
antidiuretic hormone (ADH) 53, 141
antihistamines in interstitial cystitis 79
antimuscarinic (anticholinergic) drugs 97, 156, 164–5
  elderly people and 133
  mechanism 240–1
antiproliferative factor (APF) 78
apomorphine 106
aquaporin-2 (AQP2) 54
atropine 126, 165, 283
atropine methyl nitrate 15
augmentation cystoplasty 345, 349–52, 359–67
  bacteriuria in 365
  carcinoma and 365
  choice of bowel segment 361–2

complications 363–6
definition 359
endoscopy 360
evaluation 360–1
inadequate emptying/clean intermittent
    self-catheterization 365
indications 359–60
in interstitial cystitis 367
laboratory evaluation 360
leakage 364
metabolic disturbance 363–4
mucus production 364
patient outcomes 366–7
postoperative care 363
pregnancy 365–6
preoperative considerations 360–1
radiological evaluation 360
renal function 364
spontaneous perforation 365
stone formation 364–5
surgical techniques 361
urodynamic evaluation 360
autoaugmentation 345–55, *346*
  advantages 354
  animal model studies 348
  concerns 354
  detrusor myectomy *347*, 351
  detrusor myotomy 351–2
  human studies 348–52
  laparoscopic autoaugmentation 353
  modifications of 352–3
  potential complications and morbidity 354
  pregnancy and 353–4
  seromuscular cystoplasty 352–3
  surgical technique 346–8, *347*

bacillus Calmette-Guérin 117
  in interstitial cystitis 82
baclofen 105, 106
behavioral lifestyle changes 92–3
behavioral therapies 171
  in elderly people 390
behavioral training 89–92

benign prostatic enlargement (BPE) 253
benign prostatic hyperplasia (BPH) 51, 100, 253
benign prostatic obstruction (BPO) 253
benzodiazepines 156
bioadhesion, drug 120–1
biofeedback in elderly people 390
bion® microstimulator 319–26
  battery-powered 322–6
  RF-Bion™ microstimulator 321–2, 322–3
bladder cancer 6
bladder diary 37–8, 88
bladder drill 87
bladder habits, changing 87–8
bladder outlet obstruction (BOO) 70–1
  alpha-blockers/anticholinergics combined
      therapy 254–5
  alpha-blockers/antimuscarinics combined
      therapy 256
  antimuscarinic monotherapy 255–7
  antimuscarinics, and symptoms alleviation in 256–7
  botulinum toxin injections 257
  cystoscopy 33
  doxazosin plus tolterodine in 254
  future research 258
  pharmacotherapy of 253–8
  safety of antimuscarinics in 254, 257
  tamsulosin plus tolterodine in 254
  tolterodine in 183, 184, 254, 255
bladder outlet obstruction index (BOOI) 70, 254, 401
bladder sensation 4
bladder stones, cystoscopy of 33
bladder trabeculation, cystoscopy of 33
bladder training 87–8, **89**
blood–brain barrier 247–8
botulinum toxin (Botox®; BTX-A) 14, 117, 261–71, 303
  adverse events 269
  afferent effect 264
  in bladder outlet obstruction 257
  botulinum toxin-sensitive mechanisms 103
  BTX-B 263
  clinical applications 263–4
  clinical results 265–8
  dosage 263–4
  efferent effect 264
  histological changes after BTX-A injection 267–8
  idiopathic detrusor overactivity 266
  inhibitor of growth factor release and receptor
      expression 264–5
  injection techniques 268–9
  local side effects 269
  mechanism of action 264–5, 265
  mixed neurogenic/idiopathic detrusor
      overactivity 266
  neurogenic detrusor overactivity 265–6

pathophysiology 261–2
  in pediatric patients 266–7, 381–2
  repeat BTX-A injections 267
  resiniferatoxin vs. BTX-A 267
  resistance to toxin effects 269–71
  risk of clean intermittent catheterization (CIC)
      after **270**
  in spinal cord injured patients 267
  systemic side effects 269
bowel management 93
brain imaging 20–1, 21
brain pathways 16–17
brain tumors 163
Bristol Female Lower Urinary Tract Symptoms
      (BFLUTS) 46–7
  BLFUTS-SF 46–7
Bristol Stool Scale 374
bumetanide in nocturnal polyuria 55

C-fiber bladder afferents 12
caffeine 93
  interaction with tolterodine 173
calcium channels 101
calmodulin 146
capsaicin (CAP) 12, 13, 102, 103, 117
carbachol 15, 102
cardiac issues 248
  in elderly people 389–90
central micturition reflex pathways, neurotransmitters
      in 22–3
  excitatory neurotransmitters 22
  inhibitory neurotransmitters 22
  mixed excitatory/inhibitory actions 22–3
central nervous system (CNS) as target for
      pharmacologic intervention 103–7
cerebrovascular disease 163
children, overactive bladder in 373–82, 403–4
  anticholinergic mediation 378–82
  behavioral/voiding diary/timed voiding 376–7
  biofeedback treatment 377–8
  botulinum toxin in 266–7, 381–2
  conservative treatment 376–8
  constipation and 374, 377, **378**
  diagnosis and evaluation 373–5
  neuromodulation in 381
  normal voiding frequency 373
  propiverine in 149–51, 150
  sexual abuse 374
  treatment options and outcomes 375–6
  uroflowmetry 374–5
  urinary tract infections 375
choline acetyltransferase 15
cholinergic excitatory transmission 11
chronic pelvic pain (CPP) 75

clarithromycin 206
clean intermittent catheterization (CIC) 345, 348, 365
clenbuterol 101
cognition receptor 247
cognitive dysfunction in elderly people 389
constipation 93
    in children 374, 377, **378**
continuous urinary incontinence 4
corticotropin-releasing factor 22
cost 405
    of urinary incontinence 171
craniopharyngioma 56
cyclosporine in interstitial cystitis 80, 81
cystitis
    eosinophilic 77
    tuberculosis 68, 77
    see also interstitial cystitis (IC)
cystometrography (CMG) 65, *65*, 121
cystometry 65–9
    capacity 66
    compliance 66
    detrusor contractions 66–7
    filling pressure 65–6
    leak point pressures 68–9
    sensation 66
    urodynamic stress incontinence 67–8
cystoscopy in interstitial cystitis 33
cystourethroscopy 33
cytarine 119

Danish-prostate symptom score (DAN-pss) 46
darifenacin 41, 165, 189, 203–16, 283, 381, 402
    cardiac safety 204, 215
    chemical structure *204*, 206
    chemistry 203–5, **205**
    clinical efficacy 206–13
    clinical studies **207–8**
    cognitive safety 204, 214–15, *214*
    fixed-dose studies 209, **210–11**
    flexible-dosing studies 209–11
    pharmacodynamics 203–5, **205**
    pharmacokinetics 205–6, **205**
    pharmacological profile 203–6
    quality of life improvement 216
    in subpopulations 211–13
    tolerability 213–14
    urodynamic efficacy studies 206
Data Mining Surveillance System (DMSS) scale 167–8
daunorubicin 119
daytime frequency 3
debrisoquine, interaction with tolterodine 173
defensive voiding 29
definition of overactive bladder (OAB) 4, 5–6, 27–8
delayed voiding 88

N-desethyl-oxybutynin (DEO) 115–16, 121, 165, 229
desipramine 141, 142
desmopressin 55–6
    in nocturnal polyuria 55
    polydipsia and 57
Detrunorm® 152
detrusor–external sphincter dyssynergia (DESD) 72, *72*
detrusor hyperreflexia 6, 339
detrusor instability 6
detrusor leak point pressure (DLPP) 68, *69*
detrusor overactivity (DO) **6**, 66–7, *67*, 71, *72*, 395
    diagnosis **126**
    idiopathic (IDO) 6, 125, **126**, 254, 339, 398
    neurogenic 6, 125, **126**, 339, 398
    phasic 6, *7*
    terminal 6, *7*
detrusor myectomy *347*, 351
detrusor myotomy 351–2
detrusor underactivity 69
diabetes insipidus 33
    causes 56
    desmopressin in 55, 57
    thirst and 56–7
diagnosis of overactive bladder 27–34, 397–8
    cystourethroscopy 33
    history 28–31
    imaging 33
    pad tests 31
    physical examination 31–2
    post-void residual urine measurement 32
    questionnaires 29–30, **31**
    symptom assessment 28–9
    urine analysis 32
    urodynamics 32–3
    voiding diaries 30–1
diazepam 106
dicyclomine hydrochloride (Bentyl®) 128, 133
differential diagnosis **28**
digoxin 190, 206
dihydropyrdidines 101
dimethindene 192
dimethylsulfoxide (DMSO) 117
    in interstitial cystitis 82
Ditropan XL® in pediatric overactive bladder 379–80
dopamine 22
dopamine mechanisms 106–7
doxazosin 106, 151
    tolterodine and 184
doxorubicin 119
drug absorption, barriers to, after instillation 118–22
    increased vesical residence time 120–2
    liposomes 118–20, *119*
drug comparisons 241–9
drug data presentation 249–50

drug delivery 115–16, *116*
drug–drug interactions 248
duloxetine 23, 139, 140, 141, 142, 143
  interaction with tolterodine 174
dysuria (pollakisuria) 3

economic factors in elderly people 387
edge concept 243
efficacy measures 243, **243**
elderly people 385–91, 403
  active life expectancy (ALE) 386–7
  anticholinergics and 133
  behavioral therapy 390
  biofeedback 390
  cardiac adverse events 389–90
  cognitive dysfunction 389
  economic factors 387
  electrical stimulation 390–1
  nocturia in 57
  pathophysiology 387–8
  patient education 386
  pharmacological therapy 388–90
  population 385–6
  propiverine in 149
  QTc interval 389–90
electroencephalography (EEG) 299
electromyography (EMG) 308
emepronium bromide 128
enkephalins 22
enuresis 4
  desmopressin in 55
epidermal growth factor (EGF) 78

fecal impaction 93
  see also constipation
festoterodine 283–9
  in CYP2D6 genotype deficiency 285–6
  ethnicity and 286
  in hepatic impairment 286
  metabolic pathway *284*
  pharmacodynamic profiling 283–8
  phase III analysis 288–9
  trials 287–8
finasteride 52
flavoxate hydrochloride (Urispas®) 128, **134**
flexible dosing 249
fluid management 92–3
fluorescein isothiocyanate (FITC) 122
fluoxetine (Prozac®) 139
  interaction with tolterodine 173
frequency–volume charts (FVCs) 37–40, *38*
  24–hour frequency 39
  24–hour production 39
  daytime frequency 39

incontinent episode frequency 39
interpretation 38–40
maximum voided volume 40
night-time frequency 39
nocturia 39
nocturnal urine volume 39
pad usage 39
types 37–8
urgency 39–40
functional bladder capacity (FBC) 52
functional magnetic resonance imaging (fMRI) 20, 104, 396
furosemide in nocturnal polyuria 55

G-protein 54
gabapentin 106
  in interstitial cystitis 75, 80, 83
gamma-aminobutyric acid (GABA) 22, 105–6
genitourinary pain syndromes, chronic 300
global polyuria 51
glutamic acid 22
glycine 22
glycosaminoglycan (GAG) layer 118
guarding reflex 294, *294*

half-life issues 248–9
health-related quality of life (HRQoL) 397
hemoglobin A1c (HgbA1c) 33
hemophilia A, desmopressin in 56
heparin binding epidermal growth factor (HB-EGF) 78
heparin, intravesical 76
hepatic cirrhosis 173
hexamethonium 15
Hunner's ulcers 77, 81
5-hydroxytryptamine 22, 23
hydroxyzine in interstitial cystitis 79
hyoscyamine sulfate (Levsin®)126

ICSmale (ICSmaleF) 44–6, *44–5*
  ICIQ-MLUTS 45, *45*
  ICSmaleSF 44–5
idiopathic detrusor activity (IDO) 6, 125, **126**, 254, 339, 398
imipramine 141–2, 156
  in nocturnal polyuria 55
immediate release (IR) agents 125–35
  anticholinergics as 126–7, 133
  efficacy and compliance 128–33, **129–30**
  historical background 125–6
  mixed action 127–8
  pharmacologic agents 126–34, **127**
immunosuppressive drugs in interstitial cystitis 80–1
incidence 171

Incontinence Impact Questionnaire (IIQ) 42, 193, 233, 234, 266
Indevus Urgency Severity Scale (IUSS) 42, 192
innervation of lower urinary tract 11–13, *12*
    afferent pathways 12–13
    receptors **13**
    sacral parasympathetic pathways 11–12
    sacral somatic efferent pathways 12
    thoracolumbar sympathetic efferent pathways 12
International Consultation on Incontinence Questionnaire (ICIQ) project 43
    ICIQ-FLUTS 47, *47*
    ICIQ-KHQ 43
    ICIQ-MLUTS 46, 47
    ICIQ-OAB 47
International Consultation on Incontinence (ICI) assessments 242–3, **242**
International Index of Erectile Function (IIEF) 184
International Normalized Ratio 401
International Prostate Symptom Score (IPSS) 100, 184, 254, 402
interstitial cystitis (IC) 14, 75–83, 300
    augmentation cystoplasty 367
    Bacillus Calmette-Guérin in 82
    cystoscopy 33
    diagnosis 77–8, **78**
    dimethylsulfoxide (DMSO) 82
    etiology 75–7, *76*
    hydrodistention 81–2
    invasive treatment 81–3, **81**
    Miniaturo™-I device in 332
    oral treatment 79–81, **79**
    resiniferatoxin on 82
    sacral neuromodulation 82–3
    treatment 78–83
intravesical instillation 116–18
ion channels 101–2
itraconazole 206

Kegel's exercises 31
Kerner's disease 261
ketoconazole 206, 286, 287
King's Health Questionnaire (KHQ) 42–3, 181, *215*, 216, 226

Lambert–Eaton syndrome 269
laparoscopic autoaugmentation 353
lazy bladder syndrome 378
Leicester Urinary Symptoms Questionnaire (LUSQ) 40
loop diuretics, interaction with tolterodine 174
lower urinary tract innervation 11–13, *12*
lower urinary tract symptoms (LUTS) 3–9, 47, 253, 254, 398

magnetic resonance imaging (MRI)
    as contraindication to sacral nerve stimulation devices 314
maximum cystometric capacity (MCC) 66
meningitis 56
methyllycaconitine 15
micromotion 241
Mictonorm® 152
micturition time chart 37
Miniaturo™-I device 329–34, *330*
    device description 330, *330*
    implantation procedure 311, *311*
    interstitial cystitis and 332
    overactive bladder syndrome and 332–3
    post-implantation management 331
    safety assessment 333
    screening test 330
minimal clinically important change (MCIC) 397
Miralax™ 377
mixed nocturia 51
mixed urinary incontinence 4
morphine, intrathecal 104
motor neuron disease, lower 68
Multicenter Assessment of Transdermal therapy in Overactive Bladder with Oxybutynin (MATRIX) study 236
multiple sclerosis 163, 300, 398
    desmopressin in 55
muscarinic receptors 11, 12, 97–9, 163–4, 246, 396
muscimol 105, 106
myasthenia gravis 269
myelomeningocele 149, 150, 374

naftopidil 100, 402–3
naloxone 104, 277
Name–Face Association test 215
NBC index 52
nefazodone 206
nelfinavir 206
nerve growth factor 300, 396–7
neurogenic detrusor activity (NDO) 6, 125, **126**, 339, 398
neurokinin A (NKA) 107, 395–6
neurokinin B (NKB) 107
neuroleptics 156
neuromodulation 295–8
    historical perspectives 295
    neural pathways 295–6
    neurochemistry and 300
    neurologic effects 298–300
    normal voiding 293–4, *295*
    in pediatric overactive bladder 381
    sacral, in interstitial cystitis 82–3
    urodynamic effects 298

neuropeptide Y (NPY) 12, 395
neurostimulation 404–5
nitric oxide 22
N-methyl-D-aspartate (NMDA) 22
nocturia 3, 39, 51–9
   aging and 57
   algorithm for voiding 51, 52
   behavioral training 92
   case study 57–9
   mixed causes 51, 57
nocturia index (Ni) 52
nocturnal bladder capacity (NBC) 51
   diminished 52–3, 53
nocturnal enuresis 4
nocturnal polyuria (NP) 51, 53–6
   abnormalities of arginine vasopressin
      secretion 53–4
   causes 53
   obstructive sleep apnea 54
   treatment 54–5
nocturnal urine volume (NUV) 39, 52
non-cholinergic excitatory transmission 11–12
non-steroidal anti-inflammatory drugs (NSAIDs) 75
noradrenaline mechanisms 106
norepinephrine 22
nortriptyline 142

OAB questionnaire (OAB-q) 398
OAB-Symptom Composite Score (OAB-SCS) 194, 194
obesity 93
obstructive sleep apnea 54
O'Leary-Sant questionnaire 77, 78, 332
omeprazole, interaction with tolterodine 173
Onu's nucleus 12
OPERA trial 401
opioid receptors 104
oral contraceptives, interaction with tolterodine 174
overactive bladder screener (OAB-V8) 45–6
overactive bladder symptom questionnaires 42–7, 43
overactive bladder symptoms and health-related
     quality of life 46 (OAB-q) 46, 46
overflow incontinence 4
overnight dehydration test 56, 58
Oxford Guidelines 242, 242
oxotremorine methiodide 15
oxybutynin (Oxytrol™) 98, 115, 117, 121, 127–8, 133,
     140, 189, 192, 229–36, 283, 396, 402
   adhesion 231
   adverse events 234
   clinical efficacy 231–4
      phase II study 231–2, 232
      phase III studies 232–4, 232–3
   continuation of treatment 235–6
   extended release (OXY-ER) 155–8, 165

immediate release (OXY-IR) 135, 165, 166–7
   local application site reactions 234–5
   oral, extended release 163–8
   in pediatric overactive bladder 378–9
   pharmacokinetics 230–1
   pharmacologic effects on the bladder 229
   vs. propiverine 147, 149, 150, 152–4, 158
   rationale 229–30
   safety and tolerability 234–6
   side effects 131–2
   skin tolerability 235, 235
   transdermal 230, 230
oxybutynin chloride (Ditropan®) see oxybutynin

paclitaxel 119
pad usage 39
pad tests 31
Parkinson's disease 133, 163, 300, 339
   desmopressin in 55
   dopamine receptors in 106
   idiopathic 23
patient education in elderly people 386
patient perception of bladder condition
     (PPBC) 397
PEG-PLGA-PEG 121–2
pelvic floor muscle training 88, 89–91, 90
Pelvic Pain and Urinary Frequency Questionnaire
     (PUF) 77
pentosan polysulfate sodium (PPS) 75, 76
   in interstitial cystitis 79, 83
peptidergic receptors 11
percutaneous neuromodulatory evaluation
     (PNE) 305
percutaneous sacral neuromodulation 296–8, 296
PET scanning 298
phenothiazines 156
phenoxybenzamine 140
phenylcyclohexylglycolic acid 231
phenylephrine 99
placebo response 398
pollakisuria 3
polydipsia
   dipsogenic 56, 57
   idiopathic 39
   psychogenic 56, 57
polyuria 39, 56–7, 56
positron emission tomography (PET) of brain
     20–1, 21
post-micturition symptoms 4
post-void residual urine measurement 32
post-void residual volume (PVR) 64
potassium channels 101–2
potassium sensitivity test (PST) 77
prednisone in interstitial cystitis 80–1

pregnancy
    augmentation cystoplasty in 365–6
    autoaugmentation and 353–4
    sacral nerve stimulation in 314
propantheline *see* propantheline bromide
propantheline bromide (Pro-Banthine®) 126–7, **134**,
    141, 165, 243
propiverine *see* propiverine hydrochloride
propiverine hydrochloride 128, 145–58, 165, 401–2
    benign prostatic syndrome/male overactive
        bladder 151–2
    cardiac safety 156
    cognition and psychomotor performance 155–6
    drug–drug interaction 156
    efficacy 146–52
    etiology, gender and age 152, **153–4**
    extended release (ER) formulation 156
    idiopathic detrusor overactivity 148–9
    in children 149–51, *150*
    in elderly patients 149
    long-term efficacy 152
    long-term tolerability 154–5
    neurogenic detrusor overactivity 146–8
    ophthalmological safety 156
    overall evaluation 152
    vs. oxybutynin 152–4
    pharmacology 145–6
    post-marketing drug surveillance 156–7
    post-void residual 155
    recent advances 157–8, **157**
    renal and hepatic impairment 156
    tolerability and safety 152–6
    vs. tolterodine 154, **155**
prostaglandins 396–7
prostate-specfic antigen (PSA) 33
prostatitis, chronic (CP) 75
protamine sulfate 118
protein kinase C 98
pudendal nerve stimulation 319–26
    anatomy 320–1, *321*
    battery-powered bion® microstimulator
        322–6, *323*
        explanation 326
        implantation 325, *325*
        insertion site *324*
        patient selection 322–4
        percutaneous stimulation trial 324, *324*
        post-operative follow-up 325–6
    RF-Bion™ microstimulator 321–2, *322–3*
purinergic receptors 11

QTc interval in elderly people 389–90
quality of life questionnaires 37, 397–8
questionnaires 29–30, **31**

radiation cystitis, cystoscopy 33
receptor selectivity 246
rectal laser Doppler flowmetry 300
5α-reductase inhibitors 253
reflex control of lower urinary tract 17–22
reflex sympathetic dystrophy (RSD) 76
renal concentrating capacity test (RCCT) 56, **59**
resiniferatoxin (RTX) 12, 98, 117, 119
    effects on Aδ fibres 102–3
    in interstitial cystitis 82
reverse transcriptase polymerase chain reaction
    (RTPCR) 15
RF-Bion™ microstimulator 321–2, *322–3*
Rho-kinase 98
ritonavir 206

sacral nerve stimulation (SNS) 295, **297**, **300**,
    303–15, 404–5
    anticholinergic therapy vs. 309–10, *310*
    background 303–4
    battery 313
    bellows response 311
    efficacy 308–10, 311–13
    expanding indications 310–11
    infection and 313
    mechanism of action 304–5, *304*, **304**
    MRI 314
    pain at implanted pulse generator site 313–14
    patient selection 307–8
    percutaneous neuromodulatory evaluation
        (PNE) 305
    pregnancy and 314
    technique 305–7, *305–6*
sacral parasympathetic pathways 11–12
sacral somatic efferent pathways 12
safety measures **245**
sarcoid 56
scopolamine 230
selective serotonin reuptake inhibitors (SSRIs) 105
sensory urgency 6
seromuscular cystoplasty 352–3
serotonin mechanisms 104–5
sertraline (Zoloft®) 139
Short Form McGill Pain Questionnaire
    (SF-MPQ) 332
single photon emission computed tomography,
    brain 20, 21, *21*
SNARE (soluble *N*-ethylmaleimide-sensitive fusion
    attachment protein receptor) proteins 262,
    263, 264
solifenacin *see* solifenacin succinate
solifenacin succinate 165, 189, 219–27, 283, 381, 401
    chemistry and pharmacokinetics 219–20
    clinical trials 221–6, *225*, **225**

solifenacin succinate *cont.*
   drug–drug interactions 221
   mechanism of action 220–1
   metabolism and elimination 219–20
   in nocturia 52
   STAR trial 222, *222–3*, **223**
   structure *220*
   vs. tolterodine 180
   VENUS trial 226
somatosensory evoked potentials (SEPs) 299
sphincter coordination and electromyography 71–2
spina bifida 68
   augmentation cystoplasty and 361
spinal cord tumours 68
spinal cord CNS pathways 15–16
   afferent projections in spinal cord 15
   efferent neurons 15
   spinal interneurons 15–16
spinal cord injury 163, 395
spiroperidol 106
SPM 7605 283, *284*, 286–7
SSRIs 139
stable bladder 6
Stanford Sleepiness scale 197
Stoller afferent nerve stimulation (SANS) 278, 404
stress hyperreflexia 4
stress incontinence 3–4, 68
   vs. overactive bladder (OAB) **30**
stroke 400
study comparisons 243–6
substance O 107
switch studies 251
sympathetic storage reflex 18–19
β-sympathomimetics 156
symptom questionnaires, implementation 47

tachykinin mechanisms 107
tamsulosin 100, 151
   tolterodine and 184
taxol 119
terazosin 52
terodiline 128
thiazide, interaction with tolterodine 174
thiotepa 117
thirst, disorders of 56–7
thoracolumbar sympathetic efferent pathways 12
thyroid stimulating hormone (TSH) 33
tiagabine 105
titratability 249
tolerability measures **245**
tolterodine 98, 99, 127, 133, 135, 165, 171–83, 189,
     192, 243, 283, 398–401
   037 Study Group 180–1
   5-hydroxymethyl (5-HM) metabolite 173, 174, 175

   adverse events **179**
   Antimuscarinic Clinical Effectiveness Trial
     (ACET) 179–80
   chemical structure *172*
   dosage 172
   drug interactions 173–5
   efficacy data 146, 175–81
   in elderly patients 182–3
   extended release (ER) 172, 174–5, *174*, 178–81, 401
   health related quality of life 181
   immediate release (IR) 172, 174, 175–8
   in lower urinary tract symptoms 183–4
   mechanism of action 172
   metabolism 172–3, *173*
   mixed urinary incontinence 183
   in nocturia 52–3
   OBJECT trial 177
   OPERA trial 178–9
   in pediatric patients 181–2, 380–1
   pharmacokinetic parameters **175–6**
   vs. propiverine 148, **148**, 149, 154, **155**, 158
   side effects **131–2**
   STAR study 180
tolterodine tartrate (Detrol®) *see* tolterodine
traditional Chinese medicine 278
tramadol 104
transcutaneous electrical nerve stimulation
     (TENS) 295–6
Transderm Scop™ 230
transurethral resection of the prostate (TURP) 149
   nocturia in 51
   tolterodine in 183
transvaginal denervation 339–43
   alternative treatments 339
   anesthetic block 340–1, *341*
   epidemiology 339
   historical background 339–40
   postoperative care 342
   preoperative evaluation 340–1
   surgical technique 341, *341–2*
tricyclic antidepressants 75, 76, 139–43, 156
   bladder efferent signaling 140
   central nervous system effects 139–40
   clinical studies 141–2
   in vitro studies 140
   interaction with tolterodine 174
   live animal lower urinary tract models 140–1
trospium chloride 165, 189–99, 381, 402
   adverse events **197**, **199**
   balanced selectivity for M_2/M_3 muscarinic
     receptor subtypes 191–2
   chemical structure 190
   chemistry 190
   clinical studies 192–7

efficacy 192–4, **193**
efficacy endpoints **198**
lack of CNS effects 197
lack of metabolism via hepatic cytochrome P450
    enzyme pathway 190
local activity via afferent pathways 192
muscarinic receptor (MPO) binding affinities **191**
once daily preparation 197–8
pharmacokinetic profile 190
pharmacology 190–2
post-marketing surveillance 197
role of M_2/M_3 muscarinic receptor
    subtypes 190–1
safety and tolerability 194, **195–6**
tuberculosis 56

unconscious (unaware) incontinence 4
ureteral ectopia, cystoscopy in 33
ureteroceles, cystoscopy in 33
urethral diverticulum, cystoscopy in 33
urethral sphincter storage reflex 19
urethral strictures, cystoscopy in 33
urge control techniques 88
urge incontinence 4
urge suppression strategy 91–2, **91**
urge syndrome 4, 28, 239
urge urinary incontinence (UUI) 339
urgency 3, 4–5, 339
urgency–frequency syndrome 4, 28, 239
urgency measures 40–2
  frequency of urgency 41
  intensity of urgency 40
  severity and frequency of urgency 41–2
  timing of urgency 40–1
Urgency Perception Scale (UPS) 5, 40–1
Urgency Severity Score (USS) 5
urinary incontinence 3–4
urinary retention 295
urine concentration, antimuscarinics and 247
urine storage reflexes 18–19
urodynamic OAB classification 7–8
  type 1 7, *7*
  type 2 7, *8*

type 3 7, *8*
type 4 7–8, *8*
urodynamic sphincteric incontinence 4
urodynamic stress incontinence 4
urodynamics 32–3, 63–73
urodynamic testing 64–73
uroflowmetry 64–5
Urogenital Distress Inventory 43–4, 266
Urolife BPH quality of life questionnaire 254
uroselectivity 239–40, 247
  need for 241–2
  organ selectivity 240
  receptor selectivity 240
urothelium 13–15
  receptors *14*
usage studies 249

Valsalva leak point pressure (VLPP) 68
vanilloid receptors 102–3
vanilloids 115, 117, 300
vasoactive intestinal polypeptide (VIP) 12, 22
vasopressin-regulated urea transporter (VRUT) 54
venlafaxine 140
videourodynamics 33, 63, 71, *71*, *72–3*
Visual Analog Scale 322
voiding diaries 30–1
voiding dysfunction, pathophysiology 294–5
voiding, normal, neuromodulation 293–4, *295*
voiding pressure–flow studies 69–71
voiding reflexes 19–22, *294*
  spinal micturition reflex pathway 21–2, *21*
  spinobulbospinal micturition reflex pathway
    19–20, *20*
  suprapontine control of micturition 20–1, *21*
voiding symptoms 4
von Willebrand's disease, desmopressin in 56

warfarin
  solifenacin and 221
  tolterodine interaction with 174
warning time 41
Wegener's granulomatosis 56
weight loss 93

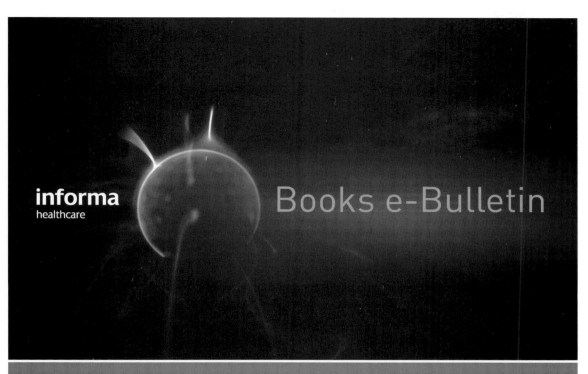
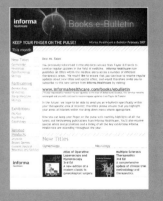